Corbin's Concepts of
Fitness and Wellness

A Comprehensive Lifestyle Approach

THIRTEENTH EDITION

Gregory J. Welk

Iowa State University

Charles B. Corbin

Arizona State University

William R. Corbin

Arizona State University

Karen A. Welk

Mary Greeley Medical Center, Ames, Iowa

Mc
Graw
Hill

CORBIN'S CONCEPTS OF FITNESS AND WELLNESS: A COMPREHENSIVE LIFESTYLE APPROACH,
THIRTEENTH EDITION

Published by McGraw Hill LLC, 1325 Avenue of the Americas, New York, NY, 10019. Copyright © 2023 by
The McGraw Hill LLC All rights reserved. Printed in the United States of America. Previous editions © 2019,
2016, 2013. No part of this publication may be reproduced or distributed in any form or by any means, or stored
in a database or retrieval system, without the prior written consent of The McGraw Hill LLC, including, but not
limited to, in any network or other electronic storage or transmission, or broadcast for distance learning.

Some ancillaries, including electronic and print components, may not be available to customers outside the
United States.

This book is printed on acid-free paper.

1 2 3 4 5 6 7 8 9 LWI 27 26 25 24 23 22

ISBN 978-1-264-06667-4 (bound edition)
MHID 1-264-06667-8 (bound edition)
ISBN 978-1-266-65513-5 (loose-leaf edition)
MHID 1-266-65513-1 (loose-leaf edition)

Portfolio Manager: *Erika Lo*
Product Development Manager: *Dawn Groundwater*
Marketing Manager: *Antoinette Moore*
Content Project Managers: *Rick Hecker/Vanessa McClune*
Buyer: *Laura Fuller*
Designer: *Beth Blech*
Content Licensing Specialist: *Sarah Flynn*
Cover Image: *Michael DeYoung/Getty Images*
Compositor: *MPS Limited*

All credits appearing at the end of the book are considered to be an extension of the copyright page.

Library of Congress Cataloging-in-Publication Data

Names: Corbin, Charles B. author. | Welk, Greg, author. | Corbin, William R., author. |
 Welk, Karen A., author.
Title: Concepts of fitness and wellness : a comprehensive lifestyle approach / Charles B. Corbin, Gregory J. Welk,
 William R. Corbin, Karen A. Welk.
Description: Thirteenth edition. | New York : McGraw Hill Education 2023. | Includes bibliographical
 references and index.
Identifiers: LCCN 2021045028 (print) | LCCN 2021045029 (ebook) | ISBN 9781264066674 (hardcover) |
 ISBN 9781266655135 (spiral bound) | ISBN 9781266655005 (ebook)
Subjects: LCSH: Physical fitness. | Exercise. | Health.
Classification: LCC RA781 .C644 2022 (print) | LCC RA781 (ebook) | DDC 613.7—dc23/eng/20211001
LC record available at https://lccn.loc.gov/2021045028
LC ebook record available at https://lccn.loc.gov/2021045029

The Internet addresses listed in the text were accurate at the time of publication. The inclusion of a website does
not indicate an endorsement by the authors or McGraw Hill, and McGraw Hill does not guarantee the accuracy
of the information presented at these sites.

Brief Contents

Section I

Lifestyles for Health, Wellness, and Fitness   1

1. Health, Wellness, Fitness, and Healthy Lifestyles: An Introduction   1
2. Determinants of Lifelong Health, Wellness, and Fitness   17
3. Self-Management Skills for Health Behavior Change   29

Section II

Foundations of Physical Activity   47

4. Preparing for Physical Activity   47
5. The Health Benefits of Physical Activity   67
6. How Much Physical Activity Is Enough?   85

Section III

Engaging in Regular Physical Activity   99

7. Adopting an Active Lifestyle   99
8. Cardiorespiratory Endurance   115
9. Vigorous Aerobic, Anaerobic, Sport, and Recreational Activities   137
10. Muscle Fitness and Resistance Exercise   155
11. Flexibility and Stretching Activities   195
12. Advanced Fitness Training   221

Section IV

Establishing Healthy Eating Habits   243

13. Body Composition and Health   243
14. Nutrition and Principles of Healthy Eating   277
15. Principles of Effective Weight Control   301

Section V

Managing Stress   315

16. Stress and Health   315
17. Stress-Management Strategies   331

Section VI

Avoiding Destructive Behaviors   351

18. The Use and Abuse of Tobacco and Other Nicotine Products   351
19. The Use and Abuse of Alcohol   363
20. The Use and Abuse of Other Drugs   379

Section VII

Adopting Preventive Habits   393

21. Preventing Sexually Transmitted Infections   393
22. Cancer, Diabetes, and Other Health Threats   407
23. Body Mechanics and Care of the Back   427
24. Making Informed Consumer Choices   463
25. Toward Optimal Health and Wellness: Planning for Healthy Lifestyle Change   479

Appendixes

A. Metric Conversion Charts   503
B. Calories of Protein, Carbohydrates, and Fats in Foods   504

References   506

Index   511

Contents

Preface   xvi

Section I

Lifestyles for Health, Wellness, and Fitness   1

1 Health, Wellness, Fitness, and Healthy Lifestyles: An Introduction   1

The HELP Philosophy   2

National Health Goals   3

Health and Wellness   6

Physical Fitness   9

Using Self-Management Skills   12

Suggested Resources and Readings   14

Lab 1A: Wellness Self-Perceptions   15

2 Determinants of Lifelong Health, Wellness, and Fitness   17

Determinants of Health, Wellness, and Fitness   18

Biological Determinants   18

Social Determinants   19

Lifestyle Determinants   21

Determinant Interactions   24

Using Self-Management Skills   24

Suggested Resources and Readings   26

Lab 2A: Healthy Habit Questionnaire   27

3 Self-Management Skills for Health Behavior Change   29

Understanding Behavior Change   30

Importance of Self-Management Skills   32

Making Lifestyle Changes   34

Using Self-Management Skills   37

Suggested Resources and Readings   42

Lab 3A: Stages of Change and Self-Management Skills   43

Section II

Foundations of Physical Activity   47

4 Preparing for Physical Activity   47

Safety Considerations for Physical Activity   48

General Considerations for Physical Activity   49

Recommendations for Typical Bouts of Physical Activity   50

Physical Activity in the Heat and Cold   52

Physical Activity in Other Environments   55

Preparing for Emergencies and Handling Injuries   56

Using Self-Management Skills   58

Suggested Resources and Readings   60

Lab 4A: Readiness for Physical Activity   61

Lab 4B: The Warm-Up   63

Lab 4C: Physical Activity Attitude Questionnaire   65

5 The Health Benefits of Physical Activity   67

Physical Activity Promotes Health, Wellness, and Fitness   68

Physical Activity Reduces Risks for Hypokinetic Diseases   70

Physical Activity Promotes Cardiovascular Health   71

Physical Activity Promotes Metabolic Health   75

Physical Activity Promotes Musculoskeletal Health   76

Physical Activity Promotes Good Mental Health   77

Physical Activity Provides Many Other Health Benefits   78

Physical Activity as Lifestyle Medicine   79

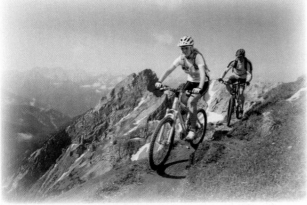

Michael Reusse/Westend61/Getty Images

Using Self-Management Skills   81

Suggested Resources and Readings   82

Lab 5A: Assessing Heart Disease Risk Factors   83

6 How Much Physical Activity Is Enough?   85

The Principles of Physical Activity   86

Application of the FIT/FITT Formula   87

The Physical Activity Pyramid   89

Physical Activity Patterns   92

Physical Fitness Standards   93

Using Self-Management Skills   94

Suggested Resources and Readings   94

Lab 6A: Self-Assessment of Physical Activity   95

Lab 6B: Estimating Your Fitness   97

Section III

Engaging in Regular Physical Activity   99

7 Adopting an Active Lifestyle   99

Fundamentals of Active Living   100

Minimizing Sedentary Behavior Is Part of an Active Lifestyle   102

The Health and Wellness Benefits of Moderate Physical Activity   104

Accumulating Moderate Physical Activity   104

Monitoring Physical Activity and Sedentary Behavior   107

Adopting and Sustaining an Active Identity   108

Using Self-Management Skills   110

Suggested Resources and Readings   110

Lab 7A: Setting Goals for Moderate Physical Activity and Self-Monitoring (Logging) Program   111

Lab 7B: Estimating Sedentary Behavior   113

8 Cardiorespiratory Endurance   115

Elements of Cardiorespiratory Endurance   116

Cardiovascular Adaptations to Physical Activity   117

Cardiorespiratory Endurance and Health Benefits   120

The FIT Formula for Cardiorespiratory Endurance   121

Threshold and Target Zones for Intensity of Activity to Build Cardiorespiratory Endurance   123

Guidelines for Heart Rate and Exercise Monitoring   126

Using Self-Management Skills   127

Suggested Resources and Readings   128

Lab Resource Materials: Evaluating Cardiorespiratory Endurance   129

Lab 8A: Counting Target Heart Rate and Ratings of Perceived Exertion   133

Lab 8B: Evaluating Cardiorespiratory Endurance   135

9 Vigorous Aerobic, Anaerobic, Sport, and Recreational Activities   137

Fundamentals of Vigorous Physical Activity   138

Vigorous Aerobic Activities   139

Vigorous Anaerobic Activities   142

Vigorous Sport Activities   142

Vigorous Recreational Activities   143

Patterns and Trends in Physical Activity Participation   144

Guidelines for Vigorous Physical Activity   146

Using Self-Management Skills   147

Suggested Resources and Readings   148

Lab 9A: The Physical Activity Adherence Questionnaire   149

Lab 9B: Planning and Logging Participation in Vigorous Physical Activity   151

Lab 9C: Combining Moderate and Vigorous Physical Activity   153

10 Muscle Fitness and Resistance Exercise   155

Factors Influencing Muscle Fitness   156

Health Benefits of Muscle Fitness Activities   158

Progressive Resistance Exercise   159

Progressive Resistance Exercise: How Much Is Enough?   162

Muscle Fitness Activities and Equipment   165

Principles of Muscle Fitness Training   167

Risks with Muscle Supplements   169

Guidelines for Safe and Effective PRE   170

Using Self-Management Skills   171

Suggested Resources and Readings   172

Lab Resource Materials: Muscles of the Body (anterior view)   173

Lab Resource Materials: Muscles of the Body (posterior view)   174

Lab Resource Materials: Muscle Fitness Tests   175

Lab 10A: Evaluating Muscle Strength: 1RM and Grip Strength   187

Lab 10B: Evaluating Muscular Endurance and Power   189

Lab 10C: Planning and Logging Muscle Fitness Exercises: Free Weights or Resistance Machines   191

Lab 10D: Planning and Logging Muscle Fitness Exercises: Calisthenics, Core Exercises, or Plyometrics   193

11   Flexibility and Stretching Activities   195

Factors Influencing Flexibility   196

Flexibility, Injuries, and Rehabilitation   198

Flexibility: How Much Is Enough?   200

Stretching Methods   201

Popular Flexibility Activities   205

Guidelines for Improving Flexibility   206

Using Self-Management Skills   207

Suggested Resources and Readings   208

Lab Resource Materials: Flexibility Tests   215

Lab 11A: Evaluating Flexibility   217

Lab 11B: Planning and Logging Stretching Exercises   219

12   Advanced Fitness Training   221

High-Level Performance and Training Characteristics   222

Training for Cardiorespiratory Endurance   224

Training for Strength, Muscular Endurance, and Power   226

Training for Speed and Power   228

Training for Functional Fitness and Flexibility   229

Training for High-Level Performance: Skill-Related Fitness and Skill   230

High-Level Performance Training   231

Performance Trends and Ergogenic Aids   232

Using Self-Management Skills   233

Suggested Resources and Readings   234

Lab Resource Materials: Skill-Related Physical Fitness   235

Lab 12A: Evaluating Skill-Related Physical Fitness   239

Lab 12B: Identifying Symptoms of Overtraining   241

Section IV

Establishing Healthy Eating Habits   243

13   Body Composition and Health   243

Understanding Obesity   244

Body Composition Indicators and Standards   245

Methods Used to Assess Body Composition   246

Health Risks Associated with Obesity   248

The Causes of Obesity   250

Treatment and Prevention of Overweight and Obesity   252

Body Image and Eating Disorders   254

Using Self-Management Skills   255

Suggested Resources and Readings   256

Lab Resource Materials: Evaluating Body Fat   257

Lab 13A: Evaluating Body Composition: Skinfold Measures   267

Lab 13B: Evaluating Body Composition: Height, Weight, and Circumference Measures   271

Lab 13C: Determining Your Daily Energy Expenditure   273

14   Nutrition and Principles of Healthy Eating   277

Guidelines and Recommendations for Healthy Eating   278

Dietary Recommendations for Carbohydrates   280

Dietary Recommendations for Fat   282

Dietary Recommendations for Proteins   283

Dietary Recommendations for Vitamins   285

Dietary Recommendations for Minerals   287

Dietary Recommendations for Water and Other Fluids   288

Understanding Contemporary Nutrition Terms, Issues, and Trends   288

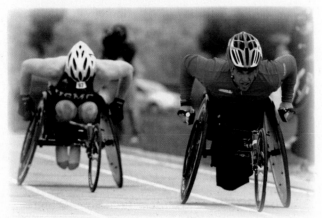

US Air Force photo by Staff Sergeant Desiree N. Palacios

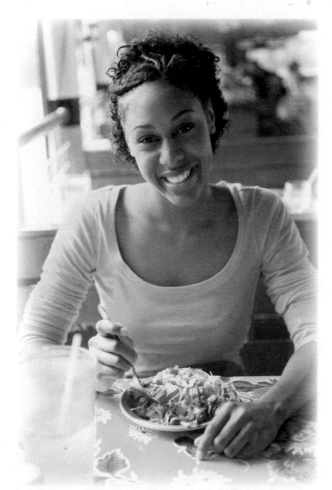

Jack Hollingsworth/Blend Images LLC

Sound Eating Practices   291

Nutrition and Physical Performance   292

Using Self-Management Skills   293

Suggested Resources and Readings   294

Lab 14A: Nutrition Analysis   295

Lab 14B: Selecting Nutritious Foods   299

15   Principles of Effective Weight Control   301

Factors Influencing Weight and Fat Control   302

Confronting an Obesogenic Environment   304

Guidelines for Losing Body Fat   305

Facts about Fad Diets and Clinical Approaches to Weight Loss   308

Using Self-Management Skills   309

Suggested Resources and Readings   310

Lab 15A: Selecting Strategies for Managing Eating   311

Lab 15B: Evaluating Fast Food Options   313

Section V

Managing Stress   315

16   Stress and Health   315

Sources of Stress   316

Stress in Contemporary Society   317

Reactions to Stress   318

Stress Effects on Health and Wellness   320

Individual Differences in the Stress Response   321

Using Self-Management Skills   324

Suggested Resources and Readings   326

Lab 16A: Evaluating Your Stress Level   327

Lab 16B: Evaluating Your Hardiness and Locus of Control   329

17   Stress-Management Strategies   331

Physical Activity and Stress Management   332

Stress, Sleep, and Recreation   333

Principles of Stress Management   334

Effective Coping Strategies   336

Effective Time-Management Skills   340

Effective Social Support   342

Using Self-Management Skills   343

Suggested Resources and Readings   344

Lab 17A: Time Management   345

Lab 17B: Relaxation Exercises   347

Lab 17C: Evaluating Levels of Social Support   349

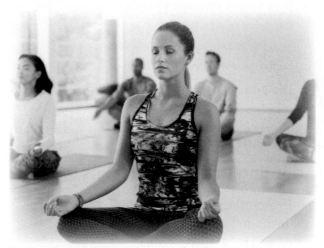

Caiaimage/Robert Daly/Getty Images

Section VI

Avoiding Destructive Behaviors   351

18 The Use and Abuse of Tobacco and Other Nicotine Products   351

Tobacco: Components and Implications of Use   352

Smoked Tobacco: Health and Economic Costs   352

Other Nicotine Products: Health and Economic Costs   355

Marketing and Use of Tobacco and Other Nicotine Products   356

Using Self-Management Skills   359

Suggested Resources and Readings   360

Lab 18A: Use and Abuse of Tobacco and Other Nicotine Products   361

19 The Use and Abuse of Alcohol   363

Alcohol and Alcoholic Beverages   364

Alcohol Consumption and Alcohol Abuse   365

Health and Behavioral Consequences of Alcohol Use   366

Risk Factors for Alcohol-Related Problems   369

Alcohol Use in Young Adults   370

Effective Approaches for Alcohol Prevention and Treatment   372

Using Self-Management Skills   373

Suggested Resources and Readings   374

Lab 19A: Blood Alcohol Level   375

Lab 19B: Perceptions about Alcohol Use   377

20 The Use and Abuse of Other Drugs   379

Classification of Illicit and Prescription Drugs   380

Prevalence and Consequences of Illicit Drug Abuse   382

Drug-Specific Prevalence and Consequences   385

Causes of Illicit Drug Abuse   388

Using Self-Management Skills   389

Suggested Resources and Readings   390

Lab 20A: Risk for Problem Drug Use   391

Section VII

Adopting Preventive Habits   393

21 Preventing Sexually Transmitted Infections   393

General Facts   394

HIV/AIDS   394

Common Sexually Transmitted Infections   398

Factors That Contribute to Sexual Risks   401

Prevention and Early Intervention of STIs   403

Using Self-Management Skills   403

Suggested Resources and Readings   404

Lab 21A: Sexually Transmitted Infection Risk Questionnaire   405

22 Cancer, Diabetes, and Other Health Threats   407

Cancer   408

Cancer Prevention   415

Diabetes   416

Alzheimer Disease and Dementia   418

Mental Health   419

Injury Prevention   419

Infectious Diseases and Other Health Threats   420

Using Self-Management Skills   421

Suggested Resources and Readings   422

Lab 22A: Determining Your Cancer Risk   423

Lab 22B: Breast and Testicular Self-Exams   425

23 Body Mechanics and Care of the Back   427

Anatomy and Function of the Spine   428

Anatomy and Function of the Core Musculature   428

Causes and Consequences of Back and Neck Pain   430

Prevention and Rehabilitation of Back and Neck Problems   433

Good Posture Is Important for Back and Neck Health   434

Good Body Mechanics Are Important for Back and Neck Health   438

Exercise Guidelines for Back and Neck Health   438

Using Self-Management Skills   442

Suggested Resources and Readings   442

Lab Resource Materials: Healthy Back Tests   455

Lab 23A: The Back/Neck Questionnaire and Healthy Back Tests   457

Lab 23B: Evaluating Posture   459

Lab 23C: Planning and Logging Core and Back Exercises   461

24 Making Informed Consumer Choices   463

Quacks and Quackery   464

Physical Activity Quackery   465

Considerations with Exercise Equipment and Fitness Programs   466

Considerations with Health Clubs and Spas   467

Body Composition Quackery   468

Nutrition Quackery   469

Consumer Protections Against Fraud and Quackery   470

Health Literacy and the Internet   472

Using Self-Management Skills   473

Suggested Resources and Readings   474

Lab 24A: Practicing Consumer Skills: Evaluating Products   475

Lab 24B: Evaluating a Health, Wellness, or Fitness Club   477

25 Toward Optimal Health and Wellness: Planning for Healthy Lifestyle Change   479

Understand Inherited Risks and Strengths   480

Make Effective Use of Health Care   481

Consider Environmental Influences on Your Health   482

Adopt and Maintain Healthy Lifestyles   484

Importance of Personal Actions and Interactions   485

Using Self-Management Skills   487

Suggested Resources and Readings   489

Lab 25A: Assessing Factors That Influence Health, Wellness, and Fitness   490

Lab 25B: Planning for Improved Health, Wellness, and Fitness   492

Lab 25C: Planning Your Personal Physical Activity Program   494

Appendixes

A Metric Conversion Charts   503

B Calories of Protein, Carbohydrates, and Fats in Foods   504

References   506

Index   511

gpointstudio/Shutterstock

Features

Corbin's Concepts of Fitness and Wellness includes magazine-like features that help students integrate and apply information they may see in the news or read about on the Internet. These features have follow-up activities available in **McGraw Hill Connect**® and can be assigned online.

- *A Closer Look* provides information about new and sometimes controversial topics related to health, wellness, and fitness and encourages critical thinking.
- *Technology Update* describes emerging health and fitness technology, innovations, and research.
- *In the News* highlights late-breaking health, wellness, and fitness events, trends, and information.
- *HELP* personalizes fitness and health issues through brief narratives that relate to the defining elements of the HELP Philosophy (H: Health, E: Everyone, L: Lifetime, P: Personal).

A CLOSER LOOK

1. Mental Health During a Pandemic 8
2. Lifestyles and COVID-19 22
3. Social Justice and the DEI Movement 32
4. AEDs 56
5. Long-Term Effects of COVID-19 on Heart Health 80
6. Exercise in a Pill? 89
7. Sedentary Behavior: How Much Is Too Much? 103
8. High-Intensity Interval Training (HIIT) 123
9. 23 and 1/2 Hours 146
10. CrossFit Controversy 166
11. Massage Rollers 207
12. "Heads Up" Concussion Awareness 223
13. What Happened to Body Positivity? 254
14. Benefits of Regenerative Farming 290
15. Food Insecurity and Obesity 305
16. Systemic Racism and Stress 319
17. Weathering the Storm 334
18. E-Cigarettes: Smoking Cessation Method or a New Path to Addiction? 358
19. Controversies over Alcohol Plus Cannabis 369
20. Cannabis/Marijuana Decriminalization 385
21. Sexual Misconduct on Campus 402
22. FDA Proposes Safety Measures for Indoor Tanning Devices 415
23. Functional Movement Tests 430
24. College Students: Victims of Misinformation 473
25. Getting Enough Sleep? Turn Off Your Phone 485

Technology Update

1. Health Websites and Podcasts 13
2. Genetic Testing 18
3. Health and Fitness Apps 39
4. Monitoring Environmental Conditions 55
5. My Life Check: A Tool to Evaluate Your Heart Health 72
6. Wearable Technology in Health Care 92
7. Standing Desks and Treadmill Desks 108
8. Pulse Oximetry Sensors 125
9. Exergaming and Virtual Racing 141
10. Online Resistance Training Options 167
11. Take-a-Break Reminders 198
12. Shoe Technology and the 2-Hour Marathon 233
13. Is Technology the Problem or the Solution? 251
14. Start Simple with MyPlate 292
15. Can Smartphone Apps Help with Weight Control? 310
16. Challenges with Interpreting Online Information 324
17. Online Stress-Management Resources 339
18. Are There "Safer" Cigarettes? 354
19. Apps to Treat Addiction? 372
20. Vaping Technology and Cannabis 389
21. "Hook-Up" Apps May Contribute to Risky Sex and STIs 402
22. Drivers of COVID-19 Vaccine Development 421
23. Breaking Bad Posture Habits 440
24. DNA Testing Services 474
25. Is the *Star Trek* Tricorder a Reality? 482

In the News

1. Healthiest Places to Live 5
2. International Health Rankings 21
3. Myths and Medical Conspiracy Theories 30
4. Sunscreens Are Not All Equally Effective 55
5. Lifestyle Medicine 80
6. Move Your Way! 93
7. Sedentary Behavior and Mental Health 101
8. Heritability and Fitness Adaptations 118
9. Youth Sports Matter 143
10. Warnings about Muscle-Building Supplements 171
11. Yoga as a Complementary Health Approach 206
12. Youth Sports: When Is It Too Much? 231
13. Quarantine 15 244
14. Boom in Plant-Based Foods 284
15. Strategies for Avoiding Emotional Eating 303
16. The News Is Stressful! 320
17. The Misinformation Superhighway 342
18. Tobacco-Use Controversies 359
19. Has COVID-19 Increased or Decreased Drinking? 366
20. The Opioid Crisis: Who Is at Fault? 387
21. Condom Use Resistance and STIs 403
22. Cancer Screening Guidelines 412
23. Digital Eye Strain and Zoom Fatigue 441
24. Operation Quack Hack: Targeting False COVID-19 Information 465
25. Healthy Lifestyles During the Pandemic 486

HELP Health is available to Everyone for a Lifetime, and it's Personal

1. COVID-19 3
2. Social Determinants and Social Justice 20
3. Do Your Friends Support or Hinder Your Efforts to Adopt Healthy Lifestyles? 38
4. Forming Physical Activity Habits 60
5. This Is Your Brain on Exercise 78
6. *Physical Activity Guidelines* Emphasize Personal Choice 87
7. Is Walking a Means to an End or an End in Itself? 105
8. Does College Make You *More* or *Less* Active? 127
9. Vigorous Exercise Boosts Metabolism Long after the Workout 139
10. Resistance Exercise Boosts Confidence and Mental Health 160
11. Functional Fitness 201
12. Extreme Exercise 224
13. Weight Discrimination 245
14. What Do *Healthy* and *Natural* Really Mean? 290
15. What Is the Secret for Long-Term Weight Control? 306
16. Telehealth Care for Stress 324
17. Dealing with College Stress 336
18. Outdoor Smoking Bans 357
19. Alcohol Treatment Navigator 372
20. Preventing Drug-Impaired Driving 388
21. CDC Campaigns to Prevent STIs 396
22. Personal Health Versus Public Health 420
23. Is Back Pain in Your Future? 432
24. Can You Help Stop Fraud? 471
25. A Planetary Health Pledge 484

Lab Activities

All end-of-chapter Lab Activities are available in **McGraw Hill Connect**® and can be assigned, completed, submitted, and graded online. Lab Resource Materials (extra materials for use in completing Lab Activities) are available for all fitness self-assessments.

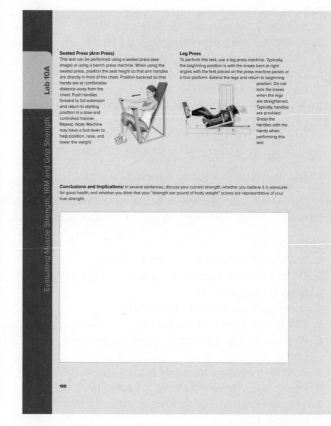

Lab 1A Wellness Self-Perceptions 15

Lab 2A Healthy Habit Questionnaire 27

Lab 3A Stages of Change and Self-Management Skills 43

Lab 4A Readiness for Physical Activity 61

Lab 4B The Warm-Up 63

Lab 4C Physical Activity Attitude Questionnaire 65

Lab 5A Assessing Heart Disease Risk Factors 83

Lab 6A Self-Assessment of Physical Activity 95

Lab 6B Estimating Your Fitness 97

Lab 7A Setting Goals for Moderate Physical Activity and Self-Monitoring (Logging) Program 111

Lab 7B Estimating Sedentary Behavior 113

Lab 8A Counting Target Heart Rate and Ratings of Perceived Exertion 133

Lab 8B Evaluating Cardiorespiratory Endurance 135

Lab 9A The Physical Activity Adherence Questionnaire 149

Lab 9B Planning and Logging Participation in Vigorous Physical Activity 151

Lab 9C Combining Moderate and Vigorous Physical Activity 153

Lab 10A Evaluating Muscle Strength: 1RM and Grip Strength 187

Lab 10B Evaluating Muscular Endurance and Power 189

Lab 10C Planning and Logging Muscle Fitness Exercises: Free Weights or Resistance Machines 191

Lab 10D Planning and Logging Muscle Fitness Exercises: Calisthenics, Core Exercises, or Plyometrics 193

Lab 11A Evaluating Flexibility 217

Lab 11B Planning and Logging Stretching Exercises 219

Lab 12A Evaluating Skill-Related Physical Fitness 239

Lab 12B Identifying Symptoms of Overtraining 241

Lab 13A Evaluating Body Composition: Skinfold Measures 267

Lab 13B Evaluating Body Composition: Height, Weight, and Circumference Measures 271

Lab 13C Determining Your Daily Energy Expenditure 273

Lab 14A Nutrition Analysis 295

Lab 14B Selecting Nutritious Foods 299

Lab 15A Selecting Strategies for Managing Eating 311

Lab 15B Evaluating Fast Food Options 313

Lab 16A Evaluating Your Stress Level 327

Lab 16B Evaluating Your Hardiness and Locus of Control 329

Lab 17A Time Management 345

Lab 17B Relaxation Exercises 347

Lab 17C Evaluating Levels of Social Support 349

Lab 18A Use and Abuse of Tobacco and Other Nicotine Products 361

Lab 19A Blood Alcohol Level 375

Lab 19B Perceptions about Alcohol Use 377

Lab 20A Risk for Problem Drug Use 391

Lab 21A Sexually Transmitted Infection Risk Questionnaire 405

Lab 22A Determining Your Cancer Risk 423

Lab 22B Breast and Testicular Self-Exams 425

Lab 23A The Back/Neck Questionnaire and Healthy Back Tests 457

Lab 23B Evaluating Posture 459

Lab 23C Planning and Logging Core and Back Exercises 461

Lab 24A Practicing Consumer Skills: Evaluating Products 475

Lab 24B Evaluating a Health, Wellness, or Fitness Club 477

Lab 25A Assessing Factors That Influence Health, Wellness, and Fitness 490

Lab 25B Planning for Improved Health, Wellness, and Fitness 492

Lab 25C Planning Your Personal Physical Activity Program 494

Building on 50 Years of Success!

The thirteenth edition ushers in a new era with a new title—*Corbin's Concepts of Fitness and Wellness*—that honors the vision and legacy of Dr. Charles (Chuck) Corbin in developing the Concepts approach over 50 years ago. Our established tradition of innovation in the fitness and wellness field continues with completely updated content, features, and online materials that are designed to support education on healthy lifestyles.

Moving into the Future

The new title also marks strategic authorship changes as Dr. Greg Welk, Professor of Kinesiology and Fellow in the National Academy of Kinesiology, takes over leadership with this new edition and its development. Dr. Welk actively teaches and conducts research in areas of fitness/wellness and health promotion and will ensure that *Corbin's Concepts of Fitness and Wellness* continues to provide instructors and students with the most current, accurate, and useful information. Dr. Chuck Corbin, lead author of all the previous *Concepts* books, continues to actively participate in all facets of authorship as a retired Emeritus Professor. Dr. Will Corbin, a professor of clinical psychology with expertise in health psychology, leads the content related to stress management, alcohol, tobacco, drugs, and sexually transmitted infections. Dr. Karen Welk, an established physical therapist, provides expertise in flexibility, strength and conditioning, back care, and contraindicated exercises. The diverse backgrounds and skills of the authors contribute to the comprehensive coverage of health, fitness, and wellness issues covered in the book. The authors work to reduce the technical jargon and focus on self-management skills and strategies to help students learn to adopt and sustain healthy lifestyles throughout life.

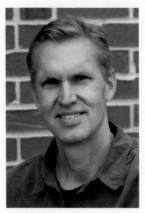
Greg Welk

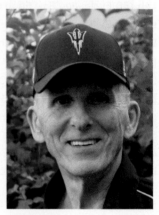
Charles Corbin

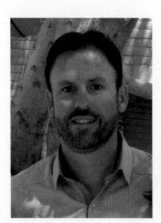
Will Corbin

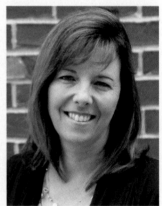
Karen Welk

Dedication

The authors would like to dedicate this edition to the millions of scientists, health-care workers, educators, and public health leaders who have directly confronted the unique challenges caused by the COVID-19 pandemic. Millions of people throughout the world lost their lives due to COVID-19, but many millions more were saved by the efforts to help people recover as well as by establishing practices to minimize its spread and through vaccine development and delivery.

Thank You

We are always listening to our users and greatly appreciate the feedback provided over the years. The insights have helped us continue to enhance instruction and improve student learning. We want to provide a special thanks to Joel Baum from Gender Spectrum for insights on revised gender terminology throughout the text. We also want to specifically thank the instructors who provided insights regarding the book and their course needs as this feedback also directly enhanced this edition's revisions:

Elizabeth Bates, *Snead State Community College*
Jennifer Brown, *Auburn University-Montgomery*
Carl Bryan, *Central Carolina Community College*
Ronnie Carda, *University of Wisconsin-Madison*
Kay Daigle, *Southeastern Oklahoma State University*
Amy Fletcher, *University of Iowa*
Rich Gennaro, *Westchester Community College*
Janene Grodesky, *Louisiana State University*
Cammie Hallmark, *Jefferson State Community College*
Kevin Harper, *Tarrant County College*
Candace Hendershot, *University of Findlay*
Heather Hudson, *University of Central Arkansas*
Brian Jenison, *Lonestar College*
Yi-Tzu Kuo, *Barry University*

Brian LaPlante, *Rochester Community and Technical College*
Kenneth Larson, *Georgia Gwinnett College*
Brandy Lynch, *University of Central Missouri*
Jordon Macht, *Campbellsville University*
Caryn Martin, *Polk State College*
Darrick Matthews, *University of Science and Arts of Oklahoma*
Jason Melnyk, *Central Connecticut State University*
Courtney Murray, *Campbellsville University*
Jason Ng, *California State University-San Bernardino*
Tom Pate, *Concordia University Texas*
Rod Porter, *Miramar College*
Kim Queri, *Rose State College*
Nicklaus Redenius, *North Dakota State University*
Mary-Anne Reid, *Michigan State University*
Kelsie Rodman, *Anderson University*
Tina Sardo, *Jamestown Community College*
Sheila M. Stepp, *State University of New York–Orange*
Kumika Toma, *Marshall University*
Zachary Townsend, *Salisbury University*
Suzanne Wambold, *The University of Toledo*
Laura V. Wheatley, *Utah Valley University*
David Wiederrecht, *Lone Star College-University Park*
Lauren Willis, *Campbellsville University*
Kendra Zenisek, *Ball State University*

To list everyone who has had an impact on the *Concepts* texts over the years would take several pages. Nevertheless, we feel that it is important to acknowledge those who have helped us. A list of the many contributors is available at **www .corbinconcepts.org**, as are additional resources we have provided that support the use of *Corbin's Concepts of Fitness and Wellness* in your course. Thank you all!

Gregory J. Welk
Charles B. Corbin
William R. Corbin
Karen A. Welk
www.corbinconcepts.org

Preface

Corbin's Concepts of Fitness and Wellness provides a comprehensive and evidence-based approach to teaching principles of health living. Foundational elements include an integrated instructional HELP philosophy that focuses on self-management skills for sustained lifestyle change, a concepts-based framework designed for achieving well-defined learning objectives, and an engaging, student-centered format that accommodates various learning preferences and methods.

Paired with **McGraw Hill Connect®,** a digital assignment and assessment platform that strengthens the link between faculty, students, and coursework, instructors and students accomplish more in less time. Connect for Fitness & Wellness is particularly useful for remote and hybrid courses and includes assignable and assessable videos, quizzes, exercises, and labs.

Integrated HELP Philosophy

Health is available to **E**veryone
for a **L**ifetime, and it's **P**ersonal.

The HELP philosophy directs the content in *Corbin's Concepts of Fitness and Wellness,* helping and empowering students to understand the personal responsibility involved in achieving sound health (including fitness and wellness) through the adoption of healthy lifestyles. Although an array of lifestyles are covered, the emphasis is on physical activity, healthy eating, and stress management (*priority lifestyles*) since they strongly impact overall health and well-being and can be obtained and sustained by using personal responsibility. Critical self-management skills, which are introduced and

detailed in Concept 3: Self-Management Skills for Health Behavior Change, are essential for making healthy decisions and lifestyle choices. Each Concept concludes with a *Using Self-Management Skills* section that reinforces key self-management skills and behaviors. Each Concept includes comprehensive *Lab Activities* that are designed to provide opportunities to learn and practice these skills. (The Lab Activities are available for online submission through **McGraw Hill Connect®.**) Ultimately, the goal is for students to learn to prepare personal programs of health behavior change that address their own needs and interests.

Concepts-Based Framework

A unique, defining aspect of *Corbin's Concepts of Fitness and Wellness* is the "concepts-based" approach to education, which begins with concise Concepts rather than lengthy chapters. Specific learning objectives are identified at the beginning of each Concept to help focus and guide students to the most important information. The *Why It Matters!* section introduces the Concept by detailing the main purpose or goal. Content within each Concept is then organized into thematic sections and each includes several more concise "concepts" or principles. Carefully worded statements introduce each of these mini-sections to help students retain the key takeaway messages in the Concept. This modularized approach to learning offers advantages for student learning and retention since the important information is introduced and then directly reinforced.

LEARNING OBJECTIVES

After completing the study of this Concept, you will be able to:

▶ Identify the determinants of health, wellness, and fitness, and explain how they each contribute to health, wellness, and fitness.

▶ Differentiate between factors over which you have lesser and greater control.

▶ Use health behavior change strategies to carry out self-assessments of personal lifestyles and wellness perceptions.

Many factors are important in developing lifetime health, wellness, and fitness, and some are more in your control than others. A factor that significantly affects your health, wellness, and fitness is referred to as a ***determinant***. Three major categories of determinants are listed in **Figure 1.** Biological factors, such as heredity, age, and sex, are shown at the bottom of the figure because they are determinants over which we have little or no control.

Learning Objectives (left) *introduce each concept, and modularized "Concept Statements"* (right, in blue) *help guide student learning.*

Student-Centered Approach to Learning

Students learn using many different types of sensory input. Accordingly, the visuals in *Corbin's Concepts of Fitness and Wellness* include photos with concept-relevant captions, figures that convey conceptual materials in an easy-to-understand format, and hundreds of detailed exercise illustrations that show exactly how to perform exercises for important dimensions of health-related fitness.

Additionally, each Concept includes four feature boxes that delve into current issues in the headlines, introduce students to ongoing research and technology, and ask students to consider how health issues affect them personally. *A Closer Look* provides information about new and sometimes controversial topics related to health, wellness, and fitness and encourages critical-thinking. *Technology Update* describes advances in health and fitness technology and prompts exploration and personal evaluation. *In the News* highlights late-breaking health, wellness, and fitness information and provides opportunities for reflection. The *HELP* feature personalizes fitness and health issues to help students internalize the information. Students have the opportunity to explore many of these topics in more detail by using the *Suggested Resources and Readings* section and additional feature-specific activities and critical thinking exercises that are accessible and assignable within **McGraw Hill Connect®**.

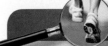

A CLOSER LOOK

Weathering the Storm

Weathering is a term used to describe health disparities that may result from cumulative socioeconomic disadvantage. Dr. Arline Geronimus first used the term to describe discrepancies in reproductive outcomes of Black versus white females, but the term is now used more broadly to refer to health disparities in Black populations. A contributing factor to this weathering is systemic racism, a topic that has garnered increased attention in the United States following the deaths of George Floyd and other Black Americans. Forms of discrimination and marginalization slowly chip away at a person, causing those who are on the receiving end to have compromised health or premature death. The concept of weathering provides a way to understand a root cause of health disparities in our society.

What steps should individuals take to address systemic racism and unjust weathering?

Feature boxes introduce and detail important societal issues, new research and technology, and opportunities for students to consider how health issues affect them personally.

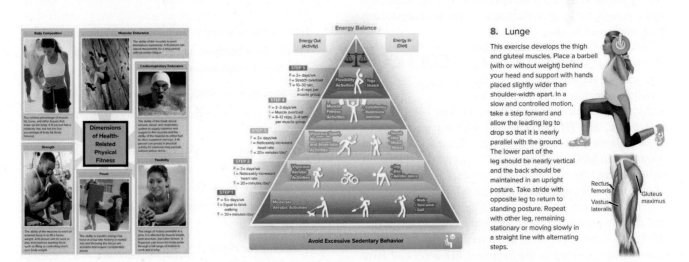

Engaging graphics, instructional diagrams (such as the unique physical activity pyramid), and detailed exercise illustrations facilitate student learning.

Source: Comstock/Getty Images; Thinkstock Images/Stockbyte/Getty Images; Stockbyte/Getty Images; Shutterstock; Ryan McVay/Getty Images; Tom Grill/Corbis/Getty Images

Highlights of the Thirteenth Edition

Concept Updates

Each revision of *Corbin's Concepts of Fitness and Wellness* incorporates new research and findings about healthy lifestyles, but the thirteenth edition was influenced by many external factors as well. This edition was conceptualized and updated during the height of the COVID-19 pandemic, which challenged all facets of our society and increased attention on the intersections of public health and personal health. While each of us needed to take responsibility for our own health, local and national mandates and laws established policies and practices needed to promote health for all. The pandemic demonstrated the role of science in medicine and health as we witnessed the rapid development of life-saving vaccines as well as the deployment of these vaccines across the world. However, the most tangible impact of COVID-19 is how it influenced our individual health and well-being.

Research conducted during the pandemic provided many new insights about health and wellness. For example, numerous studies documented the importance of healthy lifestyles (and healthy weight) for enhancing immune function and for reducing risks from COVID-19. Other studies documented the impact of the pandemic on our personal behaviors, including how it compounded stress. In this new edition, we reference many studies conducted on COVID-19 issues; however, the focus is on the implications for personal health and healthy living. Research is always evolving in the health and wellness field, but insights from new studies were particularly dramatic in recent years.

Student reflection and exploration of new trends and societal issues are particularly emphasized within the various box features that are included in each of the Concepts (*In the News, A Closer Look, Technology Update,* and *HELP*). Updated with many new topics, these features are linked to customized application assignments within **McGraw Hill Connect**® to facilitate exploration, reflection, and discussion of these complex issues. A variety of video vignettes are also embedded within the eBook and linked to Connect activities to help explain complex issues and provide opportunities for personal reflection and critical thinking. Current, accessible, and relevant resources and publications are provided in the *Suggested Resources and Readings,* while updated scientific references are provided at the end-of-text *References* section.

This new edition utilizes the most current terminology for gender and gender identity as recommended by the American Psychological Association (APA). Additionally, updates and new content illuminate the importance of *the social determinants of health* and challenges with resolving health disparities. Although our emphasis is on personal responsibility and focusing on what is within your control, mass movements against systemic racism have exposed health inequities and disparities that need to be collectively addressed by individuals, organizations, and society as a whole.

Guidelines and trends in the fitness and wellness field have also been thoroughly updated in this new edition. For example, the recent revisions from the *American College of Sports Medicine's (ACSM) Guidelines for Exercise Testing and Prescription* prompted changes in exercise recommendations for several health-related fitness areas. Other new research findings and public health updates are woven through each of the Concepts. Some of the updates are highlighted below:

1 Health, Wellness, Fitness, and Healthy Lifestyles: An Introduction
- Updated statistics about health, longevity, and wellness
- Inclusion of *Healthy People 2030* goals
- New depiction of the illness and wellness continuum
- Inclusion of equity and social justice issues within the HELP philosophy

2 Determinants of Lifelong Health, Wellness, and Fitness
- Increased coverage of the social determinants of health
- New categorization and conceptualization of lifestyle determinants
- New illustrations depicting the determinants of health, wellness, and fitness
- Integration of content on habit formation
- Distinctions between sex at birth and gender identity related to health and wellness

3 Self-Management Skills for Health Behavior Change
- Updated descriptions and depictions of social-ecological models
- Updated explanations of the Transtheoretical Model and applications
- New integrative model to explain stages of change
- More personalized explanations of self-management skills

4 Preparing for Physical Activity
- Updated safety considerations based on ACSM exercise guidelines
- New content on shoe and clothing considerations for exercise
- Enhanced coverage of guidelines for heat, cold, and treatment of injuries

5 The Health Benefits of Physical Activity

- Reorganized flow of material based on system-based adaptations

- Improved system-based depiction of the health benefits of physical activity

- Enhanced coverage of mental health

- Updated descriptions and explanations of hypokinetic conditions

- New content on lifestyle medicine and implications for health care

6 How Much Physical Activity Is Enough?

- Updated FIT principles based on ACSM guidelines for exercise testing and prescription

- Revised graphic depiction of the physical activity pyramid

- Incorporation of anaerobic exercise and high-intensity interval training (HIIT)

- Updated statistics on adults meeting the U.S. physical activity guidelines

7 Adopting an Active Lifestyle

- New title and flow to distinguish light, moderate, and vigorous physical activity

- Updated content and guidelines related to sedentary behavior

- New depiction of interactive risks of sedentary behavior and inactivity

- New content on wearable technology and applications for self-monitoring

8 Cardiorespiratory Endurance

- Updated thresholds and target zones for exercise based on new ACSM guidelines

- New calculations based on heart rate reserve and max heart rate methods

- Clarifications based on adaptations related to cardiorespiratory endurance

9 Vigorous Aerobic, Anaerobic, Sport, and Recreational Activities

- Updated title to highlight anaerobic activities

- Clearer distinctions of type of vigorous aerobic activities

- Expanded content on anaerobic activities and HIIT

- Updated data on patterns and trends in behaviors

- Refined content and strategies in self-management section

10 Muscle Fitness and Resistance Exercise

- Revised sections on differences between males and females based on sex at birth

- Clarified terminology and applications of fitness principles for resistance exercise

- New descriptions of the circuit training, plyometrics, and body weight exercises

- Updated content on the risks of supplements that tout strength and fitness enhancement

11 Flexibility and Stretching Activities

- Updated title with greater emphasis on activities promoting flexibility

- New content on injuries and rehabilitation issues

- Revised guidelines for stretching based on new research

- Updates on Pilates, yoga, and tai chi and popularity of stretching activities

12 Advanced Fitness Training

- Updated title with focus on adaptations in different metabolic systems

- Greater specification about training for different sports and activities

- New content on anaerobic capacity and training for speed/power

13 Body Composition and Health

- Updated title with greater focus on health implications of body composition

- New introduction section on societal issues and stigmatization with obesity

- Refined explanations and descriptions of body composition standards

- Updated content on causes and consequences of obesity

- Clarifications about eating disorders and implications

14 Nutrition and Principles of Healthy Eating

- Updated title with focus on principles for healthy eating

- New sections on establishing healthy eating patterns and a "total diet approach"

- Clarification on terminology and explanation of dietary guidelines

- New content on popularity of plant-based protein and vegetarian diets

- Updated content on cholesterol, trans fats, nutraceuticals, functional foods, and organic foods

- Refined section on self-management skills, focusing on self-monitoring skills

15 Principles of Effective Weight Control

- Updated title and focus on self-management skills for weight control

- Enhanced coverage of social-ecological models as related to weight control
- Updates on fad diets and clinical approaches to weight loss

16 Stress and Health

- Greater focus on stress issues unique for college students
- New content on stress associated with COVID-19 and discrimination
- Updated information on stress response and influences from personality types

17 Stress-Management Strategies

- Updated title and focus on self-management skills and strategies for stress management
- Greater coverage on social support influences
- Incorporation of SMART goals for time management

18 The Use and Abuse of Tobacco and Other Nicotine Products

- Updated title and expansion of content to cover other nicotine products
- Expanded coverage of e-cigarettes and trends with vaping
- Updated information on the economic costs to society of tobacco and nicotine use
- Updates on marketing of tobacco to increase awareness

19 The Use and Abuse of Alcohol

- Updated statistics and patterns of alcohol use and abuse
- New information on policies and environmental factors related to alcohol
- Updated data and insights on campus issues and strategies related to alcohol abuse

20 The Use and Abuse of Other Drugs

- Updated statistics and data on the prevalence of drug abuse in society
- New terminology and updates related to cannabis use in society with regard to legalization
- Updates on the independent classification of opioids
- New content on issues with misuse and risks of prescription drugs

21 Preventing Sexually Transmitted Infections

- Updated statistics on the prevalence of different sexually transmitted infections
- Revised organization and flow of content on common sexually transmitted infections
- Updates on HIV issues and treatments

22 Cancer, Diabetes, and Other Health Threats

- Updated statistics on prevalence and death rates from various cancers
- Streamlined presentation and flow of content on cancers with major updates on prostate, colon-rectal, and breast cancer
- Expanded coverage of infectious diseases and details related to COVID-19 risks

23 Body Mechanics and Care of the Back

- Relocated Concept to place it closer to chronic conditions
- Updated title with focus on posture and prevention of back and neck pain
- New graphics and explanations of degenerative disc disease and causes of back issues
- Revised explanations for the role of exercise in back and neck health
- Strategies for planning and assessment in the self-management section

24 Making Informed Consumer Choices

- Updated title with more emphasis on self-management skills and consumerism
- Streamlined recommendations on consumer considerations for exercise machines and clubs
- New information on decision making related to apps and online programs
- Updates on the FDA's efforts and strategies for curtailing fraud and quackery

25 Toward Optimal Health and Wellness: Planning for Healthy Lifestyle Change

- New organization and flow based on new conceptual model of lifestyle and social determinants of health, wellness, and fitness
- Increased emphasis on health care and health consumerism
- Updated content on strategies for healthy living, with a focus on personal responsibility

Innovations for Enhanced Learning

The thirteenth edition of *Corbin's Concepts of Fitness and Wellness* is designed to deliver a flexible and personalized approach to fitness and wellness education. The materials provide an integrated print and digital solution that enables instructors (and students) to explore options for applying the information.

Connect® Is Proven Effective

McGraw Hill Connect® is a digital teaching and learning environment that improves performance over a variety of critical outcomes; it is easy to use; and it is proven effective. Connect empowers students by continually adapting to deliver precisely what they need, when they need it, and how they need it, so your class time is more engaging and effective. *Connect for Fitness & Wellness* offers a wealth of interactive online content, including labs and self-assessments, video activities on timely health topics, and practice quizzes with immediate feedback.

New to this edition, additional Lab Activities and Self-Assessments were redesigned and added as **Application-Based Activities** to offer enhanced accessibility, a privacy option, and aggregated student self-assessment results by section. Appearing in Connect, these activities help your students assess their own health and behavior. New topics include stress and anxiety related to the outbreak of COVID-19 and adapting an exercise program for changing situations.

With just a smartphone, tablet, or webcam, students and instructors can capture video with ease. **Video Capture Powered by GoReact** doesn't require any extra equipment or complicated training. All it takes is five minutes to set up and start recording! Use Video Capture to create your own custom video capture assignment, including lab activities, exercises, presentations, self-review, and peer review. With customizable rubrics, time-coded comments, and visual markers, students will see feedback at exactly the right moment, and in context, to help improve their skills.

Also new within McGraw Hill Connect®, the **Writing Assignment tool** delivers a learning experience to help students improve their written communication skills and conceptual understanding. As an instructor you can assign, monitor, grade, and provide feedback on writing more efficiently and effectively.

Concept Clips on topics like the cardiorespiratory system and stress response are also new to this edition. Assignable and assessable through Connect, Concept Clips provide step-by-step presentations to promote student comprehension.

NewsFlash activities tie current news stories to key fitness and wellness concepts. After interacting with a contemporary news story, students are assessed on their understanding and

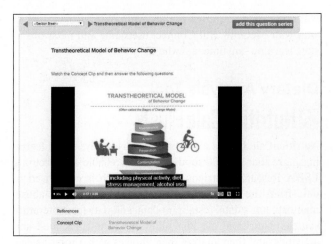

Concept Clips illustrate major topics and provide jumping-off points for class discussion.

their ability to make the connections between real-life events and course content. Examples of NewsFlash topics include addressing racial disparities during the COVID-19 pandemic, providing game-day food safety tips, and pushing the limits of human endurance.

Personalized Learning
SMARTBOOK®

Available within Connect, **SmartBook®** makes study time as productive and efficient as possible by identifying and closing knowledge gaps. SmartBook identifies what an individual student knows and doesn't know based on the student's confidence level, responses to questions, and other factors. SmartBook builds an optimal, personalized learning path for each student, so students spend less time on concepts they already understand and more time on those they don't. As a student engages with SmartBook, the reading experience continuously adapts by highlighting the most impactful content a student needs to learn at that moment in time. This ensures that every minute spent with SmartBook is returned to the student as the most value-added minute possible. The result? More confidence, better grades, and greater success.

SmartBook is optimized for smartphones and tablets and is now more accessible for students of all abilities.

ReadAnywhere

Read or study when it's convenient for you with McGraw Hill's free **ReadAnywhere** app. Available for iOS or Android smartphones or tablets, ReadAnywhere gives users access to McGraw Hill tools including the eBook and SmartBook or Adaptive Learning Assignments in Connect. Take notes, highlight, and complete assignments offline—all of your work will sync when you open the app with WiFi access. Log in with your McGraw Hill Connect username and password to start learning—anytime, anywhere!

Dietary Analysis Tool

McGraw Hill NutritionCalc Plus

NutritionCalc Plus is a powerful dietary analysis tool featuring more than 30,000 foods from the reliable and accurate ESHA Research nutrient database, which is comprised of data from the latest USDA Standard Reference database, manufacturer's data, restaurant data, and data from literature sources. NutritionCalc Plus allows users to track food and activities, and then analyze their choices with a robust selection of intuitive reports. The interface was updated to accommodate ADA requirements and a modern mobile experience native to today's students.

Your Course, Your Way

McGraw Hill Create® is a self-service website that allows you to create customized course materials using McGraw Hill Education's comprehensive, cross-disciplinary content and digital products. You can even access third-party content such as readings, articles, cases, videos, and more.

- Select and arrange content to fit your course scope and sequence.
- Upload your own course materials.
- Select the best format for your students—print or eBook.
- Select and personalize your cover.
- Edit and update your materials as often as you'd like.

Experience how McGraw Hill Education's Create empowers you to teach your students your way: *http://create.mheducation.com*

Learning Management System Integration

McGraw Hill provides a one-stop teaching and learning experience available to users of any learning management system. This institutional service allows faculty and students to enjoy single sign-on (SSO) access to McGraw Hill materials, including the award-winning **McGraw Hill Connect®** platform, from directly within the institution's website. The program provides faculty with instant access to McGraw Hill teaching materials (e.g., eTextbooks, test banks, PowerPoint slides, animations, and learning objects), allowing them to browse, search, and use any instructor ancillary content in our vast library at no additional cost to instructors or students. With this program enabled, faculty and students never need to create another account to access McGraw Hill products and services.

Instructor Resources

Instructors can access the following resources through the Library tab in **McGraw Hill Connect®**:

Instructor's Manual. The instructor's manual provides a wide variety of tools and resources for presenting the course, including learning objectives and ideas for lectures and discussions.

Test Bank. Each question has been tagged for level of difficulty, Bloom's taxonomy, and topic coverage. Organized by chapter, the questions are designed to test factual, conceptual, and higher order thinking.

Test Builder. New to this edition and available within Connect, Test Builder is a cloud-based tool that enables instructors to format tests that can be printed and administered within a Learning Management System. Test Builder offers a modern, streamlined interface for easy content configuration that matches course needs, without requiring a download.

Test Builder enables instructors to:

- Access all test bank content from a particular title.
- Easily pinpoint the most relevant content through robust filtering options.
- Manipulate the order of questions or scramble questions and/or answers.
- Pin questions to a specific location within a test.
- Determine your preferred treatment of algorithmic questions.
- Choose the layout and spacing.
- Add instructions and configure default settings.

PowerPoint. The PowerPoint presentations highlight the key points of the chapter and include supporting visuals. All slides are WCAG compliant.

Remote Proctoring. New remote proctoring and browser-locking capabilities are seamlessly integrated within Connect to offer more control over the integrity of online assessments. Instructors can enable security options that restrict browser activity, monitor student behavior, and verify the identity of each student. Instant and detailed reporting gives instructors an at-a-glance view of potential concerns, thereby avoiding personal bias and supporting evidence-based claims.

Health, Wellness, Fitness, and Healthy Lifestyles: An Introduction

LEARNING OBJECTIVES

After completing the study of this Concept, you will be able to:

▶ Describe the HELP philosophy and discuss its implications in making personal decisions about health, wellness, and fitness.

▶ Define the dimensions of health and wellness, and explain how they interact to influence health and wellness.

▶ Distinguish health-related and skill-related dimensions of physical fitness.

▶ Identify related national health goals and show how meeting personal goals can contribute to reaching national goals.

Good health, wellness, fitness, and healthy lifestyles are important for all people.

Christopher Futcher/iStock/Getty Images

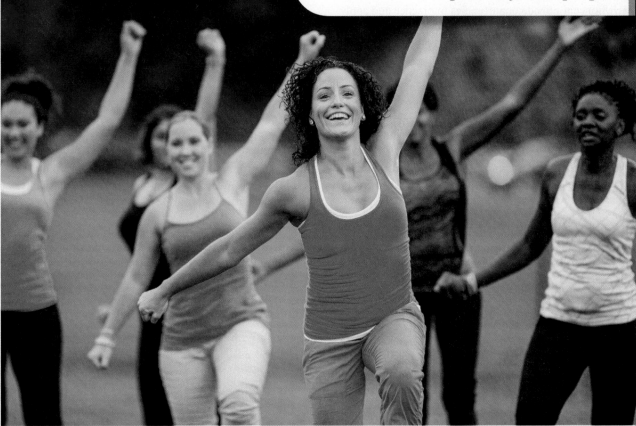

Why It Matters!

Virtually all American adults say that "being in good health" is very important, often rating it higher than money and other material things. In fact, in a recent survey of people who had taken a college fitness and wellness course 20 years prior, 92 percent considered themselves to be well informed about fitness and physical activity, and more than 50 percent remember and still use information from that class today. *Concepts of Fitness and Wellness* is specifically designed to help you learn the cognitive and behavioral skills needed to help you achieve and maintain good health, wellness, and fitness throughout life. In this first Concept, you will learn about the distinctions among health, wellness, and fitness.

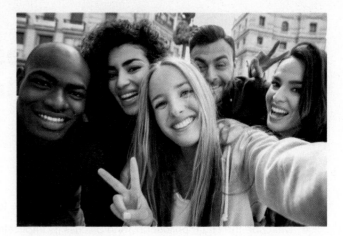

Health and wellness are available to everyone for a lifetime.
javi_indy/Shutterstock

The HELP Philosophy

The HELP philosophy provides a basis for making healthy lifestyle change possible. The acronym *HELP* characterizes an important part of the philosophy: *Health* is available to *Everyone* for a *Lifetime*, and it's *Personal*. The HELP philosophy aids you as you apply the principles and guidelines that help you adopt and sustain healthy lifestyles. Throughout this edition, you will learn a variety of *self-management skills* that are critical for healthy living. The labs in each Concept provide opportunities to practice and apply these skills so that you can use them throughout your life. An overview of basic self-management skills is provided in a later Concept.

A personal philosophy that emphasizes health can lead to behaviors that promote it. The *H* in *HELP* stands for **health**. While nearly everyone endorses the importance of good health, most people struggle to adopt and sustain healthy lifestyles. Researchers have helped advance theories related to behavior change and to determine strategies and approaches that can be learned and practiced. One theory that has been extensively tested indicates that people who believe in the benefits of healthy lifestyles are more likely to engage in healthy behaviors. The theory also suggests that people who state intentions to put their beliefs into action are likely to adopt behaviors that lead to health, wellness, and fitness.

Everyone can benefit from healthy lifestyles, but a lack of equity creates disparities. The *E* in *HELP* stands for *everyone*. While everyone *can* benefit, limited access and resources make it more challenging for some to achieve these benefits. The opportunity to develop healthy lifestyles should be available to everyone regardless of race, ethnicity, age, disability, culture, socioeconomic status, or gender identity. While it is true that issues of equality and equity are societal challenges, everyone needs to contribute to the solution by treating all members of society equally and fairly.

Healthy behaviors are most effective when practiced for a lifetime. The *L* in *HELP* stands for *lifetime*. Young people sometimes feel immortal because the harmful effects of unhealthy lifestyles are often not immediate. As we age, however, unhealthy lifestyles have cumulative negative effects. For example, compromised health status was a factor with the COVID-19 pandemic as older adults and those with chronic diseases had greater risks and higher death rates than younger and healthier individuals. Thus, adopting and sustaining healthy habits early in life is important for long-term health, wellness, and fitness.

Healthy lifestyles should be based on personal needs. The *P* in *HELP* stands for *personal*. Each person has unique needs regarding health, wellness, and fitness. People also vary in attitudes, perceptions, and personal characteristics that influence healthy lifestyles. You will be provided with information about a variety of self-management skills, but it is up to each individual to take personal responsibility for learning and using these skills.

You can adopt the HELP philosophy. As you progress through these Concepts, consider ways that you can implement the HELP philosophy. In each Concept, HELP boxes are provided to stimulate your thinking about key health issues.

Health Optimal well-being that contributes to one's quality of life. It is more than freedom from disease and illness, though freedom from disease is important to good health. Optimal health includes high-level mental, social, emotional, spiritual, and physical wellness within the limits of one's heredity and personal abilities.

HELP

Health is available to Everyone for a Lifetime, and it's Personal

COVID-19

The COVID-19 pandemic that swept the globe was caused by a novel type of virus called severe acute respiratory syndrome coronavirus 2, or SARS-CoV-2. It is specifically called a coronavirus (*corona* means "crown") because of the impression of a crown when viewed under a microscope. The disease it caused became known as COVID-19 (*CO* stands for "corona," *VI* for "virus," D for "disease," and *19* as it originated in 2019). Susceptibility, symptomology, and risks associated with COVID-19 have been highly variable, and these factors contributed to the challenges in detection and containment. Whereas one person may be asymptomatic or experience a headache or impaired taste or smell, another may lapse into respiratory failure and die. Mandates and debates on personal responsibility to wear masks, wash hands, and social distance have heightened how individuals play a critical role in containing the spread of the disease.

The HELP philosophy emphasizes that health is highly personal. What did you learn about yourself throughout the COVID-19 pandemic? How will that prepare you for future health issues and challenges?

connect ACTIVITY

National Health Goals

Healthy People 2030 **is a national public health program that establishes a comprehensive set of health promotion and disease prevention objectives with the primary intent of improving the nation's health.** The *Healthy People Initiative* began in 1980 to promote health and wellness in all Americans. The goals are revised every 10 years and, in 2020, goals for the year 2030 were established. They provide national goals for health and health promotion, but the objectives also serve as goals to motivate and guide people in making sound health decisions. A complete list of *Healthy People 2030* objectives (also referred to as goals) that relate to the content in *Concepts of Fitness and Wellness* is included in Table 1. In addition to helping change the health of society at large, the *Healthy People 2030* objectives have implications for personal health behavior change. Societal changes can occur only when individuals adjust personal behaviors and work together to make changes that benefit other people. Not all objectives will have personal implications for each individual, but increased societal awareness of the objectives may lead to future changes in the health of our country.

Table 1 ▶ *Healthy People 2030:* Health Goals and Objectives for the Nation

The following health goals are from *Healthy People 2030*, which establishes health goals for Americans. The specific goals listed below are those that are covered in *Concepts of Fitness and Wellness*. As you meet your personal goals, you contribute to the achievement of these national health goals.

Overarching Goals
- Attain healthy, thriving lives and well-being free of preventable disease, disability, injury, and premature death.
- Eliminate health disparities, achieve health equity, and attain health literacy to improve the health and well-being of all.
- Create social, physical, and economic environments that promote attaining the full potential for health and well-being for all.
- Promote health development, healthy behaviors, and well-being across all life stages.
- Engage leadership, key constituents, and the public across multiple sectors to take action and design policies that improve the health and well-being of all.

Physical Activity Objectives
- Reduce the proportion of people who do no physical activity in their free time.
- Increase the proportion of people who do enough aerobic physical activity for *substantial* and *extensive* health benefits.
- Increase the proportion of people who do enough muscle-strengthening activity.
- Increase the proportion of people who do both aerobic and muscle-strengthening activity.
- Increase the proportion of people who walk or bike to get places.
- Increase the proportion of youth who play sports.
- Increase the proportion of worksites that offer employee physical activity programs.
- Increase the proportion of older people with physical or cognitive health problems who get physical activity.
- Increase referrals of heart attack and stroke survivors for rehabilitation programs.

Hypokinetic Disease Objectives
- Improve cardiovascular health and reduce coronary heart disease and stroke deaths.
- Reduce the proportion of people with high blood pressure and high cholesterol levels.
- Reduce incidence of and overall death rate from cancer (e.g., breast, colorectal, prostate).
- Reduce incidence of sunburn.

(continued)

Table 1 ▶ *(continued)*

- Increase quality of life for cancer survivors.
- Reduce incidence of and death rate from diabetes.
- Reduce the proportion of adults who don't know they have diabetes.
- Increase diabetes screening, eye exams, and blood sugar monitoring.
- Reduce incidence of and screening for osteoporosis.
- Reduce hip fractures from and increase treatment for fractures from osteoporosis.
- Reduce the proportion of hospitalizations from dementia.
- Increase treatment for depression (including postpartum) and serious mental illness.
- Reduce suicide attempts and rate of suicide.
- Reduce the proportion of people with disabilities who experience serious psychological distress.
- Reduce pain and work limitations among those with arthritis.

Nutrition and Healthy Eating Objectives
- Increase consumption of fruits, vegetables (especially dark green, red, orange, and beans and peas), and whole grains.
- Reduce consumption of added sugars, saturated fat, and sodium.
- Increase consumption of calcium, potassium, and vitamin D.
- Reduce sales of less-than-healthy foods and drinks in schools.
- Increase the proportion of females of childbearing age who get adequate folic acid.
- Increase the proportion of worksites that offer employee nutrition programs.

Body Composition and Weight Control Objectives
- Reduce the proportion of people with obesity.
- Reduce the number of health-care visits that include counseling on weight loss, nutrition, and physical activity by people with obesity.
- Increase the proportion of females who had a healthy weight before pregnancy.

Destructive Habits Objectives
- Reduce tobacco use (cigarette, cigar, pipe).
- Increase past-year attempts to quit smoking and successful attempts.
- Increase smoke-free homes and other smoke-free environments (worksites, restaurants, bars).
- Reduce the proportion of people who don't smoke who are exposed to secondhand smoke.
- Reduce e-cigarette, flavored tobacco products, and smokeless tobacco use among youth.
- Reduce the proportion of youth exposed to tobacco marketing.
- Reduce cigarette smoking initiation among youth and young adults.
- Reduce binge drinking and alcohol use disorders.
- Reduce motor vehicle crash deaths involving a drunk driver.
- Reduce drug use over past month, marijuana use (daily or almost daily), misuse of prescription drugs, and heroin use (past year).
- Reduce drug overdoses and overdose deaths (including opioids, heroin, methadone).
- Increase the proportion of people with substance use disorders who get treatment.
- Reduce emergency room visits from prescription and nonprescription drug overdoses.
- Reduce the proportion of LGBTQ youth who use illicit drugs.

Sexually Transmitted Infections Objectives
- Reduce incidence of HPV infections prevented by vaccine in youth.
- Reduce hepatitis A, B, and C, and deaths from hepatitis.
- Increase the proportion of people who know that they have hepatitis.

Safety and Injury Prevention Objectives
- Reduce fatal injuries, unintentional injury deaths, and fatal traumatic brain injuries.
- Reduce emergency room visits for nonfatal injuries.
- Reduce motor vehicle crash deaths, deaths from crashes due to drowsy driving, and deaths of passengers not using seatbelts.
- Reduce work-related injuries and days missed from work because of injury.
- Reduce nonfatal physical assaults and fire-arms-related deaths.
- Reduce falls and fall-related deaths among older people.

Health Information and Service Objectives
- Increase electronic access to health information.
- Increase telehealth services.
- Increase access to broadband Internet.
- Increase communication with health-care providers.
- Increase the proportion of people with health and prescription drug insurance.
- Increase prevention services by community organizations.
- Increase the proportion of people who get health care when they need it.
- Reduce days exposed to unhealthy air and amount of toxic pollutants in the environment.

Source: Selected goals and objectives adapted from *Healthy People 2030.*

One overarching goal of *Healthy People 2030* is to attain healthy, thriving lives and well-being, free of preventable disease, injury, and premature death. This goal makes distinctions between **lifespan** (life expectancy) and **healthspan** (healthy life expectancy). *Lifespan* refers to the number of years you live. *Healthspan* is the number of years in your life during which you experience good health that is free of chronic diseases and debilitating conditions that limit your daily activities and your wellness (quality of life).

Prior to the COVID-19 pandemic, the lifespan (life expectancy) of Americans increased by 60 percent over the last century. During the pandemic, life expectancy in the United States decreased to its lowest level in 15 years (see Concept 2 for more information). The expected lifespan for North American countries prior to the pandemic is shown in Figure 1. The blue bars in Figure 1 depict the relative healthspan in each country and the brown bars show the number of years with poor health and low quality of life. The most recent statistics show that the United States ranks 39th to 54th in world rankings for expected lifespan (depending on the source). Among North American countries, the United States ranks behind Canada (11th to 16th) and ahead of Mexico (78th to 90th). Although unhealthy years occur more often toward the end of the lifespan, they can happen at any time. Consistent with *Healthy People 2030*, a goal of *Concepts of Fitness and Wellness* is to help you personally increase both your lifespan and your healthspan. As you meet your personal goals, you contribute to the achievement of these national health goals.

Eliminating disparities and achieving health equity is another primary goal of *Healthy People 2030*. As defined in the *Healthy People 2030* documents, a health disparity is "a particular type of health difference that is closely linked with social, economic, and/or environmental disadvantage." The goal of eliminating disparities was established because health inequities do exist. This was clearly evident

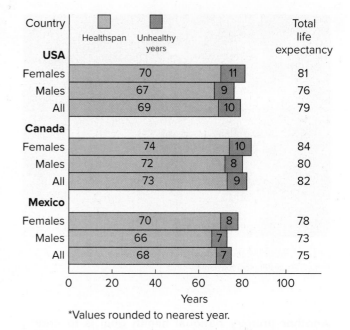

*Values rounded to nearest year.

Figure 1 ► Estimated healthspan and lifespan for many North Americans.*
Source: World Health Organization.

during the COVID-19 pandemic as some racial minorities (e.g., Blacks, Hispanics) were two to four times more likely to have confirmed cases than whites and Asian Americans. To reduce health disparities, it is important to address underlying causes.

> **Lifespan** The number of years you live (life expectancy).
>
> **Healthspan** The number of healthy years in your life. It includes years free of illness and debilitating conditions and years of wellness (years with a good quality of life).

In the News

Healthiest Places to Live

Each year a number of organizations conduct surveys to determine which American cities rate highest in well-being and/or physical fitness. The American Fitness Index from the American College of Sports Medicine (ACSM) is a prominent example, but many other organizations conduct similar surveys. A variety of criteria such as personal health behaviors, chronic health problems, recreational facilities, and community environmental factors are used in the ratings. Many news agencies also provide similar types of ratings. Search "healthiest places to live" online to find relevant links.

Do healthier people simply seek out healthier environments (and healthier cities) or are there unique attributes that help make an area or city healthier? How does your city rate?

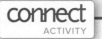

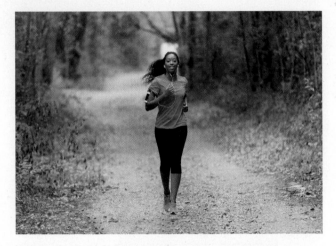

Regular physical activity can improve one's sense of well-being.
Samuel Borges Photography/Shutterstock

Another primary national health goal is to create social, physical, and economic environments that promote good health for all. The environment, both social and physical, has much to do with quality and length of life. Social environment refers to norms and values that influence our behavior, whereas physical environment refers to characteristics or features that may allow the healthier choice to be the easier choice. These features are known as "social determinants of health" and will be discussed in more detail later.

The final primary goal of the *Healthy People Initiative* is to promote health, wellness, and healthy behaviors across all stages of life. Health and wellness are products of a healthy lifestyle. Young adults generally have good health, but unhealthy lifestyles eventually take a toll and contribute to compromised health and wellness later in life. The subsequent sections will describe important distinctions among (and dimensions of) health, wellness, and fitness.

Health and Wellness

Health is more than freedom from illness and disease. The definition of health established by the World Health Organization (WHO) over 70 years ago is "a state of complete physical, mental, and social well-being." As shown in Figure 2, **illness** and **wellness** are at opposite ends of the health continuum. Healthy lifestyles contribute to both reductions in risk of illness as well as enhancements in wellness. Thus, health is much more than freedom from illness, disease, and debilitating conditions.

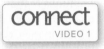

Wellness is the positive component of optimal health. Wellness is characterized by a sense of well-being reflected in optimal functioning, health-related **quality of life**, meaningful work, and a contribution to society. The term *health-related quality of life* also reflects a general sense of happiness and satisfaction with life. Wellness is often incorrectly described as something you do rather than something you have. While it is hard to directly quantify, wellness is the product of healthy lifestyles in the same way that fitness is the product of regular physical activity.

Health and wellness are personal. Every individual is unique, and health and wellness are influenced by each person's unique characteristics. Making comparisons to other people on specific characteristics may produce feelings of inadequacy that detract from one's profile of total health and wellness. Each of us has personal limitations and strengths. Focusing on strengths and learning to accommodate weaknesses are essential keys to optimal health and wellness.

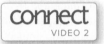

Health and wellness are multidimensional. The health and wellness dimensions include physical, emotional/mental, intellectual, social, and spiritual (see Figure 3). Each is important to optimal health and wellness.

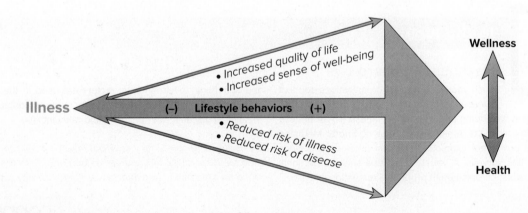

Figure 2 ▶ Wellness and illness are on opposite ends of the continuum.

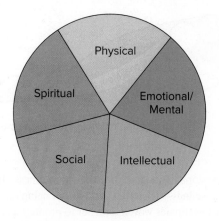

Figure 3 ▶ The dimensions of health and wellness.

Table 2 describes the various dimensions. Some people include environmental and vocational dimensions in addition to the five shown in Figure 3. Health and wellness are personal factors, so environmental and vocational health and wellness are not included in Table 2. However, the environment (including your work environment) is very important to your overall personal wellness. It is included in the conceptual model capturing determinants of health, wellness, and fitness in Concept 2.

Wellness reflects how one feels about life, as well as one's ability to function effectively. A positive total outlook on life is essential to each of the wellness dimensions. As illustrated in Table 3, a "well" person is satisfied in work, is spiritually fulfilled, enjoys leisure time, is physically fit, is socially involved, and has a positive emotional/mental outlook. The person is happy and fulfilled.

The way one perceives each dimension of wellness affects one's total outlook. Researchers use the term *self-perceptions* to describe these feelings. Many researchers believe that

Illness The ill feeling and/or symptoms associated with a disease or circumstances that upset homeostasis.

Wellness The integration of many different components (physical, emotional/mental, intellectual, social, and spiritual) that expand one's potential to live (quality of life) and work effectively and to make a significant contribution to society. Wellness reflects how one feels (a sense of well-being) about life, as well as one's ability to function effectively. Wellness, as opposed to illness (a negative), is sometimes described as the positive component of good health.

Quality of Life A term used to describe wellness. An individual with quality of life can enjoyably do the activities of life with little or no limitation and can function independently. Individual quality of life requires a pleasant and supportive community.

Table 2 ▶ Definitions of Health and Wellness Dimensions

Physical health—Freedom from illnesses that affect the physiological systems of the body, such as the heart and the nervous system. A person with physical health possesses an adequate level of physical fitness and physical wellness.

Physical wellness—The ability to function effectively in meeting the demands of the day's work and to use free time effectively. Physical wellness includes good physical fitness and the possession of useful motor skills. A person with physical wellness is generally characterized as fit instead of unfit.

Emotional/mental health—Freedom from emotional/mental illnesses, such as clinical depression, and possession of emotional wellness. The goals for the nation's health refer to mental rather than emotional health and wellness. However, mental health and wellness are conceptually the same as emotional health and wellness.

Emotional/mental wellness—The ability to cope with daily circumstances and to deal with personal feelings in a positive, optimistic, and constructive manner. A person with emotional wellness is generally characterized as happy instead of depressed.

Intellectual health—Freedom from illnesses that invade the brain and other systems that allow learning. A person with intellectual health also possesses intellectual wellness.

Intellectual wellness—The ability to learn and to use information to enhance the quality of daily living and optimal functioning. A person with intellectual wellness is generally characterized as informed instead of ignorant.

Social health—Freedom from illnesses or conditions that severely limit functioning in society, including antisocial pathologies.

Social wellness—The ability to interact with others successfully and to establish meaningful relationships that enhance the quality of life for all people involved in the interaction (including self). A person with social wellness is generally characterized as involved instead of lonely.

Spiritual health—The one component of health that is totally composed of the wellness dimension; it is synonymous with spiritual wellness.

Spiritual wellness—The ability to establish a values system and act on the system of beliefs, as well as to establish and carry out meaningful and constructive lifetime goals. Spiritual wellness is often based on a belief in a force greater than the individual that helps her or him contribute to an improved quality of life for all people. A person with spiritual wellness is generally characterized as fulfilled instead of unfulfilled.

Table 3 ▶ The Dimensions of Wellness

Wellness Dimension	Negative	Positive
Physical	Unfit	Fit
Emotional/mental	Depressed	Happy
Intellectual	Ignorant	Informed
Social	Lonely	Involved
Spiritual	Unfulfilled	Fulfilled
Total outlook	Negative	Positive

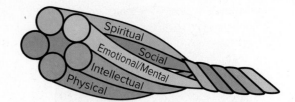

Figure 4 ▶ The integration of wellness dimensions.

self-perceptions about wellness are more important than actual circumstances or a person's actual state of being. For example, a person who has an important job may find less meaning and job satisfaction than another person with a much less important job. Apparently, one of the important factors for a person who has achieved high-level wellness and a positive outlook on life is the ability to provide self-reward. Some people, however, seem unable to give themselves credit for their successes. The development of a system that allows a person to perceive the self positively is essential, along with the adoption of positive lifestyles that encourage improved self-perceptions. The questionnaire in Lab 1A will help you assess your self-perceptions of the various wellness dimensions. For optimal wellness, aim for positive feelings about each dimension (see Table 3).

Health and wellness are integrated states of being. The segmented pictures of health and wellness shown in Figure 3 and Tables 2 and 3 are used only to illustrate the multidimensional nature of health and wellness. In reality, health and wellness are integrated states of being that can best be depicted as threads woven together to produce a larger, integrated fabric. Each dimension relates to each of the others and overlaps all the others. The overlap is so frequent and so great that the specific contribution of each thread is almost indistinguishable when looking at the total (Figure 4). The total is clearly greater than the sum of the parts.

It is possible to possess health and wellness while being ill or living with a debilitating condition. Many illnesses are curable and may have only a temporary effect on health. Others, such as Type 1 diabetes, are not curable but can be managed with proper nutrition, physical activity, and sound medical treatment. Those with manageable conditions may, however, be at risk for other health problems. For example, unmanaged diabetes is associated with a high risk for heart disease and other health problems.

Debilitating conditions, such as the loss of a limb or loss of function in a body part, can contribute to a lower level of functioning or an increased risk for illness and thus to poor health. On the other hand, such conditions need not limit wellness. A person with a debilitating condition who has a positive outlook on life may have better overall health (a longer healthspan) than a person with a poor outlook on life but no debilitating condition.

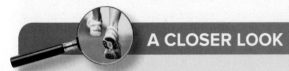

A CLOSER LOOK

Mental Health During a Pandemic

Although dealing with COVID-19 focused much of our attention on the physical risks associated with the virus, it clearly has had a dramatic impact on our mental health. Before COVID-19 impacted the United States, a national poll indicated that 87 percent of Americans were very satisfied or somewhat satisfied with their overall quality of life. However, as time passed, polls and surveys documented the toll of the pandemic on our overall well-being. One poll indicated that over 90 percent of Americans reported experiencing some form of emotional distress. Loss of jobs and financial distress, changes in schooling and childcare, canceled celebrations and social disruption, panic buying, rising death tolls and loss of loved ones, and fear of contracting the virus are many contributing factors. Living through the pandemic may have increased awareness about the frailty of life or prompted a greater appreciation for the importance of mental health and our lifestyles.

Which dimension of wellness do you think is most important for helping cope with challenges like COVID-19?

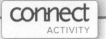

Just as wellness is possible among those with illness and disability, evidence is accumulating that people with a positive outlook are better able to resist the progress of disease and illness than are those with a negative outlook. Thinking positive thoughts has been associated with enhanced results from various medical treatments and surgical procedures.

Health and wellness products and promotions can be misleading. Because well-being is a subjective feeling, unscrupulous people can easily make claims of improved wellness for their product or service without facts to back them up. The term *holistic health* is similarly abused. Optimal health includes many dimensions; thus, the term *holistic* (total) is appropriate. In fact, the word *health* originates from a root word meaning "wholeness." Unfortunately, questionable health practices are sometimes promoted under the guise of holistic health. Care should be used when considering services and products that make claims of wellness and/or holistic health to be sure that they are legitimate.

Physical Fitness

Physical fitness is a multidimensional state of being. **Physical fitness** is the body's ability to function efficiently and effectively. It consists of at least six health-related and five skill-related dimensions (Figures 5 and 6), each of which contributes to total quality of life. Physical fitness is associated with a person's ability to 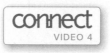 work effectively, enjoy leisure time, be healthy, resist **hypokinetic diseases or conditions**, and meet emergency situations. It is related to, but different from, health and wellness. Although the development of physical fitness is the result of many things, optimal physical fitness is not possible without regular physical activity.

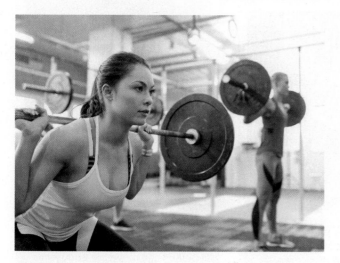

The health-related dimensions of fitness are associated with enhanced health and wellness.
Syda Productions/Shutterstock

The health-related dimensions of physical fitness are directly associated with good health. The six dimensions of health-related physical fitness are body composition, cardiorespiratory endurance, flexibility, muscular endurance, power, and strength (see Figure 5). All health-related fitness dimensions have a direct relationship to good health and reduced risk for hypokinetic diseases. This is why they are emphasized in personal fitness programs.

Possessing a moderate amount of each dimension of health-related fitness is essential to disease prevention and health promotion, but it is not essential to have exceptionally high levels of fitness to achieve health benefits. High levels of health-related fitness relate 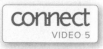 more to performance than to health benefits. For example, moderate amounts of strength are necessary to prevent back and posture problems, whereas high levels of strength contribute most to improved performance in activities such as football and jobs involving heavy lifting.

The skill-related dimensions of physical fitness are associated more with performance than with good health. The dimensions of skill-related physical fitness are agility, balance, coordination, reaction time, and speed (see Figure 6). They are called skill-related because people who possess them find it easy to achieve high levels of performance in motor skills, such as those required in sports and in specific types of jobs. Power, a dimension that requires both strength and speed, was formerly considered a skill-related dimension of fitness, but new evidence has linked power with good health.

Skill-related fitness has been called "sports fitness" or "motor fitness," but note that it is multidimensional and highly specific. For example, coordination could be hand-eye coordination, such as batting a ball; foot-eye coordination, such as kicking a ball; or many other possibilities. The five dimensions of skill-related fitness identified here are those commonly associated with successful sports and work performance. Additional information and self-assessments on skill-related fitness are included in later Concepts to help you understand the nature of total physical fitness and make important decisions about lifetime physical activity.

Physical Fitness The body's ability to function efficiently and effectively. It consists of at least 11 health-related physical fitness and skill-related physical fitness components, each of which contributes to total quality of life. Physical fitness also includes metabolic fitness and bone integrity. Optimal physical fitness is not possible without regular exercise.

Hypokinetic Diseases or Conditions *Hypo-* means "under" or "too little," and *-kinetic* means "movement" or "activity." Thus, *hypokinetic* means "too little activity." A hypokinetic disease or condition is one associated with lack of physical activity or too little regular exercise. Examples include heart disease, low back pain, Type 2 diabetes, and obesity.

Body Composition

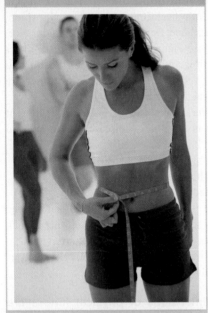

The relative percentage of muscle, fat, bone, and other tissues that make up the body. A fit person has a relatively low, but not too low, percentage of body fat (body fatness).

Muscular Endurance

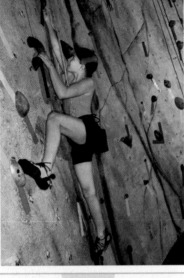

The ability of the muscles to exert themselves repeatedly. A fit person can repeat movements for a long period without undue fatigue.

Cardiorespiratory Endurance

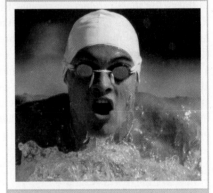

The ability of the heart, blood vessels, blood, and respiratory system to supply nutrients and oxygen to the muscles and the ability of the muscles to utilize fuel to allow sustained exercise. A fit person can persist in physical activity for relatively long periods without undue stress.

Dimensions of Health-Related Physical Fitness

Strength

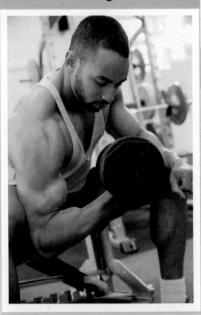

The ability of the muscles to exert an external force or to lift a heavy weight. A fit person can do work or play that involves exerting force, such as lifting or controlling one's own body weight.

Power

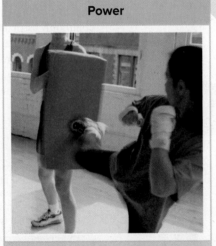

The ability to transfer energy into force at a fast rate. Kicking in martial arts and throwing the discus are activities that require considerable power.

Flexibility

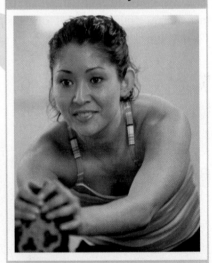

The range of motion available in a joint. It is affected by muscle length, joint structure, and other factors. A fit person can move the body joints through a full range of motion in work and in play.

Figure 5 ▶ Dimensions of health-related physical fitness.

(Body Composition): Comstock/Getty Images; (Muscular Endurance): Thinkstock Images/Stockbyte/Getty Images; (Cardiorespiratory Endurance): Stockbyte/Getty Images; (Strength): Monkey Business Images/Shutterstock; (Power): Ryan McVay/Getty Images; (Flexibility): Tom Grill/Corbis/Getty Images

Agility

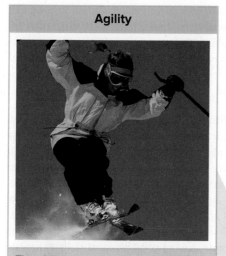

The ability to rapidly and accurately change the direction of the movement of the entire body in space. Skiing and wrestling are examples of activities that require exceptional agility.

Reaction Time

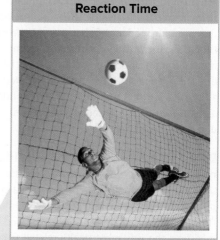

The time elapsed between stimulation and the beginning of reaction to that stimulation. Reacting to a soccer ball and starting a sprint race require good reaction time.

Dimensions of Skill-Related Physical Fitness

Coordination

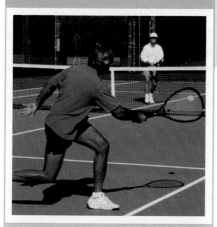

The ability to use the senses with the body parts to perform motor tasks smoothly and accurately. Juggling, hitting a tennis ball, and kicking a ball are examples of activities requiring good coordination.

Speed

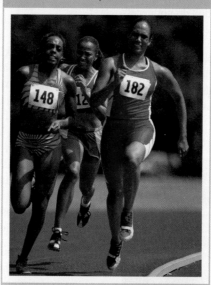

The ability to perform a movement in a short period of time. Sprinters and wide receivers in football need good foot and leg speed.

Balance

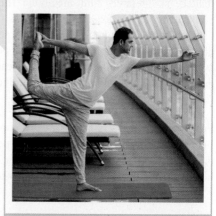

The maintenance of equilibrium while stationary or while moving. Performing tai chi movements and performing stunts on the balance beam are activities that require exceptional balance.

Figure 6 ▶ Dimensions of skill-related physical fitness.

(Agility): Karl Weatherly/Getty Images; (Reaction Time): John Lund/Drew Kelly/Blend Images LLC; (Coordination): Karl Weatherly/Getty Images; (Speed): CS Productions/Jupiterimages/Brand X/Alamy Stock Photo; (Balance): Mangostar/Shutterstock

Metabolic fitness is a nonperformance dimension of total fitness. Physical activity can provide health benefits that are independent of changes in traditional health-related fitness measures. Physical activity promotes good **metabolic fitness**, a state associated with reduced risk for many chronic diseases. People with a cluster of low metabolic fitness characteristics are said to have metabolic syndrome (also known as Syndrome X). Metabolic syndrome is discussed in more detail in a later Concept.

Bone integrity is often considered to be a nonperformance measure of fitness. Traditional definitions do not include bone integrity as a part of physical fitness, but some experts feel they should. Like metabolic fitness, bone integrity cannot be assessed with performance measures the way most health-related fitness parts can. Regardless of whether bone integrity is considered a part of fitness or a component of health, strong, healthy bones are important to optimal health and are associated with regular physical activity and sound diet.

The many components of physical fitness are specific but are also interrelated. Physical fitness is a combination of several aspects, rather than a single characteristic. A fit person possesses at least adequate levels of each of the health-related, skill-related, and metabolic fitness components. Some relationships exist among various fitness characteristics, but each component of physical fitness is separate and different from the others. For example, people who possess exceptional strength may not have good cardiorespiratory endurance and those who have good coordination do not necessarily possess good flexibility.

Functional fitness is important for people of all ages. **Functional fitness** refers to the ability to perform activities of daily life. For adults, this includes performing work and household tasks as well as leisure activities without undue

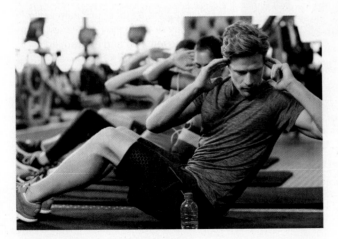

There are many ways to train to improve functional fitness.
Rido/Shutterstock

fatigue. It also includes having adequate fitness to meet the demands of emergency situations. For youth, functional fitness includes the ability to function in school and leisure activities without undue fatigue. For older adults, functional fitness plays key roles in enabling independence and in minimizing risks of falls.

Good physical fitness is important, but it is not the same as physical health and wellness. Good fitness contributes to the physical dimension of health and wellness by reducing risk for chronic diseases and by reducing the consequences of many debilitating conditions. Good fitness also contributes indirectly to other dimensions by helping us look our best, feel good, perform daily tasks, and enjoy life. However, other physical factors can also influence health and wellness. For example, having good physical skills enhances quality of life by allowing us to participate in enjoyable activities, such as tennis, golf, and bowling. Although fitness can assist us in performing these activities, regular practice is also necessary. Another example is the ability to fight off viral and bacterial infections. Although fitness can promote a strong immune system, other physical factors can influence our susceptibility to illness.

Using Self-Management Skills

Self-assessment is one of many self-management skills that can be learned to enhance lifelong healthy behaviors. Skills refer to the abilities you need in order to perform a specific task. Serving a tennis ball or typing on a computer are examples of physical or motor skills. Solving a math problem is an example of a mental or cognitive skill. A different set of skills—known as self-management skills—helps you adopt behaviors to enhance lifelong health, wellness, and fitness. *Self-assessment* (a specific self-management skill) refers to the ability to collect and evaluate personal information that will help you create a plan for improving your health, wellness, and fitness. You will conduct a variety of self-assessments as you work your way through this edition. For example, you will complete assessments for each dimension of health-related fitness and answer questionnaires to determine your wellness status, risk factors, attitudes, and health behavior patterns. To most effectively use self-assessments, consider the following guidelines:

- **Follow the same procedures each time you self-assess.** Read and follow the instructions to know how to do a self-assessment properly. Having written descriptions of the best way to perform an assessment reminds you of the proper techniques for assessment. Heeding an instructor's advice and following written descriptions of assessments helps ensure that each assessment is done the same way.

- **Use the same equipment or questionnaire each time you self-assess.** For example, when assessing your weight, use the same scale every time. Even if the scale isn't

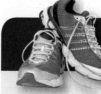

Technology Update

Health Websites and Podcasts

The Internet provides a tremendous number of sources of information about health, wellness, and fitness. However, all online sources are not equally credible or useful. The best way to get accurate information is to use reliable sources. Focus on government agencies (*.gov*), prominent medical and public health associations, and established nonprofit agencies (*.org*). The first sites that come up in searches may not be the best, so check the source. A brief list of some prominent and credible Internet sites is provided below. Additional organizations and websites are referenced in other sections.

- Academy of Nutrition and Dietetics (AND)
- American College of Sports Medicine (ACSM)
- American Council on Exercise (ACE)
- American Heart Association (AHA)
- American Medical Association (AMA)
- Center for Science in the Public Interest
- Centers for Disease Control and Prevention (CDC)
- Federal Trade Commission (FTC)
- Food and Drug Administration (FDA)
- Institute of Medicine (IOM)
- International Food Information Council (IFIC)
- Johns Hopkins Health
- Mayo Clinic Health Letter
- MedlinePlus
- National Institutes of Health (NIH)
- Pew Research Center—Health
- U.S. Consumer Information Center
- U.S. Department of Agriculture (USDA)
- WebMD
- World Health Organization (WHO)

Searching for websites or podcasts using generic terms (e.g., "health" or "fitness") will likely reveal many commercial links and sites with inaccurate or fraudulent information. Thus, when searching online, pair your search topic with the name of a credible organization (such as "vaccines and CDC" or "food allergies and International Food Information Council"). This will focus your search and lead to more credible sources.

Do you consider the quality of sources when you access health-related information on the Internet? What features should you look for to ensure credibility?

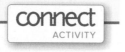

- **Practice.** Like all skills, self-assessment skills can be improved with practice. For example, if you regularly assess your fitness, you will get better at it and achieve more consistent results.
- **Be honest with yourself.** Many self-assessments require you to provide personal answers to questions. The results of your self-assessments are for you own use in establishing baseline information so that you can determine if you are improving your health, wellness, and fitness over time. The results will be meaningful only if you provide honest answers.

Use good consumer skills to evaluate information you read and hear about health, wellness, and fitness. The popularity and importance of health-related issues in our society make consumers vulnerable to misinformation, quackery, and fraud. A key to reducing your risk and to advancing your knowledge is to use good sources of information. See Technology Update for information about sound health-related websites.

Strategies for Action: Lab Information

An initial self-assessment of your wellness will provide information for future self-comparison. In Lab 1A, you will estimate your wellness using a Wellness Self-Perceptions Questionnaire, which assesses the five wellness dimensions. Assessing each dimension will help you see areas of strengths and weaknesses and determine areas of priority as you set goals and make plans for improving. Answering the same questions at a later date can help you see if you have made progress. As each person makes progress toward improving wellness, collectively we move closer to the *Healthy People* goal of living long, high-quality lives.

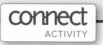

Metabolic Fitness A positive state of the physiological systems commonly associated with reduced risk for chronic diseases such as diabetes and heart disease. Metabolic fitness is evidenced by healthy blood fat (lipid) profiles, healthy blood pressure, and healthy blood sugar and insulin levels.

Functional Fitness The ability to perform activities of daily life.

completely accurate, using the same scale helps you record fluctuations in weight over time. When assessing wellness with a questionnaire, use the same form each time to achieve consistent comparisons.

Suggested Resources and Readings

The websites for the following sources can be accessed by searching online for the organization, program, or title listed. Specific scientific references are available at the end of this edition of *Concepts of Fitness and Wellness*.

- American College of Sports Medicine. (2020). *ACSM American Fitness Index: Actively Moving America to Better Health.* (pdf)
- Centers for Disease Control and Prevention. Well-Being Concepts.
- Centers for Disease Control and Prevention. About the National Health Information Survey.
- Central Intelligence Agency. (2020). *The World Factbook.* Washington, DC: Author.
- Johns Hopkins Medicine. (2018). *Reliable Health Information on the Internet.* (pdf)
- National Academies of Sciences, Engineering, and Medicine. (2019). *Integrating Social Care into the Delivery of Health Care: Moving Upstream to Improve the Nation's Health.* Washington, DC: National Academies Press.
- National Institutes of Health. MedlinePlus.
- Office of Disease Prevention and Health Promotion. Development of Healthy People 2030.
- Sharecare. Well-Being Index.
- Trust for America's Health. "The Impact of Chronic Underfunding on America's Public Health System: Trends, Risks, and Recommendations, 2020."
- U.S. Department of Health and Human Services. MyHealthfinder.
- U.S. Department of Health and Human Services. Office of Disease Prevention and Health Promotion. Health Literacy.
- U.S. Department of Health and Human Services. Office of Disease Prevention and Health Promotion. *Healthy People 2030.* Social Determinants of Health.
- World Health Organization. World Health Statistics 2020.

Lab 1A Wellness Self-Perceptions

Name	Section	Date

Purpose: To assess self-perceptions of wellness.

Procedures

1. Place an X over the appropriate circle for each question (4 = strongly agree, 3 = agree, 2 = disagree, 1 = strongly disagree).
2. Write the number found in that circle in the box to the right.
3. Sum the three boxes for each wellness dimension to get your wellness dimension totals.
4. Sum all wellness dimension totals to get your comprehensive wellness total.
5. Use the rating chart to rate each wellness area.
6. Complete the Results section and the Conclusions and Implications section.

Question	Strongly Agree	Agree	Disagree	Strongly Disagree	Score
1. I am physically fit.	4	3	2	1	
2. I am able to perform the physical tasks of my work.	4	3	2	1	
3. I am physically able to perform leisure activities.	4	3	2	1	
Physical Wellness Total =					
4. I am happy most of the time.	4	3	2	1	
5. I have good self-esteem.	4	3	2	1	
6. I do not generally feel stressed.	4	3	2	1	
Emotional/Mental Wellness Total =					
7. I am well informed about current events.	4	3	2	1	
8. I am comfortable expressing my views and opinions.	4	3	2	1	
9. I am interested in my career development.	4	3	2	1	
Intellectual Wellness Total =					
10. I have many friends and am involved socially.	4	3	2	1	
11. I have close ties with my family.	4	3	2	1	
12. I am confident in social situations.	4	3	2	1	
Social Wellness Total =					
13. I am fulfilled spiritually.	4	3	2	1	
14. I feel connected to the world around me.	4	3	2	1	
15. I have a sense of purpose in my life.	4	3	2	1	
Spiritual Wellness Total =					
Comprehensive Wellness (Sum of five wellness scores)					

Results (Record your scores from the previous page; then determine your ratings from the Wellness Rating Chart).

Wellness Dimension	Score	Rating
Physical		
Emotional/mental		
Intellectual		
Social		
Spiritual		
Comprehensive		

Wellness Rating Chart

Rating	Wellness Dimension Scores	Comprehensive Wellness Scores
High-level wellness	10–12	50–60
Good wellness	8–9	40–49
Marginal wellness	6–7	30–39
Low-level wellness	Below 6	Below 30

Conclusions and Implications: Rank each dimension of wellness. Place a 1 by the dimension you need to work on most and a 2 by the dimension needing the next most work. Rank the others as 3, 4, and 5. Then in the box below, briefly discuss your wellness ratings. Comment on your current level of wellness and dimensions that could use improvement.

◯ Physical   ◯ Emotional/mental   ◯ Intellectual   ◯ Social   ◯ Spiritual

Determinants of Lifelong Health, Wellness, and Fitness

LEARNING OBJECTIVES

After completing the study of this Concept, you will be able to:

▶ Identify the determinants of health, wellness, and fitness, and explain how they each contribute to health, wellness, and fitness.

▶ Differentiate between factors over which you have lesser and greater control.

▶ Use health behavior change strategies to carry out self-assessments of personal lifestyles and wellness perceptions.

Many factors contribute to health, wellness, and fitness, and some are more in your control than others.

Michael Reusse/Westend61/Getty Images

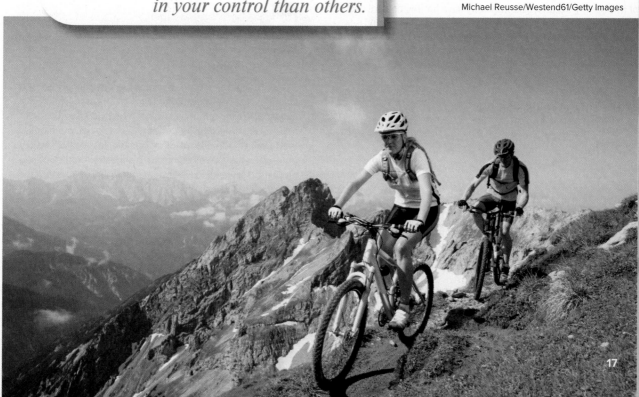

17

Determinants of Health, Wellness, and Fitness

Many factors are important in developing lifetime health, wellness, and fitness, and some are more in your control than others. A factor that significantly affects your health, wellness, and fitness is referred to as a **determinant**. Three major categories of determinants are listed in Figure 1. Biological factors, such as heredity, age, and sex, are shown at the bottom of the figure because they 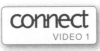 are determinants over which we have little or no control. The Centers for Disease Control and Prevention (CDC) has also emphasized the importance of various social determinants of health in public health guidelines. They are positioned at mid-level in Figure 1 because you may only have limited control over some of them (e.g., health care, education). Lifestyle

determinants are listed at the top of Figure 1. These include priority lifestyles such as being physically active, eating well, and managing stress. Lifestyle determinants are shown at the top of the figure because you have the greatest amount of control over these factors. The contributions from each of the determinants are described in subsequent sections along with insights on how they interact to influence health, wellness, and fitness. You can benefit from a knowledge of how biological determinants influence your health. You can also learn to take control over various social and lifestyle determinants by practicing and applying the **self-management skills** covered throughout this edition.

Biological Determinants

Heredity (human biology) is a determinant over which we have little control. Experts estimate that human biology, or heredity, accounts for 16 percent of all health problems, including early death. Heredity influences each dimension of health-related physical fitness, including our tendencies to build muscle and to deposit body fat. Based on their genetics, individuals also respond and adapt differently to healthy lifestyles. Even more important is that predispositions to certain diseases are inherited. Some hereditary conditions are untreatable (e.g., congenital heart defects) while others are manageable with proper medical supervision and appropriate lifestyles (e.g., diabetes). Heredity is clearly a determinant over which you have no control over, but you can take some preventive steps by being aware of your family history and by making efforts to manage factors that you can control.

Health, wellness, and fitness are influenced by your biological sex assignment at birth. Consistent with American Psychological Association (APA) terminology, the

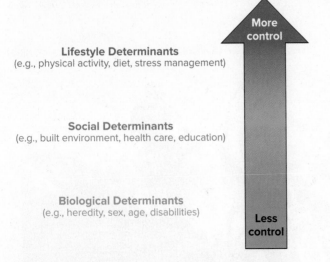

Figure 1 ▶ Determinants of health, wellness, and fitness.

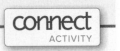

Technology Update

Genetic Testing

The interaction among our genes, environments, and lifestyles is extremely complex and the science is still evolving. While your genes do not directly *cause* you to get a disease, they can influence your risks of developing them. Many companies offer genetic testing to identify potential risks as well as produce ancestral profiles based on DNA. However, some researchers and experts have questioned the validity or utility of the profiles. (See Suggested Resources and Readings.)

Do you see value in DNA testing to identify your potential risks, or would you prefer to just focus on what you can control and not worry about things that can't be changed?

term *sex* refers to a person's sex assignment at birth. Epidemiological evidence indicates that one's sex and related biological characteristics affect disease and early mortality risk. Thus, age and sex are commonly used for evaluating fitness and health status, including various labs and activities in this edition. The fitness ratings are intended to help you determine the level of fitness necessary to achieve good health and reduce disease risk. Your sex influences how much fitness is needed for good health, but, as the APA indicates, not all people identify with their sex assignment at birth. The APA describes other important terms including *gender* ("the attitudes, feeling, and behaviors that a given culture associates with a person's biological sex") and *gender identity* ("the component of gender that describes a person's sense of their gender"). The APA emphasizes that it is important for people to be free to use the terms of their choice to describe themselves and that care should be taken by all when using pronouns in conversation. The fitness rating charts in this edition use both age and sex assignment at birth (male/female) to aid you in making informed decisions about health fitness status and are not meant to refer to a preferred gender identity.

Health, wellness, and fitness are influenced by age, but healthy lifestyles can delay and moderate the effect. In 2030, when all of the post–World War II baby boomers will be over the age of 65, adults 65 or older will make up 20 percent of the population. The number of people over 85 will triple by 2050. Data also indicate that there are more than 100,000 people over the age of 100 in the United States. The definition of *old* is clearly relative to your personal age, but societal perceptions of what constitutes "old age" are also changing. One survey reported that 25 percent of the population view that old age doesn't begin until a person hits 80 years or more.

Age is clearly a factor over which we have no control and it does directly influence our health status. The major health and wellness concerns of older adults include losing health, losing the ability to care for oneself, losing mental abilities, running out of money, being a burden to family, and being alone. Chronic pain is also a major problem among older adults with nearly 30 percent of adults over 65 experiencing chronic pain, as opposed to 3 percent of those under 30. The important message is that healthy lifestyles can dramatically reduce the effects of aging on health, wellness, and fitness. Thus, it is important to adopt and maintain healthy lifestyles to somewhat counter "normal" aging effects.

Disabilities can affect, but do not necessarily limit, health, wellness, and fitness. Disabilities typically result from factors beyond your control. Many types of disabilities affect health, wellness, and fitness. An objective disability (e.g., loss of a limb, impaired intellectual functioning) can make it difficult to function in certain circumstances but need not limit health, wellness, and fitness. All people have a limitation of one kind or another. Societal efforts to help all

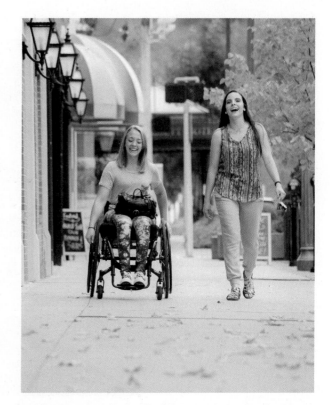

Disabilities need not limit one's ability to experience an active, fulfilling life.
PhotoAbility/Blend Images

people function within their limitations can help everyone, including people with disabilities, have a positive outlook on life and experience a high quality of life.

Social Determinants

Social determinants of health contribute to health disparities in society. Social determinants of health (SDH) are defined by the CDC and the public health service as "the conditions in the environments where people are born, live, learn, work, play, worship, and age that affect a wide range of health, functioning, and quality-of-life outcomes and risks." It is now well established that differences in these fundamental determinants contribute to the social, racial, and cultural disparities and inequities in public health. The five established dimensions of SDH include economic stability, education, the built environment, the community context, and health care (see left side of Figure 2) .

Determinant Various biological, social, environmental, or lifestyle factors that influence health status.

Self-Management Skills Skills that can be learned to support healthier decisions and adoption of healthier behaviors.

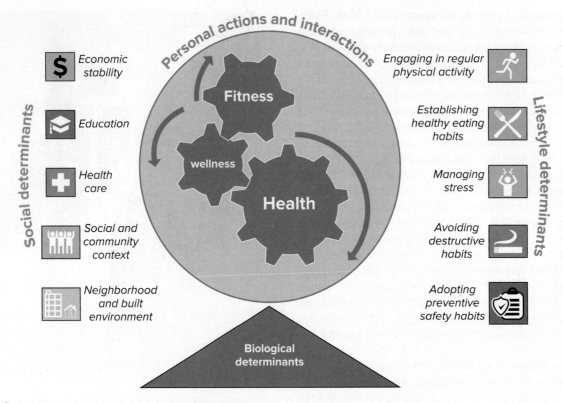

Figure 2 ▶ Influence of personal actions and interactions on health, wellness, and fitness.

The health-care system affects our ability to overcome illness and improve our quality of life. Approximately 10 percent of unnecessary deaths occur as a result of disparities in the health-care system. The quality of life for those

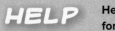

HELP   Health is available to Everyone for a Lifetime, and it's Personal

Social Determinants and Social Justice

The *Healthy People 2030* goals chart a new path for public health by increasing the focus on social determinants of health. The prioritization recognizes the greater challenges that some segments of the population have in accessing health care or in adopting healthy lifestyles. Addressing these inequities will require major changes in various systems and our society overall. The challenges parallel the need for systemic changes to address other social justice and equity issues in our society. (See Suggested Resources and Readings.)

The HELP philosophy emphasizes that health, wellness, and fitness are for everyone. Do you take aspects of your environment, health care, and your opportunities for granted? Do you think the focus on social determinants will help promote better equity in health?

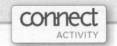

who are sick and those who tend to be sick is influenced greatly by the type of medical care they receive. As indicated in Figure 2, health care is a social determinant, one that is not equally available to all. Each year, thousands of people die because they lack health insurance. Uninsured individuals may not seek health care, and the quality of the care they do receive may not be high. Chronic conditions that go undetected can become untreatable or lead to additional complications. The passage of the Patient Protection and Affordable Care Act (shortened to the Affordable Care Act, or ACA) addressed this issue by enabling all Americans to have access to health insurance. According to the National Center for Health Statistics, the number of uninsured Americans dropped from 16 percent in 2010 to all-time lows in 2016. The percentage of uninsured American's is currently about 8.5 percent.

Even with coverage, many people fail to seek medical help when warranted, and others fail to follow medical advice. For example, they do not take prescribed medicine or do not follow up with treatments. Males are less likely to seek medical advice than females, and this is a problem since some treatable conditions lead to bigger problems or become untreatable over time. This is why it is important to follow recommendations for regular screenings and seek medical advice when warranted.

Wellness as evidenced by quality of life is also influenced by the health-care system. Traditional medicine, sometimes referred to as the **medical model**, has focused primarily on the treatment of illness with medicine, rather than illness prevention and wellness promotion. Strategies built into the ACA have placed greater emphasis on promoting healthy lifestyles within the health-care system. Examples include enhanced access to clinical preventive services, stronger referral networks to community programs, and incentives for prevention and wellness programs in the private sector. While you don't have full control over your access to quality medical care, you do have some control over your decisions to seek and follow medical advice.

The built environment and social/community context interact to influence health, wellness, and fitness. Environmental determinants account for nearly one-fourth of all early deaths and affect quality of life in many ways. While there are many facets of the environment, the notion of the *built environment* has been emphasized by public health leaders as an important predictor of lifestyle behaviors and health. The built environment includes the availability of services such as transportation, parks and trails, and food stores. Social and community context is also important and includes factors such as density of housing and neighborhood safety, as well as cohesiveness within the community.

While you don't have complete control over the built environment around you, you do have some control over how you interact with your environments and the extent with which you take advantage of available opportunities. You can seek out healthy environments that enable you to be more active or to eat healthier. You can also look to avoid unhealthy or unsafe environments. Many people actively consider aspects of their environment when considering places to live or work since it has such a strong influence on their lifestyle. Circumstances may make your preferred choices impossible, but it is important to at least be aware of the impact that your environment and the social context have on your health as well as your social, spiritual, and intellectual well-being.

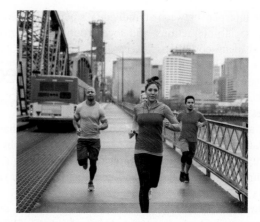

The built environment influences where and how you can be active.
FatCamera/Getty Images

Lifestyle Determinants

Your lifestyle has the most direct impact on your health and well-being. Lifestyles are more than just the way we spend our time. While lifestyles can be described simply as "patterns of living," the definition in this book (behaviors we adopt based on the context of our life circumstances) carries additional meaning. It emphasizes personal control with the use of the word *adopt,* but it also recognizes that your life circumstances can dictate your behaviors. The WHO definition of lifestyles takes an additional step by describing lifestyles as a "way of living based on identifiable patterns of behavior which are determined

Medical Model The focus of the health-care system on treating illness with medicine, with little emphasis on prevention or wellness promotion.

Lifestyles Patterns of behavior adopted within the context of personal life circumstances.

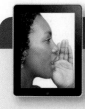

In the News

International Health Rankings

Although the United States is one of the wealthiest countries in the world, it is far from the healthiest. According to the Bloomberg Global Health Index, Americans are less healthy than people in 34 other developed countries. (Spain and Italy ranked number 1 and number 2; Canada ranked number 16.) This is attributed to a number of factors, including access to health care, environment (e.g., clean water, safe environment, economic equity), and lifestyles (e.g., sound nutrition, active living, low incidence of drug abuse). (See Suggested Resources and Readings.)

What do you think is the most significant barrier to health in the United States? Based on the factors mentioned, do you think the United States will go up or down in future rankings and why?

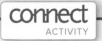
connect
ACTIVITY

by the interplay between an individual's personal characteristics, social interactions, and socioeconomic and environmental living conditions." Regardless of the definition, it is important to take control over your own lifestyle as much as possible to ensure that it guides you toward good health, wellness, and fitness. The five categories of lifestyle behaviors emphasized in this edition are engaging in regular physical activity, establishing healthy eating habits, managing stress, avoiding destructive habits, and adopting preventive safety habits (see Figure 2).

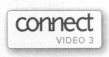

Physical activity is the behavior that contributes to improvements in physical fitness, but a broader array of lifestyle behaviors influences your overall health and wellness. The CDC uses the term *health-related quality of life* to describe the wellness benefits that result from healthy lifestyles. Public health efforts are similarly focused on enhancing the quality of life as well as the quantity. Thus, well-being, or wellness, is associated with optimal social, emotional/mental, intellectual, spiritual, and physical health.

Lifestyle choices impact risks for disease and early death. Statistics show that more than half of early deaths are the result of chronic diseases caused by unhealthy lifestyles. Scientific advances and improvements in medicine and health care have dramatically reduced the incidence of infectious diseases over the last century (see Table 1). Diphtheria

and polio, both major causes of death in the 20th century, have been virtually eliminated in Western culture. Smallpox was globally eradicated in 1977. In large measure, infectious diseases have been replaced with chronic lifestyle-related conditions as the major causes of death. Four of the top eight current causes of death (heart disease, cancer, stroke, and diabetes) fall into this category. While heart disease remains the leading killer among all adults, cancer is the leading cause for some regions and segments of the population. Until the COVID-19 outbreak, suicide was ranked 10th among leading causes of death. Six of the top ten showed recent reductions in death rates. Suicide and influenza/pneumonia were the only ones that showed increases (diabetes and kidney diseases were unchanged).

In spite of medical advances that have reduced deaths from infections, influenza and pneumonia have remained a leading killer in the United States especially among older individuals, minorities, and low-income groups. New or novel infectious diseases have affected death rates in the United States and worldwide. For example, the novel COVID-19 virus resulted in high death rates, moving it into the top 10 (number 3 in 2020). During several months in 2020 and 2021, COVID-19 was the leading cause of death. In 2020 the average life expectancy of Americans dropped by more than

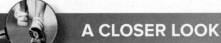

A CLOSER LOOK

Lifestyles and COVID-19

The COVID-19 pandemic revealed the important, but sometimes subtle, ways our lifestyles influence our health and well-being. Evidence accumulated quickly that older individuals and those with obesity or chronic diseases were more susceptible to COVID-19 than younger and healthier individuals. This is because underlying conditions made it harder for the body to battle the virus and less able to withstand the challenge. Research has directly documented that regular physical activity and healthy diets both improve immune function. Maintaining these habits reduces risk of chronic diseases and also enhances your body's ability to fight off microbial agents such as COVID-19. Prior to 2020, microbial agents accounted for less than 1 to 2 percent of deaths, but the impact of COVID-19 is certainly much greater. While many were able to fight off COVID-19, experts warn that we will likely face similar pandemics in the future.

How has the COVID-19 pandemic influenced your perceptions of personal health and lifestyle behaviors?

Table 1 ▶ Major Causes of Death in the United States (Based on 2020 Rankings)

Current Rank	Cause	1900 Rank	Cause
1	Heart disease	1	Pneumonia*
2	Cancer	2	Tuberculosis*
3	COVID-19*	3	Diarrhea/enteritis*
4	Unintentional injuries	4	Heart disease
5	Respiratory diseases	5	Stroke
6	Stroke	6	Liver disease
7	Alzheimer disease	7	Injuries
8	Diabetes	8	Cancer
9	Influenza/pneumonia*	9	Senility
10	Kidney disease	10	Diphtheria*

*Infectious diseases

Source: Data from the Centers for Disease Control and Prevention (CDC).

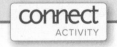

one year, to a rate that is the lowest in 15 years. As with the flu and pneumonia, older adults, minorities, and low-income groups had higher death rates from COVID-19. For example, life expectancy dropped by nearly two years for Hispanics and nearly three years for African Americans as a result of COVID-19. It is anticipated that COVID-19 will drop out of the top 10 as more people are vaccinated and other preventive methods and treatments are made available. The shifts are similar to those observed with HIV in the 1980s and 1990s when it was among the top 10 causes of death. It later dropped out of the top 10 list because of anti-retroviral treatments, early detection, and increased prevention methods.

Lifestyles interact to influence health and well-being. Although your lifestyle captures a constellation of different behaviors, some are more important than others. A report from the National Research Council and the National Academy of Medicine determined that nearly half of all deaths can be attributed to lifestyles. Inactivity and poor nutrition (combined) were identified as the leading actual cause of preventable death based on this analysis. These behaviors were likely combined since they interact to impact risks for obesity and many other chronic diseases. Tobacco use had previously been the leading cause of actual death but is now the second leading cause. Other destructive habits such as alcohol misuse, illicit drug use, and unsafe sexual behavior were also identified as prominent causes. Accidents due to firearms, toxic agents, and motor vehicles account for other premature deaths, but these may be linked to alcohol, drugs, or poor decision making.

Establishing healthy habits is important for long-term effects. Habits reflect behaviors that have become automatic or habitual. Habits can be formed for many behaviors, but Table 2 lists 10 important lifestyle habits that impact health. Emphasis in this book is on **habit formation** in three "priority" lifestyles: engaging in regular physical activity, establishing healthy eating habits, and managing stress. There are several reasons for placing priority on these lifestyles. First, they affect the lives of all people. Second, they are lifestyles in which large numbers of people can make improvement. Finally, modest changes in these behaviors can make dramatic improvements in individual and public health. Avoiding destructive habits and adopting preventive safety habits are also important but do not affect everyone as much as the first three in the table. The last five habits in Table 2 capture overall health habits that also support and enhance healthy living: social habits, prevention habits, medical habits, consumer habits, and environmental habits. Although many healthy lifestyles will be discussed in the Concepts that follow, we will focus on priority healthy lifestyles because virtually all people can achieve positive wellness benefits if they adopt and sustain them (as habits).

Physical activity A behavior that involves human movement and that results in physiological attributes including increased energy expenditure and improved physical fitness.

Habit Formation The process of making lifestyle decisions and behaviors more automatic and sustainable.

Table 2 ▶ Habits for Optimal Health

Types of Habits	Description
Physical Activity Habits	Finding ways to get regular physical activity
Nutrition Habits	Making healthy food choices
Stress Management Habits	Coping with stressful situations
Destructive Habits	Avoiding tobacco, drugs, and excessive alcohol
Safety Habits	Adopting safe practices and making safe decisions
Social Habits	Seeking out positive influences and social support
Prevention Habits	Following recommended health practices
Medical Habits	Adhering to screening guidelines/Following medical advice
Consumer Habits	Making informed choices about health, wellness, and fitness
Environmental Habits	Supporting conservation and healthy environments

Determinant Interactions

Determinants interact to influence your health, wellness, and fitness. The different determinants illustrated in Figure 2 interact to influence your health, wellness, and fitness. Biological, social, and lifestyle determinants do not operate in a vacuum. Each is influenced by the others.

Cognitions and emotions influence the choices you make. Humans have the ability to think (cognitions) and to use critical thinking to make informed choices. For example, you can use your cognitive abilities to learn about your family history and use that information to limit the negative influences of heredity. You can learn how to adapt to disabilities and personal limitations, as well as to the aging process. You can research the health-care system and seek out healthy opportunities and options even in unhealthy environments. While cognitions can be logical, we are also dramatically influenced by our moods and emotions. Learning to manage and regulate emotions is an important behavioral skill since emotions can cloud our cognitions and lead to poor decisions. Emotions also affect personal actions and interactions. A major goal of *Concepts of Fitness and Wellness* is to help you use your cognitive abilities to solve problems and make good decisions about your health, wellness, and fitness, as well as to help you be in control of your emotions when taking action and making decisions that affect your health.

Personal actions and interactions directly influence your health, wellness, and fitness. While you have no control over heredity, age, and disability (and limited control over health care and the environment), you can act (and interact) in ways to positively influence your lifestyle. Learning how to focus and prioritize your energies and actions is an important life skill and it also influences your health and well-being. Our interactions with others influence our lifestyles and the choices we make. The spread of COVID-19 dramatically illustrated how our personal actions and interactions influence each other. While you can't control all interactions, you have a choice about the environments in which you place yourself and the people with whom you interact.

Using Self-Management Skills

Manage your personal actions and interactions to overcome barriers to healthy living. There are many reasons why people with good intentions fail to be active or fail to adhere to healthy lifestyles. In this Concept, you learned that environments can either enhance or inhibit healthy behaviors. However, by planning ahead, you can take steps to address barriers and challenges imposed by your environment and become physically active.

- **Find convenient and safe places to be physically active.** Safety is a major deterrent to walking and biking for some people, but many communities have websites that provide information about safe places to participate in sports and active recreation. Search online for information about bike, walking, or jogging paths and well-lighted parks for evening activity.

- **Consider walking inside when the weather is bad.** Extremely cold or hot weather can be a significant barrier to being active. However, malls and stores can be alternative places to walk that are safe and climate controlled.

- **Advocate for safe and healthy environments.** Taking control over your health often necessitates being an advocate for change. The results may not be immediate, but advocating for parks or biking paths can lead to better opportunities for physical activity. Requesting healthier food choices at restaurants or grocery stores can also lead to gradual shifts in what is promoted or available.

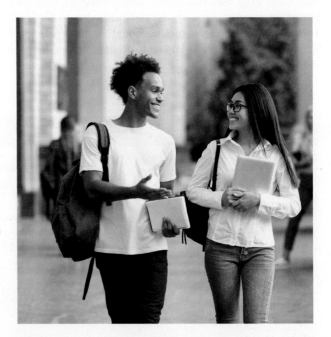

Natural areas and trails are great places for healthy recreation and relaxation.

Prostock-Studio/iStock/Getty Images

Use self-management skills to adopt and sustain a variety of healthy lifestyles. Consider how to apply these specific self-management skills to help take positive actions related to health, wellness, and fitness.

- **Manage your time effectively.** Lack of time due to busy school and work schedules may make being physically active and eating healthfully a challenge. Thus, it is important to use time wisely. Time management is a skill that can be learned to help you manage your lifestyle *and* your stress. In a later Concept, you will learn specific techniques for managing time.

- **Get help and social support from friends, family, and/ or experts.** Research shows that support from others can be helpful to eating healthfully, performing regular exercise, and adopting other healthy lifestyles. However, friends and family may not know of your interests or values regarding health and wellness. Thus, it is important to manage your personal interactions. Also, sometimes the help of an expert may be necessary. Specific information about finding help is provided in many of the Concepts.

- **Build knowledge by learning the facts.** There is considerable misinformation on the Internet and in the media, so it is important to be an informed consumer. Too often people fall prey to health fraud because they lack good information. Learning facts can help you "do it right" and avoid failure resulting from trying things that are not based on solid research.

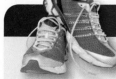

Strategies for Action: Lab Information

Self-assessments of lifestyles will help you determine areas in which you may need changes to promote optimal health, wellness, and fitness. The Healthy Habit Questionnaire in Lab 2A will help you assess your current lifestyle behaviors to determine if they are contributing positively to your health, wellness, and fitness. As you continue your study, refer back to this questionnaire to see if your lifestyles have changed.

connect
ACTIVITY

Suggested Resources and Readings

The websites for the following sources can be accessed by searching online for the organization, program, or title listed. Specific scientific references are available at the end of this edition of *Concepts of Fitness and Wellness*.

- Centers for Disease Control and Prevention. Health-Related Quality of Life.
- Centers for Disease Control and Prevention. Health, United States.
- Centers for Disease Control and Prevention. Healthy Places.
- Centers for Disease Control and Prevention. *Impact of the Built Environment on Health.* (pdf)
- Johns Hopkins Medicine. Johns Hopkins Medicine Podcasts.
- National Academies of Science, Engineering and Medicine. National Academies Press. Coronavirus Resources Collection. (pdfs)
- National Academies of Science, Engineering and Medicine. *Integrating Social Care into the Delivery of Health Care: Moving Upstream to Improve the Nation's Health.* Washington, DC: National Academies Press.
- National Academy of Medicine. *Perspectives on Health Equity and Social Determinants of Health.* Washington, DC: National Academies Press. (pdf)
- National Institutes of Health. MedlinePlus. Genetic Testing.
- National Institutes of Health. MedlinePlus. "What Is Genetic Ancestry Testing?"
- National Research Council and Institute of Medicine. *U.S. Health in International Perspective: Shorter Lives, Poorer Health.* Washington, DC: National Academies Press.
- National Research Council and Institute of Medicine. *Measuring the Risks and Causes of Premature Death: Summary of Workshops.* Washington, DC: National Academies Press.
- U.S. Department of Health and Human Services. Office of Disease Prevention and Health Promotion. *Healthy People 2030.* Social Determinants of Health.
- WorldHealth.net. Bloomberg's Global Health Index for 2020.

Lab 2A Healthy Habit Questionnaire

Name	Section	Date

Purpose: To assess the current status of various lifestyle behaviors and to help you make decisions concerning good health and wellness for the future.

Procedures

1. Complete the Healthy Habit Questionnaire by answering "Almost Never," "Sometimes," or "Almost Always" to each of the questions. If your behavior is not consistent, or you feel you are between the extremes, then choose the middle option ("Sometimes").
2. For each of the 10 lifestyle habits, sum the scores in the adjacent Total box.
3. Sum the 10 composite scores to create a Total Lifestyle Rating.
4. Record your scores in the Results section.
5. Use the Healthy Habit Rating Chart to determine your ratings. Add the ratings to the Results section.
6. Answer the question in the Conclusions and Implications section.

Results

Lifestyle Behavior	Score	Rating
Physical Activity Habits		
Nutrition Habits		
Stress-Management Habits		
Destructive Habits		
Safety Habits		
First Aid Habits		
Health Habits		
Medical Habits		
Consumer Habits		
Environmental Habits		
Total Score		

Healthy Habit Rating Chart

Habit Rating	Score
Good lifestyle	5–6
Neutral lifestyle	3–4
Needs improvement	1–2

Total Score Rating	
Good lifestyle	46–60
Neutral lifestyle	30–45
Needs improvement	<30

Note: Your scores on the Healthy Habit Questionnaire should be interpreted carefully. The statements are intended to provide a simple self-evaluation and are not designed as a screening or diagnostic tool. The various lifestyle behaviors pose different types of risks. For example, using tobacco or abusing drugs has immediate and significant negative effects on health and wellness, whereas other health lifestyles and skills, such as knowing first aid, may have subtler and less direct effects. Therefore, it is important not to compare scores on the different scales. The goal is to evaluate your overall profile and identify areas where you are doing well and areas that may need improvement.

Conclusions and Implications: In the space below, summarize the overall status of your lifestyle behaviors and indicate your strengths (areas where you are adopting healthy lifestyles) and concerns (areas where you may need to improve).

Healthy Habit Questionnaire

Directions: Use the following ratings to determine your habits: 1 = Almost Never, 2 = Sometimes, 3 = Almost Always. Place that number in the box to the right of each question. Sum the two numbers to get a score for each lifestyle habit. Sum the lifestyle habit scores to get a total lifestyle rating.

Physical Activity Habits

1. I perform physical activity most days of the week (or vigorous three days).

2. I look for ways to add physical activity into my lifestyle.

Nutrition Habits

3. I consume four to five servings of fruits and vegetables per day.

4. I make healthy food choices at stores and restaurants when possible.

Stress-Management Habits

5. I am able to identify situations in daily life that cause stress.

6. I take time out during the day to relax and recover from daily stress.

Destructive Habits

7. I do *not* smoke or use other tobacco products.

8. I do *not* binge drink or abuse alcohol or drugs.

Safety Habits

9. I use seat belts and adhere to the speed limit when I drive.

10. I practice safe sexual habits.

Social Habits

11. I seek out people and environments that support my well-being.

12. I avoid risky environments and situations.

Prevention Habits

13. I follow good hygiene practices (e.g., brushing/flossing my teeth; frequent hand washing).

14. I get an adequate amount of sleep each night.

Medical Habits

15. I do regular self-exams and have regular medical checkups.

16. I seek and follow medical advice when needed and prescribed.

Consumer Habits

17. I read product labels and make careful decisions before I buy.

18. I avoid using questionable products or programs.

Environmental Habits

19. I seek out environments that support healthy living.

20. I try to look for ways to conserve energy and protect the environment.

Total Lifestyle Rating

Note: These 10 habits capture only a sample of important lifestyle behaviors. A number of other potentially harmful behaviors are intentionally excluded due to their personal nature (such as the use and abuse of drugs, sexual practices, drinking and driving). Use the framework from this lab to think critically about your lifestyle behaviors and how you can work to improve them.

Self-Management Skills for Health Behavior Change

LEARNING OBJECTIVES

After completing the study of this Concept, you will be able to:

► Identify and define the five stages of change and explain how the stages relate to making lifestyle changes.

► Describe the four key factors that influence health behaviors, describe components in each category, and explain how the factors relate to stages of change.

► Identify and describe the self-management skills that predispose and enable you to change and to reinforce changes once you have made them.

► Identify and describe the six steps in self-planning and explain how they can be used to make personal plans for behavior change.

► Conduct self-assessments of your current stages for health behaviors and your self-management skills for making health behavior change.

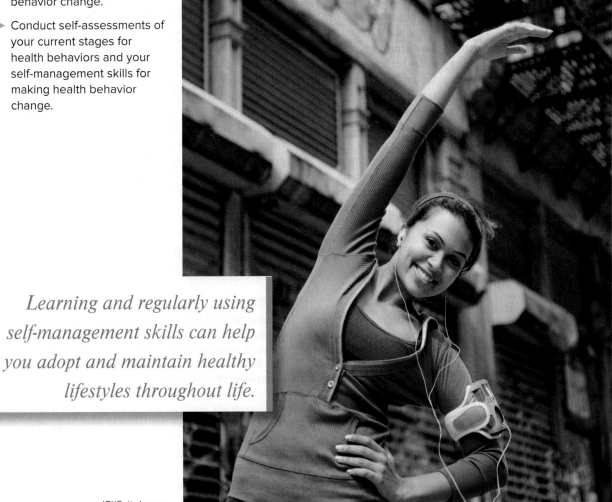

Learning and regularly using self-management skills can help you adopt and maintain healthy lifestyles throughout life.

JGI/Getty Images

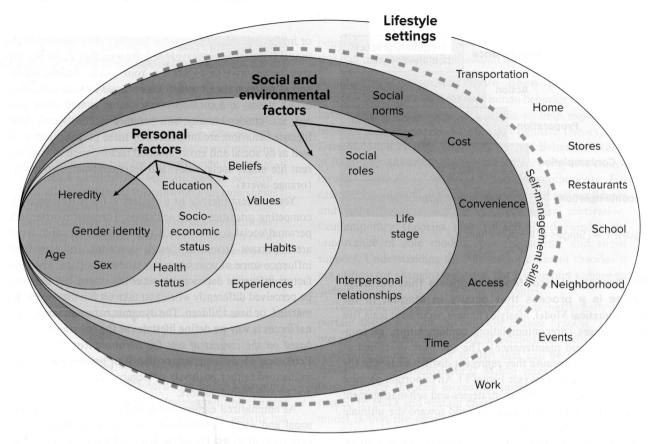

Figure 2 ▶ Layers of influence in the Social-Ecological Model.

Importance of Self-Management Skills

Learning self-management skills enhances your capacity for healthy living. The various skills needed to adopt and maintain healthy life-styles have been referred to as **self-management skills** since they

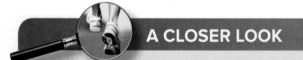

VIDEO 2

influence the way that you manage your personal lifestyles. Table 1 summarizes 15 different skills that can facilitate behavior change. As with other skills, you need to practice them to improve. In Lab 3A, you will be able to self-assess your stage of readiness for three priority lifestyles (physical activity, nutrition, and stress management) and to rate your self-management skills in each domain. Learning to apply the various skills in Table 1 is critical for healthy living.

A CLOSER LOOK

Social Justice and the DEI Movement

The notion of a "society" is that it should provide for the common interests of *all* members and protect them from outside threats. *Social justice* is a broad concept in which equity or justice is achieved in every aspect of society rather than in only some aspects or for some people. However, systemic racism, bias, and lack of tolerance for individual differences remain problematic in our larger society, making it difficult for all members to be treated equally. An increased awareness and visibility of the diversity, equity, and inclusion (DEI) movement offers some hope that this can change. *Diversity* refers to the inclusion of different types of people in

society regardless of race, ethnicity, age, disability, culture, socioeconomic status, sex, or gender identity; *equity* refers to the personal quality of being fair and impartial (free of bias or favoritism); and *inclusion* emphasizes including all people, especially those who have previously been excluded. Numerous organizations have committed to social justice and the DEI movement, but addressing the systemic challenge requires change by everyone.

How has the DEI movement influenced your attitudes and views? How can you be part of the solution?

connect
ACTIVITY

Table 1 ▶ Key Self-Management Skills

Building Knowledge and Changing Beliefs	Ability to interpret and apply information about health, wellness, and fitness. Knowledge doesn't always change beliefs, but awareness of the facts can play a role in achieving good health.
Building Self-Confidence and Motivation	Ability to act on your intentions and the discipline needed to stick to them.
Overcoming Barriers	Ability to overcome problems and challenges in adopting or maintaining healthy lifestyles. By conquering challenges, you learn skills that help you overcome other barriers.
Balancing Attitudes	Ability to balance positive and negative attitudes. Developing more favorable and optimistic outlooks can help you adhere to healthy lifestyles.
Self-Assessment Skills	Ability to assess your own health, wellness, and fitness and to learn to interpret your own self-assessment results.
Goal-Setting Skills	Ability to establish (and focus on) what you want to achieve in the future.
Self-Planning Skills	Ability to prepare and follow a plan for adopting or maintaining healthy lifestyle habits.
Performance Skills	Ability to learn lifestyle and physical skills needed to be physically active and healthy. These skills can help you feel confident and more successful in your efforts.
Consumer Skills	Ability to understand and interpret health information and make sound decisions related to health, wellness, and fitness.
Coping Skills	Ability to handle change. This set of skills helps you see situations in different perspectives and have more control over your lifestyle.
Time-Management Skills	Ability to devote time to the behaviors and activities that are most important to your personal health, wellness, and fitness.
Self-Monitoring Skills	Ability to monitor behavior and to keep records. Many people think they adhere to healthy lifestyles but, in reality, do not. Self-monitoring gives you a true picture of your behavior and helps you track progress over time.
Social Support Skills	Ability to seek out and obtain support from others. By learning to find support, you are more likely to sustain motivation and drive when faced with challenges.
Relapse Prevention Skills	Ability to return to healthy lifestyles despite challenges and setbacks. It is normal to have up and down phases, but this skill helps you avoid long-term relapses and return to healthy lifestyles when faced with barriers.
Conflict Resolution Skills	Ability to handle potential interpersonal or social conflicts that may challenge or complicate your efforts to adopt healthy lifestyles or to quit unhealthy behaviors.

Using self-management skills can help you overcome a lack of willpower. Many people reference a lack of *willpower* when explaining their lifestyle choices, but a lack of self-control may simply reflect undeveloped self-management skills. To achieve habit formation, you need to establish a personal motivation for change since that drives your decision making. Learning to set effective goals and to monitor your progress toward that goal are also important skills for behavior change. Making healthy choices can be challenging, but learning to delay gratification is part of the process. For example, resisting an extra snack often requires considerable discipline, as does resisting the temptation to relax instead of squeezing in a short bout of physical activity. It is important to be attentive to your personal needs and to not make decisions out of guilt; however,

learning to fight short-term temptations to meet your long-term goals can help build your confidence and commitment. It is important to emphasize that the ability to delay gratification is most directly determined by your underlying personal motivation for change. For habits to stick, motivations must be intrinsic (self-directed) instead of extrinsic (externally driven).

Self-Management Skills Skills that can be learned to support healthier decisions and adoption of healthier behaviors.

Making Lifestyle Changes

It takes time to change unhealthy lifestyles. People in Western cultures are used to seeing things happen quickly. We flip a switch, and the lights come on. We want food quickly, and thousands of fast food restaurants provide it. The expectation that we should have what we want when we want it has led us to also expect instantaneous changes in health, wellness, and fitness. Unfortunately, there is no quick way to health. There is no pill that can reverse the effects of a lifetime of sedentary living, poor eating, or tobacco use. Changing your lifestyle is the key. But lifestyles that have been practiced for years are not easy to change. Therefore, it is important to be both patient and persistent.

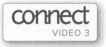

Figure 3 depicts how self-management skills can help you move through different stages of change. Consistent with the Transtheoretical Model, different strategies may be needed to move from one stage to the next. The importance of the various skills will also depend on the specific behavior and your previous experience. Consistent with the Social-Ecological Model, you should also consider the personal, social, and environmental factors that shape your values, beliefs, and decisions. You may find it easier to make positive changes if you seek out environments that are more conducive to healthy lifestyles. Similarly, you may find it easier to make changes if you make connections with people who can support these efforts. People who have friends who practice healthy habits have an easier time adopting these same behaviors. Similarly changing negative habits is harder if you are around people who practice destructive health behaviors. You may not have control over all aspects of your social circumstances or environment, but you should try to take personal responsibility for whatever is within your personal control.

Some self-management skills are especially helpful for initiating change. Using **predisposing skills** helps you initiate behavior change (e.g., move from precontemplation to contemplation and preparation). Examples of self-management skills in this category are building knowledge and changing beliefs, building self-confidence and motivation, overcoming barriers, and balancing attitudes. Self-assessments give a realistic picture of your current status and help you set goals. Knowledge provides a basis for sound decision making and can positively affect your belief that healthy lifestyles are beneficial. Confidence in your ability to change (i.e., self-efficacy) is also important—as is intrinsic or internal motivation to make change. Learning skills to overcome barriers provides encouragement that "you can do it." Adopting positive, encouraging attitudes and avoiding negative, discouraging attitudes is also important in initiating change. Table 2 provides some examples of how predisposing skills act to help you get going.

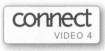

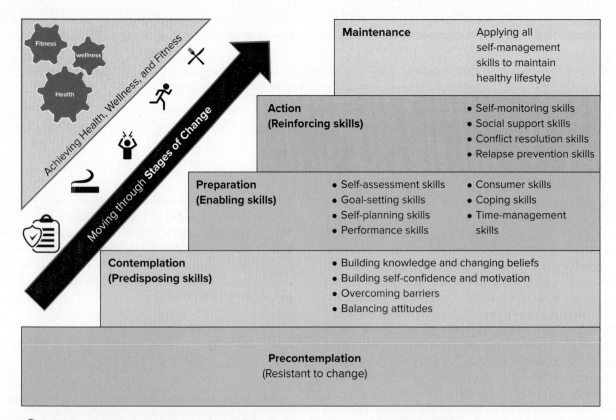

Figure 3 ▶ Relevant self-management skills to progress across the various stages of change.

Table 2 ▶ Lifestyle Examples of Predisposing Skills for Behavior Change

Predisposing Skills	Lifestyle Examples
Building Knowledge and Changing Beliefs	You may doubt that eating habits influence health and wellness, but learning about nutrition and healthy lifestyles can increase knowledge and awareness and provide the basis for changes in beliefs and behavior.
Building Confidence and Motivation	You may be tempted by snack foods and candy provided by coworkers. Resisting these foods takes discipline, but it builds confidence and motivation that helps keep focus on long-term goals.
Overcoming Barriers	You might find it hard to be physically active in the winter or bad weather. However, you can dress more appropriately or find alternate ways to be active indoors.
Balancing Attitudes	You might have negative attitudes about physical activity from sports or experiences in school. Rather than focusing on negative memories or attitudes, focus on positive outcomes (e.g., enjoyment, social interactions, or how it helps you feel). Shifting the balance to positive attitudes can help in making change.

Table 3 ▶ Lifestyle Examples of Enabling Skills for Behavior Change

Enabling Skills	Lifestyle Examples
Self-Assessment Skills	You want to know your health strengths and weaknesses. The best process is to select good tests and self-administer them. Practicing the assessments in these Concepts will help you become good at self-assessment.
Goal-Setting Skills	You decide to try to lose body fat. Setting a goal of losing 50 pounds makes success unlikely. Setting a more reasonable, behavioral goal of restricting 200 calories a day or expending 200 calories more each day for several weeks is a better strategy.
Self-Planning Skills	You want to become more active, eat better, and manage stress. Self-planning skills will help in planning programs to meet different needs.
Performance Skills	You may avoid physical activity because you do not have the physical skills equal to those of peers. Learning sports or other motor skills allows you to choose to be active.
Coping Skills	You may often feel stressed and anxious. Learning stress-management skills, such as relaxation, can help you cope. Like all skills, stress-management skills must be practiced to be effective.
Consumer Skills	You may avoid seeking medical help when you are sick and instead take an unproven remedy. Learning consumer skills provides knowledge for making sound medical decisions.
Time-Management Skills	You want to spend more quality time with family and friends. Monitoring your time can help you reallocate it in ways that are more consistent with personal priorities.

Some self-management skills are especially helpful for taking action. Using **enabling skills** can help you move from contemplation and preparation to action. Examples of self-management skills in this category are self-assessment skills, goal-setting skills, self-planning skills, performance skills, consumer skills, coping skills, and time-management skills. As shown in Figure 3, the ability to determine your needs based on self-assessments, to set goals based on needs, and to make plans based on goals are enabling skills. Performance skills enable you to enjoy yourself and to feel competent; consumer skills help you avoid making mistakes that will keep you from reaching your goals; and coping and time-management skills help you reduce the stress associated with changes in lifestyles and help you find time to take action. Table 3 provides some examples of how enabling skills can help you take action.

Some self-management skills are especially helpful in maintaining change. Using **reinforcing skills** can help you stay in the maintenance stage. Examples of self-management skills in this category are self-monitoring skills, social support, conflict resolution skills, and relapse prevention skills. Self-monitoring helps you track your behavior to see if your plans are effective (see Figure 3). Social support

Predisposing Skills Self-management skills that predispose you to adopt healthier lifestyles.

Enabling Skills Self-management skills that facilitate preparation and action steps in the behavior change process.

Reinforcing Skills Self-management skills that help sustain and reinforce healthy lifestyle behaviors.

Table 4 ▶ Lifestyle Examples of Reinforcing Skills for Behavior Change

Reinforcing Skills	Lifestyle Examples
Self-Monitoring Skills	You can't understand why you are not losing weight despite your efforts. Keeping records may show that you are not counting all the calories you consume. Learning to keep records of progress contributes to adherence.
Social Support Skills	You have developed a plan to be more active. Friends encourage the change and help develop a schedule that will allow and encourage regular activity.
Relapse Preventing Skills	You just quit smoking. To prevent relapse, you avoid situations where there is more temptation or pressure to smoke.
Conflict Resolution Skills	You find it challenging to eat healthy at work due to social pressures to snack or go to lunch, so you explain to your coworkers your preference to bring your own healthier meal from home.

from family, peers, and health professionals can be an especially important reinforcing factor. There are, however, different kinds of support and some are more helpful than others. A supportive person might ask *"How can I help you meet your goals?"* This type of support helps you take control of your own behavior and is encouraging and not controlling. However, other forms of feedback may be perceived as applying pressure and can hinder attempts to make healthy changes. For example, a statement such as *"You are not going to get anywhere if you don't stick to your diet"* is judgmental and not very encouraging. If you want to help friends and family make behavior changes, avoid applying pressure and attempt to provide positive forms of support. Learning how to seek and accept effective forms of social support from others is also important for your efforts to adopt and sustain healthy lifestyles.

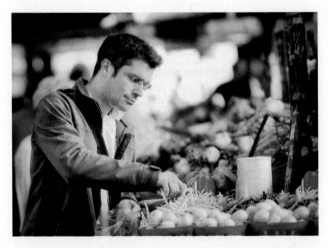

Good consumer skills enable you to select nutritious and health foods.
Nicolas McComber/Getty Images

If you change a behavior and experience success, this makes you want to keep doing the behavior. However, if attempts to change a behavior result in failure, you may conclude that the behavior cannot be achieved or isn't effective and may give up. Experts in behavior change have also determined that learning to overcome short-term setbacks or challenges is critical to long-term success. This self-management skill is often called *relapse prevention* since it is important to avoid reverting back to bad habits. With practice, you can learn to anticipate challenging situations that may make healthy lifestyles difficult. You can also learn to accept minor setbacks as temporary and return back to positive lifestyles with new insights. Using conflict resolution skills can help you maintain behaviors that involve personal or social conflicts. Prioritizing your own needs around other commitments can require communication and some degree of assertiveness at times. Learning conflict resolution skills can help you negotiate solutions and maintain your commitment. Table 4 provides specific lifestyle examples of how self-monitoring, social support, relapse prevention, and conflict resolution skills can help reinforce behavior change.

Some self-management skills interact to support adoption and maintenance of healthy lifestyles. Your ability to effectively use self-management skills will improve as you use them. The progressive steps outlined in Figure 3 highlight the unique role of some skills at specific stages. However, they each contribute to all stages of the behavior change process. For example, finding social support is listed as a reinforcing skill because support of family and friends helps you maintain a health behavior that you have changed. Social support, however, can also be important for thinking about changing your behavior and taking action. You may also need some skills more than others and the importance may vary depending on the behavior you are trying to change. Learning from your own experience is critical for adopting and maintaining healthy lifestyles.

Table 5 ▶ Self-Planning Skills

Self-Planning	Description	Self-Management Skills
1. Clarifying reasons	Knowing the general reasons for changing a behavior helps you determine the type of behavior change that is most important for you at a specific point in time. For example, if losing weight is the reason for wanting to change behavior, altering eating and activity patterns will be emphasized.	Results of the Self-Management Skills Questionnaire (Lab 3A) will help you determine which self-management skills you use regularly and the ones you might need to develop.
2. Identifying needs	Self-assessment is required to identify your needs. If you know your strengths and weaknesses, you can plan to build on your strengths and overcome weaknesses.	You will get the opportunity to practice *self-assessment* as you complete the lab activities. Examples include fitness, activity, dietary, stress, and attitude self-assessments.
3. Setting personal goals	Goal setting helps you develop a blueprint for planning.	In subsequent Concepts, you will have the opportunity to practice *setting goals* in a variety of healthy lifestyle plans as you complete the lab activities.
4. Selecting program components	A personal plan includes the specific program components that will meet your needs and goals. Examples include meal plans for nutrition and specific activities in your physical activity plan.	Several self-management skills, including *consumer skills, performance skills,* and *building knowledge*, will aid you in selecting program components.
5. Writing your plan	Your written plan provides "what" and "when" details. What are your going to do and when are you going to do it?	Effectively *managing time* is especially useful in preparing your written plan. You will get an opportunity to refine time-management skills in a lab activity later in this edition.
6. Evaluating progress	Once you have enacted your plan, you will know what works and what does not.	*Self-monitoring* is used in keeping records (logs) of your healthy behaviors (e.g., exercise, diet). Periodically *self-assessing* helps you determine if goals are met and how to modify the plan to make it better. You will get the opportunity to practice both as you complete the lab activities.

Using Self-Management Skills

Lifestyle change requires a personal commitment and the use of various self-management skills. As indicated throughout the Concept, lifestyle change is challenging and some behaviors may be harder for you to change than others. You may be in action or 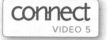 maintenance in some behaviors, but be at earlier precontemplation or preparation stages for others. Different self-management skills are important, depending on your current stage and the lifestyle behavior you are attempting to change (see Figure 3).

Self-planning is a self-management skill that requires the use of other self-management skills. The ability to set up and monitor your own lifestyle plans (i.e., self-planning skills) is particularly important in helping you take action or sustain your commitment to behavior change over time. A six-step self-planning process is introduced here to assist you in planning for lifestyle change (see Table 5). As you will note, several other self-management skills, including self-assessment, self-monitoring, and goal setting, are used within

this process. Labs in each Concept will allow you to practice these skills and in the final Concept, after you have studied a variety of concepts and self-management skills, you will develop a personal plan for several healthy lifestyles.

Step 1: Clarifying Reasons

Clarifying your reasons for behavior change is the first step in program planning. People at the precontemplation stage are not considering a change in behavior; they see no need. It's when they reach the contemplation stage that they consider changes in behavior. One of the most common and most powerful reasons for contemplating a change in a lifestyle is the recommendation of a doctor, often after a visit associated with an illness. Other common reasons are to improve personal appearance, lose weight, increase energy levels, improve the ability to perform daily tasks, and improve quality of life (wellness). Identifying your reasons for wanting to change helps you determine which behaviors to change first and helps you establish specific goals. Reflect on your reasons for wanting to make lifestyle changes before moving on to step 2.

Do Your Friends Support or Hinder Your Efforts to Adopt Healthy Lifestyles?

Learning to find positive social support is an important self-management skill. Studies of social connections over time have shown that people are more likely to become obese if they have obese friends. Similar relationships have been shown among spouses. Researchers suggest that health behaviors tend to be shared within social groups, resulting in shared outcomes.

Do your friends help you maintain a healthy lifestyle or do they make it more difficult to do so?

connect
ACTIVITY

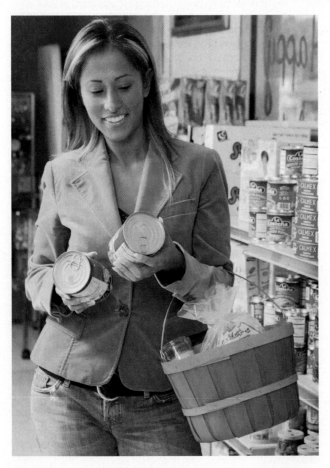

Adopting healthy lifestyle habits requires discipline and effort.
Jack Hollingsworth/Photodisc/Getty Images

Step 2: Identifying Needs

Self-assessments are useful in establishing personal needs, planning your program, and evaluating your progress. In the labs for this Concept (and others that follow), you will learn how to complete simple self-assessments of your behaviors and health/wellness status. The results of these assessments help you build personal profiles for a variety of health behaviors that can be used as the basis for program planning. With practice, self-assessments become more accurate. For this reason, it is important to repeat self-assessments and to pay careful attention to the procedures for performing them. If questions arise, get a professional opinion rather than making an error.

Periodic self-assessments can help determine if you are meeting health, wellness, and fitness standards and making progress toward personal health goals. When performed properly, self-assessments help you determine if you have met your goals and if you are meeting health standards (e.g., meeting health fitness standards, eating appropriate amounts of nutrients). Self-assessments also offer a measure of independence and can help you avoid unnecessary and expensive tests. They serve as a screening procedure to determine if you need professional assistance. However, because self-assessments may not be as accurate as tests by health and medical professionals, it is wise to have periodic tests by an expert to see if your self-assessments are accurate.

Self-assessments also have the advantage of consistent error rather than variable error. The best type of assessments are done by highly qualified experts using precise instruments. Following directions and practicing assessment techniques will reduce error significantly. Still, errors will occur. One advantage of a self-assessment is that the person doing the assessment is always the same—you. Even if you make an error in a self-assessment, it is likely to be consistent over time, especially if you use the same equipment each time you make the assessment. For example, scales have limitations for monitoring changes in weight (and fat). But if you measure your own weight using a home scale and your measurement always shows your weight to be 2 pounds higher than it really is, you have made a consistent error. You can determine if you are improving because you know the error exists. Variable errors are likely when different instruments are used, when different people make the assessments, and when procedures vary from test to test. Differences in scores are harder to explain with variable forms of error because they are not consistent.

Step 3: Setting Personal Goals

There are differences between short-term and long-term goals. Short-term goals are goals that you can accomplish in days or weeks. **Long-term goals** take longer to accomplish—sometimes months or even years.

Technology Update

Health and Fitness Apps

An array of new health products, services, and technologies continues to drive consumer interest in smartphone apps and wearable technology. While there are many different players in the market, there is also some consolidation. This is because developers build apps to take advantage of features already built into the underlying health platforms in Apple phones (Apple Health) and Android phones (Google Fit). The prominence of health and fitness technology in contemporary smartphone design demonstrates its importance to our economy as well as the health of our society. It also hints at what might be possible in the future. The acquisition of Fitbit by Google is one example.

Do you find value in health apps and wearable technology? Does it help remind you to stay active or to live healthy?

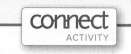

There are differences between general goals and SMART goals. **General goals** are broad statements of your reasons for wanting to accomplish something. Examples include changing a behavior such as eating better or being more active, or changing a physical characteristic such as losing weight or getting fit. **SMART goals** are less general and have several important characteristics. SMART goals are:

- **Specific:** A specific goal provides details, such as limiting calories to a specific number each day.

- **Measurable:** They allow you to perform assessments before you establish your goals and again later to see if you have met them.

- **Attainable:** They are neither too hard nor too easy. If the goal is too hard, failure is likely, which is discouraging. If the goal is too easy, it is not challenging.

- **Realistic:** They are your personal goals. If you put in the time and effort, you should have a realistic chance of meeting them. Realistic personal goals provide motivation.

- **Timely:** Timely goals are especially meaningful when you begin a program for making personal changes. Choosing goals that are timely helps you focus on the most salient changes that you want to make.

There are differences between behavioral and outcome goals. A **behavioral goal** is associated with something you do. An example of a specific short-term behavioral goal is *to perform 30 minutes of brisk walking 6 days a week for the next 2 weeks.* It is a behavioral goal because it refers to a behavior (something you do). An **outcome goal** is associated with a physical characteristic (e.g., lowering your body weight, lowering your blood pressure, building strength).

Typically, it takes weeks or months to reach outcome goals. This is because outcome goals depend on many things other than your behavior. For example, your heredity affects your body fat and muscle development.

Different factors influence your success in meeting goals. Consider these factors when setting your goals:

- *Behavioral goals are recommended for initial goal setting.* Typically, it takes weeks or months to reach outcome goals, so they make better long-term goals than short-term goals. Focus on changing behavior and outcomes will follow.

- *Outcome goals depend on many things other than your lifestyle behavior.* For example, your heredity affects your ability to achieve an outcome goal such as achieving a certain body weight and or achieving a fitness standard. The same lifestyle change program may produce different results for different people. For this reason, goals must vary from person to person, especially outcome goals. For example, two people may establish an outcome goal of losing 5 pounds over a 6-week period. Because we inherit predispositions to body composition, one person may meet the goal, while another may not, even if both strictly adhere to the same diet. A similar example can be used for fitness and physical activity. People inherit not only a predisposition to fitness but also a predisposition to benefit from training. In other words, if 10 people do the same physical activities, there will be 10 different results. One person may improve performance by 60 percent, while another might improve by only 10 percent. This makes it hard for beginners to set realistic outcome goals. Too often, people set a goal based on a comparative standard rather than on a standard that is possible for the individual to achieve in a short time.

- *Use a series of short-term goals to make progress toward long-term goals.* Once short-term behavioral goals are reached, establish new ones. After meeting a series of short-term goals, consider goal-setting guidelines for more experienced people.

Short-Term Goals Statements of intent to change a behavior or achieve an outcome in a period of days or weeks.

Long-Term Goals Statements of intent to change behavior or achieve a specific outcome in a period of months or years.

General Goals Broad statements of your reasons for wanting to accomplish something. Examples include changing a behavior such as eating better or being more active, or changing a physical characteristic such as losing weight or getting fit.

SMART Goals Goals that are Specific (*S*), Measurable (*M*), Attainable (*A*), Realistic (*R*), and Timely (*T*).

Behavioral Goal A statement of intent to perform a specific behavior (changing a lifestyle) for a specific period of time. An example is "I will walk for 15 minutes each morning before work."

Outcome Goal A statement of intent to achieve a specific test score (attainment of a specific standard) associated with good health, wellness, or fitness. An example is "I will lower my body fat by 3 percent."

Goal-setting guidelines vary depending on past history and experience with the behavior. Beginners should consider these guidelines:

- *Start with general long-term goals in mind.* It is good to have your goals in mind when you begin a program. But beginners may want to use general rather than specific long-term goals. You may choose either behavioral or outcome goals, but keep them general. For example, choose a goal of losing weight or getting fit. Getting too specific can be discouraging for reasons previously discussed.

- *Focus on SMART short-term behavioral objectives.* As noted previously, an example of a specific short-term behavioral goal is *to perform 30 minutes of brisk walking 6 days a week for the next 2 weeks.* It is a behavioral goal because it refers to a behavior (something you do). It is a SMART goal because it is specific, measurable, attainable, realistic, and timely. When using behavioral goals the principal factor associated with success is your willingness to give effort. No matter who you are, you can accomplish a behavioral goal if you give regular effort. This type of goal will help you keep your motivation level high and prevent you from being discouraged.

- *Avoid frequent outcome self-assessments; focus on self-monitoring of behavior.* A self-assessment before setting goals helps you set SMART goals. Self-assessments can also help you see if you have met your goals. For beginners, however, frequent self-assessment—especially of outcomes—is discouraged. For example, if the long-term goal is to lose weight, frequent weighing can be discouraging and even deceiving. Self-monitoring of behavior is encouraged, however. For the walking goal discussed earlier, keeping an activity log of your daily participation will help you comply.

Experienced people should consider these guidelines:

- *Start with SMART long-term goals.* Experience helps people realize that it takes time to meet long-term goals, especially outcome goals. Both SMART behavioral and outcome goals can be considered.

- *Use a series of short-term SMART goals (both behavioral and outcome) as a means of accomplishing long-term goals.* Even experienced people are more likely to achieve success if they realize that setting and meeting a series of SMART short-term goals is important. For example, a person who has high blood pressure (160 systolic) may set a long-term outcome goal of lowering systolic blood pressure to 120 over a period of 6 months. Several behavioral goals can be established for the six-month period, including taking blood pressure medication (daily), performing 30 minutes of moderate physical activity each day, and limiting salt in the diet to less than 100 percent of the recommended dietary allowance. If the long-term outcome goal is realistic, adhering to SMART short-term behavioral goals will result in achieving the outcome goal.

- *Use self-assessments and self-monitoring to determine if you are making progress.* Self-assessments can be more frequent for the experienced. Still, avoid expecting too much, especially for outcome goals. Self-monitoring of behavioral goals is good, even for the experienced. If you commit to the behavior and stick to your plan, the outcomes will follow.

Maintenance goals are also appropriate once goals have been achieved or when improvements aren't necessary. For example, the person who lowers systolic blood pressure from 160 to 120 need not continue to lower the new healthy blood pressure. Once a healthy outcome goal has been achieved, a new outcome goal of maintaining a systolic blood pressure of 120 is appropriate. Behavioral goals will also have to be modified. For the person who has reduced blood pressure to a healthy level, medication levels might be reduced for maintenance.

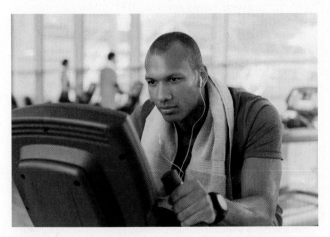

Setting and following SMART goals can help with adherence.
Jonathan Gibson/newco500/123RF

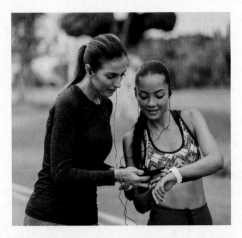

Monitoring your progress can enhance motivation.
filadendron/Getty Images

Maintenance goals are appropriate in other areas as well. For example, nutrition and exercise strategies for weight maintenance will likely be different from those for losing weight. When a person reaches a healthy level of fitness (or a healthy body weight), maintenance may be the goal rather than continued improvement. You cannot improve forever; at some point, attempting to do so may be counterproductive to health.

Making improvement can motivate you to reach long-term goals. As noted earlier, setting short-term goals that are both attainable and realistic will help you reach your long-term goals. Meeting short-term goals encourages and motivates you to continue with your healthy lifestyle plan. Don't expect to set perfect goals all the time. No matter how much self-assessing and self-monitoring you do, you may sometimes set goals too low or too high. If the goal is set too low, it is easily achieved, and a new, higher goal can be established. If the goal is set too high, you may fail to reach it, even though you have made considerable progress toward the goal.

Rather than becoming discouraged when a goal is not met, consider the improvement you have made. Improvement, no matter how small, means that you are moving toward your goal. Also, you can measure your improvement and use it to help set future goals. Of course, periodic self-assessments and good record keeping (self-monitoring) are necessary to keep track of improvements accurately.

Putting your goals in writing helps formalize them. If you don't write them down, your goals will be easy to forget. Putting goals in writing helps you establish a commitment to yourself and clearly establishes your goals. You can revise them if necessary. Written goals are not cast in concrete.

Step 4: Selecting Program Components

You can choose from many different program components to meet your goals. There are many different lifestyle changes that can be made to improve health, wellness, and fitness. They range from improving priority lifestyles (physical activity, nutrition, and stress management) to adopting positive safety and personal health habits to avoiding destructive habits. The changes you decide to make depend on your program goals. For example, if the goal is to become more fit and physically active, the program components will be the activities you choose. You will want to identify activities that match your abilities and that you enjoy. You will want to select activities that build the type of fitness you want to improve.

Other examples of program components are preparing menus for healthy eating, participating in stress-management activities, planning to attend meetings to help avoid destructive habits, and attending a series of classes to learn CPR and first aid. Preparing a list of program components that will help you meet your specific goals will prepare you for step 5, writing your plan.

Step 5: Writing Your Plan

Preparing a written plan can improve your adherence to the plan. A written plan is a pledge, or a promise, to be active. Research shows that intentions to be active are more likely to be acted on when put in writing. In the Concepts that follow, you will be given the opportunity to prepare written plans for becoming more active as well as for altering a variety of other lifestyles. A good written plan includes daily plans with scheduled times and other program details. For example, the daily written plan for stress management could include the time of day when specific program activities are conducted (e.g., 15-minute quiet time at noon; yoga class from 5:30 to 6:30). An activity plan would include a schedule of the activities for each day of the week, including starting and finishing times and specific details concerning the activities to be performed. A dietary plan would include specific menus for each meal and between-meal snacks.

In the labs that accompany the final Concept, you will write plans for several different lifestyles. By then you will have learned a variety of self-management skills that will assist you.

Step 6: Evaluating Progress

Self-assessment and self-monitoring can help you evaluate progress. Once you have written a plan, you will want to determine your effectiveness in sticking with your plan. Keeping written records is one type of self-monitoring.

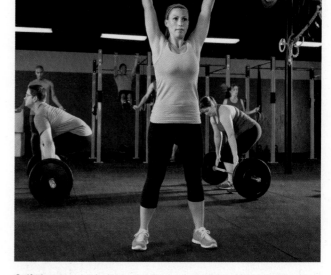

Self-planning can help you implement a variety of changes to enhance health, wellness, and fitness.
Erik Isakson/Blend Images LLC

Self-monitoring is a good way to assess success in meeting behavioral goals. Keeping a dietary log or using a pedometer to keep track of steps are examples of self-monitoring. Self-assessments are a good way to see if you have met outcome goals.

In the Concepts that follow, you will learn to self-assess a variety of outcomes (e.g., fitness, body fatness) and self-monitor behaviors (e.g., diet, physical activities, stress-management activities). In step 2 of the self-planning process, you used self-assessments to determine your needs and to help you plan your goals (step 3). Once you have tried your program, use the same self-assessments and self-monitoring strategies to evaluate the effectiveness of your program. You can see if you have met the goals you established for yourself.

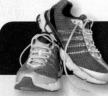

Strategies for Action: Lab Information

The lab activity worksheets that accompany each Concept will help you learn the self-management skills necessary for behavior change. Self-assessing your current health, wellness, and fitness status, as well as a self-monitoring of your current lifestyles, can help you determine your reasons for making change and help you establish SMART goals for change. The questionnaire in Lab 3A will help you identify your stages of change for various behaviors and self-management skills you can use to change the behaviors. Like all skills, practice is necessary to improve self-management skills.

connect ACTIVITY

Suggested Resources and Readings

The websites for the following sources can be accessed by searching online for the organization, program, or title listed. Specific scientific references are available at the end of this edition of *Concepts of Fitness and Wellness.*

- American Heart Association. Breaking Down Barriers to Fitness.
- Centers for Disease Control and Prevention. Overcoming Barriers to Physical Activity.
- Fogg, B. J. (2020). *Tiny Habits: The Small Changes That Change Everything.* Boston: Houghton Mifflin Harcourt.
- Hilliard, M. E. et al. (Eds.). (2018). *The Handbook of Health Behavior Change, 5th ed.* New York: Springer Publishing.
- Law, T. (2020, September 21). "COVID-19 Conspiracy Theories Are Spreading Rapidly—and They're a Public Health Risk All Their Own." *Time.*
- Lorig, K. et al. (2020). *Living a Healthy Life with Chronic Conditions: Self-Management Skills.* Boulder, CO: Bull Publishing.
- National Diversity Council. DiversityFIRST Toolkit.
- Pro-Change Behavior Systems, Inc. The Transtheoretical Model.
- Prochaska, J. O., & Prochaska, J. M. (2016). *Changing to Thrive: Using the Stages of Change to Overcome the Top Threats to Your Health and Happiness.* Center City, MN: Hazelden Publishing.

Lab 3A Stages of Change and Self-Management Skills

Name	**Section**	**Date**

Purpose: To assess your current Stage of Change for three key priority lifestyle behaviors (physical activity, nutrition, and stress management) and your self-management skills related to each one.

Procedures

1. Complete the Stages of Change Questionnaire. Check one box for each of the three priority health behaviors (physical activity, nutrition, and stress management).
2. Complete the Self-Management Skills Questionnaire. Each question reflects one of the self-management skills described in this Concept. Each of the 12 questions requires a response about three different healthy behaviors. Respond to each question by using a 3 for very true, a 2 for somewhat true, or a 1 for not true. Record the appropriate number in the box beside each question. After you have answered all 12 questions for all three healthy lifestyles, total the numbers in the three columns to get a total score for physical activity, nutrition, and stress management.
3. Record your Stages of Change for the three healthy lifestyles (the word by the box you checked) in the Results section.
4. Record your Self-Management Scores for the three healthy lifestyles in the Results section. Use the Self-Management Skills Rating Chart to determine a rating for each healthy behavior. Record your ratings in the Results section.
5. Provide the appropriate information in the Conclusions and Implications section.

Results

Health Behavior	Stage of Change	Self-Management Score	Self-Management Rating
Physical Activity			
Nutrition			
Stress Management			

Self-Management Skills Rating Chart

Rating	Score
Good	30–36
Marginal	24–29
Needs improvement	<24

Conclusions and Implications: Choose one of the three health behaviors (preferably a behavior for which you think you need improvement). In the space below, discuss your current ability to use the various self-management skills to help you change your stage for the health behavior. Which self-management skills did you score well on? Which ones could you possibly improve?

Health Behavior: _____

Stages of Change Questionnaire. Check only one box for each question.

1. **Physical Activity**

☐ Precontemplation—I am not active, and I do not plan to start.
☐ Contemplation—I am not active, but I am thinking about starting.
☐ Preparation—I am getting ready to become active.
☐ Action—I do some activity but need to do more.
☐ Maintenance—I have been active regularly for several months.

2. **Nutrition**

☐ Precontemplation—I do not eat well and don't plan to change.
☐ Contemplation—I do not eat well but am thinking about change.
☐ Preparation—I am planning to change my diet.
☐ Action—I sometimes eat well but need to do more.
☐ Maintenance—I have eaten well regularly for several months.

3. **Stress Management**

☐ Precontemplation—I do not manage stress well and plan no changes.
☐ Contemplation—I am thinking about making changes to manage stress.
☐ Preparation—I am planning to change to manage stress better.
☐ Action—I sometimes take steps to manage stress better but need to do more.
☐ Maintenance—I have used good stress-management techniques for several months.

Self-Management Skills Questionnaire	Very True	Somewhat True	Not True	Activity Score	Nutrition Score	Stress Score
1. I regularly self-assess: (self-assessment)						
personal physical fitness and physical activity levels	3	2	1	▢		
the contents of my diet	3	2	1		▢	
personal stress levels	3	2	1			▢
2. I self-monitor and keep records concerning: (self-monitoring)						
physical activity	3	2	1	▢		
diet	3	2	1		▢	
stress in my life	3	2	1			▢
3. I set realistic and attainable goals for: (goal setting)						
physical activity	3	2	1	▢		
eating behaviors	3	2	1		▢	
reducing stress in my life	3	2	1			▢
4. I have a personal written or formal plan for: (self-planning)						
regular physical activity	3	2	1	▢		
what I eat	3	2	1		▢	
managing stress in my life	3	2	1			▢
5. I possess the skills to: (performance skills)						
perform a variety of physical activities	3	2	1	▢		
analyze my diet	3	2	1		▢	
manage stress (e.g., progressive relaxation)	3	2	1			▢
6. I have positive attitudes about: (balancing attitudes)						
my ability to stick with an activity plan	3	2	1	▢		
my ability to stick to a nutrition plan	3	2	1		▢	
my ability to manage stress in my life	3	2	1			▢
7. I can overcome barriers that I encounter: (overcoming barriers)						
in my attempts to be physically active	3	2	1	▢		
in my attempts to stick to a nutrition plan	3	2	1		▢	
in my attempts to manage stress in my life	3	2	1			▢

Self-Management Skills Questionnaire (cont.)	Very True	Somewhat True	Not True	Activity Score	Nutrition Score	Stress Score
8. I know how to identify misinformation: (consumer skills)						
relating to fitness and physical activity	3	2	1			
relating to nutrition	3	2	1			
relating to stress management	3	2	1			
9. I am able to get social support for my efforts to: (social support)						
be active	3	2	1			
stick to a healthy nutrition plan	3	2	1			
manage stress in my life	3	2	1			
10. When I have problems, I can get back to: (relapse prevention)						
my regular physical activity	3	2	1			
my nutrition plan	3	2	1			
my plan for managing stress	3	2	1			
11. I am able to adapt my thinking to: (coping strategies)						
stick with my activity plan	3	2	1			
stick with my nutrition plan	3	2	1			
stick with my stress-management plan	3	2	1			
12. I am able to manage my time to: (time management)						
stick with my physical activity plan	3	2	1			
shop for and prepare nutritious food	3	2	1			
perform stress-management activities	3	2	1			
Total Activity Score						
Total Nutrition Score						
Total Stress Score						

Preparing for Physical Activity

LEARNING OBJECTIVES

After completing the study of this Concept, you will be able to:

▶ Identify and describe key factors for safely participating in a moderate to vigorous physical activity program.

▶ Describe the warm-up, the workout, and the cool-down and explain why each is important.

▶ Explain the potential risks associated with exposure to heat, cold, and altitude and describe precautions that can be taken to prevent problems.

▶ Identify the factors that contribute to soreness and injury from physical activity and describe steps that can be taken to recover from them.

▶ Identify and describe the common positive and negative attitudes about physical activity and explain how they relate to regular participation.

▶ Assess your readiness for physical activity and demonstrate appropriate warm-up activities.

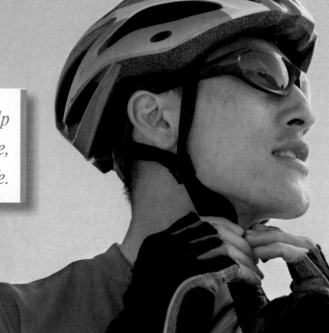

Proper preparation can help make physical activity enjoyable, effective, and safe.

John Lund/Drew Kelly/Blend Images LLC

47

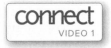

Why It Matters!

Engaging in physical activity is a priority lifestyle because it positively impacts multiple dimensions of health, wellness, and fitness. There are few risks involved with moderate-intensity physical activity, but it is important to start slowly and follow appropriate guidelines if you perform more vigorous activity or if you participate in outdoor activities. This Concept will provide guidelines for safe and effective physical activity. The information will help you prepare for and make physical activity a part of your normal routine.

Safety Considerations for Physical Activity

Physical activity is safe for almost everyone. There are risks associated with physical activity, but the risks of physical inactivity are far greater. Most people are not likely to be injured when doing moderate-intensity physical activity; however, injuries and other adverse events do sometimes happen. Musculoskeletal injuries are the most common, but rates are relatively low and many are preventable. People who are physically fit have a lower risk of injury than people who are not, so one prevention strategy is to slowly build up a good base of fitness. The type, intensity, and volume of physical activity also affect risk of injuries and adverse events. Therefore, it is still important to follow guidelines to reduce your risks.

Self-screening using the PAR-Q+ can identify potential risk. In recent years, the American College of Sports Medicine (ACSM) revised screening guidelines to remove unnecessary barriers to adopting physically active lifestyles. Individuals are encouraged to self-screen using the Physical Activity Readiness Questionnaire for Everyone (**PAR-Q+**). This questionnaire was developed by the PAR-Q+ Collaboration team of investigators, with support from the Public Health Agency of Canada and the British Columbia Ministry of Health Services. It includes a seven-item screening questionnaire (see Lab 4A) and a two-page follow-up questionnaire with questions about medical conditions. People who answer "no" to all seven screening questions on the PAR-Q+ can skip the additional medical questions and begin participation as long as they follow the guidelines on the questionnaire. However, people who answer "yes" to one or more questions should complete the follow-up questions on pages 2 and 3 of the PAR-Q+ and consult a qualified exercise professional and/or a physician based on the nature of the medical condition. Many clinical, commercial, and worksite fitness programs also use the PAR-Q+ as a form of screening, but they may also ask participants to sign a "participant declaration," included in the questionnaire. Although the PAR-Q+ is included as part of Lab 4A to enable self-screening, a more comprehensive version is available online at http://eparmedx.com.

Professional screening can help establish medical readiness for exercise. While moderate physical activity is relatively safe, additional screening can be warranted before performing structured **exercise** or higher-intensity physical activity. In addition to the PAR-Q+, the ACSM recommends that exercise professionals use a pre-participation screening system (professional screening) that considers a person's current and desired level of physical activity levels as well as the presence of signs or symptoms of cardiovascular, metabolic, or renal disease. There is insufficient evidence to indicate that risk factors (e.g., high blood pressure, high cholesterol, high BMI) increase risk of adverse events in physical activity in those who do not have an actual disease, so risk factors are no longer of primary consideration by professionals when performing pre-participation screening. However, other indicators may cause the exercise professional to refer a participant to a physician for additional evaluation. The ACSM guidelines may warrant a physical exam, additional laboratory tests, and/or a **clinical exercise test** to evaluate readiness for structured exercise or more intense levels of physical activity.

There is no way to be absolutely sure that you are medically ready to begin a physical activity program. Even a thorough exam by a physician cannot guarantee that a person has no limitations that may cause a problem during exercise. However, new screening methods have been implemented because overly stringent methods used in the past have excluded some individuals from exercise unnecessarily. Use of the PAR-Q+ (see Lab 4A) and

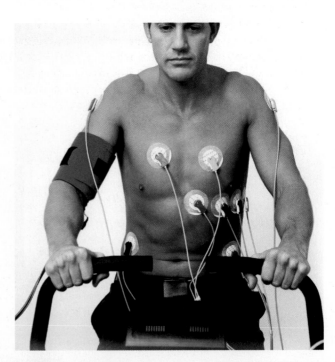

A standard exercise test—an example of professionally guided screening—is recommended for some individuals to ensure they can exercise safely.
Digital Vision/Punchstock/Getty Images

adherence to the ACSM guidelines are advised to help minimize the risk while encouraging maximum participation. Note that people over the age of 45 who are *not* accustomed to vigorous to maximal effort exercise are still encouraged to consult a qualified exercise professional before engaging in this intensity of exercise.

General Considerations for Physical Activity

Shoes play a critical role for performance and injury prevention. Although shoes are designed based on the needs of a given activity, they all share some common features. The four primary features of shoes are flexibility, support, cushioning, and traction. What makes a shoe unique for a given sport is how each of those four features are integrated into the design of the shoe (see Figure 1):

- *Flexibility* refers to the amount of give in the shoe's outsole (the bottom part of the shoe that makes contact with the ground). Some activities benefit from more flexibility in the sole than others. A highly flexible sole is important for permitting quick movements in activities such as tennis, lacrosse, and dance. However, a stiffer sole is preferable in other activities (e.g., basketball and running) to enhance propulsion and to protect the foot from excess motion.

- *Support* refers to how much stability a shoe provides in order to reduce an unwanted amount of inward or outward roll of the foot and ankle. Excess inward roll (pronation) is controlled mainly by the midsole while outward roll (supination) is controlled by the upper (the part of the shoe that wraps around the top and sides of the foot). A more rigid upper is important for protecting the ankle from a rolling injury during activities such as tennis and basketball.

- *Cushioning* reflects a shoe's ability to absorb shock and protect the heel and midfoot from impact with the ground. Extra cushioning is important in activities that involve jumping and leaping (e.g., basketball and volleyball) since the impact forces are greater on landing. Running shoes tend to have more cushioning than walking shoes for this same reason.

- *Traction* delivers the degree of grip needed to be safe and to perform effectively. Shoes like trail running or hiking shoes require more tread to navigate uneven ground or handle wet or muddy conditions. Court shoes have specialized soles designed to perform well on either hard or soft court surfaces, improving traction and preventing unwanted sliding or slipping. Many athletic shoes use specially designed cleats to further enhance traction.

Hybrid shoes, known as cross-trainers, can be a versatile option, but they typically don't provide the needed features for

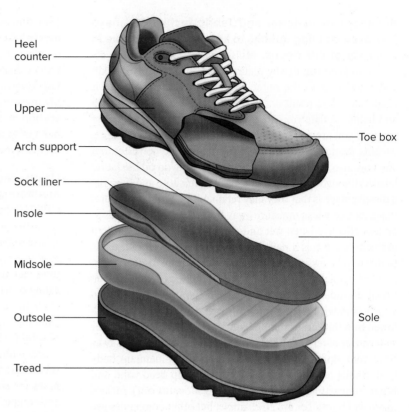

Figure 1 ▶ Anatomy of an activity shoe.

specific activities. For example, they may lack the cushioning and support needed for running and the ankle support for activities such as basketball. Most shoes have very thin sock liners, but supplemental inserts can be purchased to provide more cushioning and/or support. Custom orthotics can also be used to correct alignment problems or minimize foot injuries (such as plantar fasciitis). A very important, and frequently neglected, consideration is to replace shoes after extended use. Runners typically replace shoes every four to six months (or 400–600 miles), even if the outer appearance of the shoe is still good. The main functions of athletic shoes are to reduce shock from impact and protect the foot. One of the best prevention strategies for avoiding injuries is to replace your shoes on a regular basis. (See the Concept on performance for additional insights on sport-specific shoes.)

PAR-Q+ An acronym for Physical Activity Readiness Questionnaire for Everyone; designed to help determine if you are medically suited to begin an exercise program.

Exercise Physical activity done for the purpose of getting physically fit.

Clinical Exercise Test A test, typically administered on a treadmill, in which exercise is gradually increased in intensity while the heart is monitored using an electrocardiogram (ECG) device that monitors heart functionality. Symptoms not present at rest may be evident as exercise intensity is increased.

Advances in material and fabric technology have improved clothing options to keep you comfortable in a variety of conditions. Moisture-wicking fabrics are designed to keep you dry by pulling sweat away from your skin and drawing it to the outer layer of the material where it evaporates. The result is a fabric that feels dry to the touch and helps regulate your core body temperature, regardless of whether you are working out on a hot or cold day. Moisture-wicking fabrics are often made from synthetic polyester, but you may also see polypropylene, nylon, or rayon on the fabric label. Although synthetic materials are versatile and durable, a disadvantage is that they may retain odors. Wool is a natural material that wicks moisture away from the body but tends to be less effective when wet and can add bulk and weight to a garment. Cotton is a naturally absorbent material that tends to dry more slowly, making it a poor choice for athletic wear.

Physical activity in cold or wet conditions requires additional considerations. For activity in the cold, it is best to wear a thin wickable material as your base (inner) layer, followed by a thicker insulating layer, and finally, a windproof or waterproof outer layer. The base layer helps move sweat away from your skin while the middle layer helps maintain body heat. Shells or outerwear layers should help keep wind and water from getting in (while still letting moisture out). Jackets made with Gore-Tex are an example, but other companies use different fabrics to achieve the same objective. Table 1 provides some guidelines for dressing for physical activity.

Planning for physical activity should include steps to check and maintain equipment. Some activities are more equipment intensive than others. To ensure a safe and effective outing on a bike, it is important to wear a helmet and ensure that the bike is working properly (e.g., well-inflated tires, functioning brakes, and lubricated chain). Wearing protective gear while rollerblading (e.g., wrist guards, knee pads) or playing racquetball (e.g., eyewear) is also important to reduce risks of injury. Water sports such as canoeing and kayaking also present unique considerations and wearing life preservers is always recommended. The adoption of prevention strategies during physical activity is similar to the habit of wearing a seat belt in a car. The chances of having an accident may be small, but it is better to be safe.

Using technology can help with planning and monitoring physical activity. Smartphones have built-in GPS (Global Positioning System) technology and this can assist with navigation as well as with monitoring. Many individuals use web-based apps, such as MapMyRun/Ride or TrailLink, to plan routes for walking, biking, or hiking. The location features can also provide safety advantages by helping with navigating or letting family or friends keep tabs on where you are at. Many commercial activity monitors can also assist with planning, tracking, and monitoring physical activity. An array of subscription-based services are also available to facilitate or support physical activity programming. For example, online subscriptions to services like Zwift or Peleton provide opportunities for engaging indoor cycling by providing virtual routes and competition. All these types of technology-based resources and tools can facilitate or support physical activity but are certainly not essential. Some individuals find value in these functions but others may not perceive the same benefits.

Drink fluids before, during, and after physical activity. Remember to drink fluids before activity and about 1 cup for each 15–20 minutes during activity. After activity, drink about 2 cups for each pound of weight lost. The thirst mechanism lags behind the body's actual need for fluid, so drink even if you don't feel thirsty. Fluids are needed for exercise in the cold as well as exercise in the heat. The color of your urine can reveal hydration status. Clear (almost colorless) urine produced in large volumes indicates that you are hydrated. As water in the body is reduced, the urine becomes more concentrated and is a darker yellow color. This indicates dehydration and a need for fluid replacement.

Water is generally the best choice for replacing fluids since it is less expensive and doesn't contain extra calories. Fluid-replacement beverages (e.g., Gatorade, Powerade) are designed to provide added energy (from carbohydrates) without impeding hydration. If you choose to use one of these beverages, select one that contains electrolytes and no more than 4 to 8 percent carbohydrates. Additional details are provided in the Concept on performance.

Recommendations for Typical Bouts of Physical Activity

The warm-up phase prepares the body for more vigorous activity. According to the ACSM, the **warm-up** can improve range of motion and may reduce injury risk. It increases

---

Table 1 ▶ Selecting Appropriate Clothing for Activity

General Guidelines
- Avoid clothing that is too tight or that restricts movement.
- Material in contact with skin should be porous.
- Clothing should protect against wind and rain but allow for heat loss and evaporation (e.g., Gore-Tex, Coolmax).
- Wear layers so that a layer can be removed if not needed.
- Wear socks for most activities to prevent blisters, abrasions, odor, and excessive shoe wear.
- Socks should be absorbent and fit properly.
- Do not use nonporous clothing that traps sweat; these garments prevent evaporation and cooling.

Special Considerations
- Consider eye protection for racquetball and other sports.
- Females should wear an exercise bra for support.
- Males should consider an athletic supporter for support.
- Wear helmets and padding for activities with risk of falling, such as biking or inline skating.
- Wear reflective clothing for night activities.
- Wear water shoes for some aquatic activities.
- Consider lace-up ankle braces to prevent injury.
- Consider a mouthpiece for basketball and other contact sports.

body temperature, decreases risk of irregular heartbeats, and allows the body to transition into the workout that follows. The ACSM recommends a warm-up of *light to moderate intensity activities specific to the muscle groups employed during exercise.* However, some individuals (and athletes engaged in specific sports or activities) may benefit from different types of warm-up routines. A structured **stretch warm-up** includes exercises designed to stretch the muscles beyond their normal length. This is a traditional form of warm-up that is an enjoyable part of the regular exercise routine for many. In general, recent research has not confirmed the long-standing notion that a stretch warm-up reduces injury risk. Evidence that a stretch warm-up reduces post-exercise soreness is also uncertain. Athletes who participate in sports and activities requiring a larger-than-normal range of motion (e.g., gymnastics and diving) typically perform a stretch warm-up (after a general warm-up) as part of their pre-exercise routine. In these activities, the stretching is important for their performance. The stretch warm-up, however, can reduce strength, power, and/or speed performance, especially if the stretches last more than 60 seconds. For athletes and those concerned with high-level performance in activities that require strength, power, or speed, a stretch warm-up is not recommended. Typical exercisers who are not concerned with high-level performance, and who enjoy a stretch warm-up, may choose to perform a stretch warm-up after a general warm-up.

An alternative to a stretch warm-up is a **dynamic warm-up** that includes moderate-intensity, calisthenic-type activities (see Lab 4B for examples). Unlike the stretch warm-up, the goal is not to lengthen the muscles, but to move the joints through a full range of motion. The ACSM recommends a dynamic warm-up when preparing for *cardiorespiratory endurance, aerobic exercise, sports, or resistance exercise, especially activities that are of long duration or with many repetitions.* A specific type of dynamic warm-up known as the *sport-specific warm-up* is recommended prior to sports. Examples include performing layups or shooting baskets before a basketball game or swinging a golf club or tennis racket before playing the actual game.

It is important to note that the stretch warm-up and dynamic warm-up are not the same as a workout to improve flexibility. A stretch warm-up prepares you for your workout, but stretching exercises designed to improve flexibility are considered part of a workout. (Additional information about stretching exercises is included in the Concept on flexibility.) Depending on intensity of the workout or conditioning phase, the warm-up can last from 5 to 15 minutes. The ACSM recommends that the warm-up last no more than 15 minutes. Table 2 provides information about types of warm-up activities for various types of physical activity.

Warm-Up Light to moderate physical activity performed to prepare for a more vigorous workout (also referred to as the 'initiation phase).

Stretch Warm-Up The performance of stretching exercises prior to a vigorous workout.

Dynamic Warm-Up The performance of calisthenics of gradually increasing intensity prior to a vigorous workout (e.g., jumping jacks, jumping, skipping).

Table 2 ▶ Warm-Up Guidelines for Different Physical Activities

Activity	Guidelines
Moderate Activity	• For walking and activities of equal intensity, no warm-up is necessary. • For moderate recreation, such as golf, a sport-specific warm-up may be performed. • A dynamic warm-up and a stretch warm-up can be performed but it is not typically necessary for most moderate activities
Vigorous Aerobics	• For most vigorous activities a dynamic warm-up is recommended (see Lab 4B). • For jogging, biking, swimming, and similar aerobic activities, performing the activity slowly and then with increased intensity can serve as a dynamic warm-up.
Vigorous Anaerobic Activities and Sports	• A dynamic warm-up is recommended to prepare the body for high intensity (anaerobic) activities. A stretch warm-up can be performed after the dynamic warm-up, but it may limit performance in activities requiring strength, speed, and power. • For sports, a dynamic warm-up is recommended and can include sport specific movements. A stretch warm-up is not recommended for sports requiring strength, speed or power.
Muscle Fitness Exercises	• Prior to training for or competing in events requiring muscle fitness or speed, a dynamic warm-up is recommended. If stretching is performed it should be after the workout while the muscles are warm.
Flexibility Exercises and Activities Requiring Flexibility	• Prior to activities such as gymnastics, diving, dance and other similar activities, a dynamic warm-up or general warm-up (jogging, brisk walking) should be performed followed by a stretching warm-up). • Prior to performing activities such as gymnastics, diving, and dance, a stretch warm-up is recommended after the general warm-up.

The workout is the principal component of an activity program and occurs after the warm-up and before the cool-down. A **workout** can refer to physical activities designed as training for fitness and health, participation in sport or recreation for fun and enjoyment, or participation in moderate exercise for general health and wellness. If performed as part of a more structured exercise routine, it is the component that provides the stimulus for adaptations and improved conditioning. The specific benefits from a workout depend on the type and intensity of activity that is performed (see the Concept on the health benefits of physical activity). Information about appropriate frequency, intensity, and length of time for different types of physical activities is included in subsequent Concepts (look for descriptions of the "physical activity pyramid").

A cool-down after the workout promotes an effective recovery from physical activity. After a vigorous workout a **cool-down** can pe performed to help the body transition back to a resting state. The cool-down can consist of light to moderate physical activity such as walking or slow jogging. Some may prefer to include stretching while the muscles are warm. The moderate aerobic activity promotes effective recovery by aiding the return of blood from the working muscles to the heart. In addition to helping reduce metabolic by-products, the general cool-down helps the cardiovascular system (heart rate and blood pressure) return to a normal state. The cool-down phase typically lasts for 5-10 minutes but may be longer if stretching exercises are included.

Figure 2 depicts how muscle contractions influence circulation and why it is important to perform a cool-down following vigorous activity. During physical 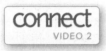 activity, the heart pumps a large amount of blood to supply the working muscles with the oxygen needed to keep moving. The muscles squeeze the veins, which forces the blood back to the heart. Valves in the veins prevent the blood from flowing backward. As long as exercise continues, muscles move the blood back to the heart, where it is once again pumped to the body. If exercise is stopped abruptly, the blood is left in the area of the working muscles and has no way to get back to the heart. In the case of a runner, the blood pools in the legs. Because the heart has less blood to pump, blood pressure may drop. This can result in dizziness and can even cause a person to pass out. The best way to prevent this problem is to slow down gradually after exercise and keep moving until blood pressure and heart rate have returned to near resting values. This phase is especially important for those with cardiovascular risk factors or disease.

Physical Activity in the Heat and Cold

Physical activity in hot and humid environments challenges the body's heat loss mechanisms. During vigorous activity, the body produces heat, which must be

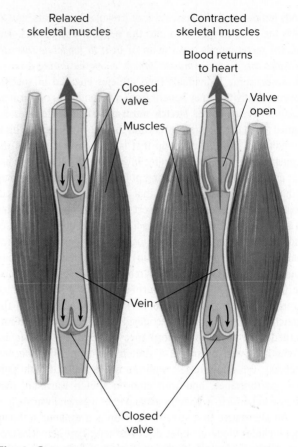

Figure 2 ▶ Muscle contractions help the veins return blood to the heart.

dissipated to regulate body temperature. The body has several ways to dissipate heat. *Conduction* is the transfer of heat from a hot body to a cold body. *Convection* is the transfer of heat through the air or any other medium. Fans and wind can facilitate heat loss by convection and help regulate temperature. The primary method of cooling is through *evaporation* of sweat. The chemical process involved in evaporation transfers heat from the body and reduces the body temperature. When conditions are humid, the effectiveness of evaporation is reduced, since the air is already saturated with moisture. This is why it is difficult to regulate body temperature when conditions are hot and humid.

Acclimatization improves the body's tolerance in the heat. Individuals with good fitness respond better to activity in the heat than individuals with poor fitness. However, with regular exposure, your body can adapt to tolerate heat more effectively. With adaptation, your body becomes conditioned to sweat earlier, to sweat more profusely, and to distribute the sweat more effectively around the body, and the composition of sweat is also altered. This process makes it easier for your body to maintain a safe body temperature. Gradually expose yourself to physical activity in hot and humid environments to facilitate acclimatization.

Table 3 ▶ Types of Heat-Related Problems

Problem	Symptoms	Severity
Heat cramps	Muscle cramps, especially in muscles most used in exercise	Least severe
Heat exhaustion	Muscle cramps, weakness, dizziness, headache, nausea, clammy skin, paleness	Moderately severe
Heatstroke	Hot, flushed skin; dry skin (lack of sweating); dizziness; fast pulse; unconsciousness; high temperature	Extremely severe

Heat-related illness can occur if proper hydration is not maintained. Maximum sweat rates during physical activity in the heat can approach 1–2 quarts per hour. If this fluid is not replaced, **dehydration** can occur. If dehydration is not corrected with water or other fluid-replacement drinks, it becomes increasingly difficult for the body to maintain normal body temperatures. At some point, the rate of sweating decreases as the body begins to conserve its remaining water. It shunts blood to the skin to transfer excess heat directly to the environment (conduction), but this is less effective than evaporation. **Hyperthermia** and associated heat-related problems can result (see Table 3).

Precautions should be taken when doing physical activity in hot and humid environments. The **heat index** (also referred to as apparent temperature) combines temperature and humidity to help you determine when an environment is safe for activity. The combination of high temperature and humidity presents the greatest risk of heat-related

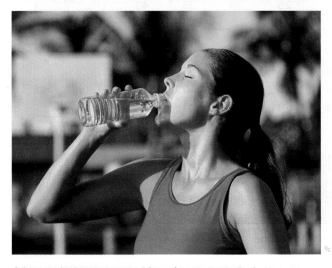

Adequate hydration is critical for safe exercise in the heat.
Liquidlibrary/PictureQuest

problems in exercise. Physical activity is safe when the apparent temperature is below 80°F (26.7°C). Figure 3 shows the risk of exercise at progressively higher apparent temperatures. Limit or cancel activity if the apparent temperature reaches the danger zone.

Physical activity in exceptionally cold and windy weather can be dangerous. Activity in the cold presents the opposite problems of exercise in the heat. In the cold, the primary goal is to retain the body's heat and avoid **hypothermia** and frostbite. Early signs of hypothermia include shivering and cold extremities caused by blood shunted to the body core to conserve heat. As the core temperature continues to drop, heart rate, respiration, and reflexes are depressed. Subsequently, cognitive functions decrease, speech and movement become impaired, and bizarre behavior may occur. Frostbite results from water crystallizing in the tissues, causing cell destruction.

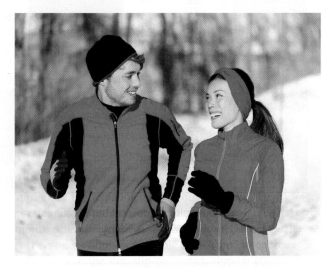

Wind, cold, and altitude present some additional challenges for winter exercise.
Mariclav/Getty Images

Workout The component of a total physical activity program designed to produce health, wellness, fitness, and other benefits using appropriate amounts of different types of physical activity.

Cool-Down Light to moderate activity performed after a more vigorous workout to help the body recover.

Dehydration Excessive loss of water from the body, usually through perspiration, urination, or evaporation.

Hyperthermia Excessively high body temperature caused by excessive heat production or impaired heat loss capacity. Heatstroke is a hyperthermic condition.

Heat Index An index based on a combination of temperature and humidity that is used to determine if it is dangerous to perform physical activity in hot, humid weather (also called apparent temperature).

Hypothermia Excessively low body temperature (less than 95°F), characterized by uncontrollable shivering, loss of coordination, and mental confusion.

Sunscreen should be applied 20–30 minutes before going outside and then reapplied every 2 hours and after swimming, sweating heavily, or using a towel. It is important to use sunscreen even on cloudy days as 80 percent of the sun's rays penetrate the clouds and reach the skin. This is the reason why people can become surprised with a sunburn after being outside on a cool, cloudy day. Using a quality sunscreen product is also important. Products that pass the test for protecting against both UVA and UVB rays can be called broad spectrum sunscreens. The designation of Sun Protection Factor (SPF) indicates how long a sunscreen will protect you from the more harmful UVA rays. A product with an SPF 15 indicates that you are exposed to the equivalent of 1 minute of UVB rays for each 15 minutes you spend in the sun. So, 1 hour in the sun wearing SPF 15 sunscreen is the same as spending 4 minutes totally unprotected. A sunscreen with an SPF of at least 15 (often labeled as broad spectrum) provides a base level of protection, but products with higher SPF numbers are generally recommended.

Preparing for Emergencies and Handling Injuries

Learning and practicing CPR skills can save someone's life. To be prepared for physical activity, you also need to be prepared for emergencies. Active people in particular should know cardiopulmonary resuscitation (CPR). Many people feel confused about CPR and worry that they may do something wrong; but evidence suggests that the simple steps can save people's lives. Guidelines from the American Heart Association (AHA) use the letters C-A-B to guide a rescuer to remember the three key steps in CPR (C = Compressions; A = Airway; B = Breathing). If a person is unresponsive, a trained rescuer should first call for help (including dialing 911) and then begin chest compression immediately (30 times at a rate of 100 times per minute). Then open the airway and give mouth-to-mouth rescue breaths (2 times). Repeat the 30-2 compression-to-breath cycle. If you aren't comfortable with the procedure, a "hands-only" approach (compression only) is still recommended. The availability of automated external defibrillators (AEDs) is increasingly common, but you still need to be prepared to use one (see the A Closer Look feature to review the steps for CPR).

Knowing the basic types of injuries can help in treatment and recovery. The most common injuries incurred in physical activity are strains and sprains. A strain refers to an injury to muscle fibers. For example, the hamstring muscle can be strained after a vigorous sprint if you are not prepared or conditioned. A sprain is an injury to ligaments, a connective tissue that connects bones to bones. A sprained ankle is a common injury that occurs when the ankle is rolled to the outside (inversion) after jumping or running. Other common sprains are to the knee, the shoulder, and the wrist. Although these basic distinctions can help you understand injuries, a physician should be consulted for an appropriate diagnosis.

Overuse injuries are also common among those who exercise regularly, a result of doing too much exercise or not providing sufficient time for the body to recover and adapt. These injuries often start as minor aches and pains but, if ignored, can turn into

 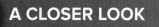
A CLOSER LOOK

AEDs

The availability of automated external defibrillators (AEDs) is increasingly common in public places and they have been shown to save lives. The use of new drone technology offers the potential to deploy AEDs to the scene of an emergency to increase access to this support. With this technology, a 911 dispatcher would be able to deploy a drone to the scene faster than other medical units could arrive and could even use a drone's camera to provide virtual assistance. Even with this support, knowing the basics of CPR and how to use an AED is still important. Visit the AHA website (www.cpr.heart.org) to take a closer look so that you are prepared. (See link in Suggested Resources and Readings.)

How confident are you that you would be ready in an emergency? What steps will you take (or have you taken) to be ready to perform CPR or use an AED if an emergency arises?

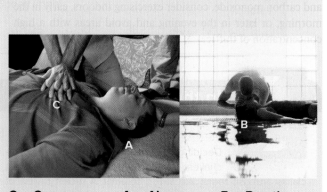

C = Compress
Push hard and fast in the center of the chest

A = Airway
Tip head back and lift the chin to open airway

B = Breath
Give mouth-to-mouth breaths

(left): Walter Lockwood/Photolibrary/Getty Images; (right): Steven Taylor/The Image Bank/Getty Images

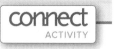

overuse injuries that may require rest and time off from physical activity. A common injury in runners is plantar fasciitis, an inflammation of the fibrous tissue (plantar fascia) that connects your heel bone to your toes. Another common running injury is a *shin splint,* which is associated with pain on the front of the shin. The key to preventing overuse injuries is to build up slowly and to allow time to recover between workouts. If you feel discomfort or pain during or following exercise sessions, skip a session to let your body recover.

Knowing how to treat minor injuries can help you reduce their negative effects. Most minor soft tissue injuries, such as muscle strains and ligamentous sprains, lead to rapid swelling and inflammation in the injured area. Although swelling is a normal part of the body's response, reducing the swelling is important for more effective recovery. The simple acronym *RICE* can help you remember a basic first aid strategy for minor injuries (see Table 4): *R* stands for *rest; I* stands for *ice*; *C* stands for *compression*; and *E* stands for *elevation*. There are different versions of this acronym, but the basic notion is to try to reduce swelling and inflammation.

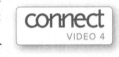

Some over-the-counter pain remedies can help reduce the pain of muscle strains and ligamentous sprains. There are important differences in their effects. For example, nonsteroidal anti-inflammatory drugs (NSAIDs) such as ibuprofen (e.g., Motrin, Advil) or naproxen (Aleve) have anti-inflammatory properties, but acetaminophen (e.g., Tylenol) does not. NSAIDs and acetaminophen also work differently to relieve pain. NSAIDs relieve pain by reducing the production of hormones called prostaglandins that cause pain, while acetaminophen works on the parts of the brain that receive the pain messages.

Understanding soreness can help you persist in physical activity and avoid problems. A common experience for many exercisers is a certain degree of muscle soreness that begins 12-24 hours after an intense workout and peaks 2-3 days later. This soreness, termed *delayed-onset*

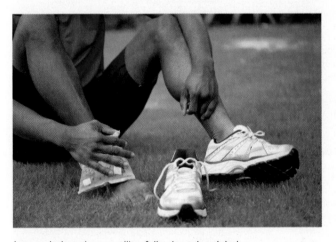

Ice can help reduce swelling following minor injuries.
Science Photo Library/Getty Images

Table 4 ▶ The RICE Formula for Treating Minor Injuries	
RICE Components	**Application of Components**
Rest	For a day or two, rest helps you avoid further damage to the tissues. During this period, it is important to *protect* the injured body part using crutches and stabilizing devices (e.g., ankle brace). After a day or two, passive movement can begin to help retain (or prevent loss of) range of motion. This can be followed by light exercise over the next few days as appropriate (*optimal loading*). Gradually increasing the load can speed recovery.
Ice	The quick application of cold (ice or ice water) to a minor injury minimizes swelling and speeds recovery. Cold should be applied to as large a surface area as possible (soaking is best). If ice is used, it should be wrapped to avoid direct contact with the skin. Apply cold for 20 minutes, three times a day, allowing 1 hour between applications.
Compression	Wrapping or compressing the injured area also helps minimize swelling and speeds recovery. Elastic bandages or elastic socks are good for applying compression. Care should be taken to avoid wrapping an injury too tightly because this can result in loss of circulation to the area.
Elevation	Keeping the injured area elevated (above the level of the heart) is effective in minimizing swelling. If pain or swelling does not diminish after 24–48 hours, or if there is any doubt about the seriousness of an injury, seek medical help.

muscle soreness (DOMS), typically occurs anytime you push your limits or begin a new exercise. DOMS is caused by microscopic muscle tears that result from the excessive loads on the muscles. Some people mistakenly believe that lactic acid is the cause of muscle soreness. Lactic acid (a by-product of anaerobic metabolism) is produced during vigorous exercise, but levels return to normal within 30 minutes after exercise, while the onset of DOMS is much later. DOMS can affect people in all stages of fitness, from beginners to elite athletes, and relates to the principle of progression. You can minimize the risk of DOMS by making more gradual increments in the volume and intensity of activity and by including a dynamic warm-up and low-intensity cool-down in your routine. With incremental training, your body will adapt and you will find that the same exercise bout no longer makes you sore.

While it may be uncomfortable to some, there are no long-term consequences of DOMS and it does not predispose one to muscle injury. While you are waiting for your body to heal (usually 2–3 days), it is a good idea to participate in some form of gentle movement and avoid further high-intensity activities. Research findings are mixed on treatment recommendations for DOMS. There is some indication that massage, warm or cool baths, or topical analgesics may ease the stiffness and pain. While DOMS does not typically require medical attention, according to the ACSM you should seek medical attention if it persists more than 7 days, your urine becomes abnormally dark, or you have swelling in your arms or legs.

Muscle cramps can be relieved by statically stretching a muscle. Muscle cramps are pains in the large muscles that result when the muscles contract vigorously for a continued period of time. Muscle cramps are usually not considered to be an injury, but they are painful and may seem like an injury. They are usually short in duration and can often be relieved with proper treatment. Cramps can result from lack of fluid replacement (dehydration), from fatigue, and from a blow directly to a muscle. Static stretching can help relieve some cramps. For example, the calf muscle, which often cramps among runners and other sports participants, can be relieved using the calf stretcher exercise, which is part of the warm-up in this Concept.

Using Self-Management Skills

Building knowledge is important for making informed decisions about physical activity. The choices you make can influence the risk of injuries and adverse events during physical activity. Wear reflective clothing and lights when doing outdoor activities in the early morning or evenings to increase visibility. Use recommended safety equipment and follow guidelines for exercising in extremes of heat and cold, paying particular attention to hydration status. Following principles of progression and getting sufficient rest between workouts is also important for reducing risks of injuries. By adopting a long-term perspective with physical activity, your body will adapt and your fitness level will improve.

Balancing attitudes can help you get started and stick with a physical activity program. Active people generally have more positive attitudes than negative ones. This is referred to as a "positive balance of attitudes." Practicing self-management skills can help you develop more positive attitudes and limit the impact of negative attitudes. The first step in changing attitudes is becoming aware of your personal attitudes toward physical activity, both positive and negative (See Tables 5 and 6). Awareness of

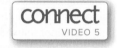

Table 5 ▶ Negative Attitudes about Physical Activity		
Negative Attitudes	**Importance for Physical Activity Behavior**	**Application Strategies**
I don't have the time.	Time is a convenient excuse but lifestyle decisions are a matter of priorities.	Planning a daily schedule can help you find the time for activity and avoid wasting time on things that are less important.
I find it to be inconvenient.	Some people might focus on the burden instead of the benefit (e.g., "It takes too long to get to the gym"; "It makes me sweaty and messes up my hair").	Finding ways to build activity into your schedule can help. Moderate activity can be done without getting too hot or sweaty.
I just don't enjoy it.	Some people do not find activity to be enjoyable or invigorating. They may assume that it has to be strenuous and fatiguing.	There are many activities to choose from. If you don't enjoy vigorous activity, try more moderate forms of activity, such as walking.
I am not good at physical activity.	Some people are self-conscious and worry about being judged (e.g., "People might laugh at me," "Sports make me nervous").	Selecting activities properly, avoiding comparisons to others, and learning skills can help anyone be more active.
I am not fit enough to do it.	Some people avoid exercise because of health reasons or because they lack the energy or fitness to do it.	Moderate activity can be safe for most people, and fitness can improve if you build up gradually.
I have no place to be active.	Some people lack access to facilities or find it hard to stay active in bad weather.	Many popular activities don't require equipment. Finding ways to be active at home can also help.
I am too old.	Some people begin to feel that activity is something they cannot do as they get older.	Everyone can benefit from properly planned activity. Older people who are just beginning activity should start slowly and set realistic goals to get started.

Table 6 ▶ Positive Attitudes about Physical Activity

Positive Attitudes	Importance for Physical Activity Behavior	Application Strategies
I simply enjoy being active.	The sense of fun, well-being, and general enjoyment associated with physical activity is well documented.	Find activities that you enjoy. Many people find walking to be a simple and enjoyable activity because it doesn't require skill.
I value how it enhances my health.	Improving health is a primary reason for many people, and it takes only moderate amounts to benefit.	Learning about the powerful benefits of fitness can provide motivation to start.
I want to look my best.	Improving appearance is a major reason some people participate in regular exercise. Regular activity can help you look your best.	Activity can help with weight control but set realistic goals and avoiding comparisons with others.
I like how I feel after I am active.	Physical activity provides an outlet from daily frustrations and can help reduce depression and anxiety.	Build in time to take short activity breaks and allow your mind to be freed up from daily hassles while you are active.
I like to challenge myself.	The engaging challenges can build a sense of personal accomplishment. This is a powerful motivator for physical activity.	Seek opportunities to learn new skills and try new things. Reward yourself for accepting challenges and for trying.
I like the social benefits it provides.	Physical activity provides opportunities to spend quality time with friends and family.	Find ways to be active with family and friends. Select partner or team activities that deemphasize competition.
I find it fun to compete against others.	Many people find "the thrill of victory" and "sports competition" very satisfying.	If you don't enjoy the "competing" aspect, focus on how you are improving versus winning or losing.
I find it helps me feel good about myself.	Participation in physical activity can be an important part of your identity. It can help you feel good about yourself, build your confidence, and increase self-esteem.	Physical activity is something that is self-determined and within your control. Schedule activity just as you would any important priority to accomplish during the week.
I value time to enjoy the outdoors.	Spending time outside and experiencing nature pair well with many physical activities.	Seek out parks, bike and walking trails, and other outdoor settings for your activities.

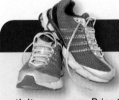

Strategies for Action: Lab Information

Pre-participation screening can help you safely participate in a physical activity program. Prior to participation, the use of the PAR-Q+ is recommended. In Lab 4A, answer the seven questions in the Par-Q+ to see if you are ready for participation. If you answer "yes" to any of the seven questions, you should follow up as indicated. Athletes and people who plan very vigorous training may require additional screening.

A proper warm-up can prepare your body for activity and a gradual cool-down can improve recovery. Lab 4B provides examples of dynamic exercises and stretching exercises that can

be considered when performing a warm-up. You can try these exercises and use the warm-up guidelines presented in the previous pages of this Concept to determine what works best for your needs.

Assessing your attitudes concerning physical activity can help you change them. Active people generally have more positive attitudes than negative ones. This is referred to as a "positive balance of attitudes." The questionnaire in Lab 4C gives you the opportunity to assess your balance of attitudes. If you have a "negative balance" score, you can analyze your attitudes and determine how you can change them to view activity more favorably.

connect
ACTIVITY

your attitudes can help you capitalize on strengths while minimizing known barriers or challenges.

- *Knowing the most common negative attitudes can help you avoid them.* Most people want to be active but negative attitudes can get in the way of regular physical activity adherence. The most common negative attitudes (excuses) for avoiding regular physical activity are listed in Table 5. Experts consider many of these attitudes to be barriers that can be overcome. Use the self-management strategies in Table 5 to overcome negative attitudes and limit excuses for being inactive.

- *Knowing the most common positive attitudes can motivate you to adopt them.* Just as there are negative attitudes that limit activity, there are positive attitudes that encourage it. The most common reasons people give for being physically active are highlighted in Table 6. Use the application strategies to develop positive attitudes that can help you stay active.

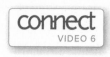

VIDEO 6

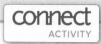

ACTIVITY

HELP   Health is available to Everyone for a Lifetime, and it's Personal

Forming Physical Activity Habits

To establish habits for physical activity, it is critical to find intrinsic reasons for doing it, such as alleviating stress, rather than solely for extrinsic rewards, such as weight loss. A habit doesn't require doing something at the same time or have a specific routine, but it does imply that it is somewhat automatic for you. If exercise is not a habit, the act of doing it becomes effortful, and extrinsic motives will likely not be enough to keep you doing it. Developing an intrinsic reward system takes time and experience, but it helps to gradually identify the personal reasons why you value it. You may not love exercise when you first start, but it can become more habitual and part of your lifestyle.

Do you have intrinsic reasons for being physically active? What strategies can you use to make physical activity more of a habit?

Suggested Resources and Readings

The websites for the following sources can be accessed by searching online for the organization, program, or title listed. Specific scientific references are available at the end of this edition of *Concepts of Fitness and Wellness.*

- AirNow. Air Quality Index (AQI).
- American Cancer Society. Be Safe in the Sun.
- American College of Sports Medicine. ACSM Position Stands:
  - Exertional Heat Illness During Training and Competition
  - Exercise and Fluid Replacement
  - Prevention of Cold Injuries During Exercise

- American Heart Association. Online First Aid CPR AED Course Options.
- Environmental Working Group (EWG). Guide to Sunscreens.
- Miller, R. (2019, May 23). "State of Sunscreen: Lotions Lacking." *USA Today.*
- PAR-Q+ Collaboration. Physical Activity Readiness Questionnaire for Everyone (PAR-Q+) and Medical Examination (ePARmed-X+).
- WebMD. Understanding Heat-Related Illness—Symptoms.

Lab 4A Readiness for Physical Activity

Name	Section	Date

Purpose: To help you determine your physical readiness for physical activity.

Procedures

1. Read the entire PAR-Q+ that follows.
2. After reading the PAR-Q+, answer the seven questions in the area bordered by the black box.
3. Record the number of "yes" answers in the Results section.
4. Discuss your medical readiness in the Conclusions and Implications section.

Results

Determine your PAR-Q+ score. Place an X over the circle that includes the number of "yes" answers that you had for the PAR-Q+.

(0) (1) (2) (3) (4) (5) (6) (7)

1. If you answered "no" to all seven questions, you are cleared for physical activity.
2. Follow the guidelines in the second section (inside the green border) of the PAR-Q+ before beginning physical activity.
3. If you answered "yes" to any of the questions, go to http://eparmedx.com to answer follow-up questions about medical conditions (pages 2 and 3 of the questionnaire) and inform your instructor of any limitations. If you have a temporary illness, are pregnant, or if your health changes delay activity (see information inside the yellow border at the bottom of the form).
4. If you plan to participate in physical activity at a fitness center or a health club, you may be asked to sign a separate declaration such as the one shown in the green area or on page 4 of the full PAR-Q+ form (see http://eparmedx.com).

Conclusions and Implications: In several sentences, discuss your readiness for physical activity. Base your comments on your questionnaire results and the types of physical activities you plan to perform in the future.

2020 PAR-Q+

The Physical Activity Readiness Questionnaire for Everyone

The health benefits of regular physical activity are clear; more people should engage in physical activity every day of the week. Participating in physical activity is very safe for MOST people. This questionnaire will tell you whether it is necessary for you to seek further advice from your doctor OR a qualified exercise professional before becoming more physically active.

GENERAL HEALTH QUESTIONS

Please read the 7 questions below carefully and answer each one honestly: check YES or NO.	YES	NO
1) Has your doctor ever said that you have a heart condition ☐ OR high blood pressure ☐?	☐	☐
2) Do you feel pain in your chest at rest, during your daily activities of living, **OR** when you do physical activity?	☐	☐
3) Do you lose balance because of dizziness **OR** have you lost consciousness in the last 12 months? Please answer **NO** if your dizziness was associated with over-breathing (including during vigorous exercise).	☐	☐
4) Have you ever been diagnosed with another chronic medical condition (other than heart disease or high blood pressure)? **PLEASE LIST CONDITION(S) HERE:** _____	☐	☐
5) Are you currently taking prescribed medications for a chronic medical condition? **PLEASE LIST CONDITION(S) AND MEDICATIONS HERE:** _____	☐	☐
6) Do you currently have (or have had within the past 12 months) a bone, joint, or soft tissue (muscle, ligament, or tendon) problem that could be made worse by becoming more physically active? Please answer **NO** if you had a problem in the past, but it *does not limit your current ability* to be physically active. **PLEASE LIST CONDITION(S) HERE:** _____	☐	☐
7) Has your doctor ever said that you should only do medically supervised physical activity?	☐	☐

☑ **If you answered NO to all of the questions above, you are cleared for physical activity.**
Please sign the PARTICIPANT DECLARATION. You do not need to complete Pages 2 and 3.

- ▶ Start becoming much more physically active – start slowly and build up gradually.
- ▶ Follow Global Physical Activity Guidelines for your age (https://apps.who.int/iris/handle/10665/44399).
- ▶ You may take part in a health and fitness appraisal.
- ▶ If you are over the age of 45 yr and NOT accustomed to regular vigorous to maximal effort exercise, consult a qualified exercise professional before engaging in this intensity of exercise.
- ▶ If you have any further questions, contact a qualified exercise professional.

PARTICIPANT DECLARATION
If you are less than the legal age required for consent or require the assent of a care provider, your parent, guardian or care provider must also sign this form.

I, the undersigned, have read, understood to my full satisfaction and completed this questionnaire. I acknowledge that this physical activity clearance is valid for a maximum of 12 months from the date it is completed and becomes invalid if my condition changes. I also acknowledge that the community/fitness centre may retain a copy of this form for its records. In these instances, it will maintain the confidentiality of the same, complying with applicable law.

NAME _____ DATE _____

SIGNATURE _____ WITNESS _____

SIGNATURE OF PARENT/GUARDIAN/CARE PROVIDER _____

🛑 **If you answered YES to one or more of the questions above, COMPLETE PAGES 2 AND 3.**

⚠️ **Delay becoming more active if:**

- ✓ You have a temporary illness such as a cold or fever; it is best to wait until you feel better.
- ✓ You are pregnant - talk to your health care practitioner, your physician, a qualified exercise professional, and/or complete the ePARmed-X+ at **http://eparmedx.com** before becoming more physically active.
- ✓ Your health changes - answer the questions on Pages 2 and 3 of this document and/or talk to your doctor or a qualified exercise professional before continuing with any physical activity program.

Copyright © 2020 PAR-Q+

01-11-2017

Note: It is important that you answer all questions honestly. The PAR-Q+ is a scientifically and medically researched pre-exercise selection device. It complements exercise programs, exercise testing procedures, and the liability considerations attendant with such programs and testing procedures. PAR-Q+, like any other pre-exercise screening device, will misclassify a small percentage of prospective participants, but no pre-exercise screening method can entirely avoid this problem.

Lab 4B The Warm-Up

Name	**Section**	**Date**

Purpose: To familiarize you with possible warm-up and cool-down exercises.

Procedures

1. Consider the specific type of workout you are planning to perform and place a check in the Results section (e.g., moderate activity, vigorous activity). When completed, place a check in the box in the Results section that corresponds to your planned workout.
2. Perform a general cardiovascular warm-up.
3. Perform each of the exercises in Chart 1. Perform dynamic exercises several times. Perform stretching exercises three times for 15–30 seconds each.
4. After you perform the specific warm-up exercises, place a check beside the warm-up exercises that you think you would most likely include in your personal warm-up for the workout you checked (See Table 2 for details).
5. Answer the question in the Conclusions and Implications section.

Results

Type of Workout (check one):

☐ Moderate Activity

☐ Vigorous Activity

☐ Vigorous Anaerobics and Sports

☐ Muscle Fitness Exercise

☐ Activities Requiring Flexibility

Warm-Up Exercises (check those that you would include in your warm-up):

Dynamic Warm-Up

☐ Grapevine

☐ Knee stride and reach

☐ High skip and reach

☐ Inchworm

☐ Backward jog

Stretch Warm-Up

☐ Calf stretch

☐ Hamstring stretch

☐ Seated side stretch

☐ Leg hug

Conclusions and Implications: In several sentences, explain the reasons for your selections.

Chart 1 The Warm-Up

Lab 4B

The Warm-Up

Dynamic Exercises. If you choose a dynamic exercise warm-up, perform the five exercises below and/or exercises from the Basic 8 for Calisthenics in the Concept on muscle fitness.

Grapevine

With feet at shoulder width and arms out at shoulder height, move sideways. With right leg, step across left leg, then step to left with left leg, right leg step behind left leg, step left leg to left. Repeat in the opposite direction, starting with left leg. Repeat several times.

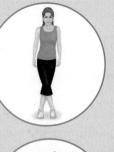

Inchworm

From push-up position, walk the feet toward the hands several steps, keeping the hands still. Then walk the hands forward keeping the feet still. Repeat several times.

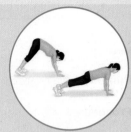

Knee Stride and Reach

Take a long stride forward with the right leg, touch the left knee to the floor. Reach up with both arms as you stride. Stand and repeat with left stride and right knee touch. Repeat 10–20 times.

Backward Jog

Jog backward slowly using moderately long steps. Pump your arms back and forth. Cover a distance of 10 yards, turn around, and backward jog in opposite direction. Repeat several times.

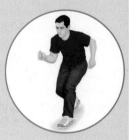

High Skip and Reach

Do a slow high skip. Alternate swinging one arm up and high above the head. Right arm up when on the right foot; left arm up when on the left foot. Repeat 10–20 times.

When performing a dynamic warm-up in the future you may want to consider the exercises from the Basic 8 for Calisthenics in the Concept on muscle fitness, as well as the exercises here.

Stretching Exercises. If you choose to do a stretch warm-up, perform the four stretching exercises below and/or other stretching exercises from the Concept on flexibility. Perform each stretch for at least 15–30 seconds.

Calf Stretch

This exercise stretches the calf muscles (gastrocnemius and soleus). Face a wall with your feet 2–3 feet away. Step forward on your left foot to allow both hands to touch the wall. Keep the heel of your right foot on the ground, toe turned in slightly, knee straight, and buttocks tucked in. Lean forward by bending your front knee and arms and allowing your head to move nearer the wall. Hold. Repeat with the other leg.

Seated Side Stretch

This exercise stretches the muscles of the trunk. Begin in a seated position with the legs crossed. Stretch the left arm over the head to the right. Bend at the waist (to right), reaching as far as possible to the left with the right arm. Hold. Do not let the trunk rotate. Repeat to the opposite side. This exercise can be done in the standing position but is less effective.

Hamstring Stretch

This exercise stretches the muscles of the back of the upper leg (hamstrings) as well as those of the hip, knee, and ankle. Lie on your back. Bring the right knee to your chest and grasp the toes with the right hand. Place the left hand on the back of the right thigh. Pull the knee toward the chest, push the heel toward the ceiling, and pull the toes toward the shin. Attempt to straighten the knee. Stretch and hold. Repeat with the other leg.

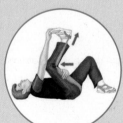

Leg Hug

This exercise stretches the hip and back extensor muscles. Lie on your back. Bend one leg and grasp your thigh under the knee. Hug it to your chest. Keep the other leg straight and on the floor. Hold. Repeat with the opposite leg.

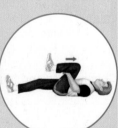

When performing a stretch warm-up in the future, consider the four stretching exercises above and/or other stretching exercises from the Concept on flexibility.

Lab 4C Physical Activity Attitude Questionnaire

Name	Section	Date

Purpose: To evaluate your feelings about physical activity and to determine the specific reasons you do or do not participate in regular physical activity.

Directions: The term *physical activity* in the following statements refers to all kinds of activities, including sports, formal exercises, and informal activities such as jogging and cycling. Make an X over the circle that best represents your answer to each question.

	Strongly Disagree	Disagree	Undecided	Agree	Strongly Agree	Item Score	Attitude Score
1. I should do physical activity regularly for my health.	1	2	3	4	5		Health and Fitness Score
2. Doing regular physical activity is good for my fitness and wellness.	1	2	3	4	5	+ =	
3. Regular exercise helps me look my best.	1	2	3	4	5		Appearance Score
4. I feel more physically attractive when I do regular physical activity.	1	2	3	4	5	+ =	
5. One of the main reasons I do regular physical activity is that it is fun.	1	2	3	4	5		Enjoyment Score
6. The most enjoyable part of my day is when I am exercising or doing a sport.	1	2	3	4	5	+ =	
7. Taking part in physical activity helps me relax.	1	2	3	4	5		Relaxation Score
8. Physical activity helps me get away from the pressures of daily living.	1	2	3	4	5	+ =	
9. The challenge of physical training is one reason I do physical activity.	1	2	3	4	5		Challenge Score
10. I like to see if I can master sports and activities that are new to me.	1	2	3	4	5	+ =	
11. I like to do physical activity that involves other people.	1	2	3	4	5		Social Score
12. Exercise offers me the opportunity to meet other people.	1	2	3	4	5	+ =	
13. Competition is a good way to make physical activity fun.	1	2	3	4	5		Competition Score
14. I like to see how my physical abilities compare with those of others.	1	2	3	4	5	+ =	
15. When I do regular exercise, I feel better than when I don't.	1	2	3	4	5		Feeling Good Score
16. My ability to do physical activity is something that makes me proud.	1	2	3	4	5	+ =	
17. I like to do outdoor activities.	1	2	3	4	5		Outdoor Score
18. Experiencing nature is something I look forward to when exercising.	1	2	3	4	5	+ =	

Procedures

1. Read and answer each question in the questionnaire.
2. Write the number in the circle of your answer in the box labeled "Item Score."
3. Add scores for each pair of scores and record in the "Attitude Score" box.
4. Record each attitude score and a rating for each score (use Rating Chart) in the following chart.
5. Record the number of good and excellent scores in the box provided. Use the score in the box to determine your rating using the Balance of Attitudes Rating Chart.

Results: Record your results as indicated in the Procedures section.

Physical Activity Attitude Questionnaire Results

Attitude	Score	Rating
Health and fitness		
Appearance		
Enjoyment		
Relaxation		
Challenge		
Social		
Competition		
Feeling good		
Outdoor		

How many good or excellent scores do you have?

Balance of Feeling Score

Having 5 or more in the box above indicates that you have a positive balance of attitudes (more positive than negative attitudes).

Attitude Rating Chart

Rating Category	Attitude Score
Excellent	9–10
Good	7–8
Fair	5–6
Poor	3–4
Very poor	2

Balance of Attitudes Rating Chart

Excellent	6–9
Good	5
Fair	4
Poor	2–3
Very poor	0–1

In a few sentences, discuss your "balance of attitudes" rating. Having more positive than negative scores (positive balance of attitudes) increases the probability of being active. Include comments on whether you think your ratings suggest that you will be active or inactive and whether your ratings are really indicative of your attitudes. Do you think that the scores on which you were rated poor or very poor might be reasons you would avoid physical activity? Explain.

The Health Benefits of Physical Activity

LEARNING OBJECTIVES

After completing the study of this Concept, you will be able to:

▶ Define the term *hypokinetic* and explain how physical activity can reduce risk of hypokinetic diseases and conditions.

▶ Identify several cardiovascular diseases/conditions associated with physical inactivity and explain how physical activity can help reduce risk.

▶ Describe metabolic syndrome and explain how physical activity can help reduce risk of this hypokinetic condition.

▶ Explain how physical activity can help reduce risk of other hypokinetic conditions.

▶ Explain the role of physical activity in preventing conditions associated with aging.

▶ Explain the role of physical activity in promoting optimal wellness.

▶ Present an overview of the health and wellness benefits of physical activity and fitness.

▶ Identify related national health goals and show how meeting personal goals can contribute to reaching national goals.

▶ Assess your heart disease risk factors.

Physical activity and good physical fitness can reduce the risk of illness and contribute to optimal health, wellness, and fitness.

JoseGirarte/E+/Getty Images

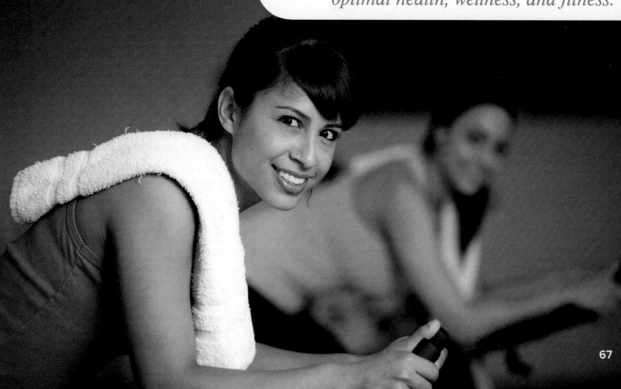

Why It Matters!

The overarching goal of the *Healthy People 2030* national health objectives is to help all people have high-quality, longer lives free of preventable disease, injury, and premature death. You can personally achieve these goals by committing to being physically active your entire life. Physical activity improves physical fitness and contributes to high-quality life (wellness, the positive component of good health). Regular physical activity also contributes to a longer life (lifespan) free of preventable disease and injury (healthspan). Physical activity is certainly not a panacea for all health issues, but it is likely the most important thing you can do to achieve good health, wellness, and fitness. This Concept will reinforce the importance of these tangible benefits associated with a physically active lifestyle.

"Physical fitness is not only one of the most important keys to a healthy body; it is the basis of dynamic and creative intellectual activity. The relationship between the soundness of the body and the activities of the mind is subtle and complex. Much is not yet understood. But we do know what the Greeks knew: that intelligence and skill can only function at the peak of their capacity when the body is healthy and strong; that hardy spirits and tough minds usually inhabit sound bodies."

—**President John F. Kennedy, "The Soft American,"**
***Sports Illustrated*, 1960**

Physical Activity Promotes Health, Wellness, and Fitness

Physical activity enhances many body systems. The human body is amazing for many reasons, but a unique feature is that it gets better with use! The body is designed for movement and adapts by making exercise easier on various body systems. Adaptations are summarized here and are depicted conceptually in the blue boxes in Figure 1.

- *Cardiorespiratory System:* The circulatory and respiratory systems work together to distribute oxygen throughout the body. The heart gets stronger with use and the improved oxygen carrying capacity of the system improves performance and work efficiency. The adaptations also reduce risks for various cardiovascular diseases.

- *Musculoskeletal System:* The muscular and skeletal systems work together to enable our bodies to move. With regular activity, muscles, bones, and associated tissues adapt to work more effectively and efficiently. Muscles and bones both get stronger with use and the adaptations contribute to improved sports performance, reduced risks of injury, and improved mobility in older adults.

- *Metabolic System:* The digestive and endocrine systems work together to help our bodies convert food into energy and maintain a healthy body composition. Improvements in lipid profiles and glucose control contribute to enhanced metabolic fitness and reduced risk for diabetes and many chronic diseases.

- *Immune System:* The immune system helps the body fight off infection and improves recovery from illness (as evidenced by the differential susceptibility to COVID-19 for fit versus unfit individuals). Physical activity contributes to healthier body systems and reductions in many forms of cancer.

- *Nervous System:* The brain and nervous system link our mind and body. As emphasized in the quote by President Kennedy, "Hardy spirits and tough minds usually inhabit sound bodies." Physical activity improves many aspects of brain and nervous functions and directly contributes to mental health and reduced risks of mental illness.

Physical activity contributes to good physical fitness. Physical activity is a behavior (something that you do) while physical fitness is something that you have. The specific gains in health-related physical fitness (cardiorespiratory endurance, muscular endurance, strength, power, flexibility, and body composition) depend on the type and amount of physical activity performed. If you do the process (regular physical activity), the product (physical fitness) follows! Guidelines are provided in separate Concepts, but the generalized benefits of improved fitness are summarized below (see green boxes in Figure 1).

- *Enjoying Leisure:* Good physical fitness enhances the quality of leisure time. Active forms of recreation also provide opportunities to socialize and interact with others. Enjoying your leisure time may not add years to your life, but it can add life to your years.

- *Functioning Effectively:* Good physical fitness helps you function more effectively in your daily tasks. Although the need for each component of physical fitness is specific to each individual, every person requires enough fitness to perform normal daily activities without undue fatigue. Whether it be walking, performing household chores, or merely enjoying the simple things in life without pain or fear of injury, good fitness is important to all people.

- *Working Efficiently:* Good physical fitness can help an individual work more efficiently. A person who can resist fatigue, muscle soreness, back problems, and other symptoms associated with poor health-related fitness is capable of working productively and still has energy at the end of the day.

- *Handling Emergencies:* Unexpected emergencies often demand performance that requires good fitness. For example, flood victims may need to fill sandbags for hours without rest, and accident victims may be required to walk or run long distances for help.

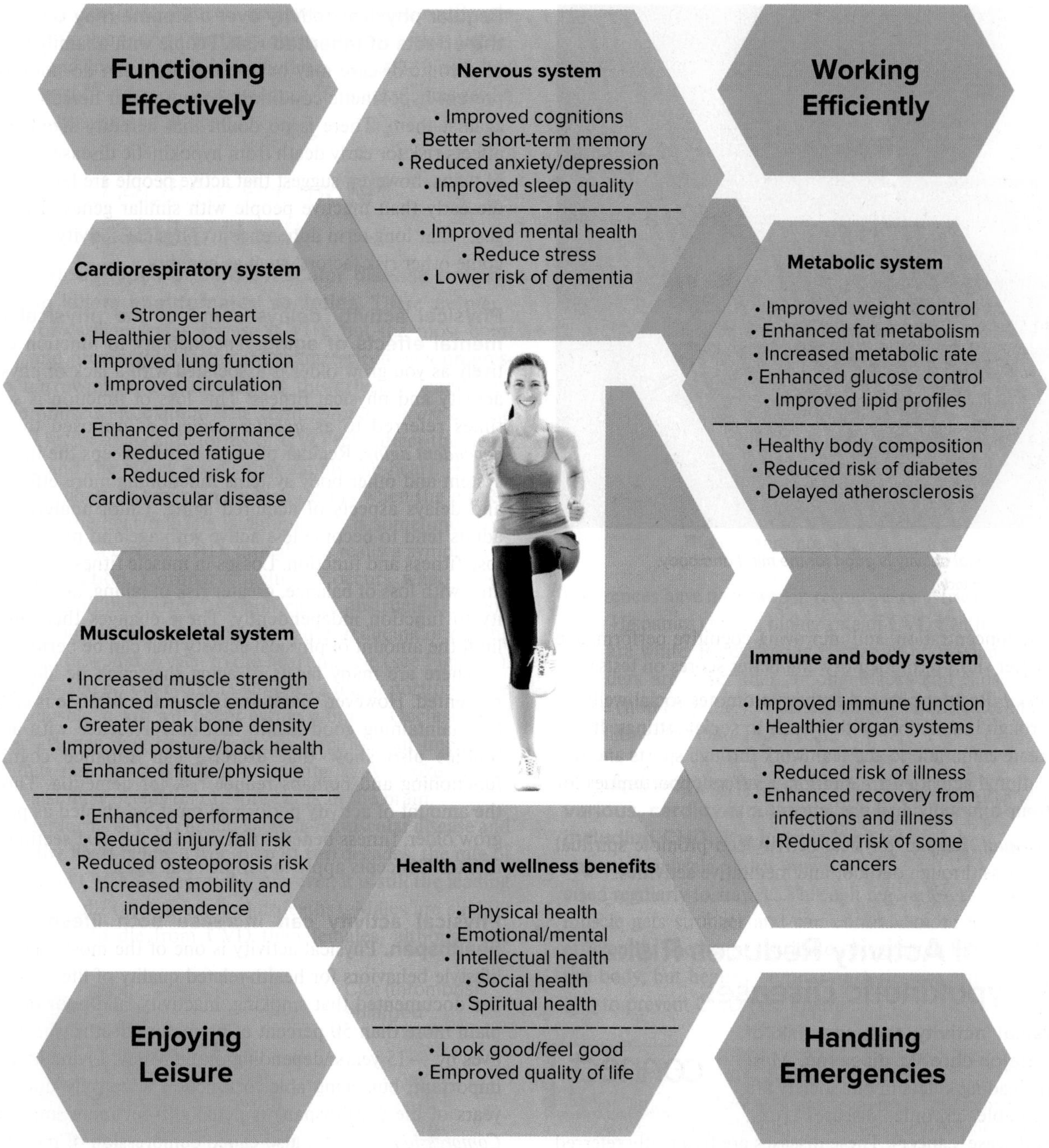

Functioning Effectively

Nervous system

- Improved cognitions
- Better short-term memory
- Reduced anxiety/depression
- Improved sleep quality

- Improved mental health
- Reduce stress
- Lower risk of dementia

Working Efficiently

Cardiorespiratory system

- Stronger heart
- Healthier blood vessels
- Improved lung function
- Improved circulation

- Enhanced performance
- Reduced fatigue
- Reduced risk for cardiovascular disease

Metabolic system

- Improved weight control
- Enhanced fat metabolism
- Increased metabolic rate
- Enhanced glucose control
- Improved lipid profiles

- Healthy body composition
- Reduced risk of diabetes
- Delayed atherosclerosis

Musculoskeletal system

- Increased muscle strength
- Enhanced muscle endurance
- Greater peak bone density
- Improved posture/back health
- Enhanced fiture/physique

- Enhanced performance
- Reduced injury/fall risk
- Reduced osteoporosis risk
- Increased mobility and independence

Immune and body system

- Improved immune function
- Healthier organ systems

- Reduced risk of illness
- Enhanced recovery from infections and illness
- Reduced risk of some cancers

Health and wellness benefits

- Physical health
- Emotional/mental
- Intellectual health
- Social health
- Spiritual health

- Look good/feel good
- Emproved quality of life

Enjoying Leisure

Handling Emergencies

Figure 1 ▶ Health, wellness, and fitness benefits of physical activity.

(photo): Neustockimages/Getty Images

Physical activity contributes to optimal wellness. As mentioned in previous Concepts, wellness is considered to be the positive dimension of health. Regular physical activity promotes a high quality of life by contributing to each of the five dimensions of health and wellness (see orange box in Figure 1).

- *Physical:* Regular physical activity enhances physical wellness by promoting good physical fitness (see previous section). Active people are less likely to miss work or

school. Good fitness from regular physical activity helps you look your best.

- *Emotional/Mental:* Regular physical activity promotes emotional/mental wellness as evidenced by positive mood states, reduced anxiety and depression, improved self-concept, and greater independence.

- *Intellectual:* Regular physical activity fosters intellectual wellness by stimulating new brain cell development, enhancing higher-order brain functions such as attention

The importance of exercise for heart health and reducing risks of cardiovascular disease is well established. The American Heart Association (AHA) recognizes physical inactivity as one of the five modifiable risk factors for CHD along with smoking, high blood cholesterol, hypertension, and overweight/obesity. Risks of CHD are higher in males and increase with age, but adopting healthy lifestyles and managing hereditary risks can greatly reduce overall risks. Since practicing healthy eating habits and avoiding diabetes are also central for cardiovascular health, the AHA developed Life's Simple 7, which targets smoking, inactivity, poor nutrition, overweight/obesity, high blood cholesterol, high blood pressure, and high blood sugar.

Campaigns such as Life's Simple 7 (and the associated My Life Check assessment) are designed to promote awareness of CHD risks and contribute to reducing health-care costs in society (see Technology Update). The CDC indicates that eliminating the three risk factors of smoking, inactivity, and poor eating could prevent 80 percent of heart disease and stroke, 80 percent of Type 2 diabetes, and 40 percent of cancer cases. The economic costs of CHD are high. In fact, one of every six dollars spent on health care goes to CHD treatment. While physical activity has independent benefits for cardiovascular health, it also directly addresses and reverses some of the other risk factors. These are described in the next two sections.

Physical Activity Improves Lipid Profiles to Improve Cardiovascular Health

Atherosclerosis, which begins early in life, is implicated in many cardiovascular diseases. Atherosclerosis is a condition that contributes to heart attack, hypertension, stroke and peripheral vascular disease. Deposits on the walls of arteries restrict blood flow and oxygen supply to the tissues. **Arteriosclerosis** refers to the hardening of the plaque, which further impairs circulation. Atherosclerosis can precipitate heart attacks and strokes because a fibrous clot is more likely to obstruct a narrowed artery than a healthy, open one.

Current theory suggests that atherosclerosis begins when damage occurs to the cells of the inner wall, or endothelium, of the artery (see Figure 4). Substances associated with blood clotting are attracted to the damaged area. These substances seem to cause the migration of smooth muscle cells, commonly found only in the middle wall of the artery (media), to the endothelium. In the later stages, fats and other substances form plaques, or protrusions, that progressively diminish the internal diameter of the artery.

Physical activity can help prevent atherosclerosis by lowering blood lipid levels. While physical activity directly reduces risks of heart attack and stroke, it also improves lipid profiles. There are several kinds of **lipids** (fats) in the bloodstream, including **lipoproteins**, phospholipids, triglycerides, and cholesterol. Cholesterol is the most well known, but it is not the only culprit. Many blood fats are manufactured by the body itself, whereas others are ingested in high-fat foods, particularly saturated fats (fats that are solid at room temperature).

As noted earlier, blood lipids are thought to contribute to the development of atherosclerotic deposits on the inner walls of the artery. One substance, called **low-density lipoprotein (LDL)**, is a major contributor to the development of atherosclerosis. LDL is basically a core of cholesterol surrounded by protein and another substance that makes it water soluble. The benefit of regular exercise is that it can reduce blood lipid levels, including LDL-C (the cholesterol core of LDL). People with high total cholesterol and LDL levels

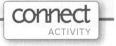

Technology Update

My Life Check: A Tool to Evaluate Your Heart Health

While the risk factors for cardiovascular disease are well established, many people still struggle to make the needed changes to improve their health. The American Heart Association has developed a simple, effective, and free assessment called My Life Check that gives you a quick "heart score" based on your lifestyles. The assessment focuses on what are referred to as the "Simple 7" key risk indicators/behaviors: manage blood pressure, control cholesterol, reduce blood sugar, get active, eat better, lose weight, and stop smoking. (Search "My Life Check" or see the link in Suggested Resources and Readings.)

Would tracking these indicators help you maintain a healthy lifestyle? If these data were linked to your physician's office, would it help you be more accountable for your lifestyle?

connect
ACTIVITY

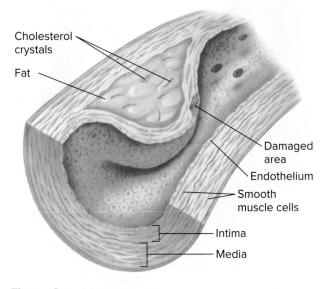

Figure 4 ▶ Atherosclerosis.

Table 1 ▶ Cholesterol Classifications (mg/dL)

	Total (TC)	LDL-C	HDL-C	TC/HDL-C
Optimal	——	<100	——	
Near optimal	——	100–129	——	——
Desirable	<200	——	60+	——
Borderline	200–239	130–159	40–59	3.6–5.0
High risk	240+	160–189	<40	5.0+
Very high risk	——	>190	——	——

Source: Third Report of the National Cholesterol Education Program.

have a higher than normal risk for heart disease (see Table 1). However, there are subtypes of LDL cholesterol (characterized by their small size and high density) that pose even greater risks. These subtypes are hard to measure and not included in most current blood tests, but future research will no doubt help us better understand and measure them.

Triglycerides are another type of blood lipid. Elevated levels of triglycerides are related to heart disease. Triglycerides lose some of their ability to predict heart disease with the presence of other risk factors, so high levels are more difficult to interpret than other blood lipids. Normal levels are considered to be 150 mg/dL or less. Values of 151–199 are borderline, 200–499 are high, and above 500 are very high. It would be wise to include triglycerides in a blood lipid profile. Physical activity is often prescribed as part of a treatment for high triglyceride levels.

Physical activity can help prevent atherosclerosis by increasing HDL in the blood. Whereas LDLs carry a core of cholesterol that is involved in the development of atherosclerosis, **high-density lipoprotein (HDL)** picks up cholesterol and carries it to the liver, where it is eliminated from the body. HDL is often called the "good cholesterol" and is desirable. When having a blood test, ask for information about HDL as well as the other measures included in Table 1. Individuals who have regular physical activity usually have lower total cholesterol, lower LDL, and higher HDL levels than inactive people.

Physical activity can help prevent atherosclerosis by reducing blood coagulants. Fibrin and platelets (types of cells involved in blood coagulation) deposit at the site of an injury on the wall of the artery, contributing to the process of plaque buildup, or atherosclerosis. Regular physical activity has been shown to reduce fibrin levels in the blood. The breakdown of fibrin seems to reduce platelet adhesiveness and the concentration of platelets in the blood.

Monitoring lipid profiles can help identify risks for atherosclerosis. Lipid profiles can help determine the relative proportion of LDL and HDL as well as levels of circulating triglycerides. However, a number of other constituents in the blood have been shown to be associated with risk for cardiovascular disease. These compounds are not necessarily causes of atherosclerosis, but they are indicators of inflammatory processes that lead to plaque formation. Inflammatory processes also soften existing plaque and increase the likelihood of plaque rupture or the formation of clots, which can directly precipitate heart attacks.

A number of inflammatory markers have been studied, but a recent AHA/CDC position statement indicates that most are not yet applicable for routine risk assessment for a variety of reasons. The position statement indicates that C-reactive protein (CRP) is the one inflammatory marker recommended for use in screening. CRP values above 3.0 mg/L are considered high risk and values below 1.0 mg/L are considered low risk. You may want to ask your physician about inflammatory markers at your next physical exam.

Physical Activity Reduces Hypertension and Improves Circulation

Hypertension is a separate form of cardiovascular disease, but it is also a major risk for heart attack and stroke. High blood pressure **(hypertension)** scars the vessel walls, promotes plaque formation, and increases the risks for heart attack, stroke, kidney damage, and other health problems. Normal **systolic blood pressure** is less than 120 mm Hg, and normal **diastolic blood pressure** is less than 80 mm Hg. Guidelines from the American Heart

Atherosclerosis The deposition of materials along the arterial walls; a type of arteriosclerosis.

Arteriosclerosis Hardening of the arteries due to conditions that cause the arterial walls to become thick, hard, and nonelastic.

Lipids All fats and fatty substances.

Lipoproteins Fat-carrying proteins in the blood.

Low-Density Lipoprotein (LDL) A core of cholesterol surrounded by protein; the core is often called "bad cholesterol."

Triglycerides A type of blood fat associated with increased risk for heart disease.

High-Density Lipoprotein (HDL) A blood substance that picks up cholesterol and helps remove it from the body; often called "good cholesterol."

Fibrin A sticky, threadlike substance that, in combination with blood cells, forms a blood clot.

Hypertension High blood pressure; excessive pressure against the walls of the arteries that can damage the heart, kidneys, and other organs of the body.

Systolic Blood Pressure The upper blood pressure number, often called working blood pressure. It represents the pressure in the arteries at its highest level just after the heart beats.

Diastolic Blood Pressure The lower blood pressure number, often called resting pressure. It is the pressure in the arteries at its lowest level just before the next beat of the heart.

Table 2 ▶ Blood Pressure Classifications for Adults

Category	Systolic Blood Pressure (mm Hg)		Diastolic Blood Pressure (mm Hg)
Normal	<120	and	<80
Elevated	120–129	and	<80
Stage 1 Hypertension	130–139	or	80–89
Stage 2 Hypertension	140 and up	or	90 and up
Hypertensive Crisis	>180	and/or	>120

Source: www.heart.org/hbp.

Association and the American Stroke Association distinguish levels of hypertension based on stages to characterize the progressively greater risks with higher values (see Table 2). The term *prehypertension* was previously used to characterize an elevated value between 120/80 and 140/90. However, research has shown that risks are already doubled by the time readings reach 130/80. The stage-based guidelines provide a more effective way to characterize levels of risk. *Stage 1 Hypertension* is define as an elevated blood pressure between 130/80 and 139/89, while *Stage 2 Hypertension* is defined as systolic BP at 140 or higher, or diastolic at 90 or higher. Excessively high blood pressure (above 180) is considered to be a "hypertensive crisis" that requires immediate medical attention.

Hypertension is sometimes referred to as the "silent killer" because many people do not know they have it. More than 50 percent of African Americans have high blood pressure, more than twice the rate of Hispanics and white non-Hispanics. Native Americans have a 10 percent greater incidence compared to Hispanics and white non-Hispanics. Males have higher rates of hypertension than females. Incidence increases for all groups with age. Exceptionally low blood pressures (below 100 systolic and 60 diastolic) do not pose the same risks to health as high blood pressure but can cause dizziness, fainting, and lack of tolerance to change in body positions.

It is important to be aware of your blood pressure levels and to monitor them over time, particularly with age. With practice and good equipment, you can accurately measure your own blood pressure. Because blood pressure can be elevated by emotions and circumstances, a single measurement may not be accurate. At least two separate measurements are recommended. While self-assessments can be helpful, they are not a substitute for periodic assessments by a qualified medical person.

Physical activity strengthens the heart and can help manage hypertension. Regular physical activity helps keep blood pressure in healthy levels and can reduce levels for individuals with hypertension. Exercise increases blood pressure on a short-term basis, but it imposes a positive stress

on the heart by challenging it to pump higher volumes of blood. This leads to desirable adaptations that improve cardiac function and lower resting heart rate and blood pressure.

Although resting heart rate is not considered to be a good measure of health or fitness, decreases in individual heart rate following training reflect positive adaptations. It indicates that the heart can pump the same amount of blood with fewer beats. Normal resting heart rate values may range from 50 to 80, but people who regularly do physical activity typically have lower resting heart rates than people who do no regular activity. Some endurance athletes have heart rates in the 30-50 beats per minute (bpm) range, which is still considered healthy or normal. Changes in heart rate are not directly related to changes in blood pressure, so it is important to monitor it independently. However, it is well established that inactive, less fit individuals have a greater chance of being hypertensive than active, fit people.

Physical activity improves circulation and reduces risks of having a heart attack (or dying from one). Within the heart, many tiny branches extend from the major coronary arteries. All of these vessels supply blood to the heart muscle. Active people are likely to have greater blood-carrying capacity in these vessels, probably because the vessels are larger and more elastic. Also, active people may have more profuse distribution of arteries within the heart muscle (see Figure 5), which results in greater blood flow. There is evidence that physical activity may promote the growth of "extra" blood vessels, which are thought to open up to provide the heart muscle with the necessary blood and oxygen when the oxygen supply is diminished, as in a heart attack. Blood flow from extra blood vessels is referred to as **coronary collateral circulation**.

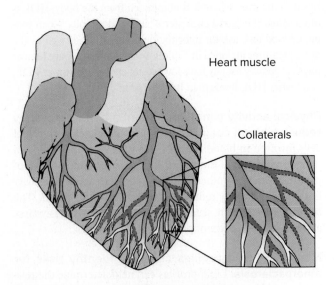

Heart muscle

Collaterals

Figure 5 ▶ Coronary collateral circulation.

Improved coronary circulation provides protection against heart attacks since healthier vessels are larger and less occluded. The development of collateral blood vessels supplying the heart may also diminish the effects of a heart attack, as these extra (or collateral) blood vessels may take over the function of regular blood vessels if another vessel gets clogged. Regular physical activity is also helpful in preventing peripheral vascular disease. People who exercise regularly have better blood flow to the working muscles and other tissues than inactive, unfit people. Since peripheral vascular disease is associated with poor circulation to the extremities, regular exercise can be considered one method of preventing this condition.

Physical activity improves circulatory control and regulation. The heart of an inactive person is less able to resist stress and is more susceptible to an emotional storm that may precipitate a heart attack. The heart is rendered inefficient by one or more of the following circumstances: high heart rate, high blood pressure, and excessive stimulation. All of these conditions require the heart to use more oxygen than is normal and decrease its ability to adapt to stressful situations.

The inefficient heart beats rapidly because it is dominated by the sympathetic nervous system, which speeds up the heart rate. Thus, the heart continuously beats rapidly, even at rest, and never has a true rest period. High blood pressure also makes the heart work harder and contributes to its inefficiency.

Research indicates that regular physical activity can:

- lead to dominance of the parasympathetic nervous system, which slows the heart rate and helps the heart work efficiently;
- help the heart rate return to normal faster after emotional stress;
- strengthen the heart muscle, making it better able to weather an emotional storm;
- reduce hormonal effects on the heart, thus lessening the chances of circulatory problems; and
- reduce the risk of sudden death from ventricular fibrillation (arrhythmic heartbeat).

Physical Activity Promotes Metabolic Health

Metabolic syndrome is a condition characterized by poor metabolic fitness. Metabolic syndrome is a metabolic disorder that is characterized by a clustering of various metabolic risk factors (see Figure 6). People with at least three of the following characteristics are considered to have metabolic syndrome: blood pressure above 130/85, a fasting blood sugar level of 100 or higher, blood triglycerides of 150 or above, a low blood HDL level (less than 40 for males and less than 50 for females), and/or a high abdominal

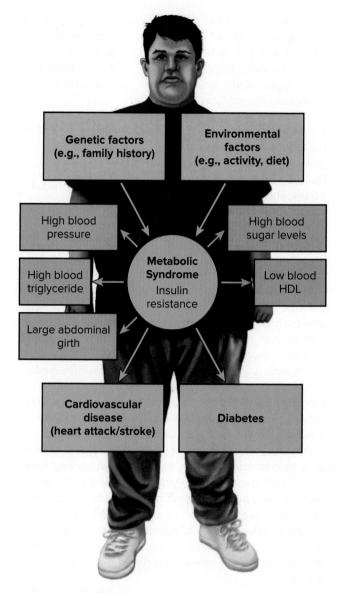

Figure 6 ▶ Mechanism and effects of metabolic syndrome.
Source: www.heart.org/hbp.

circumference (equal to or above 40 inches for males or 35 inches for females). Collectively, these risk factors contribute to insulin resistance (i.e., the body does not use insulin effectively) and associated risks for diabetes (see next section) as well as cardiovascular disease.

Family history and other genetic factors can predispose a person to obesity and metabolic syndrome; however, it is also influenced directly by lifestyle factors such as physical activity and diet (see blue boxes in Figure 6). Physical activity

Coronary Collateral Circulation Circulation of blood to the heart muscle associated with the blood-carrying capacity of a specific vessel or development of collateral vessels (extra blood vessels).

positively impacts all of the underlying precursors of metabolic syndrome as well as the various chronic conditions associated with it. Lab 5A can be used to screen for possible
risk of metabolic syndrome. A periodic physical exam with
blood profiles and a metabolic syndrome assessment is recommended, especially as you get older.

**Diabetes is a prevalent metabolic disease linked to
metabolic syndrome.** Diabetes mellitus (diabetes) is a
group of disorders that results when
there is too much sugar in the blood. It
occurs when the body does not make
enough insulin or when the body is not
able to use insulin effectively.

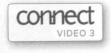

Type 1 diabetes, or insulin-dependent diabetes, accounts
for a relatively small number of the diabetes cases and is not
considered to be a hypokinetic condition. Type 2 diabetes
(often not insulin-dependent) was formerly called "adult-onset
diabetes." Reports indicate more cases of Type 2 diabetes
among children than in the past, in part because of better record keeping but also because of increases in obesity among
children in recent years.

Diabetes is the seventh leading cause of death. According
to the American Diabetes Association (ADA), there are
more than 34 million people who have been diagnosed as diabetic. Unfortunately, another 7 million are diabetic and do
not know it. An estimated additional 88 million are pre-
diabetic. Diabetes accounts for at least 10 percent of all short-
term hospital stays and has a major impact on health-care
costs in Western society. African Americans, Hispanics,
Native Americans, and Asian Americans all have higher rates
of diabetes than white Non-Hispanics. People over 65 have
more than twice the rate of diabetes as those below 65, and
males have higher rates of undiagnosed diabetes than
females. Males of all groups have higher diabetes rates than
females.

There are several tests for diabetes and pre-diabetes. The
most commonly used are the oral glucose tolerance test
(OGTT) that assesses your ability to regulate blood sugar. A
blood test (A1C) that assesses your blood sugar levels over
the past two to three months is considered to be a good indicator of blood sugar regulation. A1C levels below 5.7 percent
are normal, between 5.7 percent and 6.5 percent are in the
pre-diabetes range, and values above 6.5 percent are in the
diabetes range. Consult your physician to see what test is
most appropriate for you.

Medical intervention is clearly essential for people with
Type 2 diabetes, but healthy lifestyles are important for effective treatment. Regular physical activity can help reduce body
fatness, decrease insulin resistance, improve insulin sensitivity, and improve the body's ability to clear sugar from the
blood in a reasonable time. With sound nutritional habits and
proper medication, physical activity can be useful in the management of both types of diabetes. Additional details on diabetes are provided in the Concept on other health threats.

**Physical activity contributes to maintaining a healthy
body weight and improved metabolic fitness.** Excess
body weight is one of the contributing factors to metabolic
syndrome and diabetes. Although physical activity is critical
for both prevention and treatment of overweight and obesity,
evidence suggests that risk of diabetes and metabolic syndrome can be reduced by physical activity regardless of
weight status. Thus, the benefits of physical activity on metabolic fitness are so robust that they are largely independent of
whether weight loss occurs or not. This evidence is consistent
with research showing that fat people who are fit are not at
especially high risk for early death. However, it is still critical
to maintain a healthy body composition. When high body
fatness is accompanied by low cardiorespiratory endurance
and low metabolic fitness, risk for early death increases
substantially. Additional details on body composition are
provided in the Concept on body composition.

Physical Activity Promotes Musculoskeletal Health

**Physical activity is important to maintaining bone
density and decreasing risk for osteoporosis.** Some
experts consider bone integrity to be a health-related component of physical fitness. Bone density cannot be self-
assessed. It is measured using a dual X-ray absorptiometry
(DXA) machine, an expensive and sophisticated form of
X-ray machine that can also be used to measure body fatness.
Healthy bones are dense and strong. When bones lose calcium and become less dense, they become porous and are at
risk for fracture. The bones of young children are not especially dense, but during adolescence and early adulthood
(see Figure 7), bones increase in density to a level higher
than at any other time in life (peak bone density). Though
bone density often begins to decrease in young adulthood,
it is not until older adulthood that bone loss becomes
dramatic. Over time, if bone loss continues, older adults
become susceptible to a condition called osteoporosis (bone

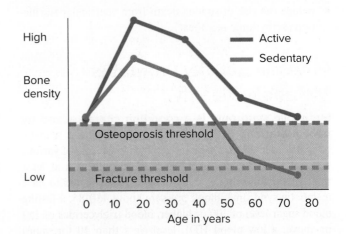

Figure 7 ▶ Changes in bone density with age.

density drops below the osteoporosis threshold). Some will have crossed the fracture threshold, putting them at risk for fractures, especially to the hip, vertebrae, and other "soft" or "spongy" bones of the skeletal system. Active people have a higher peak bone mass and are more resistant to osteoporosis (see the blue line in Figure 7) than sedentary people (see the red line in Figure 7).

Females, especially postmenopausal females, have a higher risk of osteoporosis than males, but it is a disease of both sexes. Although Figure 7 reflects the combined bone density status for males and females, males typically have a higher peak bone mass than females, and for this reason, males can lose more bone density over time without reaching the osteoporosis or fracture threshold. More females reach the osteoporosis and fracture thresholds at earlier ages than males. Whites and Asians have higher risk of osteoporosis than other racial/ethnic groups. Other risk factors for osteoporosis are age, family history/heredity, frame size, smoking, caffeine use, alcohol use, current or previous eating disorders, early menstruation, low dietary calcium intake, low body fat, amenorrhea, and extended bed rest.

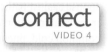

Physical activity reduces risks of back problems. Active people who possess good muscle fitness are less likely to have back and musculoskeletal problems than are inactive, unfit people. Because few people die from it, back pain does not receive the attention given to such medical problems as heart disease and cancer. But back pain is the second leading medical complaint in the United States, second only to headaches. Only the common cold and the flu cause more days lost from work. At some point in our lives, approximately 80 percent of all adults experience back pain that limits the ability to function normally. It is by far the most frequently injured of all body parts.

The great majority of back ailments are the result of poor muscle strength, low levels of endurance, and poor flexibility. Tests on patients with back problems show weakness and lack of flexibility in key muscle groups. Lack of fitness is probably the leading reason for back pain in Western society. Other factors also increase the risk of back ailments, including poor posture, improper lifting and work habits, heredity, and diseases such as scoliosis and arthritis. Muscle fitness is particularly important for reducing risks of back problems. Targeted exercises to improve core strength and endurance can help promote good posture and reduce risks of back problems later in life (see Concept on posture and back care).

Physical Activity Promotes Good Mental Health

Physical activity can help with prevention and treatment of mental health disorders. Nearly half of adult Americans will report having a mental health disorder at

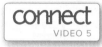

some point in life. There is increasing awareness and acceptance of mental health issues in society and considerable research has been done to identify causes and to test appropriate treatments. Although the conditions are complex and can't be fully addressed here, evidence supports the importance of healthy lifestyles for both prevention and treatment of many mental health conditions.

Depression is a stress-related condition experienced by many adults. Thirty-three percent of inactive adults report that they often feel depressed. For some, depression is a serious disorder that physical activity alone will not cure; however, research indicates that activity, combined with other forms of therapy, can be effective.

Anxiety is an emotional condition characterized by worry, self-doubt, and apprehension. More than a few studies have shown that symptoms of anxiety can be reduced by regular activity. Less fit people who do regular aerobic activity seem to benefit the most. In one study, one-third of active people felt that regular activity helped them cope better with life's pressures.

An additional benefit of regular exercise is increased self-esteem. Improvements in fitness, appearance, and the ability to perform new tasks can improve self-confidence.

Physical activity is associated with better and more restful sleep. Increased attention has been paid to the importance of sleep for optimal mental (and physical) health. National guidelines for physical activity in Canada incorporate sleep and minimizing sedentary time to document that these three distinct Yes, behaviors interact to promote good health and well-being. People with insomnia (the inability to sleep) seem to benefit from regular activity if it is not done too vigorously right before going to bed. Regular aerobic activity is associated with reduced brain activation, which can result in greater ability to relax or fall asleep.

Physical activity reduces risk of dementia and Alzheimer disease. More than a few studies indicate that factors relating to heart health also contribute to brain health. The studies indicate that physical and challenging mental activities are especially important for preventing decline in cognitive function and reducing the risk of developing Alzheimer disease and dementia. Although additional research is needed, this is important news for physicians and public health officials looking for ways to reduce the prevalence of Alzheimer disease. (*Note:* Although many organizations retain the use of the term *Alzheimer's disease,* leading scholars and journals in the field use *Alzheimer disease* because the German physician and scientist for whom the disease was named discovered the disease but did not have it. We use *Alzheimer disease* in deference to the recommendation of the experts.)

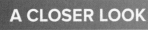

A CLOSER LOOK

Long-Term Effects of COVID-19 on Heart Health

Extensive research on the SARS-CoV-2 virus that causes COVID-19 has documented potential long-term risks of exposure, including an increased risk of myocarditis, or inflammation of the heart tissue. Estimates suggest that 40 to 80 percent of people with COVID-19 may show signs of myocarditis. Although it often resolves naturally with time, studies have documented that individuals are susceptible even after the symptoms of COVID-19 are gone. Athletes and active individuals should be aware of the risk since myocarditis can cause complications such as abnormal heart rhythms, chronic heart failure, and even sudden death. Experts suggest that increased rates of heart failure may be an unfortunate long-term result of having COVID-19.

Do the long-term risks change your perceptions about the implications of COVID-19?

connect ACTIVITY

Physical activity is a major part of worksite and school health promotion programs. Companies realize the importance of promoting healthy lifestyles among their employees. Worksite health promotion programs typically focus broadly on promoting a variety of healthy lifestyles, but physical activity is considered the mainstay of most programs. To facilitate active lifestyles, many companies build their own fitness centers inside the workplace or provide free or reduced-cost memberships for employees. Worksite programs that promote activity can reduce risk factors in employees and help companies save money and control the high cost of health care. Employees miss less work (i.e., reduced absenteeism), are more productive while at work (i.e., increased "presenteeism"), and have higher morale. Schools, including many universities, also recognize the importance of physical activity, resulting in the expansion of fitness centers on many campuses. The expansion of worksite and school health physical activity programming can provide benefits to individuals while also advancing public health.

Many factors promote health and wellness and reduce the risk for disease. Inactivity, poor nutrition, smoking, and inability to cope with stress are all risk factors associated with various chronic diseases. These factors are in your control, and changing them can dramatically reduce your risk for chronic diseases. Other risk factors over which you have some control include weight/body composition, blood lipids and other blood constituents, and blood pressure. You also have some control over your health care. Recent reductions in chronic disease have resulted because of improved health care. For example, heart disease rates have decreased dramatically in recent years because of better detection (e.g., exercise tests, angiograms, CT scans), better emergency care, and improved medications.

Some risk factors, however, are not within your control (e.g., age, heredity, and gender). Table 4 summarizes the risk factors that are within your control as well as those that are

patient's physical activity program at every visit." The initiative has taken off both in the United States and internationally. The website (www.exerciseismedicine.org) provides information to the general public, health-care providers, health and fitness professionals, and the media.

A complementary organization called the American College of Lifestyle Medicine has sought to extend the EIM mission by promoting a broader lifestyle-based approach. They have focused considerable attention on promoting primary prevention strategies into mainstream medical care. See In the News for more details.

In the News

Lifestyle Medicine

To reduce the burden on the health-care system, clinical practices are placing a greater emphasis on health promotion and prevention. Historically, the standard approach in medicine has been to treat the symptoms of disease instead of the underlying cause. However, a new movement toward lifestyle medicine is shifting the focus to behavioral approaches. As defined by the American College of Lifestyle Medicine (ACLM), lifestyle medicine is *"the evidence-based practice of helping individuals and families adopt and sustain healthy behaviors that affect health and quality of life."*

The primary behaviors emphasized include doing physical activity, eating healthy foods, managing stress, avoiding risky substances, forming positive relationships, and improving sleep. The focus on prevention is also consistent with trends in insurance and health care; however, it will take time to become standard practice.

Would you be more inclined to seek out a physician if he or she had specific training or credentials in "lifestyle medicine"?

connect ACTIVITY

Table 4 ▶ Hypokinetic Disease Risk Factors

Factors That Cannot Be Altered

1. *Age*. As you grow older, your risk of contracting hypokinetic diseases increases. For example, the risk for heart disease is approximately three times as great after 60 as before. The risk of back pain is considerably greater after 40.
2. *Heredity*. People who have a family history of hypokinetic disease are more likely to develop a hypokinetic condition, such as heart disease, hypertension, back problems, obesity, high blood lipid levels, and other problems. African Americans are 45 percent more likely to have high blood pressure than white individuals; therefore, they suffer strokes at an earlier age with more severe consequences.
3. *Biological sex at birth*. Individuals designated as "male" based on their sex at birth have a higher incidence of many hypokinetic conditions than individuals designated as "female" at birth. However, differences in incidence of hypokinetic conditions between individuals designated male at birth and individuals designated female at birth have decreased recently. Postmenopausal individuals have a higher heart disease risk than premenopausal individuals.

Factors That Can Be Altered

4. *Regular physical activity*. Regular exercise can help reduce the risk for hypokinetic disease.
5. *Diet*. A clear association exists between hypokinetic disease and certain types of diets. The excessive intake of saturated fats, such as animal fats, is linked to atherosclerosis and other forms of heart disease. Excessive salt in the diet is associated with high blood pressure.
6. *Stress*. People who are subject to excessive stress are predisposed to various hypokinetic diseases, including heart disease and back pain. Statistics indicate that hypokinetic conditions are common among those in certain high-stress jobs and those having Type A personality profiles.
7. *Tobacco use*. Smokers have five times the risk of heart attack as nonsmokers. Most striking is the difference in risk between older female smokers and nonsmokers. Tobacco use is also associated with the increased risk for high blood pressure, cancer, and several other medical conditions. Apparently, the more you use, the greater the risk. Stopping tobacco use even after many years can significantly reduce the hypokinetic disease risk.
8. *Body (fatness)*. Having too much body fat is a primary risk factor for heart disease and is a risk factor for other hypokinetic conditions as well. For example, loss of fat can result in relief from symptoms of Type 2 diabetes, can reduce problems associated with certain types of back pain, and can reduce the risks of surgery.
9. *Blood lipids, blood glucose, and blood pressure levels*. High scores on these factors are associated with health problems, such as heart disease and diabetes. Risk increases considerably when several of these measures are high.
10. *Diseases*. People who have one hypokinetic disease are more likely to develop a second or even a third condition. For example, if you have diabetes,* your risk of having a heart attack or stroke increases dramatically. Although you may not be entirely able to alter the extent to which you develop certain diseases and conditions, reducing your risk and following your doctor's advice can improve your odds significantly.

*Some types of diabetes cannot be altered.

not. By adopting healthy lifestyles, you can take control over some of the preventable disease risks. For example, by being physically active you can reduce your risk for heart disease and diabetes (even if you are overweight). Altering your diet can reduce the chances of developing high levels of blood lipids and reduce the risk for atherosclerosis (even if you have a family history of the condition). Adopting healthy lifestyles is a proactive approach to health and wellness but it does not ensure disease immunity. Even so, studies of twins suggest that active people are less likely to die early than inactive people with similar genes. This finding suggests that long-term adherence to physical activity can overcome risk factors considered to be out of your control, such as heredity. Lab 5A helps you assess your heart disease risk factors, both those not in your control and those in your control. Although the lab focuses on heart disease risk factors, many of the factors are also risk factors for other chronic diseases.

Too much activity can lead to hyperkinetic conditions. The information presented in this Concept points out the health benefits of physical activity performed in appropriate amounts. When done in excess or incorrectly, physical activity can result in **hyperkinetic conditions**, the most common being overuse injury

to muscles, connective tissue, and bones. Recently, anorexia nervosa and body neurosis have been identified as conditions associated with inappropriate amounts of physical activity. These conditions are discussed in the Concept on performance.

Using Self-Management Skills

Building knowledge is important to making sound decisions about health, wellness, and fitness. Acquiring knowledge can help you become motivated to make change and be sure that the changes you make are effective. Changes based on bad information can produce poor results and loss of motivation and confidence. The information in this Concept is based on sound scientific evidence and provides you with information for making good decisions about fitness and health. However, every day new information becomes available. For this reason, it is important to keep your "knowledge" up to date by accessing accurate information. All fitness and health information

Hyperkinetic Conditions Diseases/illnesses or health conditions caused, or contributed to, by too much physical activity.

is not equal. For example, one of the most common sources of fitness and health information on the Web is Wikipedia. Yet studies show that information on Wikipedia is often incorrect—especially information about drugs, medicines, and supplements. There is much misinformation in the media as well. Be skillful in acquiring knowledge. When selecting sources (e.g., books, articles, Internet links) use your investigative skills. Check the credentials of the authors, the organization sponsoring the website, and so on. Additional information is provided in the Concept on consumerism and at websites such as MedlinePlus (search "evaluating health information" online).

Changing your beliefs is important to behavior change. Experts indicate that in addition to acquiring knowledge it is important to examine our beliefs if we are to make behavior (lifestyle) changes. If we hold beliefs that are inconsistent with the facts, what are the reasons? Why are we resisting the facts? Why do we do things that are against our health interests? For example, many people know that smoking is bad for them but still smoke. The "facts" may seem abstract leading to statements such as, "It takes a long time for smoking to cause cancer and I can stop anytime I want to." Some actually believe that they are special, that smoking affects others but not "me."

More than a few prominent people have made similar statements about exercise. Mark Twain is credited with the saying, "whenever I get the urge to exercise, I lie down until the feeling passes" and astronaut Neil Armstrong is credited with saying, "I believe that every human has a finite number of heartbeats. I don't intend to waste any of mine running around doing exercises." There is some question about the origin of these statements but, regardless, they have been widely circulated. They illustrate the point that well-informed people can still hold beliefs that are counter to the facts and that limit healthy lifestyle change. In some cases, help from others (social support) is necessary (e.g., smoking cessation assistance) to make positive changes.

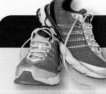

Strategies for Action: Lab Information

A self-assessment of risk factors can help you modify your lifestyle to reduce risk for heart disease. The Heart Disease Risk Factor Questionnaire in Lab 5A will help you assess your personal risk factors for heart disease. It is not a substitute, however, for a regular medical exam that includes an assessment of other cardiovascular disease risk factors, such as cholesterol and blood glucose. This will allow you to use more sophisticated and accurate risk factor assessments (see the My Life Check tool highlighted in the Technology Update feature).

It is never too early to start being active to improve health. Many of the studies presented in this Concept indicate that being "active for a lifetime" prevents health problems. Young adults often think "I'll worry about these problems when I get older." But what you do early in life has much to do with your current health, as well as your health later in life.

Subsequent Concepts cover the different components of health-related fitness and the type and amount of activity needed to improve these components. The lab activities in each of these Concepts are designed to help you begin planning *now* for lifelong physical activity.

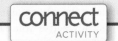
connect
ACTIVITY

Suggested Resources and Readings

The websites for the following sources can be accessed by searching online for the organization, program, or title listed. Specific scientific references are available at the end of this edition of *Concepts of Fitness and Wellness*.

- American College of Sports Medicine. ACSM Scientific Pronouncements: Physical Activity Guidelines for Americans:
  - Physical Activity, Cognition and Brain Outcomes
  - Physical Activity in Cancer Prevention and Survival
  - Physical Activity, All-Cause and Cardiovascular Mortality, and Cardiovascular Disease
  - Benefits of Physical Activity During Pregnancy and Postpartum
  - Physical Activity to Prevent and Treat Hypertension
  - Effects of Physical Activity in Knee and Hip Osteoarthritis

- American College of Sports Medicine. Exercise is Medicine®: A Global Health Initiative.
- American Heart Association. My Life Check/Life's Simple 7.
- American Heart Association. Recommendations for Physical Activity in Adults and Kids.
- Centers for Disease Control and Prevention. Health and Academic Achievement. (pdf)
- Centers for Disease Control and Prevention. Racial and Ethnic Disparities in Heart Disease. (pdf)
- Harvard School of Public Health. Simple Steps to Preventing Diabetes.
- Moore, G., Durstine, J. L., & Painter, P. (eds.). (2016). *ACSM'S Exercise Management for Persons with Chronic Diseases and Disabilities.* Champaign, IL: Human Kinetics.
- National Institutes of Health. All of Us Research Program.
- PAR-Q+ Collaboration. Physical Activity Readiness Questionnaire for Everyone (PAR-Q+) and Medical Examination (ePARmed-X+).
- U.S. Department of Health and Human Services. (2018). *Physical Activity Guidelines for Americans.*

Design Element: (*magnifying glass*): Siede Preis/Getty Images; (*runners shoes*): Maridav/Getty Images; (*tablet*): McGraw Hill; (*woman*): GlobalStock/Getty Images; (*blue sports shoes*): chictype/Getty Images; (*smartphone*): Alexey Boldin/Shutterstock; (*Why It Matters*): MHHE

Lab 5A Assessing Heart Disease Risk Factors

Name	**Section**	**Date**

Purpose: To assess your risk of developing coronary heart disease. See next page for directions.

Heart Disease Risk Factor Questionnaire

Risk Points

	① 1	② 2	③ 3	④ 4	Score
Unalterable Factors					
1. How old are you?	30 or less	31–40	41–54	55+	
2. Do you have a history of heart disease in your family?	None	Grandparent with heart disease	Parent with heart disease	More than one with heart disease	
3. What is your biological sex at birth?	Female		Male		
				Total Unalterable Risk Score	
Alterable Factors					
4. Do you get regular physical activity?	4–5 days a week	3 days a week	Fewer than 3 days a week	No	
5. Do you have a high-fat diet?	No	Slightly high in fat	Above normal in fat	Eat a lot of meat and fried and fatty foods	
6. Are you under much stress?	Less than normal	Normal	Slightly above normal	Quite high	
7. Do you use tobacco?	No	Cigar or pipe	Less than 1/2 pack a day or use smokeless tobacco	More than 1/2 pack a day	
8. What is your percentage of body fat?*	F = 17–28% M = 10–20%	29–31% 21–23%	32–35% 24–30%	>35% >30%	
9. What is the systolic number in your blood pressure?	<120	121–140	141–160	>160	
10. Do you have other diseases?	No	Ulcer	Diabetes**	Both	

Extra Points: Add points for as many of the following test results as you have available: 1 point for CRP above 3, 1 point for homocysteine above 100, 3 points for LDL above 130, 3 points for TC/HDL-C above 4. If only total cholesterol is available, add 1 point for a score of 200–240 or 3 points for scores above 240.

Total Alterable Risk Score	
Extra Points	
Grand Total Risk Score	

*If unknown, estimate your body fat percentage or see Lab 13A.

**Diabetes is a risk factor that is often not alterable.

Source: Adapted from *CAD Risk Assessor*, William J. Stone.

Procedures

1. Answer the 10 questions in the Heart Disease Risk Factor Questionnaire and determine whether you should add the extra points by circling the answer that is most appropriate for *you*.
2. For each of your answers, look at the top of the column. In the box provided at the right of each question, write down the number of risk points for that answer.
3. Determine your unalterable risk score by adding the risk points for questions 1, 2, and 3.
4. Determine your alterable risk score by adding the risk points for questions 4 through 10.
5. Determine your total heart disease risk score by adding the scores obtained in steps 3 and 4.
6. Look up your risk ratings on the Heart Disease Risk Rating Chart and record them in the Results section. Answer the questions in the Conclusions and Implications section.

Results: Write your risk scores and risk ratings in the appropriate boxes below.

Heart Disease Risk Scores and Ratings

	Score	Rating
Unalterable risk		
Alterable risk		
Total heart disease risk		

Heart Disease Risk Rating Chart

Rating	Unalterable Score	Alterable Score	Total Score
Very high	9 or more	21 or more	31 or more
High	7–8	15–20	26–30
Average	5–6	11–14	16–25
Low	4 or less	10 or less	15 or less

Conclusions and Implications: The higher your score on the Heart Disease Risk Factor Questionnaire, the greater your heart disease risk. In several sentences, discuss your risk for heart disease. Which of the risk factors do you need to control to reduce your risk for heart disease? Why?

How Much Physical Activity Is Enough?

LEARNING OBJECTIVES

After completing the study of this Concept, you will be able to:

▶ Describe each of the key principles of physical activity and explain how the principles relate to each other in helping you achieve health, wellness, and fitness.

▶ Name the four elements of the FITT formula and explain how the formula relates to the concepts of *threshold of training* and *target zones* for different types of physical activity.

▶ List the five steps in the physical activity pyramid and identify the FIT formula for each.

▶ Describe the physical activity patterns of adults, differentiating among groups based on age, sex, gender identity, and ethnicity.

▶ Describe the four fitness zones used for self-assessments of physical fitness and explain how each level relates to health and performance.

▶ Identify related national health goals and show how meeting personal goals can contribute to reaching national goals.

▶ Self-assess your current activity level for each step of the physical activity pyramid and estimate your current health and skill-related physical fitness.

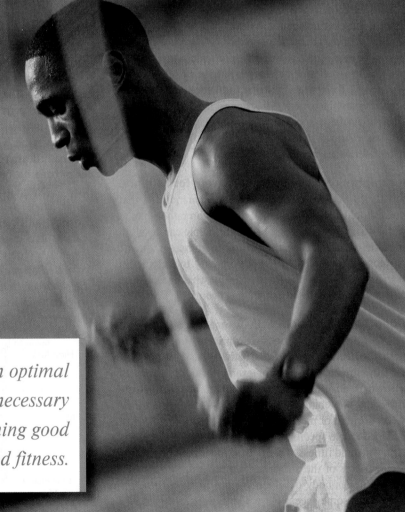

There is a minimal and an optimal amount of physical activity necessary for developing and maintaining good health, wellness, and fitness.

Eyewire/Getty Images

to produce benefits. The appropriate intensity varies with the desired benefit. Health benefits from metabolic fitness require only moderate activity, but performance benefits require more vigorous activity.

Time (how long)—Physical activity must be done for an adequate length of time to be effective. The length of the activity session depends on the type of activity and the expected benefit.

Type (kind of activity)—The benefits derived depend on the type of activity performed. For example, moderate activity must be done at least 5 days a week, while muscle fitness activity may be done as few as 2 days a week.

When determining the formula for each type of activity, the shorter acronym (FIT) can be used because you have already determined the activity type. In the following section, you will learn more about the **FIT** formula for each type of activity in the physical activity pyramid. In subsequent Concepts, each formula is described in greater detail.

The volume and progression of physical activity are important considerations. The American College of Sports Medicine (ACSM) indicates that volume and progression should be considered in planning your physical activity program. *Volume* refers to the total amount of physical activity that you perform 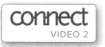 each day. It is a combination of the frequency, intensity, and total amount of time spent in exercise. For example, a short but more intense bout of activity can provide a volume of activity similar to a longer, moderate exercise bout. Various combinations of frequency, intensity, and time of physical activity (volume) can be used in a gradual progression to reach personal goals based on individual needs. *Progression* refers to the application of the principle of progression described earlier in this Concept. Essentially, to continue to improve you have to progress (i.e., increase) any or all of the FIT components. However, being patient is important, too. Attempts to get fit fast will probably be counterproductive, so the key is to start slowly and progress gradually using the FITT formula.

Consistent patterns of physical activity are recommended. The recommended daily volume of exercise for achieving health benefits is approximately 30 minutes per day, but this can be accumulated in several short bouts or in one longer 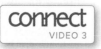 bout. In studying the benefits of physical activity, scientists also distinguish between the acute and chronic benefits of physical activity. Following guidelines for physical activity and performing regular physical activity over time will lead to an array of adaptations and improvements in physical fitness (chronic benefits). However, there are also benefits associated with each individual bout of physical activity (acute benefits). For example, regular physical activity is important for glucose regulation and maintenance of metabolic health. Consistent patterns are also critical for stress management, relaxation, and mental health.

The threshold of training and target zone depend on your fitness and goals. Regular physical activity provides significant **health benefits,** but improving fitness and achieving performance benefits can require more intentional and specific forms of exercise. The **threshold of training** is the minimum amount of activity (frequency, intensity, and time) necessary to produce benefits. The threshold depends on your current level of fitness as well as on the benefit expected.

The **target zone** begins at the threshold of training and stops at the point where the activity becomes excessive or counterproductive. While lack of physical activity contributes to hypokinetic diseases, there are also risks associated with doing too much activity (hyperkinetic) such as overtraining or increased risks of injury. The various body systems adapt best when physical activity is progressive and not too extreme. For example, evidence has clearly documented that excessive exercise hampers the immune system and increases risks of illness. Thus, too much exercise can also a problem. Figure 2 illustrates the threshold of training and target zone concepts.

Some people incorrectly associate threshold of training and target zones with only cardiorespiratory endurance. As the principle of specificity suggests, the type of physical activity for improving each component of fitness (including metabolic fitness), has its own FIT formula and its own threshold and target zone.

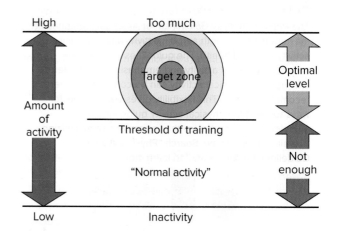

Figure 2 ▶ Physical activity target zone.

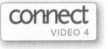

A CLOSER LOOK

Exercise in a Pill?

Some people wish that the benefits of exercise could be bottled up in a pill. This challenge has intrigued scientists for decades and considerable research has been done to try to develop medicines that mimic some of the associated benefits. The basic notion is to try to identify molecules or processes that are activated when we exercise and then to figure out ways to activate them. One effort is focused on trying to influence a metabolic pathway that promotes improved muscle function and cardiorespiratory endurance. Another effort is focused on trying to modify enzymes to speed up metabolism and increase sugar uptake. Previous reports of "exercise in a pill" have not panned out, so it is prudent to be skeptical. Vitamins cannot capture the benefits of a healthy diet, and pills likely cannot capture the full benefits of exercise.

Are you intrigued or troubled by the concepts of trying to develop an "exercise pill"?

connect
ACTIVITY

The Physical Activity Pyramid

The *Physical Activity Guidelines for Americans* indicate that a variety of types of physical activity are needed for good health. The guidelines recommend that adults perform weekly minimums of 150 minutes of moderate-intensity aerobic activity or 75 minutes of vigorous-intensity aerobic activity to achieve health benefits. The

connect
VIDEO 4

guidelines also indicate that increasing weekly activity to 300 minutes of moderate activity or 150 provides substantial additional benefits. A combination of moderate and vigorous activities can be used to meet guidelines with each minute of vigorous activity providing benefits equal to those for performing 2 minutes of moderate activity. Muscle fitness exercises, performed 2 or more days a week, should be included in meeting the moderate to vigorous activity guidelines. Performing a variety of types of activity helps build all dimensions of fitness as well as ensuring that all of the many health benefits of activity are achieved.

The guidelines provide recommendations for personalizing activity plans by helping people "*progress toward and beyond physical activity targets.*" The notion of moving beyond the guidelines is consistent with the dose-response principle by encouraging additional activity. However, the statement also emphasizes the principle of individuality by trying to help all individuals move toward the guidelines. Recommendations for people at different levels of engagement are listed:

- People who are inactive (perform little or no moderate to vigorous activity) are encouraged to replace sedentary behavior (such as sitting) with light-intensity physical activity.

- People who are insufficiently active (don't meet national guidelines) should aim to increase participation in moderate activity and to reduce time spent being sedentary.

- People who are active (meet national guidelines) can gain additional benefits by doing additional moderate to vigorous physical activity or reducing sedentary behavior.

The physical activity pyramid classifies activities by type and associated benefits. The physical activity pyramid (see Figure 3) was created to help readers better understand the different *types* of physical activity (e.g., the last *T* in FITT). Over the years, it has proven to be a useful model for illustrating how each type of activity contributes to the development of health, wellness, and fitness. The pyramid depicts five different steps. Each step represents a step toward achieving health, wellness, and fitness. Inactivity is shown below the pyramid because it does not represent a step toward active living. Placement in the pyramid is not meant to suggest that higher steps are more important than lower steps. Activities from all steps are important for optimal health, wellness, and fitness. Key concepts illustrated by the physical activity pyramid include the following:

- Each type of activity has its own FIT formula and unique health, wellness, and fitness benefits.

- The different types of physical activity can be combined to meet activity guidelines.

- Extended periods of inactivity can be harmful to your health.

- Eating well (sound nutrition) is an important companion behavior to physical activity (see energy balance scale at the top of Figure 3).

Each of the five steps of the physical activity pyramid are discussed in greater detail in the paragraphs that follow as well as in later Concepts.

Inactivity can be hazardous to your health. The steps in the physical activity pyramid show the five different types of physical activity (Figure 3). The phrase "Avoid Excessive Sedentary Behavior" appears below the pyramid in bold black letters. This is important because current evidence indicates that excess amounts of prolonged sedentary behavior can increase risk of chronic disease. Even active people are at risk if they are sedentary for long periods of time when not involved in activity. (See the Concept on adopting an active lifestyle for additional information.)

Health Benefits The results of physical activity that provide protection from hypokinetic disease or early death.

Threshold of Training The minimum amount of physical activity that will produce health and fitness benefits.

Target Zone The amounts of physical activity that produce optimal health and fitness benefits.

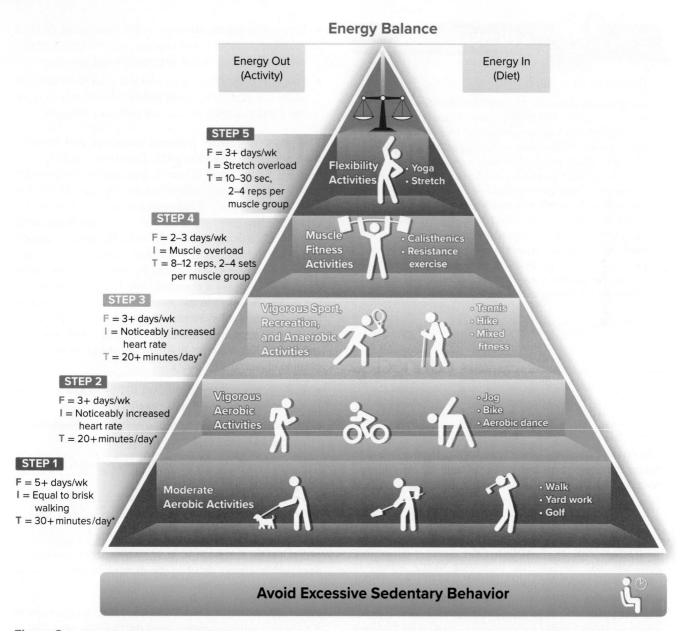

Figure 3 ▶ The physical activity pyramid.
*150 minutes of moderate or 75 minutes of vigorous activity per week is recommended; moderate and vigorous activity can be combined to meet guidelines.
Source: Charles B. Corbin.

Moderate aerobic activities provide many benefits for modest amounts of effort. Moderate aerobic activities equal in intensity to brisk walking provide significant health benefits. For a variety of reasons, they are depicted as step 1 of the physical activity pyramid (see Figure 3). The broad bottom of the pyramid illustrates that moderate activities are the most widely performed activities among adults. For optimal benefits, moderate activities are performed 5 or more days per week compared to 2–3 days per week for activities in steps 2–5. Finally, and perhaps most important, moderate activities provide many benefits for a modest amount of effort (see Figure 1). Moderate aerobic activities, such as walking to and from work, climbing the stairs rather than taking

an elevator, or doing brisk housework when done as part of the normal daily routine are often referred to as lifestyle physical activities. Moderate activities that are not part of the normal daily routine, such as taking a walk or a bike ride, can also be planned specifically to increase activity levels.

Studies indicate that individuals with active jobs have reduced risks for many chronic conditions. Those who actively commute (bike or walk) to work or to run errands have also been found to have better health profiles. The regular accumulation of activity as a part of one's lifestyle is sufficient to promote positive improvements in metabolic fitness, and these improvements can positively impact health. Additional activity from the other layers of the pyramid are strongly recommended.

Moderate activity can be viewed as the baseline, or minimal, activity that should be performed. A summary of the FIT formula for moderate activity is illustrated in step 1 of Figure 3.

Vigorous aerobic activities provides additional health benefits. **Vigorous aerobic activities** (step 2) are of greater intensity than moderate activities (step 1). The greater intensity results in significantly higher heart rates and higher oxygen consumption. Because of its greater intensity, vigorous aerobics can be performed as few as 3 days a week and are especially good for building cardiorespiratory endurance and helping control body fatness. Examples of vigorous aerobic activities, sometimes referred to as active aerobics, are jogging, biking, and aerobic dance. Vigorous aerobic activities can provide metabolic fitness and health benefits similar to moderate activities and can be performed instead of, or in combination with, moderate activities to meet national activity guidelines.

Vigorous sports, recreation, and anaerobic activities can provide similar benefits as vigorous aerobic activity. **Vigorous sports, recreation, and anaerobic activities** captures a range of sport, recreation, and fitness activities that generally feature intermittent bouts of higher-intensity activity (step 3). Sports such as soccer, tennis, and basketball have a vigorous aerobic component but also involve intermittent sprints that require anaerobic bursts of energy. Recreation activities like hiking also can include periods of intermittent, high-intensity movement. Fitness regimens such as high-intensity interval training (HIIT) and high-intensity circuit training (HICT) are also included at this level since they involve short bursts of vigorous, anaerobic activity. HIIT and HICT have become popular alternatives to traditional exercise routines since they provide variety and can build both cardiorespiratory fitness and muscular fitness. Also included at step 3 are mixed fitness activities that include combinations of dance, calisthenics, martial arts, and aerobics.

Muscle fitness activities are important for optimal fitness and health. There are muscle fitness benefits from many different activities, including vocational activities that require lifting, active sports such as gymnastics and wrestling, and recreational activities such as rock climbing. Various **muscle fitness activities**, such as resistance training, plyometrics, and calisthenics, are included at step 4 of the pyramid and they contribute to strength, muscular endurance, and power. The many health and performance benefits of muscle fitness exercises are described in the Concept on muscle fitness. A general description of the FIT formula for muscle fitness exercises is included in Figure 3 (step 4).

Flexibility activities are important for building and maintaining flexibility. There are flexibility benefits from many different activities, including sports such as gymnastics and diving. The **flexibility activities** included at step 5 of the pyramid are those that are planned specifically to build flexibility, such as stretching exercises and yoga. The many

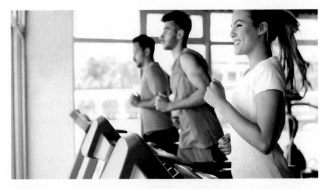

Meeting the physical activity guidelines can help you look and feel your best.
nd3000/Shutterstock

benefits of flexibility exercises and stretching activities are described in a separate Concept on flexibility. A general description of the FIT formula for flexibility exercises is included in Figure 3 (step 5).

Energy balance is important for maintaining a healthy body composition. Weight management requires that energy intake be matched by energy expenditure. The FIT formula messages in the physical activity pyramid provide general information about the amounts of activity (energy expenditure) necessary for general health and fitness benefits. But these amounts may not be enough for weight management (or weight loss). Current physical activity guidelines suggest that 45–60 minutes of daily moderate activity may be necessary (as opposed to 30 minutes).

The balance scale at the top of the pyramid in Figure 3 illustrates the importance of balancing energy intake with energy expenditure. (More information about maintaining energy balance for body composition is included in the Concept on nutrition and the Concept on diet.)

Some important factors should be considered when using the physical activity pyramid. The physical activity pyramid is a useful model for describing different types of activity as well as the benefits and FIT formula for each type.

Moderate Aerobic Activities Aerobic activities equal in intensity to a brisk walk are referred to as moderate activities.

Vigorous Aerobic Activities Aerobic activities that elevate the heart rate and are greater in intensity than a brisk walk.

Vigorous Sports, Recreation, and Anaerobic Activities Vigorous activities characterized by short, intermittent bursts of movement and alternating rest. (See step 3 of the physical activity pyramid.)

Muscle Fitness Activities Higher-intensity resistance activities that contribute to improved muscle strength, muscle endurance, and power. (See step 4 of the physical activity pyramid.)

Flexibility Activities Lower-intensity stretching movements that contribute to improved flexibility and range of motion. (See step 5 of the activity pyramid.)

However, it shouldn't be interpreted too rigidly. The following statements summarize the most important points:

- *No single activity provides all of the benefits.* Many people wonder, "What is the perfect form of physical activity?" There is no single activity that can provide all of the health, wellness, and fitness benefits. It is best to perform activities from all steps of the pyramid because each type of activity has different benefits.

- *Something is better than nothing.* Some people may say, "I just don't have time to do all of the activities in the pyramid." This could lead some to throw up their hands in despair, concluding, "I just won't do anything at all." Evidence indicates that something is better than nothing, so try to do a little activity and add more as time allows.

- *Activities from steps 2 and 3 can be used instead of, or in combination with, those from step 1 to achieve health and fitness benefits.* While more people typically perform moderate activities (step 1), many prefer more vigorous activities from steps 2 and 3 of the pyramid. Both provide health benefits and the two can be combined to meet activity guidelines.

- *Activities from steps 4 and 5 are useful even if you are limited in performing activities at other levels.* It is best to include some activities from steps 1, 2, and 3, but muscle fitness exercise and flexibility exercise do provide benefits on their own.

- *Good planning will allow you to schedule activities from all steps in a reasonable amount of time.* In subsequent Concepts, you will learn more about each step of the pyramid, as well as how to plan a total physical activity program.

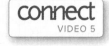

Technology Update

Wearable Technology in Health Care

Many consumers use physical activity monitors and apps on their smartwatches to get real-time reports of their physical activity behaviors. However, new medical applications are also being developed that use integrated sensors in smartwatches and other biosensors to provide clinicians with information that can support patient care. For example, wearable devices can now record blood pressure or electrocardiogram (ECG or EKG) data related to heart rhythms. Other sensors can record blood pressure. Wearable technology will continue to transform health care in years to come.

Would this type of technology be important to you in selecting a smartwatch? Would you be open to sharing data from a smartwatch to potentially improve health monitoring at some point in your life?

Physical Activity Patterns

The percentage of adults who meet physical activity goals varies by sex at birth, age, and ethnicity. National physical activity goals have been established for moderate to vigorous aerobic physical activity as well as for muscle fitness exercise. As noted in Table 1, only about half of Americans meet national goals for aerobic activity and less than a third meet national goals for muscle fitness activity (30 percent). For aerobic activity, males are more active than females and non-Hispanic whites are more active than non-Hispanic Blacks and Hispanics. The age groups that are most likely to meet aerobic activity goals are the youngest group (18–24) and the oldest (65+). For muscle fitness activity, non-Hispanic Blacks meet the goal more often than non-Hispanic whites and Hispanics. Muscle fitness activity decreases with age, with young people being twice as likely to meet the national goals. The good news is that the numbers in Table 1 show higher percentages of adults meeting aerobic activity goals than in the past: 51 percent as compared to 43 percent 10–15 years earlier.

Too many Americans (26 percent) still report performing no regular leisure-time activity. This pattern is more common in females (27 percent) than males (25 percent), more likely in non-Hispanic Blacks (31 percent) and Hispanics (31 percent) than non-Hispanic whites (24 percent), and more likely with increases with age (17 percent for 18–24 compared with 31 percent for 65+).

Table 1 ▶ Percentages of Adults Who Meet National Activity Goals

Classification	Aerobic Activity	Both Aerobic and Muscle Fitness Activity
Gender	Percentage	Percentage
Male	52%	35%
Female	50	26
Age	Percentage	Percentage
18–24	53%	47%
25–34	49	37
35–44	49	31
45–54	50	27
55–64	51	24
65+	49	23
Ethnicity	Percentage	Percentage
Non-Hispanic White	53%	30%
Non-Hispanic Black	44	32
Hispanic	45	29

Source: National Health Interview Survey.

In the News

Move Your Way!

The "Move Your Way" campaign from the U.S. Department of Health and Human Services is designed to help Americans take incremental steps toward becoming more active. One of the major findings reported in the latest *Physical Activity Guidelines for Americans* is that "the benefits of physical activity can be achieved in a variety of ways." "Move Your Way" reinforces this important message, while also acknowledging the challenges that some people face in finding ways to be active. The program provides guidelines and strategies for different segments of the population. A particularly useful assessment tool is the online Activity Planner that guides individuals toward creating their own personal plan. (See Suggested Resources and Readings.)

Does the "Move Your Way" campaign message resonate with you? Will it help promote broader engagement in physical activity in society?

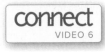

The "weekend warrior" approach to physical activity is not recommended. While guidelines emphasize regular (preferably daily) physical activity, some prefer to pack all of their activity into one or two sessions. These individuals are often called "weekend warriors" since they may get all of their activity on the weekend. A study in *JAMA Internal Medicine* reported that people who exercised regularly on only 1–2 days a week had many of the same benefits as those who exercised more frequently as long as they met the overall goal (i.e., 150 minutes of moderate activity or 75 minutes of vigorous activity per week). The results could lead some to believe that the weekend warrior approach is a sound strategy. However, it is important to note that physical activity in this study was assessed only at the beginning of the study and researchers assumed that participants continued the same level of activity over the many years of the study. More important is the fact that the weekend warriors in this study reported that they regularly met the recommended standards for minutes of moderate and vigorous physical activity per week. They just did the activity (frequently sporting activities) on fewer days per week (1–2 days) instead of the recommended (3 or more days per week). More than half (55 percent) were active on 2 days, so the total volume of activity was likely sufficient to maintain a level of fitness needed to safely perform their activities. The researchers concluded that both approaches had similar outcomes, but the preponderance of evidence supports the recommendation for regular (more frequent) activity. Performing aerobic activity on a more regular basis not too many days apart provides a better approach to fitness, health, and injury prevention. While some activity is better than none, evidence does not support the use of occasional vigorous activity for those who are unfit and those who have not been regularly active.

Physical Fitness Standards

Health-based criterion-referenced standards are recommended for rating your fitness. This Concept has focused on the amount of physical activity necessary to get health and fitness benefits. Another question to be answered is

"How much physical fitness is enough?" Most experts recommend **health-based criterion-referenced standards** to rate your current fitness. These standards are based on how much fitness is needed for good health. Other standards use norms or percentiles that compare a person's fitness against a reference population. Knowing how you compare with other people is not that important. In fact, such comparisons have been shown to be discouraging to many

Strategies for Action: Lab Information

A self-assessment of your current activity at each level of the pyramid can help you determine future activity goals. Lab 6A provides you with the opportunity to assess your physical activity at each level of the pyramid.

Self-assessments of physical fitness can help you prepare a fitness profile that can be used in program planning. In the Concepts that follow, you will learn to perform a variety of self-assessments of fitness and will learn the scores that are necessary on these assessments to reach the good fitness zone, as described in Table 2. In the meantime, you can complete Lab 6B. This lab will help you understand the nature of each part of fitness and allow you to see your personal strengths and weaknesses in fitness. When you complete the more detailed self-assessments later in this edition, you will be able to determine the accuracy of your estimates.

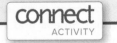

Health-Based Criterion-Referenced Standards The amount of a specific type of fitness necessary to gain a health or wellness benefit.

Table 2 ▶ The Four Fitness Zones

High-Performance Zone

Reaching this zone provides additional health benefits and is important to high-level performance. However, high performance scores are hard for some people to achieve, and for many people high-level performance is not important. So reaching this zone may be more important to some than others.

Good Fitness Zone

If you reach the good fitness zone, you have enough of a specific fitness component to help reduce health risk. However, staying active (in addition to reaching this fitness zone) is important.

Marginal Fitness Zone

Marginal scores indicate that some improvement is in order, but you are nearing minimal health standards set by experts.

Low Fitness Zone

If you score low in fitness, you are probably less fit than you should be for your own good health and wellness.

people. Determining if your fitness is adequate to enhance your health and wellness is more relevant.

In the Concepts that follow, you will perform many different self-assessments to determine your fitness zone for each dimension of fitness. Four different rating zones are used (see Table 2). The long-term goal is to achieve the "good fitness zone," a standard associ- 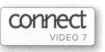 ated with good health. People in the low fitness zone have a higher risk than those in the other three zones and a goal should be to first strive to move out of the low zone into the marginal fitness zone. Those in the marginal zone are at lower risk than those in the low fitness zone, but they should strive to move into the good fitness zone.

With reasonable amounts of physical activity over time, most people should be able to improve their fitness enough to make it into the good fitness zone. For personal reasons, some may wish to aim for the high-performance zone. Reaching the high-performance zone is important for those interested in high-level performance, but should not be a goal of those in the low or marginal fitness zones until the good fitness zone is reached. Reaching this level provides additional health benefits, but considerable effort is necessary to reach it.

Using Self-Management Skills

Knowledge is important to making sound decisions about fitness and health. Building knowledge is a self-management skill needed to help you make good decisions about healthy lifestyles. The information in this Concept is based on the most recent research and guidelines from professional and governmental organizations. Keep up-to-date on current and new recommendations, such as those in the most recent *Physical Activity Guidelines for Americans*. Knowing and applying the physical activity guidelines, such as those described in this Concept, can help you get and stay active.

Self-confidence is especially important in becoming more active. People who lack self-confidence typically don't think they can do something that they actually can do. To build self-confidence, set small, realistic goals that ensure success in order to encourage effort. Basically, "the little train that could" was right. If you set a realistic goal ("I think I can") and achieve several small goals, you gradually accomplish larger goals ("I know I can"). The example used in an earlier Concept applies here. A person says, "I would like to be more active, but I have never been good at physical activities." By starting with a small but reasonable goal, a 10-minute walk, the person sees that "I can do it." Over time, the person becomes confident and increases activity. Getting positive feedback from others (social support) is also effective in building self-confidence.

Intrinsic motivation increases exercise adherence. Intrinsic motivation refers to doing a behavior because it is satisfying to you rather than doing it for an external reward (extrinsic motivation). People who are intrinsically motivated will participate because they enjoy it or because it provides them with a level of satisfaction. For some, previous experiences in physical activity have not been satisfying and this has reduced their intrinsic motivation. Some things that can be done to improve intrinsic motivation include examining your attitudes in order to reduce negative attitudes and increase positive attitudes. You can also do an assessment of your current activities and then try new activities that provide a fresh perspective. Building self-confidence through meeting small and manageable goals can also boost intrinsic motivation by improving your self-perceptions.

Suggested Resources and Readings

The websites for the following sources can be accessed by searching online for the organization, program, or title listed. Specific scientific references are available at the end of this edition of *Concepts of Fitness and Wellness*.

- American College of Sports Medicine. (2021). *ACSM's Guidelines for Exercise Testing and Prescription* (11th ed.). Philadelphia: Wolters Kluwer.
- American Heart Association. AHA Recommendations for Physical Activity in Adults and Kids.
- Centers for Disease Control and Prevention. CDC Physical Activity Trend Maps.
- U.S. Department of Health and Human Services. Move Your Way Activity Planner.
- U.S. Department of Health and Human Services. (2018). *Physical Activity Guidelines for Americans*.

Lab 6A Self-Assessment of Physical Activity

Name	Section	Date

Purpose: To estimate your current levels of physical activity from each category of the physical activity pyramid.

Procedures

1. Place an X over the circle that characterizes your participation in each category in the pyramid. Place an X over one circle, at the bottom of the pyramid, to indicate days of inactivity.
2. Determine if you met the national goal for each type of activity. In the Results section, place an X over the "yes" circle if you meet the goal in each area or an X over the "no" circle if you do not meet the goal.

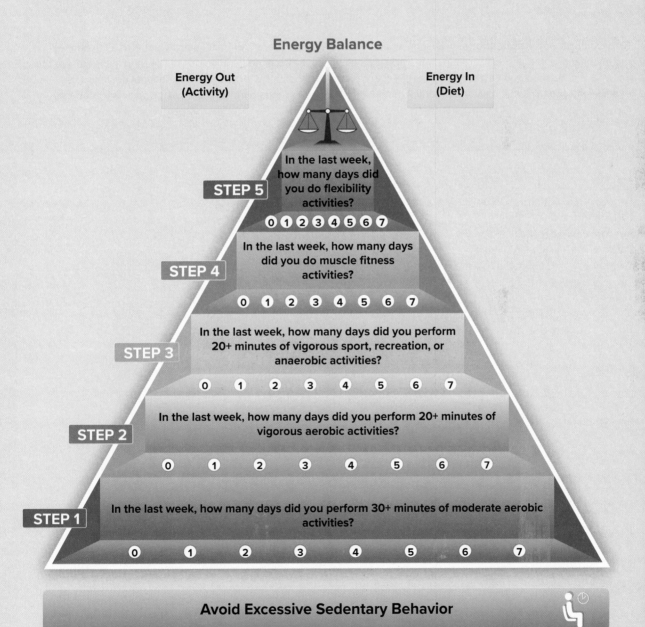

Energy Balance

Energy Out (Activity)   **Energy In (Diet)**

STEP 5 In the last week, how many days did you do flexibility activities?
0 1 2 3 4 5 6 7

STEP 4 In the last week, how many days did you do muscle fitness activities?
0 1 2 3 4 5 6 7

STEP 3 In the last week, how many days did you perform 20+ minutes of vigorous sport, recreation, or anaerobic activities?
0 1 2 3 4 5 6 7

STEP 2 In the last week, how many days did you perform 20+ minutes of vigorous aerobic activities?
0 1 2 3 4 5 6 7

STEP 1 In the last week, how many days did you perform 30+ minutes of moderate aerobic activities?
0 1 2 3 4 5 6 7

Avoid Excessive Sedentary Behavior

Results

Activity Type	Step	National Goal	Did You Meet the National Health Goal?	
Moderate activity	1	5 days or more	Yes	No
Vigorous activity	2 and 3	3 days or more	Yes	No
Muscle fitness	4	2 days or more	Yes	No
Flexibility exercises	5	3 days or more	Yes	No
Inactivity	—	Avoid total inactivity	Yes	No

Conclusions and Implications: In the space below, describe your current physical activity patterns. Do you meet the national health goals in all areas? If not, in what types of activity from the pyramid do you need to improve? Are the answers you gave for the past week typical of your regular activity patterns? If you meet all national health goals, explain why you think this is so. Do you think that meeting the goals in the pyramid indicates good activity patterns for you?

Lab 6B Estimating Your Fitness

Name	Section	Date

Purpose: To help you better understand each of the 11 dimensions of health-related and skill-related physical fitness.

Procedures

1. Consider a warm-up before and cool-down after. Perform each of the activities described in Chart 1.
2. Estimate your current fitness levels. Place a check in the appropriate circle for each fitness dimension in the Results section. If the activity was difficult or if past tests suggest it, check the "low fitness" circle; if the activity was somewhat difficult or if you think you need improvement, check the "marginal fitness" circle; if the task was relatively easy or if past tests indicate it, check the "good fitness" circle; and if you think your fitness in an area is sufficient, check the "high performance" circle.

Special Note: The activities performed in this lab *are not intended as valid tests of physical fitness*. Completing the activities will help you better understand each dimension of fitness. You should not rely primarily on the results of the activities to make your estimates. Consider previous fitness tests you have taken and your own best judgment of your current fitness. In later Concepts, you will learn how to perform accurate assessments of each fitness dimension that will help you assess the accuracy of your estimates.

Results

Fitness Zones

Fitness Component	Low Fitness	Marginal Fitness	Good Fitness	High Performance
Body Composition	◯	◯	◯	◯
Cardiorespiratory Endurance	◯	◯	◯	◯
Flexibility	◯	◯	◯	◯
Muscular Endurance	◯	◯	◯	◯
Power	◯	◯	◯	◯
Strength	◯	◯	◯	◯
Agility	◯	◯	◯	◯
Balance	◯	◯	◯	◯
Coordination	◯	◯	◯	◯
Reaction Time	◯	◯	◯	◯
Speed	◯	◯	◯	◯

Conclusions and Implications: Describe the information you used to make your estimates of physical fitness. How confident are you that these estimates are accurate?

Directions: Attempt each of the activities in Chart 1. Place a check in the circle next to each component of physical fitness to indicate that you have attempted the activity.

Chart 1 Physical Fitness Activities

Body Composition ◯

1. *The pinch.* Have a partner pinch a fold of fat on the back of your upper arm (body fatness), halfway between the tip of the elbow and the tip of the shoulder.

   Men: no greater than 3/4 inch

   Women: no greater than 1 inch

Cardiorespiratory Endurance ◯

2. *Run in place.* Run in place for 1.5 minutes (120 steps per minute). Rest for 1 minute and count the heart rate for 30 seconds. A heart rate of 60 (for 30 sec.) or lower passes. A step is counted each time the right foot hits the floor.

Flexibility ◯

3. *Backsaver toe touch.* Sit on the floor with one foot against a wall. Bend the other knee. Bend forward at the hips. After three warm-up trials, reach forward and touch your closed fists to the wall. Bend forward slowly; do not bounce. Repeat with the other leg straight. Pass if fists touch the wall with each leg straight.

Muscular Endurance ◯

4. *Side leg raise.* Lie on the floor on your side. Lift your leg up and to the side of the body until your feet are 24–36 inches apart. Keep the knee and pelvis facing forward. Do not rotate so that the knees face the ceiling. Perform 10 with each leg.

Power ◯

5. *Standing long jump.* Stand with the toes behind a line. Using no run or hop step, jump as far as possible. Men must jump their height plus 6 inches. Women must jump their height only.

Strength ◯

6. *Push-up.* Lie face down on the floor. Place the hands under the shoulders. Keeping the legs and body straight, press off the floor until the arms are fully extended. Women repeat once; men, three times.

Agility ◯

7. *Paper ball pickup.* Place two wadded paper balls on the floor 5 feet away. Run until both feet cross the line, pick up the first ball, and return both feet behind the starting line. Repeat with the second ball. Finish in 5 seconds.

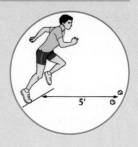
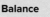

Balance ◯

8. *One-foot balance.* Stand on one foot; press up so that the weight is on the ball of the foot with the heel off the floor. Hold the hands and the other leg straight out in front for 10 seconds.

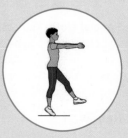

Coordination ◯

9. *Paper ball bounce.* Wad up a sheet of notebook paper into a ball. Bounce the ball back and forth between the right and left hands. Keep the hands open and palms up. Bounce the ball three times with each hand (six times total), alternating hands for each bounce.

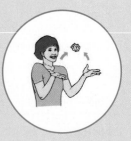

Reaction Time ◯

10. *Paper drop.* Have a partner hold a sheet of notebook paper so that the side edge is between your thumb and index finger, about the width of your hand from the top of the page. When your partner drops the paper, catch it before it slips through the thumb and finger. Do not lower your hand to catch the paper.

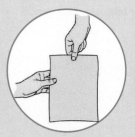

Speed ◯

11. *Double-heel click.* With the feet apart, jump up and tap the heels together twice before you hit the ground. You must land with your feet at least 3 inches apart.

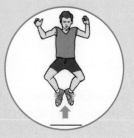
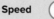

Adopting an Active Lifestyle

LEARNING OBJECTIVES

After completing the study of this Concept, you will be able to:

▶ Define moderate physical activity and differentiate it from light and vigorous physical activity.

▶ Describe the health benefits of moderate physical activity, and explain why moderate physical activity is the most popular form of physical activity.

▶ Describe and explain the FIT formula for moderate physical activity.

▶ Plan a personal moderate physical activity program based on SMART goals, and self-monitor your plan.

▶ Evaluate your current environment and determine ways to modify it to encourage moderate physical activity.

▶ Describe the risks associated with inactivity, including excessive sitting.

Inactivity has many health risks that can be overcome with regular moderate-intensity physical activity.

Blend Images/Michael DeYoung/Getty Images

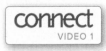

Why It Matters!

Humans are clearly meant to move, but the nature of our society has made it difficult for many people to lead active lifestyles. Cars, motorized golf carts, riding lawn mowers, elevators, remote control devices, and email are just some of the modern conveniences that have reduced the amount of activity in our daily lives.

Finding ways to get regular physical activity is critical for optimal health, wellness, and fitness; but it is now clear that avoiding inactivity is also important. In fact, evidence suggests that sedentary living (i.e., too much sitting) puts your health at risk even if you are physically active. In this Concept, you will learn about the risks associated with excessive sedentary behavior as well as the benefits of moderate activity (sometimes referred to as moderate-intensity activity). You will also learn strategies to help you avoid sedentary living and incorporate moderate activity into your daily routine.

Fundamentals of Active Living

Various behaviors constitute an active lifestyle. Most people have an intuitive understanding of what constitutes physical activity but may not be aware that it refers to an array of behaviors. The five steps in the physical activity pyramid illustrate the different types of physical activity (Figure 1). As described in a previous Concept, there is a unique FIT formula for each type of activity in the pyramid. All of the activities in the pyramid provide health, wellness, and fitness benefits; however, each type of activity has some unique benefits, as described in this and subsequent Concepts.

Both sedentary living and inactive behavior should be avoided. The terms *inactive* and *sedentary* are seemingly similar but have quite different meanings. *Inactivity* refers to a lack of physical activity as indicated by the failure to meet national physical activity goals. *Sedentary* refers to behaviors that are of low intensity, such as lying or sitting. A person can meet guidelines for physical activity but still spend too much time being sedentary. It is now clear that sedentary behavior presents risks to a person's health, independent of the level of activity. In other words, there are health risks even for active people who sit too much. The phrase "Avoid Excessive Sedentary Behavior" is included in bold black type below the pyramid to emphasize the independent risks associated with sedentary lifestyles. It is important to note that some sedentary behavior is important to productive and healthy living. Work and leisure activities are appropriate forms of sedentary behaviors; but it is still important to still minimize extended periods of sitting by taking intermittent breaks.

Moderate physical activity is the foundation of an active lifestyle. Moderate physical activity is included at the base of the physical activity pyramid (see Figure 1) because it can be performed by virtually all people, regardless of fitness level or age. Moderate activities include some activities of daily living as well as less intense sports and recreational activities. Taking a brisk walk is a simple and logical way to incorporate moderate activity into daily living. However, activities of daily living, such as walking the dog, gardening, mowing the lawn, doing carpentry, or doing housework, can count as moderate activities.

Walking is the most popular of all leisure-time activities among adults. Females walk more than males, and young adults (aged 18–29) walk less than older adults, probably because of more involvement in sports and other vigorous activities. As many as 40–50 percent of

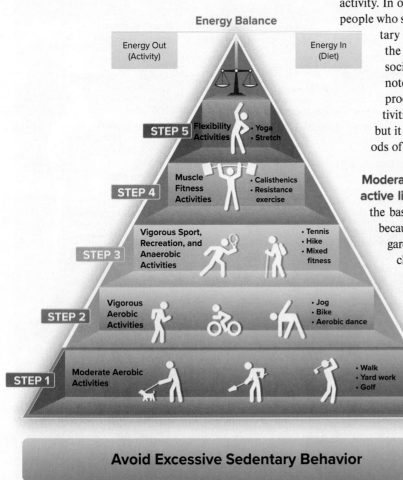

Energy Balance

Energy Out (Activity)

Energy In (Diet)

STEP 5 Flexibility Activities
• Yoga
• Stretch

STEP 4 Muscle Fitness Activities
• Calisthenics
• Resistance exercise

STEP 3 Vigorous Sport, Recreation, and Anaerobic Activities
• Tennis
• Hike
• Mixed fitness

STEP 2 Vigorous Aerobic Activities
• Jog
• Bike
• Aerobic dance

STEP 1 Moderate Aerobic Activities
• Walk
• Yard work
• Golf

Avoid Excessive Sedentary Behavior

Figure 1 ▶ The physical activity pyramid, step 1: Moderate Aerobic Activities.

In the News

Sedentary Behavior and Mental Health

The COVID-19 pandemic exposed many issues and challenges associated with mental health in society. While uncertainty, stress, and isolation are key contributors, a sedentary lifestyle may also influence malaise and depression. Excess sedentary time has been found to exaggerate mood problems, so experts have been concerned that it may compound or amplify mental health problems associated with COVID-19. Many people have found physical activity to be a valuable release, but minimizing sedentary activities is also important. A recent study documented that substituting prolonged sedentary time with sleep was associated with lower stress and better mood. Substituting sedentary activity with light physical activity was also associated with improved mood.

Do you currently take steps to intentionally limit sedentary behavior? Do you consider the "quality" of your sedentary behavior?

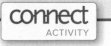
connect
ACTIVITY

adults say they walk, but less than half that number report walking 30 minutes or more at least 5 days a week.

While overall activity levels tend to decline with age, involvement in lifestyle activity actually tends to increase. This is because many older adults move away from vigorous sports and recreation and spend more time in lifestyle activities, such as gardening and golf. Older adults tend to have more time and money for these types of recreational activities, and the lower intensity may be appealing. The advantage of moderate activity is that there are many opportunities to be active. Finding enjoyable activities that fit into your daily routine is the key to adopting a more active lifestyle.

Physical activity can be characterized by intensity. Scientists classify activities based on how they compare to the amount of energy expended at rest. Resting energy expenditure is defined as 1 metabolic equivalent, or 1 MET. Other activities are then assigned values in multiples of METs. For generally healthy adults, an activity that requires an energy expenditure of 3.0–6.0 METs is classified as a moderate-intensity activity. This means that it requires between three and six times the energy expended while at rest. Forms of **moderate physical activity (MPA)** are often referred to as aerobic physical activities because the aerobic metabolism can typically meet the energy demand of the activity. This allows moderate activities to be performed comfortably for extended periods of time by most people.

Activities above 6 METs are categorized as **vigorous physical activity (VPA)**, and these cannot usually be maintained as easily unless a person has a good level of fitness. Examples include more structured aerobic activities (e.g., jogging, biking, swimming) or vigorous sports (e.g., soccer). Activities below 3.0 METs can be classified as light intensity, but researchers now distinguish **light physical activity (LPA)** from sedentary behavior. Examples of LPA include lower-intensity activities of daily living such as showering, grocery shopping, washing dishes, and casual walking, and these activities range from 1.5 to 3.0 METs. Sedentary behavior is characterized by sitting and lying postures and have MET values ranging from 1.0 to

1.5. While sleeping involves lying and is a resting activity, it is considered as a separate activity and is not considered as sedentary behavior in this type of classification. Distinctions among the types of activities are summarized in Table 1.

Table 1 ▶ Classification of Physical Activity Intensities for Generally Healthy Adults

Classification	Intensity Range	Examples
Sedentary	1.0–1.5 METs	Sitting, lying
Light	1.5–3.0 METs	Showering, grocery shopping, playing musical instrument, washing dishes
Moderate	3.0–6.0 METs	Walking briskly, mowing lawn, playing table tennis, doing carpentry
Vigorous	>6.0 METs	Hiking, jogging, digging ditches, playing soccer

Moderate Physical Activity (MPA) An activity that can be comfortably sustained (similar to brisk walking) with intensities 3.0 to 6.0 three times as intense as lying or sitting at rest (3–6 METs).

Vigorous Physical Activity (VPA) An activity that is more vigorous than a moderate activity, with intensities at least six times as intense as lying or sitting at rest (>6 METs).

Light Physical Activity (LPA) An activity that involves standing and/or slow movements with intensities 1.5 to 3.0 times as intense as lying or sitting at rest (1.5–3.0 METs).

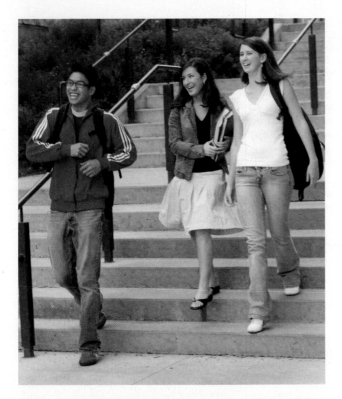

Brief walks throughout the day can help you meet recommended levels of moderate activity.
Purestock/Superstock

Activity classifications vary depending on one's level of fitness. Normal walking is considered light activity for a person with good fitness (see Table 2), but for a person with low to marginal fitness the same activity is considered moderate. Similarly, brisk walking may be a vigorous activity (rather than moderate) for individuals with low fitness. Table 2 helps you determine the type of lifestyle activity considered moderate for you. Beginners with low fitness should start with normal rather than brisk walking, for example. In later Concepts, you will learn to assess your current fitness level. You may want to refer back to Table 2 after you have made self-assessments of your fitness.

Minimizing Sedentary Behavior Is Part of an Active Lifestyle

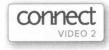

Sedentary behavior is an established risk factor for many chronic diseases. Extended periods of sedentary time have been associated with obesity, diabetes risk, and a number of other conditions, even if a person gets sufficient amounts of physical activity. Numerous studies have documented these effects, but perhaps the strongest evidence to date to support a direct relationship between time spent sitting and risk of early mortality is from a large longitudinal study of over 8,000 adults. The study monitored lifestyle patterns using objective activity monitors that captured both the total sedentary time as well as the extent of prolonged sitting. By monitoring the same participants over time, the researchers were able to examine associations between sedentary behavior and various health risks. In the primary analyses, risk of death was greater for those with more sitting time (and longer sedentary bouts) even after controlling for age, weight status, and exercise habits.

Research has also clarified the biochemical mechanisms that explain health risks associated with sedentary living. Interestingly, the mechanisms are similar to the established pathways that link hypertension and high cholesterol to cardiovascular disease. In both cases, blood vessel inflammation is a precursor to impaired arterial health which then contributes to cardiovascular disease. Reducing or minimizing extended bouts of sedentary time is important for reducing common health risks.

Reducing sedentary behavior is important to good health and wellness. Public health guidelines now specifically emphasize the importance of minimizing sedentary behavior. But how much is excessive? Evidence suggests that both the total amount of time spent in sedentary behavior and the length of continuous periods of sitting are associated with health risks. For example, studies indicate that taking breaks in sedentary time leads to improvements in metabolic

Table 2 ▶ Classification of Moderate Physical Activities for People of Different Fitness Levels				
	Activity Classification by Fitness Level			
Sample Lifestyle Activities	**Low Fitness**	**Marginal Fitness**	**Good Fitness**	**High Performance**
Washing face, dressing, typing, driving	Light	Very light or light	Very light	Very light
Normal walking, bowling, mopping	Moderate	Moderate	Light	Light
Brisk walking, shoveling, social dancing	Vigorous	Moderate/vigorous	Moderate	Moderate

health profiles (i.e., better glucose/insulin regulation) even if the total amount of sedentary time is the same. Therefore, minimizing the total amount of sedentary time and taking periodic breaks to avoid extended periods of sitting are recommended.

The type of sedentary behavior also matters. Studies have documented that mentally passive activities such as watching television are more likely to be associated with depression and low mood than more stimulating sedentary activities such as working on a computer, playing a game, or doing puzzles. The COVID-19 pandemic has brought greater attention to issues of isolation and sedentary behavior. While binge-watching television is a common way to pass time, it probably is best to mix up and alter your choices of sedentary activities to support mental health.

Although the research is still evolving, there is consensus that sedentary behavior detracts from health in multiple ways. An international collaboration called the Sedentary Behavior Research Network is focused on studying sedentary behavior, and the World Health Organization (WHO) has recently released updated international guidelines on physical activity and sedentary behaviors. The guidelines provide the basis for implementing the *Global Action Plan on Physical Activity 2030*. See A Closer Look for details.

Light activity is better than no activity. National physical activity guidelines focus on the accumulation of MPA and VPA as shown in the physical activity pyramid. However, the national guidelines also make it clear that some activity is better than no activity. Even shifting sedentary time to forms of LPA can have positive effects. The main advantage of the accumulation of light activity is that it likely reflects less time spent in sedentary activities. The *Canadian 24-Hour Movement Guidelines* specifically reference the importance of making daily choices to balance physical activity, sedentary behavior, and sleep as part of an active lifestyle. The guidelines provide an important message since time spent in one category influences the available time for others. Adopting a 24-hour perspective on your daily lifestyle choices is a sound strategy for active and healthy living.

Minimizing sedentary time can also have implications for weight control. The bulk of our day is typically spent in sedentary behaviors, but incorporating LPA into your day can help burn more calories. Some researchers refer to LPA as non-exercise activity thermogenesis (NEAT) to emphasize the substantial number of calories that can be burned by performing more LPA. The use of a standing desk is one way to minimize harmful effects of sedentary behavior while also helping burn more calories.

While LPA is better than no activity, it is not sufficient to obtain the health benefits associated with MPA or VPA. The independence of physical activity and sedentary behavior is captured in the heat-map image in Figure 2. The section in the upper left corner (red area) is the high-risk zone since that area reflects low physical activity and high sedentary behavior. The area in the lower right corner (green area) is the low-risk zone since it reflects high physical activity and low sedentary behavior. Efforts to minimize sedentary time move you down the *y*-axis toward the green zone. Similarly, adding moderate or vigorous activity to your routine also

A CLOSER LOOK

Sedentary Behavior: How Much Is Too Much?

Bold and direct statements such as "sitting is the new smoking" have helped promote awareness about the harmful effects of sedentary behavior. New international guidelines by the World Health Organization support that sedentary behavior is a significant public health threat. Many organizations are also working to change societal perceptions and habits related to sedentary behavior. A group called JustStand.org says its mission is to lead the "uprising (literally and figuratively) to sit less, stand up and move more." (See Suggested Resources and Readings to further explore the harmful effects of sedentary behavior.)

Has the emphasis on sedentary behavior in the popular press influenced your behavior? Do you believe "sitting is the new smoking" or do you think this is overstated?

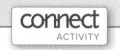

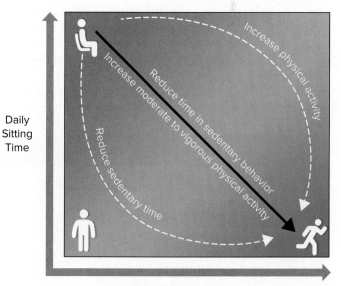

Moderate-to-Vigorous Physical Activity

Risk of all-cause mortality decreases as one moves from red to green.

Figure 2 ▶ Conceptual model showing combined health risks of high levels of sedentary behavior and low levels of physical activity.

moves you toward the green zone by moving you to the right on the *x*-axis. The best option is to replace sedentary time with physical activity, but replacing sedentary time with LPA can contribute to good health.

The Health and Wellness Benefits of Moderate Physical Activity

Moderate physical activity provides significant health benefits. Research has clearly shown that even modest amounts of MPA have significant health benefits. Two early studies paved the way for this line of research. One study reported that postal workers who delivered mail had fewer health problems than workers who sorted mail. Another study reported that drivers of double-decker buses in the United Kingdom had more health problems than conductors who climbed the stairs during the day to collect the tickets. The studies controlled for other lifestyle factors, so the improved health was attributed to the extra activity accumulated throughout the day. Since then, hundreds of studies have further confirmed the importance of MPA for good health.

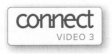

Moderate physical activity promotes metabolic fitness. Metabolic fitness is fitness of the systems that provide the energy for effective daily living. Indicators of good metabolic fitness include normal blood lipid levels, normal blood pressure, normal blood sugar levels, and healthy body fat levels. Moderate physical activity promotes metabolic fitness by keeping the metabolic system active. Building and maintaining cardiorespiratory endurance requires a regular challenge to the cardiovascular system, and building metabolic fitness requires a similar regular challenge to the metabolic system. Individuals with good levels of fitness will receive primarily **metabolic fitness benefits** from moderate activity, but those with low fitness will likely receive metabolic and cardiorespiratory endurance benefits. Moderate activity is particularly important for the large segments of the population that do not participate in other forms of regular exercise. As previously described, some activity is clearly better than none.

Moderate physical activity has wellness benefits. The health benefits from physical activity are impressive, but the **wellness benefits** may have a bigger impact on our daily lives. Numerous studies have shown that physical activity is associated with improved quality of life, but it has proven difficult to determine the contributing factors or underlying mechanisms. The influence may be due to reduced stress, improved cognition, better sleep, improved self-esteem, reduced fatigue, or (more likely) a combination of many different effects. Research suggests that college students who are more physically active have more positive feeling states ("pleasant-activated feelings") than students who are less physically active, even after controlling for sleep and previous days' activity and feeling states. They also noted that feeling states improved on days when people reported performing more activity than normal. Multiple studies documented the importance of physical activity as a coping strategy during the COVID-19 pandemic.

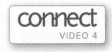

Accumulating Moderate Physical Activity

There is a FIT formula for moderate physical activity. Public health guidelines for physical activity have recommended that adults accumulate 150 minutes of moderate-intensity activity each week, an amount equal to 30 minutes 5 days a week. Although these are considered minimal levels, or threshold levels, for health, performing more can provide additional benefits. Thus, to achieve the target zone you should aim for the accumulation of 30–60 minutes (or more) per day. Table 3 summarizes the frequency, intensity, and time (duration) guidelines to meet the threshold levels or to achieve the target zone for MPA.

Table 3 ▶ The FIT Formula for Moderate Physical Activity		
	Threshold of Training (minimum)[a]	**Target Zone (optimal)**
Frequency	At least 5 days a week	5–7 days a week
Intensity[b]	• Equal to brisk walking[b] • 3–5 METs[b]	• Equal to brisk to fast walking[b] • 3–6 METs[b]
Time (duration)[c]	Accumulation of 30 minutes	Accumulation of 30–60 minutes or more
Volume[d]	• Total of 500 MET-minutes per day • Expend about 150 calories per day	• Total of 1,000 or more MET-minutes • Expend up to 300 calories or more per day

[a]The recommendation of 150 minutes can be accumulated throughout the week, but these thresholds provide a good target.
[b]Heart rate and relative perceived exertion can also be used to determine intensity.
[c]Depends on fitness level.
[d]MET-minutes are standardized, but energy expenditure levels are based on a 70 kg person (see Table 4).

Vigorous activity can substitute for moderate activity.
The *Physical Activity Guidelines for Americans* focus on the volume of physical activity performed. Moderate activity is sufficient to meet the guidelines, but VPA can also be substituted to meet the weekly targets. According to the guidelines, each minute of VPA counts as 2 minutes of MPA. Therefore, the guideline can also be met by performing 75 minutes of VPA instead of 150 minutes of MPA. It is common to see guidelines emphasize moderate or vigorous physical activity (MVPA) to reflect the notion that they both count in meeting guidelines.

Another effective way to compute an overall volume of physical activity is to focus on the total number of *MET-minutes* of physical activity you perform. To compute MET-minutes, you simply multiply the MET level of the activity you performed by the number of minutes. For example, a 30-minute brisk walk (approximately 3 METs) would yield 90 MET-minutes (3 METs × 30 minutes). However, note that this same volume can also be achieved with a 15-minute run that requires approximately 6 METs (6 METs × 15 minutes). The threshold of training is set at accumulating 500 MET-minutes per week through combinations of MPA or VPA while the target zone is set at 1,000 MET-minutes per week (see Table 3). Some people might prefer to perform longer and more relaxed bouts of MPA while others may prefer to perform shorter sessions of VPA. Both can contribute to meeting the physical activity guidelines.

Moderate activity can be accumulated throughout the day to meet guidelines. Sustained bouts of activity are recommended, but accumulating MPA throughout the day also provides benefits. Previous guidelines suggested that bouts of activity should be 10 minutes in length or longer to be meaningful. However, the evidence has not supported the importance of the specific 10-minute bout recommendation. Aiming for extended bouts of activity is best, but short-duration moderate activity accumulated throughout the day is also beneficial. The intermittent activity can also be helpful for breaking up sedentary time.

Figure 3 illustrates the activity profiles for three different people that accumulate MPA in different ways. The pink line profiles a person who is inactive except for brief walks from the car to the office in the morning and from the office to the car in the evening. This person is sedentary and does not meet the MPA guideline. Because some activity is better than none, the brief walks are better than no activity at all. The green line represents the activity of a person who meets the MPA standard in multiple bouts, including lifestyle activities such as walking to and from work, walking to lunch, and climbing the stairs. In contrast, the blue line represents a person who is sedentary most of the day but

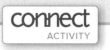
meets the MPA by taking a long walk on a treadmill during the noon hour. You can accumulate activity using the method that you prefer while working to achieve the recommended guidelines.

Individual needs are more important than population guidelines. Guidelines for physical activity depend on the unique needs of the target population. Special guidelines have been developed for children since they need more physical activity than adults. Youth are encouraged to obtain at least 60 minutes and up to several hours of activity each day since it is important for optimal growth and development. Unique guidelines may be appropriate for older adults and adults with chronic conditions. As previously described (see Table 2), activity that is moderate for young adults may be too intense for some older individuals or those with health problems. Because of this, recommendations for these individuals generally focus on tracking minutes of activity. This allows the intensity to be a self-determined level that corresponds to a person's relative level of fitness. Although guidelines provide useful public health targets, ultimately each individual must establish a personal commitment to be physically active.

Metabolic Fitness Benefits Improvements in metabolic function that reduce risks of diabetes and metabolic syndrome.

Wellness Benefits Increases in quality of life and well-being.

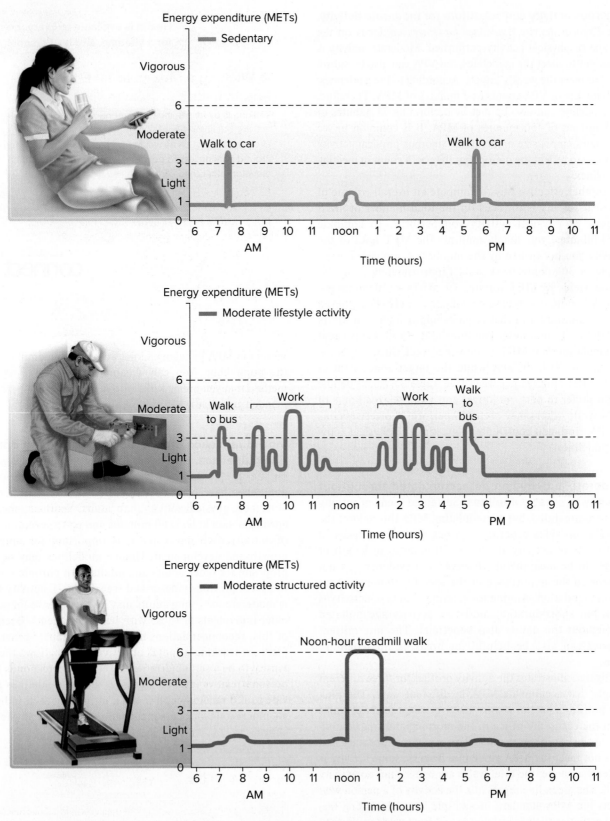

Figure 3 ▶ Comparison of people performing moderate activity in different ways.

Monitoring Physical Activity and Sedentary Behavior

Step counts can help monitor physical activity patterns. Steps have become a popular and well-understood metric to quantify physical activity. Digital pedometers have been used for years to provide an easy way for people to track steps, but step counts can be reported on other monitoring devices, including various consumer activity monitors and smartphone apps. Steps provide a good indicator of activity for most people since most forms of activity involve some locomotor movement (major exceptions would be swimming and cycling). The ability to easily monitor daily step counts provides a helpful reminder to many people about the importance of being active during the day.

Studies on large numbers of people provide data to help classify people into activity categories based on step counts (see Table 4), but it is beneficial to set goals on your own baseline. Wear the pedometer (or similar monitoring device) for 1 week to establish a baseline step count (average steps per day). Then, set a goal of increasing steps per day by 1,000 to 3,000 steps. Walking a mile is approximately 1,500–2,000 steps for most people, so this increment would provide a reasonable short-term goal. Keep records of daily step counts to help you determine if you are meeting your goal. Setting a goal that you are likely to meet will help you find success. As you meet your goal, increase your step counts gradually.

There are some limitations in using steps as indicators of total physical activity. A person with longer legs will accumulate fewer steps over the same distance than someone with shorter strides (due to a longer stride length). A person running will also accumulate fewer steps over the same distance than a person who walks. There is considerable variability in the quality (and accuracy) of monitors and step counting apps, so it is also important to consider this when interpreting data.

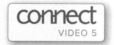

Activity monitors and cell phone apps can track and promote physical activity. The marketplace is flooded with an array of consumer activity monitors that provide estimates of time spent in physical activity. Most devices are now designed to be worn on the wrist since it is a comfortable location. This has also enabled features to be directly built into smartwatches that automatically link to associated cell phone apps. The leading devices in the marketplace include Fitbit (now owned by Google), Garmin, and Apple Watch. The devices vary in accuracy, but studies have consistently found consumer monitors to be less accurate than similar types of monitoring devices used by researchers. This isn't surprising since the need for precision isn't as important to most consumers. However, the algorithms built into these devices continue to improve over time. Many devices now integrate data from embedded heart rate sensors in the wrist bands to improve the accuracy of the estimates and the utility of the data. The heart rate data, for example, help monitors detect activities that may not involve motion at the wrist such as biking. The utility and functionality of the monitor for your particular lifestyle is an important consideration when selecting a monitor for personal use.

Behavioral feedback from monitors (and associated phone apps) can also promote physical activity and remind users to stand up and move more during the day (thereby minimizing sedentary time). Some have prompts or start vibrating if the monitor has been stationary for more than 60 minutes. Other devices provide visual cues or feedback on the screen. While consumer devices have many features designed to prompt behavior, acting on the prompts still requires personal decision making and self-management skills. Some evidence has also documented that excessive monitoring can add pressure or lead to compulsive exercise. The features in these devices and apps can help some make behavior changes but may not be effective or practical for others.

Energy expenditure can be used to monitor physical activity. The overall volume of physical activity can be evaluated by computing the energy cost of different activities that you perform. The recommendation highlighted in the original *Surgeon General's Report on Physical Activity* in 1996 focused on energy expenditure and called for adults to accumulate about 1,000 kcal/week (or about 150 kcal/day). Thus, as shown in Table 3, an energy expenditure of between 150 and 300 kcal/day from physical activity is also sufficient for meeting physical activity guidelines. While not as simple as tracking time, calories expended from physical activity can be estimated if the approximate MET value of the activity is known. The energy cost of resting energy expenditure (1 MET) is approximately 1 calorie per kilogram of body weight per hour (1 kcal/kg/hr). An activity such as brisk walking (4 mph) requires an energy expenditure of about 4 METs, or 4 kcal/kg/hr. A 150-lb person (~70 kg) walking for an hour would expend about 280 kcal (4 kcal/hr × 70 kg × 1 hr). Note that a 30-minute walk would burn approximately 150 calories and satisfy the guideline.

Table 4 ▶ Activity Classification for Pedometer Step Counts in Healthy Adults

Category		Steps/Day
Sedentary		<5,000
Low active		5,000–6,999
Somewhat active	Threshold	7,000–9,999
Active	Target Zone	10,000–12,500
Very active		>12,500

Source: Based on values from Tudor-Locke.

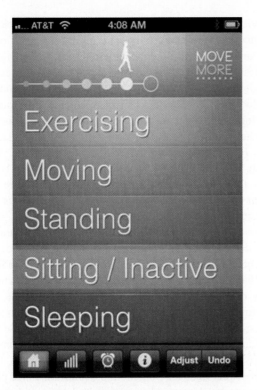

Smartphone apps provide feedback to help track active and sedentary time.
©Apgeo Design, LLC.

Commercial fitness equipment can provide energy expenditure estimates. The devices use an estimated MET level based on the selected intensity or a measured heart rate (if a heart rate sensor is used). The timer on the machine then tracks the time of the workout, and this allows calories to be estimated during the workout. The accuracy of the estimate will depend on the internal calculations, but energy expenditure can't be estimated unless body weight is entered during the setup process. If this wasn't obtained, the calorie estimates are probably based on some reference value of weight and therefore may not be accurate. Table 5 lists estimated METs for different activities, along with calorie estimates (per hour of exercise) for people of different body weights.

Adopting and Sustaining an Active Identity

Seek ways to reduce and/or break up sedentary time. Much time in our daily lives is spent being sedentary (e.g., reading/studying, working at computers, driving in cars, eating). A key for healthy living (and weight control) is to minimize time spent being sedentary. The popularity of standing desks has increased in recent years as a way to promote more activity at work (see the Technology Update). Minimizing time spent watching television or standing while on the phone can also help reduce total sedentary time. The negative effects of sedentary time can also be minimized with periodic

Technology Update

Standing Desks and Treadmill Desks

Many office workers now embrace flexible and active workstations that enable them to stand or move more freely while working. However, most people don't have access to the same type of furniture at home and may gravitate back to sitting if they work from home. Flexible work environments, online meetings, and telecommuting have changed how we live and work. However, minimizing sedentary time and maintaining good posture are important regardless of location. Home-based workers can consider options for customizing or updating existing desks to facilitate standing while working at their computer. (See link in Suggested Resources and Readings.)

Do you consciously try to minimize excess sedentary time while working or studying? Would you take advantage of an active workstation if it was available on campus or at your work/home office? Why or why not?

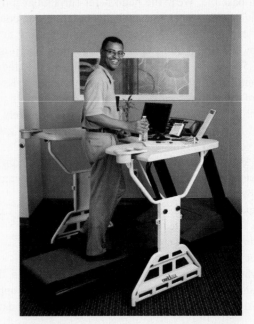

©TrekDesk

connect
ACTIVITY

breaks. Research suggests that the risks are due to prolonged sitting, so take periodic standing breaks.

Seek out ways to add physical activity into your day. Active commuting is one way to add physical activity to your lifestyle. It takes additional preparation and the logistics can be challenging, but it is a great way to build activity into your day. In addition to providing beneficial amounts of physical activity, this can save time, reduce gas, save money, and help the environment. Another option

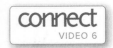

connect
VIDEO 6

Table 5 ▶ Calories Expended in Lifestyle Physical Activities

Activity Classification/Description	METs[a]	Calories Used per Hour for Different Body Weights					
		100 lb (45 kg)	120 lb (55 kg)	150 lb (70 kg)	180 lb (82 kg)	200 lb (91 kg)	220 lb (100 kg)
Gardening Activities							
Gardening (general)	5.0	227	273	341	409	455	502
Mowing lawn (hand mower)	6.0	273	327	409	491	545	599
Mowing lawn (power mower)	4.5	205	245	307	368	409	450
Raking leaves	4.0	182	218	273	327	364	401
Shoveling snow	6.0	273	327	409	491	545	599
Home Activities							
Child care	3.5	159	191	239	286	318	350
Cleaning, washing dishes	2.5	114	136	170	205	227	249
Cooking/food preparation	2.5	114	136	170	205	227	249
Home/auto repair	3.0	136	164	205	245	273	301
Painting	4.5	205	245	307	368	409	450
Strolling with child	2.5	114	136	170	205	227	249
Sweeping/vacuuming	2.5	114	136	170	205	227	249
Washing/waxing car	4.5	205	245	307	368	409	450
Leisure Activities							
Bocci ball/croquet	2.5	114	136	170	205	227	249
Bowling	3.0	136	164	205	245	273	301
Canoeing	5.0	227	273	341	409	455	501
Cross-country skiing (leisure)	7.0	318	382	477	573	636	699
Cycling (<10 mph)	4.0	182	218	273	327	364	401
Cycling (12–14 mph)	8.0	364	436	545	655	727	799
Dancing (social)	4.5	205	245	307	368	409	450
Fishing	4.0	182	218	273	327	364	401
Golf (riding)	3.5	159	191	239	286	318	350
Golf (walking)	5.5	250	300	375	450	500	550
Horseback riding	4.0	182	218	273	327	364	401
Swimming (leisure)	6.0	273	327	409	491	545	599
Table tennis	4.0	182	218	273	327	364	401
Walking (3.5 mph)	3.8	173	207	259	311	346	387
Occupational Activities							
Bricklaying/masonry	7.0	318	382	477	573	636	699
Carpentry	3.5	159	191	239	286	318	350
Construction	5.5	250	300	375	450	500	550
Electrical work/plumbing	3.5	159	191	239	286	318	350
Digging	7.0	318	382	477	573	636	699
Farming	5.5	250	300	375	450	500	550
Store clerk	3.5	159	191	239	286	318	350
Waiter/waitress	4.0	182	218	273	327	364	401

Note: MET values and caloric estimates are based on values listed in *Compendium of Physical Activities.*
[a]*Based* on values of those with "good fitness" ratings.
Source: Ainsworth et al. (2011). "2011 Compendium of Physical Activities: A Second Update of Codes and MET Values." *Medicine and Science in Sports and Exercise,* 43(8), 1575–1581.

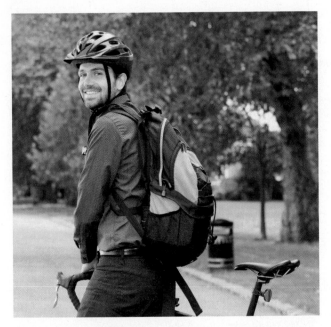

Bike commuting is an effective way to add physical activity to your day.
©Image Source/CORBIS

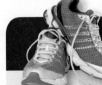

Strategies for Action: Lab Information

Preparing a plan of moderate physical activity plan, including SMART goals, is a good place to start. Moderate physical activity is something that virtually anyone can do. In Lab 7A, you will set moderate physical activity goals and plan a 1-week moderate physical activity program. As you prepare your goals and plan, keep in mind the guidelines on SMART goals. For some people, this plan may be the main component of a lifetime plan. For others, it may be only a beginning that leads to the selection of activities from other levels of the physical activity pyramid. Even the most active people should consider regular moderate physical activity because it is a type of activity that can be done throughout life.

Self-monitoring moderate physical activity can help you stick with it. The self-monitoring chart in Lab 7A not only helps you keep a log of moderate activities (or step counts), but it also lets you hone your self-management skills. Charts like this can be copied to make a log book for long-term activity self-monitoring.

Self-monitoring of sedentary behavior can help you minimize sedentary time. In Lab 7B, you will conduct an assessment of your sedentary behavior. You will determine time spent being inactive and also calculate a Sedentary Behavior Index based on the ratio of your sedentary to light activity. Reducing time spent in sedentary behavior takes conscious effort, but the lab will provide a way to examine it.

connect
ACTIVITY

is to take more active trips to the store. Research suggests that the overwhelming majority of our car trips are 1 mile or less. Walking or biking even a few of these trips can have a big impact. The ability to walk or bike to work or to the store may not be possible for you because of the nature of your community or the safety of the roads. However, there are a number of other strategies you can use to get more activity in your day. Consider parking farther away from store entrances, using the stairs rather than the elevator, taking walking breaks, and even standing (instead of sitting) when convenient. Adopting an active lifestyle in a sedentary society is challenging, but it is within your control.

Using Self-Management Skills

Preparing a moderate physical activity plan requires the use of multiple self-management skills. You can use the six steps in program planning outlined in the Concept on self-management skills to prepare a moderate physical activity plan. Preparing a plan requires the use of a variety of self-management skills including self-assessment, goal setting, and self-monitoring. Preparing a plan also gives you a chance to practice using these skills.

Self-monitoring your sedentary behaviors can aid in reducing them and increasing activity levels. The advent of activity monitors has made it easy to objectively self-monitor physical activity patterns. The monitors also provide information about the amount of time spent doing nothing (being inactive). (See the Strategies for Action: Lab Information for alternate methods of assessing sedentary behavior.)

Suggested Resources and Readings

The websites for the following sources can be accessed by searching online for the organization, program, or title listed. Specific scientific references are available at the end of this edition of *Concepts of Fitness and Wellness.*

- Active Living Research. MOVE! A Blog About Active Living.
- American College of Sports Medicine. *Reducing Sedentary Behaviors: Sit Less and Move More.* (pdf)
- JustStand.org. The Facts: The Human Body Is Designed to Move.
- Sedentary Behaviour Research Network. Terminology Consensus Project.
- Scott, L. & Stanten, M. (2020). *The Walking Solution.* Champaign, IL: Human Kinetics.
- Tremblay, M. S., et al. (Eds.). (2016, June). "Canadian 24-Hour Movement Guidelines for Children and Youth: An Integration of Physical Activity, Sedentary Behaviour, and Sleep." *Applied Physiology Nutrition and Metabolism;* 41:S311–27
- U.S. Department of Health and Human Services. (2018). *Physical Activity Guidelines for Americans.*
- World Health Organization. *WHO Guidelines on Physical Activity and Sedentary Behaviour.* (pdf)

Lab 7A Setting Goals for Moderate Physical Activity and Self-Monitoring (Logging) Program

Name	**Section**	**Date**

Purpose: To set moderate activity goals and to self-monitor (log) physical activity.

Procedures

1. Read the five stages of change questions. Place a check by the stage that best represents your current moderate physical activity level. If you are at stages 1–3 (precontemplation, contemplation, or preparation), you may want to set goals below the threshold of 30 minutes per day to get started. Those at the action or maintenance stage should consider goals of 30 minutes or more per day.
2. Determine moderate activity goals for each day of a 1-week period. In the columns (Chart 1) under the heading "Moderate Activity Goals," record the total minutes per day that you expect to perform **OR** the total steps per day that you expect to perform. Record the specific date for each day of the week in the "Date" column.
3. The goals should be realistic for you, but try to set goals that would meet current physical activity guidelines. If you choose step goals, you will need a pedometer. Use Table 5 in this Concept to help you choose daily step goals.
4. If you choose minutes per day as your goals, use Chart 2 to keep track of the number of minutes of activity that you perform on each day of the 7-day period. Record the number of minutes for each bout of activity of at least 10 minutes in length performed during each day (Chart 2). Determine a total number of minutes for the day and record this total in the last column of Chart 2 and in the "Minutes Performed" column of Chart 1.
5. If you choose steps per day as your goals, determine the total steps per day accumulated on the pedometer and record that number of steps in the "Steps Performed" column for each day of the week (Chart 1).
6. Answer the questions in the Conclusions and Implications section (use full sentences for your answers).

Determine your stage for moderate physical activity. Check only the stage that represents your current moderate activity level.

☐ Precontemplation: I do not meet moderate activity guidelines and have not been thinking about starting.

☐ Contemplation: I do not meet moderate activity guidelines but have been thinking about starting.

☐ Preparation: I am planning to start doing regular moderate activity to meet guidelines.

☐ Action: I do moderate activity, but I am not as regular as I should be.

☐ Maintenance: I regularly meet national goals for moderate activity.

Chart 1 Moderate Physical Activity Goals and Summary Performance Log

Select a goal for each day in a 1-week plan. Keep a log of the activities performed to determine if your goals are met.

	Date	Moderate Activity Goals		Summary Performance Log	
		Minutes/Day	Steps/Day	Minutes Performed	Steps Performed
Day 1					
Day 2					
Day 3					
Day 4					
Day 5					
Day 6					
Day 7					

111

Chart 2 Moderate Physical Activity Log (Daily Minutes Performed)

If you choose minutes per day as goals, write the number of minutes for each bout of moderate activity performed each day. Record a daily total (total minutes of moderate activity per day) in the "Daily Total" column. Record daily totals in Chart 1.

	Date	Moderate Activity Bouts					Daily Total
		Bout 1	**Bout 2**	**Bout 3**	**Bout 4**	**Bout 5**	
Day 1							
Day 2							
Day 3							
Day 4							
Day 5							
Day 6							
Day 7							

Did you meet your moderate activity goals for at least 5 days of the week?   (Yes)   (No)

Do you think you can consistently meet your moderate activity goals?   (Yes)   (No)

What activities did you perform most often when doing moderate activity?
List the most common activities in the spaces below.

Conclusions and Implications

1. Do you feel that you will use moderate physical activity as a regular part of your lifetime physical activity plan, either now or in the future? Use several sentences to explain your answer.

2. Did setting goals and logging activity make you more aware of your daily moderate physical activity patterns? Explain why or why not.

Lab 7B Estimating Sedentary Behavior

Name	**Section**	**Date**

Purpose: To estimate time spent in sedentary behavior.

Procedures

1. Pick a day of the week to evaluate.
2. Use the Sedentary Behavior Assessment to estimate the time spent in different intensities of activity during the day.
3. Summarize the results for the time spent in each category and be sure your daily total = 24 hours.
4. Calculate the ratio of sedentary to light activity and use the Rating Chart to determine your Sedentary Behavior Index. *Note:* There are no absolute guidelines, but a smaller ratio is desirable.
5. Calculate the average breaks in sedentary time across the five categories and use the Rating Chart to determine your Sedentary Break Index. *Note:* There are no absolute guidelines, but a larger number of average breaks is desirable.
6. Record your scores and the indexes in the Results section.
7. Answer the questions in the Conclusions and Implications section.

Sedentary Behavior Index Rating Chart

Sedentary Behavior Index	Sedentary/Light Ratio
Low Sedentary	<1
Moderate Sedentary	1.0–2.0
High Sedentary	>2.0

Sedentary Break Index	Average Break Score
Frequent Breaks	4–5
Moderate Breaks	2–3
Infrequent Breaks	0–1

Results: Summarize your activity/inactivity profile by completing the following:

Sleep Time (hr)	=	_____	Sleep %	=	_____
Sedentary Time (hr)	=	_____	Sedentary %	=	_____
Light Time (hr)	=	_____	Light %	=	_____
Moderate Activity Time (hr)	=	_____	Moderate %	=	_____
Vigorous Activity Time (hr)	=	_____	Vigorous %	=	_____
Total Hours	=	_____			
Sedentary/Light Ratio	=	_____	Average Break Score	=	_____
Sedentary Behavior Index	=	_____	Sedentary Break Index	=	_____

Conclusions and Implications: Summarize the overall assessment of your sedentary behaviors by describing both the total time you spend sedentary and the calculated sedentary/light ratio. Comment on the frequency of breaks in sedentary behavior and explain how changing the frequency of your breaks would influence your Sedentary Behavior Index. Do you feel you are effectively minimizing sedentary time, or do you think you may have room for improvement?

Based on categories and constructs used in the Workforce Sitting Questionnaire (Chau et al., 2011).

Sedentary Behavior Assessment (complete these steps in order):

1. Estimate the total time you spend in sedentary or light activity (Sedentary + Light) by subtracting from 24 (hours) the estimated time you spend (in hours) sleeping, engaged in moderate physical activity (MPA), and engaged in vigorous physical activity (VPA). The formula below will give you an estimate of the combined time spent in sedentary or light activities.

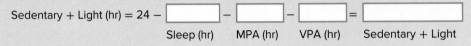

Sedentary + Light (hr) = 24 − [   ] − [   ] − [   ] = [   ]

Sleep (hr)   MPA (hr)   VPA (hr)   Sedentary + Light

2. Estimate the time you spend being sedentary (i.e., sitting or lying) in five major categories or settings and then sum for the whole day. For each category, estimate the frequency of breaks in the sedentary behavior for that category.

The following categories represent key time periods when people spend significant time being sedentary.	Estimate the total time spent sitting or lying in each of these categories throughout the day (not sleeping).		Estimate how many breaks from sitting you take during 1 hour of sitting in each of these settings (e.g., standing up, stretching, walking). Put an X that best captures the frequency of breaks.
	(hr)	(min)	
Traveling to/from places (e.g., bus/car)	[ ]	[ ]	5 4 3 2 1 0
At school and work (e.g., class, meetings, presentations, work)	[ ]	[ ]	5 4 3 2 1 0
Watching TV or using other media (e.g., TV, video games)	[ ]	[ ]	5 4 3 2 1 0
Computer use at home (e.g., homework, Web searching, email)	[ ]	[ ]	5 4 3 2 1 0
Other leisure activities (e.g., reading, relaxing, talking)	[ ]	[ ]	5 4 3 2 1 0

Total Sedentary Time =   = _____ hr + _____ min   Average Break Score = _____

3. Calculate the time spent in light activity by subtracting your estimated sedentary time (step 2) from the estimated time spent in Sedentary + Light (step 1).

Estimated Light Activity = [   ] − [   ] = [   ]

Sedentary + Light (step 1)   Sedentary Time (step 2)   Light Time

4. Calculate a ratio of sedentary to light activity by dividing Sedentary Time (step 2) by Light Time (step 3). Use the formula below to make your calculations.

Estimated Sedentary/Light Ratio = [   ] / [   ] = [   ]

Sedentary Time (step 2)   Light Time (step 3)   Sedentary/Light Ratio

Based on categories and constructs used in the Workforce Sitting Questionnaire (Chau et al., 2011).

Cardiorespiratory Endurance

LEARNING OBJECTIVES

After completing the study of this Concept, you will be able to:

- ▶ Describe the different components of the cardiovascular and respiratory systems.

- ▶ List the health benefits of cardiorespiratory endurance.

- ▶ Outline the FIT formula for moderate to vigorous physical activity designed to promote cardiorespiratory endurance.

- ▶ Identify several methods of determining exercise intensity levels for promoting cardiorespiratory endurance, select the method you think is most useful to you, and explain the reasons for your choice.

- ▶ Describe key guidelines for monitoring aerobic exercise, including self-monitoring heart rate.

- ▶ Indicate several self-assessments for cardiorespiratory endurance, select the self-assessment you feel is most useful to you, and explain the reasons for your choice.

Cardiorespiratory endurance influences physical performance in many activities and contributes to optimal health.

Maridav/Shutterstock

Why It Matters!

Cardiorespiratory endurance is generally considered to be the most important aspect of physical fitness. The fitness of the cardiovascular and respiratory systems is central to good health since your heart and lungs need to be healthy to efficiently pump blood and oxygen through your entire body. The heart is a muscle and, like other muscles, it gets stronger and more efficient if it is regularly trained. Healthy blood vessels are also critical for carrying blood and nutrients to the tissues; but without a healthy respiratory system, the circulatory system would be ineffective in providing oxygen to the body. Regular physical activity is essential for keeping both the cardiovascular and respiratory systems working properly, reducing the risk of heart disease and stroke as well as providing additional health and wellness benefits that extend well beyond reducing risks for disease. This Concept describes the function of the cardiovascular and respiratory systems and explains how to determine the appropriate intensity of exercise needed to promote cardiorespiratory endurance. Thus, it can be viewed as an owner's manual for your cardiovascular and respiratory systems.

Elements of Cardiorespiratory Endurance

The term *cardiorespiratory endurance* has several synonyms. Cardiorespiratory endurance is the ability of the heart, blood vessels, blood, and respiratory system to supply nutrients and oxygen to the muscles, and the ability of the muscles to utilize fuel to allow 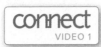 sustained exercise. A person with good cardiorespiratory endurance can persist in physical activity for relatively long periods without undue stress. Cardiorespiratory endurance is the preferred name for this component of fitness, but it is sometimes referred to as cardiovascular fitness, cardiovascular endurance, or aerobic fitness.

Good cardiorespiratory endurance requires a fit heart muscle. The heart is a powerful muscle that pumps blood through the body. The heart of a normal individual beats reflexively about 40 million times a year. In a single day, the heart pumps over 4,000 gallons of blood through the body. To keep the cardiovascular system working effectively, it is crucial to have a strong and fit heart.

Like other muscles in the body, the heart becomes stronger if it is exercised. The size and strength of the heart increases, and it can pump more blood with each beat, accomplishing the same amount of work with fewer beats. Typical resting heart rate (RHR) values are around 70–80 beats per minute, but a highly trained endurance athlete may have an RHR in the 40s or 50s. There is some individual variability in RHR, but a decrease in your RHR with training indicates clear improvements in cardiorespiratory endurance.

Good cardiorespiratory endurance requires a fit vascular system. The heart has four chambers that pump and receive blood in a rhythmical fashion to maintain good circulation (see Figure 1). Blood containing a high concentration of oxygen is pumped by the left ventricle through the aorta (a major artery), where it is carried to the tissues. Blood flows through a sequence of arteries to capillaries and to veins. Veins carry the blood containing lesser amounts of oxygen back to the right side of the heart, first to the atrium and then to the ventricle. The right ventricle pumps the blood to the lungs. In the lungs, the blood picks up oxygen (O_2), and carbon dioxide (CO_2) is removed. From the lungs, the oxygenated blood travels back to the heart, first to the left atrium and then to the left ventricle where it is pumped out to the rest of the body.

A dense network of arteries distributes the oxygenated blood to the muscles, tissues, and organs. Healthy arteries are elastic, are free of obstruction, and expand to permit the flow of blood. Muscle layers line the arteries and control the size of the arterial opening upon the impulse from nerve fibers. Unfit arteries may have a reduced internal diameter (atherosclerosis) because of deposits on the interior of their walls, or they may have hardened, nonelastic walls (arteriosclerosis).

The blood in the four chambers of the heart does not directly nourish the heart. Rather, numerous small arteries within the heart muscle provide for coronary circulation. Poor coronary circulation precipitated by unhealthy arteries can be the cause of a heart attack.

Deoxygenated blood flows back to the heart through a series of veins. The veins are intertwined in the skeletal muscle, and this allows normal muscle action to facilitate the return of blood to the heart. When a muscle is contracted, the vein is squeezed, and this pushes the blood back to the heart. Small valves in the veins prevent the backward flow of the blood, but defects in the valves can lead to pooling of blood in the veins. Regular physical activity keeps the valves of the veins healthy and helps reduce pooling of blood in the veins.

Capillaries are the transfer stations where oxygen and fuel are released, and waste products, such as carbon dioxide, are removed from the tissues. The veins receive the blood from the capillaries for the return trip to the heart.

Good cardiorespiratory endurance requires healthy blood and a fit respiratory system. The process of taking in oxygen (through the mouth and nose) and delivering it to the lungs, where it is picked up by the blood, is called external respiration. External respiration requires fit lungs as well as blood with adequate **hemoglobin.** Hemoglobin carries oxygen through the bloodstream. Lack of hemoglobin reduces oxygen-carrying capacity—a condition known as **anemia.**

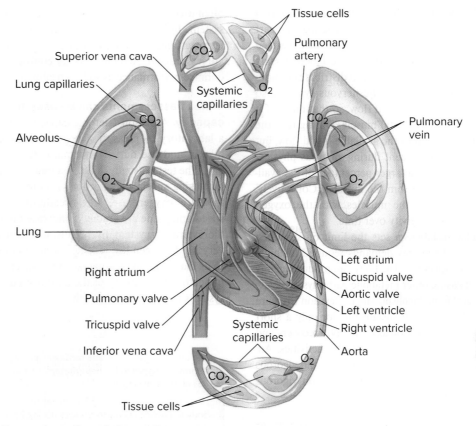

Figure 1 ▶ Cardiovascular and respiratory systems.

Delivering oxygen to the tissues from the blood is called internal respiration. Internal respiration requires an adequate number of healthy capillaries. In addition to delivering oxygen to the tissues, these systems remove carbon dioxide. Good cardiorespiratory endurance requires fitness of both the external and internal respiratory systems.

Good cardiorespiratory endurance requires fit muscle tissue capable of using oxygen. Once the oxygen is delivered, the muscle tissues must be able to use oxygen to sustain physical performance. Physical activity that promotes cardiorespiratory endurance stimulates changes in muscle fibers that make them more effective in using oxygen. Outstanding distance runners have high numbers of well-conditioned muscle fibers that can readily use oxygen to produce energy for sustained running. Training in other activities would elicit similar adaptations in the specific muscles used in those activities.

Cardiovascular Adaptations to Physical Activity

Physical activity challenges the cardiovascular and respiratory systems to deliver oxygen. When you perform physical activity, a number of changes occur to increase the availability of oxygen to the muscles (see Table 1). Breathing rate and depth increase, allowing the body to take

Table 1 ▶ Changes in Cardiovascular and Respiratory Function Between Rest and Exercise for a Person with Good Cardiorespiratory Endurance

		Rest	Maximal Exercise
Lungs	Breathing Rate (breaths/min)	12	30
Heart	Heart Rate (beats/min)	70	190–200
	Stroke Volume (mL/beat)	75	150
	Cardiac Output[a] (L/min)	5.2	28.5
Arteries	Blood Flow Distribution (%)	20%	70%
Muscle	Oxygen Extraction (%)	5%	20%
System	$\dot{V}O_2$ (mL/kg/min)[b]	3.5	60

[a]Cardiac output = heart rate × stroke volume.
[b]$\dot{V}O_2$-oxygen consumption = cardiac output × oxygen extraction.

Hemoglobin The oxygen-carrying protein (molecule) of red blood cells.

Anemia A condition in which hemoglobin and the blood's oxygen-carrying capacity are below normal.

Elite endurance athletes can extract 5-6 liters of oxygen per minute from the environment, and this high aerobic capacity is what allows them to maintain high speeds in both training and competition without becoming excessively tired. In comparison, an average person typically extracts about 2-3 liters per minute. $\dot{V}O_2$ max is typically adjusted to account for a person's body size because bigger people may have higher scores due to their larger size. Values are reported in milliliters (mL) of oxygen (O_2) per kilogram (kg) of body weight per minute (mL/kg/min).

The field tests in Lab 8B are designed to estimate your cardiorespiratory endurance. They are functional fitness tests that determine your ability to persist in exercise for relatively long periods of time. Some, such as the Bicycle Test, allow you to estimate your aerobic capacity in terms of $\dot{V}O_2$ max.

Cardiorespiratory Endurance and Health Benefits

Good cardiorespiratory endurance reduces risk for heart disease, other hypokinetic conditions, and early death. Numerous studies have confirmed that good cardiorespiratory endurance is associated with a reduced risk for heart disease as well as a number of other chronic, hypokinetic conditions. The consensus is that individuals with low fitness are three to six times more likely to develop symptoms of heart disease, metabolic syndrome, or diabetes than individuals with high fitness. While the specific amount of fitness needed to reduce risks varies by condition and population, evidence clearly supports the need for at least a moderate level of fitness. As shown in Figure 3, there are dramatic reductions in risk in moving from the low fitness category to the moderate fitness category for both males and females. Thus, this should be the goal for most people.

The drop in risk associated with moving from moderate to high fitness is not as great as the drop from low to moderate fitness. However, the gains are tangible and still clinically important. Doing some activity is clearly better than doing none; but doing more than the minimum has added benefits.

The benefits of cardiorespiratory endurance are independent of its beneficial effect on other risk factors. Physical activity has been shown to have beneficial effects on some other established heart disease risk factors, such as cholesterol, blood pressure, and body fat. It is important to note that the beneficial effects of cardiorespiratory endurance on risk for heart disease and early death are considered to be independent of these other effects. This means that active/fit people would still have lower health risks even if their cholesterol, blood pressure, and body fat levels were identical to those in a matched set of inactive/unfit people. This evidence has contributed to the labeling of physical inactivity as a major, independent risk factor for heart disease. The independent risk associated with physical inactivity is as large as (or larger than) risks associated with any of the other established risk factors. However, the added benefit of performing physical activity is that it also helps reverse or control other major risk factors such as high cholesterol and high blood pressure.

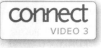

Good fitness reduces risks regardless of weight status. Some people think they cannot be fit if they are overweight. It is now known that appropriate physical activity can build cardiorespiratory endurance in all types of people, including those with excess body fat. In fact, numerous studies have demonstrated that a fit, overweight person is at lower risk of chronic disease than an unfit person who is normal weight. These findings demonstrate that low fitness is a greater risk than excess body fatness for chronic disease prevention. The greatest risk is among people who are both unfit and overfat.

Good cardiorespiratory endurance contributes to enhanced physical functioning. Moving out of the low fitness zone is of obvious importance to disease risk reduction. Achieving the good fitness zone on tests further reduces disease and early death risk and provides wellness benefits, including the ability to enjoy leisure activities and meet emergency situations. In older adults, achievement of good fitness results in an improved ability to function and maintain independence. Cardiorespiratory endurance in the high-performance zone provides benefits that may be important for success in certain athletic events and in occupations that require high performance levels (e.g., firefighters).

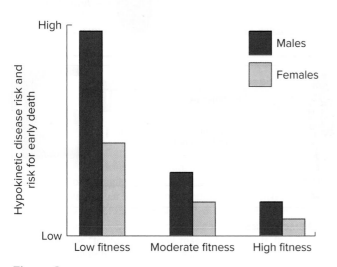

Figure 3 ▶ Risk reduction associated with cardiorespiratory endurance.

Source: Adapted from Blair et al.

The FIT Formula for Cardiorespiratory Endurance

The FIT formula for cardiorespiratory endurance varies for people of different activity levels. Adaptations to physical activity are based on the overload principle and the principle of progression. It is important to provide an appropriate challenge to the cardiovascular and respiratory systems (overload), but the challenge should be progressive, increasing gradually as fitness improves. For most people, vigorous physical activity from steps 2 and 3 (see Figure 4) is necessary to improve cardiorespiratory endurance. However, for people with low fitness, moderate physical activity (step 1) produces improvements.

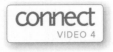

The ACSM Guidelines for Exercise Testing and Prescription provide generalized recommendations for building cardiorespiratory endurance. The guidelines are periodically updated to help clinicians and exercise specialists prescribe exercise for their clients. The most recent (11th) edition specifically references the importance of tailoring prescriptions to meet individual needs. To facilitate the application of the principle of progression, the FIT formula is customized for people of five different fitness and activity levels (See Table 2). While the *frequency* of exercise is similar for the different levels, the *intensity* and amount of *time* spent in activity vary considerably. Individuals with lower fitness levels should use lower intensities since their maximal capacity is also lower. As fitness improves, the intensity should be increased to maintain or improve fitness. The fitness assessments at the end of the Concept can help you determine the

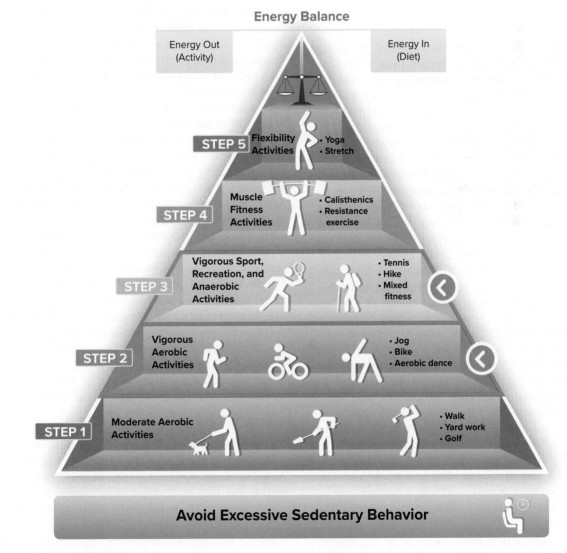

Figure 4 ▶ Select activities from steps 2 and 3 of the pyramid for optimal cardiorespiratory endurance.

Source: Charles B. Corbin.

Fitness Level	**Very Low**	**Low**	**Marginal**	**Good**	**High Performance**
Activity Level	Sedentary	Some light to moderate activity	Moderate and some Vigorous Activity	Regular moderate to vigorous activity	Habitual moderate to vigorous activity
F = Frequency (days per week)	3–5	3–5	3–5	3–5	3–5
I = Intensity					
Heart Rate Reserve (HRR)	30–40%	40–55%	55–70%	60–74	75–89
Max. Heart Rate (maxHR)	57–67%	64–74%	74–84%	77–86	87–95
Relative Perceived Exertion (RPE)	12–13	12–13	13–14	14–15	15–17
T = Time (minutes per day)	20–30	30–60	30–90	30–90	30–90

Table 2 ▶ FIT Formula for Cardiorespiratory Endurance for People of Different Fitness and Activity Levels

most appropriate guidelines for your current level of fitness. The sections that follow provide added information about the FIT formula.

The frequency (F) of physical activity to build cardiorespiratory endurance ranges from 3 to 5 or more days a week. Moderate activity can be safely performed every day, but additional considerations are important for vigorous physical activity. Vigorous physical activity provides additional benefits (compared to moderate activity); however, it can increase risk for orthopedic injury if it is done too frequently. Therefore, 5 days a week is the maximal recommended dose for most people. Healthy people who are fit and regularly active and have no evidence of joint problems or injuries may train up to 6 days a week, but most experts agree that at least 1 day off a week is beneficial. The ACSM recommendation of 3–5 days per week is appropriate for all levels of fitness; however, the optimal amount for you may depend on your fitness and on the associated intensity and time (duration) of the exercise sessions you perform. Also, remember that activity on 1 or 2 days is better than none at all.

The intensity (I) of physical activity necessary to produce cardiorespiratory endurance depends on a person's level of fitness. Consistent with the overload principle and the principle of progression, you need to exercise at a gradually increasing level of intensity that is higher than normal to improve cardiorespiratory endurance. To determine the appropriate intensity, it is important to have some indicator of a person's overall fitness. If the maximal aerobic capacity is known, an appropriate intensity can be set at a percentage of the maximum level. Because these values cannot be calculated without special equipment, other indicators of relative intensity are more commonly used.

Heart rate provides a good indicator of the relative challenge presented by a given bout of exercise. Therefore, guidelines for the intensity of physical activity to build

cardiorespiratory endurance are typically based on percentages of **heart rate reserve (HRR)** or maximal heart rate (maxHR). The latest ACSM guidelines suggest a range of 60–89 percent of HRR (or 77–95 percent of maxHR). However, as outlined in Table 2, individuals with lower levels of fitness can achieve improvements with lower intensity ranges.

A **rating of perceived exertion (RPE)** refers to the assessment of the intensity of exercise based on how the participant feels; a subjective assessment of effort. RPE has been shown to be useful in assessing the intensity of aerobic physical activity. The RPE scale ranges from 6 (very, very light) to 20 (very, very hard), with 1-point increments in between. If the values are multiplied by 10, the RPE values loosely correspond to HR values (e.g., 60 = rest HR and 200 = maxHR). The ACSM guidelines recommend an RPE range from 14–17 for vigorous aerobic activity, but values of 12–14 can be appropriate for individuals with low levels of fitness (see Table 2).

Regardless of what method is used, the important point is that lower intensities provide a cardiorespiratory endurance benefit for low-fit inactive and/or sedentary people, but higher intensities are needed for more fit people. The use of high-intensity interval training (HIIT) is promoted in some fitness centers as a way to increase the exercise stimulus and challenge; however, it also increases risk of injury and may cause exercise to be less pleasurable. See A Closer Look to learn the debates about the merits of HIIT. Use Table 2 to determine the appropriate *intensity of exercise* based on your current activity and fitness level.

The amount of time (T) for building cardiorespiratory endurance depends on the intensity. The ACSM, the American Heart Association, and the U.S. Department of Health and Human Services all recommend a minimum of 150 minutes of moderate activity per week, or 75 minutes of vigorous activity per week (or a combination of minutes from moderate and vigorous activity). Extending the length of time for exercise bouts has additional benefits for health and wellness, as well as cardiorespiratory endurance. For example,

A CLOSER LOOK

High-Intensity Interval Training (HIIT)

Although high-intensity interval training (HIIT) continues to be a popular topic among fitness enthusiasts, most consumers don't understand the basis for it. Interval training has been used by athletes for many years to increase the intensity of training and to help elicit stronger gains in performance. However, it is now widely accepted by the general public as a way to squeeze exercise into a busy schedule. The alternating bouts of high-intensity exercise with low-intensity rest periods can provide a greater fitness benefit in shorter periods of time—an important benefit for busy people. However, experts caution that it may increase risk of injury, particularly for beginning exercisers, low-fit individuals, and older adults. The high intensity may also detract from the enjoyment of exercise and limit long-term adherence. Research "HIIT" to learn more about the pros and cons.

Does this type of routine make exercise seem like work rather than play? Does this type of routine appeal to you or not?

connect
ACTIVITY

150–300 minutes of moderate activity per week is beneficial in losing body fat and maintaining a healthy body weight. For fit and active people, extending bouts of vigorous activity from 20 up to 90 minutes provides health and wellness benefits and enhances cardiorespiratory endurance. The updated ACSM guidelines suggest a basic range of 20–60 minutes, but a broader set of ranges are provided in Table 2. This facilitates use for individuals with higher levels of fitness or for individuals that choose to emphasize moderate intensity activity.

Different patterns of activity can be used to achieve the recommended dose of exercise. Some people may prefer to perform regular 30-minute bouts of exercise but others may prefer to accumulate it throughout the day. A pattern of three 10-minute bouts provides similar benefits to one 30-minute session. The number of days per week can vary from 3 to 6 days per week, but exercising 1 day a week with no regular activity in between (i.e., being a weekend warrior) is discouraged. The prescriptions in Table 2 are aimed at improving cardiorespiratory endurance based on individual characteristics of typical people. Specialized training regimens are typically needed for those interested in high-performance events (e.g., running races, triathlons) and competitive sports.

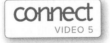

connect
VIDEO 5

Threshold and Target Zones for Intensity of Activity to Build Cardiorespiratory Endurance

There is a minimum intensity and an optimal intensity range for activity designed to develop cardiorespiratory endurance. As noted earlier, monitoring heart rate and making ratings of perceived exertion are the most practical methods of determining the intensity of activity necessary to build cardiorespiratory endurance. The threshold of training (minimum intensity) and the target zone (optimal intensity range) can be determined using several methods. Most methods are based on heart rate, so the target zone is typically referred to as *target heart rate zone*. Ratings of perceived exertion (RPEs) can also be used to define the target zone for exercise intensity. This section provides details of using these methods.

An estimate of maximal heart rate (maxHR) is needed to determine appropriate target heart rate zones for aerobic exercise. Your maxHR is the highest heart rate attained in maximal exercise. It could be determined using an electrocardiogram while exercising to exhaustion; however, it can also be estimated with formulas. MaxHR is known to decrease with age, so one simple and commonly used approach is to subtract your age from 220 (i.e., maxHR = 220 − age). However, studies have shown that this formula leads to inaccurate estimates for most people. A number of more specialized, nonlinear equations have been developed to

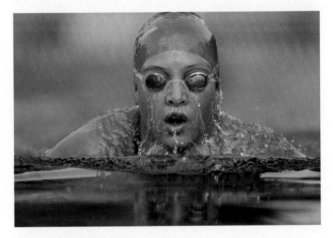

Aerobic activities provide an ideal stimulus for improving cardiorespiratory endurance.
Purestock/SuperStock

Heart Rate Reserve (HRR) The difference between maximal heart rate (highest heart rate in vigorous activity) and resting heart rate (lowest heart rate at rest).

Rating of Perceived Exertion (RPE) The assessment of the intensity of exercise based on how the participant feels; a subjective assessment of effort.

avoid this problem. For example, a new formula for women was recently developed (maxHR = 206 × [0.88 × age]). There is currently no consensus on the most accurate method, but evidence supports the utility of a relatively simple nonlinear method known as the Tanaka formula: maxHR = 208 − (0.7 × age). Calculations made at a variety of ages show little, if any, differences between the formulas, so it is recommended for most applications. Table 3 illustrates the calculations for determining maxHR for a 22-year-old.

The heart rate reserve (HRR) method is the preferred way to calculate target heart rate zones. Table 2 provides five different intensity ranges for activity designed to build cardiorespiratory endurance. After you have assessed your fitness using fitness tests (see the Lab Resource Materials section and Lab 8B), determine which of the five intensity ranges is best for you based on your current activity and fitness.

Table 3 provides a worked example for calculating heart rate target zones using the HRR method. The example is for a 22-year-old with good cardiorespiratory endurance who does regular moderate to vigorous physical activity and who has a resting heart rate of 68 beats per minute. The target heart rate zone for this hypothetical person is 60–89 percent. To determine the threshold of training (minimum heart rate for building cardiorespiratory endurance), use 60 percent of the working heart rate, and then add that value to the resting

heart rate. To determine the upper limit of the target zone, use 89 percent of the working heart rate and add that value to the resting heart rate.

Because target zone heart rates vary for people of different fitness and activity levels and because resting and maximal heart rates vary, each person will have a unique range of heart rates defining the target heart rate zone. The chart in Figure 5 allows you to look up your threshold and target heart rate zones for the HRR method. Locate your resting heart rate on the left and your age across the top (up to age 65). The values at the point where they intersect represent your target heart rate (based on 60 percent and 89 percent of HR reserve). Look across the columns for a given row to see how the target zone changes with age. Look down the rows for a certain column and see how the target zone changes with resting heart rate. The chart shows that fit individuals (lower rest HR values) have lower target heart rate zones than unfit individuals (higher rest HR values). This may seem somewhat paradoxical, but the reason is that fit individuals start exercise with a lower HR value and therefore have a larger HRR.

The percentage of maximal heart rate method is an alternative way to calculate target heart rate zones. The percentage of maxHR method is simpler to use than the HRR method, but it is not as accurate. This procedure takes maximal heart rate into account but does not factor in individual differences in resting heart rate. People with a typical resting HR of 60–70 bpm will tend to get similar values with both methods, but the percentage of maxHR method tends to be less accurate for people with high or low resting heart rates.

To use the percentage of maxHR method, first find your maximum HR with the formula (maxHR = 208 − [0.7 × age]). Then multiply your maxHR by the appropriate percentages from Table 2. For a person with good fitness and who performs regular moderate to vigorous activity, the percentages would be 80 to 91 percent. The maxHR for a 22-year-old is 193, so the target heart rate zone would be 149–183 using this method (.77 × 193 = 149 and 0.95 × 193 = 183). This procedure yields similar but slightly higher values than for the HRR method. The differences between the two methods vary for people of different ages, resting heart rates, and fitness/activity levels. The percentage of maxHR method is considered an acceptable alternative method, but the HRR method is more precise as it takes fitness level and resting heart rate into account.

Regardless of method, the threshold and target zone heart rates should be used only as general guidelines for aerobic exercise. By bringing your heart rate above the threshold and into the target zone, you will provide an optimal challenge to your cardiovascular and respiratory systems and maintain/improve your cardiorespiratory endurance. Guidelines for heart rate monitoring are provided in the next section.

Ratings of perceived exertion can be used to monitor the intensity of physical activity. The ACSM suggests that regularly active people can use RPE to determine if they

Table 3 ▶ Sample Target Heart Zone Calculations for a 22-Year-Old, Using the Percentage of Heart Rate Reserve Method

Calculating Maximal Heart Rate

Maximal heart rate	= 208 − (0.7 × age)
	= 208 − (0.7 × 22)
	= 208 − 15.4
	193

Calculating Heart Rate Reserve

Maximal heart rate	193 bpm
Minus resting heart rate	− 68 bpm
Equals heart rate reserve (HRR)	125 bpm

Calculating Threshold Heart Rate

HRR	125 bpm
×60%	×0.60
Equals	75 bpm
Plus resting heart rate	+68 bpm
Equals threshold heart rate	143 bpm

Calculating Upper Limit Heart Rate

HRR	125 bpm
×89%	×0.89
Equals	111 bpm
Plus resting heart rate	+68 bpm
Equals upper limit heart rate	179 bpm

Rest HR	Threshold	Age 20	25	30	35	40	45	50	55	60	65
50	60%	136	134	132	130	128	126	124	122	120	118
	89%	178	175	172	169	166	163	159	156	153	150
55	60%	138	136	134	132	130	128	126	124	122	120
	89%	179	176	172	169	166	163	160	157	154	151
60	60%	140	138	136	134	132	130	128	126	124	122
	89%	179	176	173	170	167	164	161	157	154	151
65	60%	142	140	138	136	134	132	130	128	126	124
	89%	180	177	174	170	167	164	161	158	155	152
70	60%	144	142	140	138	136	134	132	130	128	126
	89%	180	177	174	171	168	165	162	159	155	152
75	60%	146	144	142	140	138	136	134	132	130	128
	89%	181	178	175	172	168	165	162	159	156	153

Figure 5 ▶ Effect of age and resting heart rate on target heart range.

are exercising in the target zone (see Table 4). Ratings of perceived exertion have been shown to correlate well with HRR. For this reason, RPE can be used to estimate exercise intensity, avoiding the need to stop and count heart rate during exercise. A rating of 14 is equal to threshold, and a rating of 17 is equal to the upper limit of the target zone. As shown in Table 2, beginners may start with moderate activity and an RPE target zone of 12–13. Anaerobic activities such

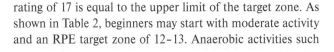

Technology Update

Pulse Oximetry Sensors

The use of pulse oximeters increased dramatically in response to the COVID-19 pandemic. The SARS-CoV-2 virus directly attacks the lungs, which is why coughing and difficulty in breathing are major symptoms. A low-oxygen saturation level can also be an indicator since it reflects inadequate oxygenation in the lungs. Sales of inexpensive pulse oximeters to consumers jumped in response to individuals' interests in monitoring potential risks or symptoms. These devices clip on your fingertip and provide readings of blood oxygen levels as well a heart rate count. Medical experts stated that most people do not typically need to have an oximeter but have acknowledged that they were helpful in detecting symptoms of COVID-19.

How has the COVID-19 pandemic increased your awareness of cardiorespiratory health and how viruses can impact different body systems?

connect ACTIVITY

Table 4 ▶ Ratings of Perceived Exertion (RPEs)

Rating	Description	Target Zone
6		
7	Very, very light	
8		
9	Very light	
10		
11	Fairly light	
12		
13	Somewhat hard	
14		X
15	Hard	X
16		X
17	Very hard	X
18		
19	Very, very hard	
20		

Source: Data from Borg.

fitness expert to do this test properly. It does allow you to estimate your aerobic capacity ($\dot{V}O_2$ max). The swim test is especially useful to those with musculoskeletal problems and other disabilities. The running test is the most vigorous and for this reason may be best for more advanced exercisers with high levels of motivation.

Results on the walking, running, and swimming tests are greatly influenced by the motivation of the test taker. If the test taker does not try hard, fitness results are underestimated. The bicycle and step tests are influenced less by motivation because one must exercise at a specified workload and at a regular pace. Because heart rate can be influenced by emotional factors, by exercise prior to the test, and other factors, tests using heart rate can sometimes give incorrect results. Thus, do your self-assessments when you are relatively free from stress and are rested. Prior to performing any of

these tests, be sure that you are physically and medically ready. Prepare yourself by doing some regular physical activity for 3–6 weeks before actually taking the tests.

Building knowledge and changing beliefs can help you sustain physical activity. Getting started with a physical activity program is relatively easy, but sticking with it over time can be challenging. Many factors contribute to poor adherence. Lack of knowledge is an important one. Many people have misconceptions about exercise or lack the knowledge needed to plan an effective program. Learning the facts about exercise and making a personal commitment to regular physical activity can help to improve adherence. The information in this Concept can help you know how to exercise properly and provide you with expectations that you can reasonably attempt to meet.

Strategies for Action: Lab Information

Practicing self-monitoring of physical activity intensity can help you make sure that activity improves cardiorespiratory endurance. In Lab 8A you will have the opportunity to practice counting heart rate at rest and after exercise to see if the exercise bout gets you into the heart rate target zone. You will also get the opportunity to practice using RPE to determine if the exercise is of adequate intensity to build cardiorespiratory endurance. Practice increases the accuracy of your self-monitoring and provides information that will allow you to select one or both of these techniques for use in the future.

Practicing self-assessments for cardiorespiratory endurance can help you choose a test that is best for you. In Lab 8B you will have the opportunity to self-assess your cardiorespiratory endurance using one or more tests. Trying several tests will help you make an informed choice about which test will be most useful to you in the future. A non-exercise estimate of cardiorespiratory endurance is also provided for comparison. Although this self-report tool has limitations, it is increasingly being used as a screening tool by physicians to determine if patients have risks associated with poor fitness.

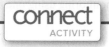

Suggested Resources and Readings

The websites for the following sources can be accessed by searching online for the organization, program, or title listed. Specific scientific references are available at the end of this edition of *Concepts of Fitness and Wellness*.

- American College of Sports Medicine. (2022). *ACSM's Guidelines for Exercise Testing and Prescription*. Philadelphia: Wolters Kluwer, Chapter 5.
- American Heart Association. *How Much Physical Activity Do You Need?* (pdf)

- Frey, M. (2020, October 31). "How to Improve Your Cardiorespiratory Endurance." *Verywell Fit.*
- Healthline. "What Is Cardiorespiratory Endurance and How Can You Improve It?"
- Ito, S. (2019). "High-Intensity Interval Training for Health Benefits and Care of Cardiac Diseases: The Key to an Efficient Exercise Protocol." *World Journal of Cardiology*, 11(7), 171–188.
- Livestrong. "7 Amazing Things Cardio Can Do for Your Brain and Body."
- Quindry, J. C., et al. (2019). "Benefits and Risks of High-Intensity Interval Patients with Coronary Artery Disease." *American Journal of Cardiology*, 123(8), 1370–1377.

Lab Resource Materials: Evaluating Cardiorespiratory Endurance

The Walking Test

- Warm up; then walk 1 mile as fast as you can without straining. Record your time to the nearest second.
- Immediately after the walk, count your heart rate for 15 seconds; then multiply by four to get a 1-minute heart rate. Record your heart rate.
- Use your walking time and your postexercise heart rate to determine your rating using Chart 1.

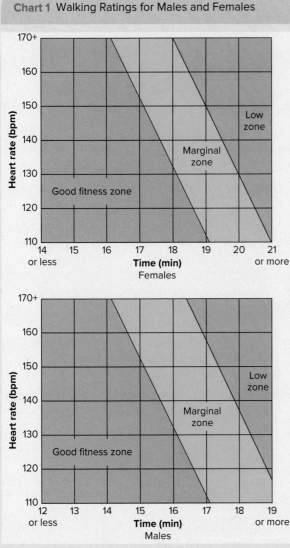

Chart 1 Walking Ratings for Males and Females

Source: James M. Rippe, M.D.

The ratings in Chart 1 are for ages 20–29. They provide reasonable ratings for people of all ages.

Note: The walking test is not a good indicator of high performance; the running and bicycle tests are recommended.

The Step Test

- Step up and down on a 12-inch-tall bench for 3 minutes at a rate of 24 steps per minute. One step consists of four beats—that is, "up with the left foot, up with the right foot, down with the left foot, down with the right foot."
- Immediately after the exercise, sit down on the bench and relax. Don't talk.
- Locate your pulse or have someone locate it for you.
- Five seconds after the exercise ends, begin counting your pulse. Count the pulse for 60 seconds.
- Your score is your 60-second heart rate. Locate your score and your rating on Chart 2.

Chart 2 Step Test Rating Chart

Classification	60-Second Heart Rate
High-performance zone	84 or less
Good fitness zone	85–95
Marginal fitness zone	96–119
Low fitness zone	120 and above

Source: Kasch and Boyer.

As you grow older, you will want to continue to score well on this rating chart. Because your maximal heart rate decreases as you age, you should be able to score well if you exercise regularly.

The Astrand-Ryhming Bicycle Test

- Ride a stationary bicycle ergometer for 6 minutes at a rate of 50 pedal cycles per minute (one push with each foot per cycle). Cool down after the test.
- Set the bicycle at a workload between 300 and 1,200 kpm. For less fit or smaller people, a setting in the range of 300–600 is appropriate. Larger or fitter people will need to use a setting of 750–1,200. The workload should be enough to elevate the heart rate to at least 125 bpm but no more than 170 bpm during the ride. The ideal range is 140–150 bpm.
- During the sixth minute of the ride (if the heart rate is in the correct range—see previous step), count the heart rate for the entire sixth minute. The carotid or radial pulse may be used.
- Use Chart 3 (males) or 4 (females) to determine your predicted oxygen uptake score in liters per minute. Locate your heart rate for the sixth minute of the ride in the left column and the work rate in kp · m/min across the top. The number in the chart where the heart rate and work rate intersect represents your predicted O_2 uptake in liters per minute. The bicycle you use must allow you to easily and accurately determine the work rate in kp · m/min.

- Ratings are typically assigned based on milliliters per kilogram of body weight per minute. To convert your score to milliliters per kilogram per minute (mL/kg/min), the first step is to multiply your score from Chart 3 or 4 by 1,000. This converts your score from liters to milliliters. Then divide your weight in pounds by 2.2. This converts your weight to kilograms. Finally, divide your score in milliliters by your weight in kilograms. This gives you your score in mL/kg/min.

- Example: An oxygen uptake score of 3.5 liters is equal to a 3,500-milliliter score (3.5 × 1,000). If the person with this score weighed 150 pounds, his or her weight in kilograms would be 68.18 kilograms (150 divided by 2.2). The person's oxygen uptake would be 51.3 mL/kg/min (3,500 divided by 68.18).

- Use your score in mL/kg/min to determine your rating (Chart 5).

Chart 3 Determining Maximal Oxygen Uptake ($\dot{V}O_2$ max) Using the Bicycle Test—Males (liters O_2/min)

Heart Rate	Work Rate (kp·m/min) 450	600	900	1,200	Heart Rate	Work Rate (kp·m/min) 450	600	900	1,200	1,500	Heart Rate	Work Rate (kp·m/min) 450	600	900	1,200	1,500
123	3.3	3.4	4.6	6.0	139	2.5	2.6	3.6	4.8	6.0	155	2.0	2.2	3.0	4.0	5.0
124	3.3	3.3	4.5	6.0	140	2.5	2.6	3.6	4.8	6.0	156	1.9	2.2	2.9	4.0	5.0
125	3.2	3.2	4.4	5.9	141	2.4	2.6	3.5	4.7	5.9	157	1.9	2.1	2.9	3.9	4.9
126	3.1	3.2	4.4	5.8	142	2.4	2.5	3.5	4.6	5.8	158	1.8	2.1	2.9	3.9	4.9
127	3.0	3.1	4.3	5.7	143	2.4	2.5	3.4	4.6	5.7	159	1.8	2.1	2.8	3.8	4.8
128	3.0	3.1	4.2	5.6	144	2.3	2.5	3.4	4.5	5.7	160	1.8	2.1	2.8	3.8	4.8
129	2.9	3.0	4.2	5.6	145	2.3	2.4	3.4	4.5	5.6	161	1.7	2.0	2.8	3.7	4.7
130	2.9	3.0	4.1	5.5	146	2.3	2.4	3.3	4.4	5.6	162	1.7	2.0	2.8	3.7	4.6
131	2.8	2.9	4.0	5.4	147	2.3	2.4	3.3	4.4	5.5	163	1.7	2.0	2.8	3.7	4.6
132	2.8	2.9	4.0	5.3	148	2.2	2.4	3.2	4.3	5.4	164	1.6	2.0	2.7	3.6	4.5
133	2.7	2.8	3.9	5.3	149	2.2	2.3	3.2	4.3	5.4	165	1.6	1.9	2.7	3.6	4.5
134	2.7	2.8	3.9	5.2	150	2.2	2.3	3.2	4.2	5.3	166	1.6	1.9	2.7	3.6	4.5
135	2.7	2.8	3.8	5.1	151	2.2	2.3	3.1	4.2	5.2	167	1.5	1.9	2.6	3.5	4.4
136	2.6	2.7	3.8	5.0	152	2.1	2.3	3.1	4.1	5.2	168	1.5	1.9	2.6	3.5	4.4
137	2.6	2.7	3.7	5.0	153	2.1	2.2	3.0	4.1	5.1	169	1.5	1.9	2.6	3.5	4.3
138	2.5	2.7	3.7	4.9	154	2.0	2.2	3.0	4.0	5.1	170	1.4	1.8	2.6	3.4	4.3

Chart 4 Determining Maximal Oxygen Uptake ($\dot{V}O_2$ max) Using the Bicycle Test—Females (liters O_2/min)

Heart Rate	Work Rate (kp·m/min) 300	450	600	750	900	Heart Rate	Work Rate (kp·m/min) 300	450	600	750	900	Heart Rate	Work Rate (kp·m/min) 400	600	750	900
123	2.4	3.1	3.9	4.6	5.1	139	1.8	2.4	2.9	3.5	4.0	155	1.9	2.4	2.8	3.2
124	2.4	3.1	3.8	4.5	5.1	140	1.8	2.4	2.8	3.4	4.0	156	1.9	2.4	2.8	3.2
125	2.3	3.0	3.7	4.4	5.0	141	1.8	2.3	2.8	3.4	3.9	157	1.8	2.3	2.7	3.2
126	2.3	3.0	3.6	4.3	5.0	142	1.7	2.3	2.8	3.3	3.9	158	1.8	2.3	2.7	3.1
127	2.2	2.9	3.5	4.2	4.8	143	1.7	2.2	2.7	3.3	3.8	159	1.8	2.3	2.7	3.1
128	2.2	2.8	3.5	4.2	4.8	144	1.7	2.2	2.7	3.2	3.8	160	1.8	2.2	2.6	3.0
129	2.2	2.8	3.4	4.1	4.8	145	1.6	2.2	2.7	3.2	3.7	161	1.8	2.2	2.6	3.0
130	2.1	2.7	3.4	4.0	4.7	146	1.6	2.2	2.6	3.2	3.7	162	1.8	2.2	2.6	3.0
131	2.1	2.7	3.4	4.0	4.6	147	1.6	2.1	2.6	3.1	3.6	163	1.7	2.2	2.5	2.9
132	2.0	2.7	3.3	3.9	4.6	148	1.6	2.1	2.6	3.1	3.6	164	1.7	2.1	2.5	2.9
133	2.0	2.6	3.2	3.8	4.5	149	1.5	2.1	2.6	3.0	3.5	165	1.7	2.1	2.5	2.9
134	2.0	2.6	3.2	3.8	4.4	150	1.5	2.0	2.5	3.0	3.5	166	1.7	2.1	2.5	2.8
135	2.0	2.6	3.1	3.7	4.4	151	1.5	2.0	2.5	3.0	3.4	167	1.6	2.0	2.4	2.8
136	1.9	2.5	3.1	3.6	4.3	152	1.4	2.0	2.5	2.9	3.4	168	1.6	2.0	2.4	2.8
137	1.9	2.5	3.0	3.6	4.2	153	1.4	2.0	2.4	2.9	3.3	169	1.6	2.0	2.4	2.8
138	1.8	2.4	3.0	3.5	4.2	154	1.4	2.0	2.4	2.8	3.3	170	1.6	2.0	2.4	2.7

Chart 5 Bicycle Test Rating Scale (mL/O$_2$/kg/min)

Age	Males				
	17–26	27–39	40–49	50–59	60–69
High-performance zone	50+	46+	42+	39+	35+
Good fitness zone	43–49	35–45	32–41	29–38	26–34
Marginal fitness zone	35–42	30–34	27–31	25–28	22–25
Low fitness zone	<35	<30	<27	<25	<22

Age	Females				
	17–26	27–39	40–49	50–59	60–69
High-performance zone	46+	40+	38+	35+	32+
Good fitness zone	36–45	33–39	30–37	28–34	24–31
Marginal fitness zone	30–35	28–32	24–29	21–27	18–23
Low fitness zone	<30	<28	<24	<21	<18

The 12-Minute Run Test

- Locate an area where a specific distance is already marked, such as a school track or football field, or measure a specific distance using a bicycle or automobile odometer.
- Use a stopwatch or wristwatch to accurately time a 12-minute period.
- For best results, warm up prior to the test; then run at a steady pace for the entire 12 minutes (cool down after the test).
- Determine the distance you can run in 12 minutes in fractions of a mile. Depending on your age, locate your score and rating in Chart 6.

Chart 6 Twelve-Minute Run Test Rating Chart

Classification—Males	Males (Age)							
	17–26		27–39		40–49		50+	
	Miles	Km	Miles	Km	Miles	Km	Miles	Km
High-performance zone	1.80+	2.90+	1.60+	2.60+	1.50+	2.40+	1.40+	2.25+
Good fitness zone	1.55–1.79	2.50–2.89	1.45–1.59	2.35–2.59	1.40–1.49	2.25–2.39	1.25–1.39	2.00–2.24
Marginal fitness zone	1.35–1.54	2.20–2.49	1.30–1.44	2.10–2.34	1.25–1.39	2.00–2.24	1.10–1.24	1.75–1.99
Low fitness zone	<1.35	<2.20	<1.30	<2.10	<1.25	<2.00	<1.1	<1.75

Classification—Females	Females (Age)							
	17–26		27–39		40–49		50+	
	Miles	Km	Miles	Km	Miles	Km	Miles	Km
High-performance zone	1.45+	2.35+	1.35+	2.20+	1.25+	2.00+	1.15+	1.85+
Good fitness zone	1.25–1.44	2.00–2.34	2.20–1.34	1.95–2.19	1.15–1.24	1.85–1.99	1.05–1.14	1.70–1.84
Marginal fitness zone	1.15–1.24	1.85–1.99	1.05–1.19	1.70–1.94	1.00–1.14	1.60–1.84	.95–1.04	1.55–1.69
Low fitness zone	<1.15	<1.85	<1.05	<1.70	<1.00	<1.60	<.95	<1.55

Source: Based on data from Cooper.

The 12-Minute Swim Test

- Locate a swimming area with premeasured distances, preferably 20 yards or longer.
- After a warm-up, swim as far as possible in 12 minutes using the stroke of your choice.

- For best results, have a partner keep track of your time and distance. A degree of swimming competence is a prerequisite for this test.
- Determine your score and rating using Chart 7.

Chart 7 Twelve-Minute Swim Rating Chart

	Males (Age)							
	17–26		**27–39**		**40–49**		**50+**	
Classification—Males	Yards	Meters	Yards	Meters	Yards	Meters	Yards	Meters
High-performance zone	700+	650+	650+	600+	600+	550+	550+	500+
Good fitness zone	600–699	550–649	550–649	500–599	500–599	475–549	450–549	425–499
Marginal fitness zone	500–599	450–549	450–459	400–499	400–499	375–475	350–449	325–424
Low fitness zone	Below 500	Below 450	Below 450	Below 400	Below 400	Below 375	Below 350	Below 325

	Females (Age)							
	17–26		**27–39**		**40–49**		**50+**	
Classification—Females	Yards	Meters	Yards	Meters	Yards	Meters	Yards	Meters
High-performance zone	600+	550+	550+	500+	500+	450+	450+	400+
Good fitness zone	500–599	450–549	450–549	400–499	400–499	375–449	350–449	325–400
Marginal fitness zone	400–499	350–449	350–449	325–399	300–399	275–375	250–349	225–324
Low fitness zone	Below 400	Below 350	Below 350	Below 325	Below 300	Below 275	Below 250	Below 225

Source: Based on data from Cooper.

Non-Exercise Estimate of Cardiorespiratory Endurance

- Follow the steps in Lab 8B to determine your score.
- Use Chart 8 to determine your rating.

Chart 8 Non-Exercise Fitness Assessment Rating Chart

Rating	Score
Needs Improvement	1–4
Marginal	5–9
Good Conditioning	10–13
Highly Conditioned	131+

Lab 8A Counting Target Heart Rate and Ratings of Perceived Exertion

Name	Section	Date

Purpose: To learn to count heart rate accurately and to use heart rate and/or ratings of perceived exertion (RPEs) to establish the threshold of training and target zones.

Procedure

1. *Resting Heart Rate:* Practice counting the number of pulses felt for a given period of time at both the carotid and radial locations while sitting still. Then, use a clock or watch to count for 15, 30, and 60 seconds using both sites. Record the values in the Results section and complete calculations of heart rate. *Note:* The practice in locating your carotid and radial pulses quickly is important when trying to count your pulse after exercise.
2. *Run 1:* Run a quarter mile at a comfortable pace; then count your heart rate at the end of the run. Use 15-second pulse counts (choose either carotid or radial) and multiply by four to get heart rate in beats per minute (bpm).
   - Rate your rating of perceived exertion (RPE) for the run (see RPE chart). Record your results.
   - Record the bpm in the Results section.
3. *Run 2:* Repeat the run a second time. This time, try to intentionally run at a speed that gets you in the heart rate and RPE target zone. Record your heart rate and RPE results.

Results: Record your *resting* heart rates in the boxes below.

Carotid Pulse   **Heart Rate per Minute**   **Radial Pulse**   **Heart Rate per Minute**

Carotid Pulse		Heart Rate per Minute	Radial Pulse		Heart Rate per Minute
	15 seconds × 4 =			15 seconds × 4 =	
	30 seconds × 2 =			30 seconds × 2 =	
	60 seconds × 1 =			60 seconds × 1 =	

Record your heart rate and rating of perceived exertion for run 1.

Pulse Count   **Heart Rate per Minute**

Pulse Count		Heart Rate per Minute
	15 seconds × 4 =	

Rating of Perceived Exertion

Record your heart rate and rating of perceived exertion for run 2.

Pulse Count   **Heart Rate per Minute**

Pulse Count		Heart Rate per Minute
	15 seconds × 4 =	

Rating of Perceived Exertion

Ratings of Perceived Exertion (RPEs)

Rating	Description	Target Zone
6		
7	Very, very light	
8		
9	Very light	
10		
11	Fairly light	
12		
13	Somewhat hard	
14		X
15	Hard	X
16		X
17	Very hard	X
18		
19	Very, very hard	
20		

Source: Data from Borg.

Answer the following questions:

Which pulse-counting technique did you use after the runs? Carotid ◯ Radial ◯

What is your target zone based on %HRR (to calculate, see Table 3)? [＿＿＿＿＿] bpm

Was your heart rate for run 1 enough to get in the heart rate target zone? Yes ◯ No ◯

Was your RPE for run 1 enough to get in the target zone (14–17)? Yes ◯ No ◯

Was your heart rate for run 2 enough to get in the heart rate target zone? Yes ◯ No ◯

Was your RPE for run 2 enough to get in the target zone (14–17)? Yes ◯ No ◯

Conclusions and Implications: In several sentences, discuss your results, including which method you would use to count heart rate and why. Also discuss heart rate versus RPE for determining the target zone.

Lab Supplement:* You may want to keep track of your exercise heart rate over a week's time or longer to see if you are reaching the target zone in your workouts. Shade your target zone with a highlight pen and plot your exercise heart rate for each day of the week (see sample).

Exercise Heart Rate								Sample	
200									
190									
180									
170									
160									
150									
140									
130									
120									
110									
100									
90									
80									
	Monday	Tuesday	Wednesday	Thursday	Friday	Saturday	Sunday	Day 1	Day 2
								155	162

Write in your daily exercise heart rate in the boxes above.

Lab 8B Evaluating Cardiorespiratory Endurance

| Name | | Section | | Date | |

Purpose: To acquaint you with several methods for evaluating cardiorespiratory endurance and to help you evaluate and rate your own cardiorespiratory endurance.

Procedure

1. Perform one or more of the five cardiorespiratory endurance tests and determine your ratings using the information in the Lab Resource Materials.
2. Perform each of the steps for the Non-Exercise Estimate of Cardiorespiratory Endurance, using the information in the Lab Resource materials. Learning this technique will allow you to estimate your fitness when you are injured or for some other reason cannot do a performance test.

Results

1. Record the information from your cardiorespiratory endurance test(s) in the spaces provided.
2. After you have completed the steps for the Non-Exercise Estimate of Cardiorespiratory Endurance, use Chart 8 in the Lab Resource Materials to determine your fitness rating.

Walking Test

Time _____ minutes

Heart rate _____ bpm

Rating _____ (see Chart 1)

Bicycle Test

Workload _____ kpm

Heart rate _____ bpm

Weight in lb. _____ pounds

Weight in kg _____ kg (Divide pounds by 2.2)

$\dot{V}O_2$ max _____ mL/O_2/kg (see Chart 3 and 4)

Rating _____ (see Chart 5)

Non-Exercise Test

Score _____

Rating _____ (see Chart 8)

Step Test

Heart rate _____ bpm

Rating _____ (see Chart 2)

12-Minute Run Test

Distance _____ miles

Rating _____ (see Chart 6)

12-Minute Swim Test

Distance _____ yards

Rating _____ (see Chart 7)

Non-Exercise Estimate of Cardiorespiratory Endurance

Record your scores and do the calculations to determine scores for A to E.

- Look up your activity score on Chart 1. Record score in box A. ☐ (A)

- Record your gender (female = 0/male = 1) _____ × 2.77 = ☐ (B)

- Determine your resting heart rate (Lab 8A). Record here. _____ × 0.03= ☐ (C)

- Calculate your BMI (see Lab 13B). Record here. _____ × 0.17 = ☐ (D)

- Record your age in years. _____ × 0.10 = ☐ (E)

Use the following formula to calculate your score. Use Chart 8 to get your rating; record this below.

| 18.07 | + | **A** | + | **B** | − | **C** | − | **D** | − | **E** | = | **Estimated Cardiorespiratory Endurance (METs)** |

18.07 + ☐ + ☐ − ☐ − ☐ − ☐ = ☐

| **Chart 1** Self-Reported Activity Score (for Step 1) |

Activity Score	Choose the Score That Best Describes Your Physical Activity Level
0.00	I am inactive or do little activity other than usual daily activities.
0.32	I regularly (>5 days/week) participate in physical activities requiring low levels of exertion that result in slight increases in breathing and heart rate for at least **10 minutes** at a time.
1.06	I participate in aerobic exercises (e.g., brisk walking, jogging) or other activities (e.g., sports or active recreation) requiring similar levels of exertion for **20–60 minutes per week.**
1.76	I participate in aerobic exercises (e.g., brisk walking, jogging) or other activities (e.g., sports or active recreation) requiring similar levels of exertion for **1–3 hours per week.**
3.03	I participate in aerobic exercises (e.g., brisk walking, jogging) or other activities (e.g., sports or active recreation) requiring similar levels of exertion for **over 3 hours per week.**

Conclusions and Implications

1. In several sentences, explain why you selected the tests you selected. Discuss your current level of cardiorespiratory endurance and steps you will need to take to maintain or improve it. Comment on the effectiveness of the tests you selected.

2. In several sentences, explain your results from the non-exercise assessment by comparing the results with the other test(s). Did the self-report version classify you into the same fitness category? Try to explain any differences you noted.

Vigorous Aerobic, Anaerobic, Sport, and Recreational Activities

LEARNING OBJECTIVES

After completing the study of this Concept, you will be able to:

► Explain the difference between moderate and vigorous physical activity and describe the unique benefits of vigorous physical activity.

► Identify several different types of vigorous aerobic activities and describe the advantages of each as possible activities in a personal activity program.

► Identify several different types of vigorous anaerobic activities and describe the advantages of each as possible activities in a personal activity program.

► Identify several different types of vigorous sport activities, describe the advantages of sport activities in a personal activity program, and explain the importance of skill learning to sports performance.

► Plan and self-monitor a vigorous physical activity program, and evaluate the factors that will help you adhere to it.

Vigorous aerobic, anaerobic, sport, and recreational activities promote health, wellness, fitness, and enhanced performance.

Ingram Publishing

Why It Matters!

Vigorous activities provide numerous health benefits and there are many ways to be active. Some people enjoy the challenge and thrill of sports while others prefer the independence and freedom of individual aerobic or anaerobic exercise. Some people like exercising with friends or in groups while others like to exercise alone. In this Concept, you will learn about the different types of vigorous physical activity as well as strategies to help you adopt and maintain an active identity over time.

Fundamentals of Vigorous Physical Activity

Vigorous activity builds fitness and promotes health and wellness. The physical activity pyramid is designed to help people better understand the many types of physical activity that can produce health, wellness, and fitness benefits. Moderate physical activity provides the foundation for an active and healthy lifestyle, but vigorous physical activity is important in building cardiorespiratory endurance (see Figure 1). Vigorous physical activity is characterized as having an intensity that is at least six times more intense than resting (i.e., 6 METs). Brisk walking is often used as an example of moderate activity while running is a good example of a vigorous activity. However, there are many options and ways to perform vigorous physical activity.

Four different types of vigorous physical activity are described in this Concept: vigorous aerobic activities, vigorous sport activities, vigorous recreational activities, and vigorous anaerobic activities. The higher intensity of these vigorous activities provides a good stimulus to the cardiorespiratory system and promotes positive training adaptations if performed regularly. However, many people pursue these activities for reasons other than health. For example, they also provide quality recreation, fun challenges, friendly competition, and enjoyable social interactions.

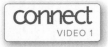

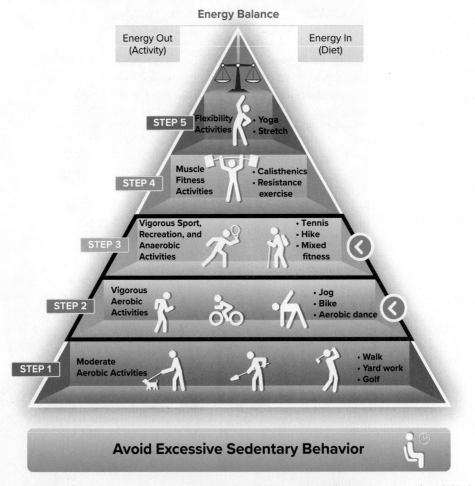

Figure 1 ▶ Vigorous aerobic, anaerobic, sport, and recreational activities are included at the second and third steps of the physical activity pyramid.

Table 1 ▶ Benefits of Vigorous Physical Activity*

- Vigorous activity meets national guidelines for physical activity and reduces risk of many chronic diseases and early death.

- Vigorous activity provides greater health benefits than moderate activity even when the total volume or calorie expenditure is the same.

- Vigorous activity provides additional health benefits (in a dose-response manner) when performed beyond the minimal guidelines.

- Vigorous activity contributes to many wellness benefits including improved quality of life, reduced risk of depression, reduced anxiety, and improved cognitions.

- Vigorous activity improves cardiorespiratory endurance and enhances ability to perform activities that require good cardiorespiratory endurance.

*Benefits depend on regular participation (at least 3 days a week) and appropriate intensity and duration (at least 20 minutes at target intensity).

Vigorous physical activity provides additional health benefits over moderate physical activity. Participation in moderate activity provides important health benefits, but an advantage of vigorous activity is that you can meet the public health guidelines in fewer days or with less overall time. A minute of vigorous physical activity essentially counts as 2 minutes of moderate physical activity since it is twice as intense. However, participation in vigorous physical activity also provides additional benefits, such as improved cardiorespiratory endurance and improved performance. These benefits are additive even if you already perform moderate-intensity activity (see Table 1).

HELP **Health is available to Everyone for a Lifetime, and it's Personal**

Vigorous Exercise Boosts Metabolism Long after the Workout

The benefits of vigorous exercise persist even after the workout is over. Research indicates that even a single bout of vigorous exercise helps you burn calories long after the exercise session is over. For example, a vigorous 45-minute bike workout burns approximately 330 calories, but you can expect to burn perhaps 500 total calories (a 37 percent increase) due to the heightened metabolism in the hours following the workout. This extra boost to the metabolism can have important implications for energy balance and weight control.

How does this information influence your perception about the importance of vigorous exercise?

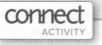

To get the benefits outlined in Table 1, vigorous activity should be performed at least 3 days a week for 20 minutes at the appropriate target intensity. Additional activity above this minimum amount has added benefits, but the amount depends on the specific health 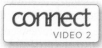 indicator, your baseline level of fitness, and other factors. The point of maximum health benefits has not been established, but the added benefits from additional vigorous exercise were emphasized by the expert panel that developed the 2018 *Physical Activity Guidelines for Americans.* Distinctions and examples of the different types of vigorous physical activity are provided in the subsequent sections along with strategies for incorporating them into your lifestyle.

Vigorous Aerobic Activities

Vigorous aerobic activities provide an effective stimulus for building cardiorespiratory endurance. The word *aerobic* literally means "with oxygen." Dr. Ken Cooper of the Cooper Institute in Dallas popularized the term in his book *Aerobics,* published in 1968. His book emphasized the importance of **vigorous aerobic activities** such as those in step 2 of the physical activity pyramid (e.g., jogging, aerobic dance, and cycling). The higher intensity of these activities provides a good stimulus to build cardiorespiratory endurance. The term **aerobic exercise** is used to reflect the specific and intentional use of vigorous aerobic activities to promote fitness. Many people also refer to these types of exercise sessions as cardio workouts.

Vigorous aerobic activities share some common characteristics. They are often rhythmical and typically involve the large muscle groups of the legs. The rhythmical nature allows it to be performed continuously and the activation of large muscle groups is important in providing an appropriate challenge to the cardiovascular and respiratory systems. As the name implies, the body relies on aerobic (oxidative) metabolic pathways to provide the needed energy for aerobic exercise. This system uses glucose and stored forms of glucose called glycogen to provide the sustained energy needed to perform aerobic activity. With training, individuals can perform vigorous physical activity aerobically and maintain high intensities for extended periods of time (i.e., hours).

A variety of vigorous aerobic activities are available for meeting individual needs and interests. Because there are so many choices, many beginning exercisers want to

Vigorous Aerobic Activities Aerobic activities that elevate the heart rate and are greater in intensity than a brisk walk.

Aerobic Exercise A structured and intentional form of aerobic physical activity intended to maintain or improve cardiorespiratory fitness.

know which type of aerobic exercise is best. The best form of exercise is clearly whatever form you enjoy and will do regularly. All forms of aerobic activity provide the same generalized benefits for the cardiovascular system. However, a recent review concluded that running may be particularly beneficial. In one major study, runners were found to have a 45 percent lower risk of death from heart disease or stroke and a 30 percent lower risk of early death than non-runners, after controlling for overall levels and intensity of activity. Runners were also found to live 3 years longer than non-runners but the most important observation was that even short bouts of running (5–10 minutes) have health benefits. The results demonstrate that there are many benefits of running, but there are also greater risks of injury associated with running. Thus, the more important message is that participation in vigorous physical activity provides additive benefits over participation in moderate-intensity activities.

Many exercise enthusiasts embrace cross training, in which a number of different activities are used to meet the aerobic exercise guidelines. It is normal to also vary patterns depending on the season. Many people choose to remain indoors during very hot or very cold weather and only perform outdoor activities when temperatures are more moderate.

Vigorous aerobic activities can be done either continuously or intermittently. The rhythmical nature of activities such as running, swimming, cycling, skiing, and in-line skating allow them to be performed as a **continuous aerobic activity**. However, evidence suggests that the benefits are similar if performed intermittently as an **intermittent aerobic activity**. For example, studies have shown that three 10-minute exercise sessions in the target zone are as effective as one 30-minute exercise session. Still, experts recommend bouts of 20–60 minutes in length, with several 10- to 15-minute bouts being an acceptable alternative when longer sessions are not possible.

Vigorous aerobic activity in a group setting provides opportunities for social interaction. Although most vigorous aerobics can be done individually, many people prefer the social interactions and challenge of group exercise classes. A number of fitness and community recreation centers offer group exercise classes. While large commercial fitness centers remain popular, many small private fitness centers provide an appealing alternative for some people. An example is the Curves franchise that provides a structured group exercise format, allowing people to exercise in a more convenient, small-group setting. A similar line of centers branded under the name Kosama offers shorter enrollments and personalized attention over a set period of time rather than an ongoing membership.

An advantage of fitness centers and group exercise classes is that there is a social component, which helps increase motivation and promote consistency. A disadvantage is that all participants are generally guided through the same exercise.

A vigorous routine can cause unfit people to overextend themselves, while an easy routine may not be intense enough for experienced exercisers. A well-trained group exercise leader can help participants adjust the exercise to their own level and ability. Check the qualifications of the exercise leader to verify credentials and certifications for leading group exercise. Descriptions of some common forms of vigorous aerobics offered in health and fitness centers are provided below:

- *Dance aerobics: A choreographed series of movements done to music.* There are a variety of forms of dance aerobics. In *high-impact dance aerobics,* both feet leave the ground simultaneously for a good part of the routine. Although this provides a good workout, it may not be ideal for everyone. In *low-impact dance aerobics,* one foot stays on the floor at all times, making risk of injury lower and a good choice for beginners or older exercisers. In *step aerobics,* the participant steps up and down on a bench while doing various dance steps. Step aerobics is typically low impact but relatively higher in intensity due to the stepping.

- *Rhythmic dance: A more fluid dance-oriented form of aerobics.* Rhythmic dance evolved naturally out of the aerobic dance movement, and there are many examples of dance-based classes. Jazzercise is one of the more long-lasting and well-known forms, and it paved the way for more hybridized group exercise classes. Classes in hip-hop aerobics have been popular for a while as well as Zumba and other Latin-based dance classes.

- *Martial arts: Popular, vigorous aerobic activities.* In addition to traditional martial arts, such as karate and tae kwon do, a number of other alternative forms have been developed, including kickboxing, aerobic boxing, cardio karate, box fitness, and Tae Bo. These activities involve intermittent bouts of high-intensity movements and lower-intensity recovery. Because martial arts involve a lot of arm work, they can be effective in promoting good overall fitness. Some activities are more intense than others, so consider the alternatives to find the best fit for you.

- *Spinning classes: Attracting new people to bicycling.* A spinning class is a group cycling class performed on specialized indoor bike trainers. A group leader typically leads participants through routines that involve intermittent bursts of high-intensity intervals followed by spinning at lower resistance to recover. While specific to cycling, the format has appealed to a broader set of fitness enthusiasts who just enjoy the challenge it provides.

- *Water-based classes: Taking advantage of the resistive properties of water.* Water walking and water exercise classes are popular alternatives to swimming. Although these activities can be done alone, they are typically conducted in group settings and are especially good for people with arthritis, musculoskeletal problems, or high body fat. The body's buoyancy in water assists the participant and reduces injury risk. The resistance of the water provides an overload that

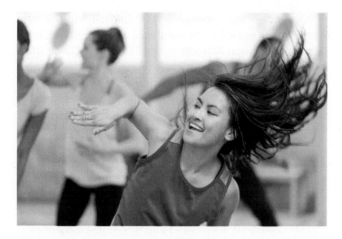

Many people enjoy the social interactions of group exercise classes.
Christopher Futcher/E+/Getty Images

helps the activity promote health and cardiorespiratory benefits. Exercises done in shallow water tend to be low in impact, while deeper-water exercises are considered to be higher-impact activities. Neither type requires the ability to swim. Water activity also serves as a way of rehabilitating from injury.

- *Combo aerobic classes: Cross-training applications.* Hybrid combo classes combine aerobics, resistance exercise, plyometrics, and/or calisthenics. They offer a complete workout in a structured and engaging group environment. Classes are marketed with customized names to reflect the nature of the activities involved (e.g., CardioPump, PowerPump, Cardio Sculpt, BodyJam, BodyAttack). There are a number of certification programs for combo classes designed to ensure consistency and quality of programming.

Exercise machines can provide an engaging indoor alternative to traditional aerobic exercises. Many people prefer aerobic exercise machines because of their ease of use, safety, and convenience. Treadmills have historically been the most commonly used exercise machine, but elliptical devices and an array of stair-climbing devices are also extremely popular. Bike, rowing, and skiing machines are also commonly used but they may be most popular among individuals that specifically enjoy these activities.

A drawback of exercise machines is that interest and novelty may wear off over time. However, new features have been developed to enhance interest and ease of use. For example, some machines have personalized key systems, which automatically record your settings and the details of your workout each time you use the machine. This information can then be downloaded onto computers for automatic logging. Newer machines have also started to utilize gaming technology to further enhance the user experience. Interactive displays in these machines allow you to feel like you are exercising outdoors and you can compete against virtual or real

Technology Update

Exergaming and Virtual Racing

The COVID-19 pandemic led to creative solutions to maintain our interest in sports and fitness. Sporting events at all levels were modified to promote safety of both athletes and spectators. Organizations also shifted to hosting virtual running and biking events that allowed people to post their routes and times using available fitness tracking apps and technology. The most prominent example of this was the online Tour de France bike race that used a virtual training software platform called Zwift. Biking enthusiasts from all over the world routinely use Zwift to bike with each other on virtual routes. The sophistication of bike technology enabled professional riders to compete virtually while allowing fans to watch online. Interactive fitness technology and gamification provide novel ways to make exercise more interesting and engaging. The applications of exergaming will continue to evolve and become more sophisticated over time.

Do these types of technology motivate you to exercise? Why or why not?

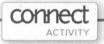

opponents. Through wireless computer networks, it is possible for users to save their data on websites and/or share their results through social media applications. See Technology Update to explore interactive machines.

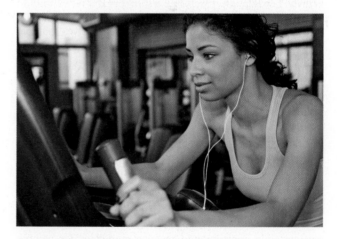

Smart exercise equipment can connect to your phone apps and link to related social media applications.
Blend Images/Alamy Stock Photo

Continuous Aerobic Activity Aerobic activities that are slow enough to be sustained for relatively long periods without frequent rest periods.

Intermittent Aerobic Activity Aerobic activities, relatively high in intensity, alternated with frequent rest periods.

Vigorous Anaerobic Activities

Anaerobic activities can promote cardiorespiratory endurance and fitness. **Vigorous anaerobic activities** are high-intensity conditioning activities with energy demands that can't be met with the aerobic metabolism. The body uses anaerobic metabolic processes (i.e., processes that do not require oxygen) to meet the energy demands of these activities. Pure anaerobic activities, such as sprinting, rely on stored supply of fuel that can be readily converted into energy, but this high-energy (ATP-PC) system) can provide energy only for approximately 10 seconds. The body can also use a glycolytic pathway that relies on glucose to produce energy for longer bouts, but a by-product of this process (**lactic acid**) eventually causes the muscles to fatigue. While the energy needs are met anaerobically, oxygen consumption is also maximal. Following a bout of anaerobic activity, you keep breathing fast because the body needs the extra oxygen to rebuild energy stores and to break down the lactic acid. This is sometimes called **oxygen debt**. The body essentially pays back the oxygen debt by supplying extra oxygen after the anaerobic exercise. In some ways, it is like using a credit card to borrow money that is paid back later. Repeated bouts of anaerobic exercise provide a good stimulus to improve both **aerobic capacity** and **anaerobic capacity**.

Anaerobic exercise has become more popular in recent years. Because anaerobic activity is typically performed as a means of improving fitness and enhancing performance, it is often referred to as anaerobic exercise. Interval training, the most common form of anaerobic exercise, involves multiple bouts of very high-intensity exercise followed by rest periods. Interval training has been used by athletes for years, but it is now popular among fitness enthusiasts through various forms of high-intensity interval training (HIIT). Fitness centers now promote HIIT and other forms of **anaerobic exercise** as being more efficient and effective ways to exercise. Proponents suggest that HIIT helps people by providing them with a way to get maximal benefit in the shortest possible time. However, many experts are concerned that the high-intensity "work-like" regimens make exercise less enjoyable and may discourage long-term adherence. There are also greater risks for injury from this form of exercise. Performing vigorous anaerobic activity can certainly contribute to meeting guidelines for aerobic activity since the cardiorespiratory system is also engaged and challenged. However, it isn't necessary to exercise to high intensity to get benefits. Additional detail on anaerobic activities is provided in the Concept on muscle fitness and resistance exercise.

Mixed fitness and hybrid activities include a range of aerobic and anaerobic activities. The nature of fitness-related activities continually evolves as people invent and discover new ways to engage in physical activity. The term *mixed fitness activities* has been used to describe workouts that include several different types of activities. Circuit training, for example, includes multiple exercise stations at which different types of activities are performed. For example, stair stepping (vigorous aerobics), resistance exercises (muscle fitness exercise), sprints (anaerobic exercise), and stretching (flexibility exercise) are sometimes used in circuits. The term *hybrid exercise* has similarly been coined to describe exercises that flow together to allow for a whole-body workout. These routines or regimens aren't really new forms of physical activity, but rather different ways to combine types of physical activity. Other examples of mixed fitness activities are those that combine martial arts and vigorous aerobics and CrossFit activities. Additional detail is provided in the Concept on muscle fitness and resistance exercise.

Vigorous Sport Activities

Participation in vigorous sport activities can build cardiorespiratory endurance. Sports typically involve brief intermittent periods of sprinting or high-intensity activity but they vary in the type, nature, and intensity of movement involved. The action in soccer, basketball, and tennis involves bursts of activity followed by rest; thus, they share characteristics of anaerobic activities described earlier. They are classified as **vigorous sports** and can provide benefits similar to those from vigorous aerobic activities and vigorous anaerobic activities if performed regularly and at a vigorous intensity (i.e., at least 6 METS). Of course, any sport can be more or less active, depending on how you perform it. Shooting baskets or even playing half-court basketball is not as vigorous as playing a full-court game. Swimming and cycling are popular activities that can also be considered sports. However, most people do these activities noncompetitively, so they are typically considered as vigorous aerobic activities. Sports such as golf, bowling, and billiards/pool are aerobic, but are light to moderate in intensity. For this reason, they are classified as moderate physical activities.

Sports are popular for a variety of reasons. While team sports are common activities for children and adolescents, there are fewer options 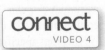 for adults. Intramural sports on college campuses are popular since they provide opportunities for casual or competitive sports experiences. In recent years, there has been a boom in e-sports (electronic sports), which essentially is competitive video-gaming, especially on college campuses. These sports do not involve physical activity but do meet other criteria of sport activities: they follow rules, are competitive, and require skill. While critics argue that these activities promote sedentary behavior, individuals can enjoy these activities and still find ways to get sufficient physical activity in their lifestyle.

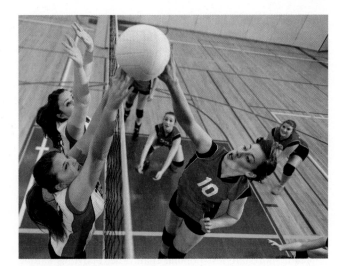

Volleyball is a popular competitive and recreational sport that can be played for a lifetime.
Christopher Futcher/iStock/Getty Images

The competitive nature of sport is attractive to many people, but it can also be a deterrent. Focusing on the enjoyment of the activity can help reduce the emphasis on competition. Slow-pitch softball is much more popular than fast-pitch softball or baseball because it allows people of all abilities to play successfully. Lifetime sports such as bowling and golf use a handicap system to allow people with a wide range of abilities to compete.

For the greatest enjoyment, try to participate with others who have the same goals and skill level. If you choose to play against a person with lesser skill, you will not be challenged. On the other hand, if you lack skill or your opponent has considerably more skill, the activity will be frustrating. For optimal challenge and enjoyment, learn the skills of a given sport before competing. Additional information on sports and learning skills is provided later in this Concept.

Vigorous Recreational Activities

Some recreational activities can also be classified as vigorous. Activities that you do in your free time for personal enjoyment or to "re-create" yourself are considered recreational activities. Recreational activities that exceed threshold intensity for cardiorespiratory endurance are considered **vigorous recreational activities**. They are more vigorous than activities

Vigorous Anaerobic Activities Anaerobic activities require energy beyond what can be provided by the aerobic metabolism. Vigorous anaerobic activities are generally short and intermittent in nature and typically higher intensity than vigorous aerobic activities.

Lactic Acid Substance that results from the process of supplying energy during anaerobic exercise; a cause of muscle fatigue.

Oxygen Debt The oxygen consumed following anaerobic exercise that is used to rebuild the supply of high-energy fuel.

Aerobic Capacity A measure of the ability of the heart and lungs to get oxygen to the muscles. Typically expressed as the maximum amount of oxygen that can be consumed in one minute of high intensity aerobic activity.

Anaerobic Capacity A measure of the ability of the body to perform high intensity, intermittent activity. Performance reflects the ability to produce energy using the anaerobic (without oxygen) energy systems

Anaerobic Exercise A structured and intentional form of exercise characterized by repeated, short bouts of high-intensity physical activity intended to maintain or improve cardiorespiratory and muscular fitness.

Vigorous Sports Sports are competitive activities that have an organized set of rules, along with winners and losers. Vigorous sports are those of similar intensity to vigorous aerobic activities.

Vigorous Recreational Activities Recreational activities are those that are done during leisure time that do not meet the characteristics of sports. Vigorous recreational activities are of similar intensity to vigorous aerobic activities.

In the News

Youth Sports Matter

The Science Board of the President's Council on Sports, Fitness, and Nutrition released a new report on the importance of youth sports. The report documents 10 ways in which youth sports contribute to positive mental health, including enjoyment, increased life satisfaction, less risky behavior, and enhanced self-confidence and self-esteem, to name a few. The report is part of a broader National Youth Sport Strategy (NYSS) developed by the U.S. Department of Health and Human Services to promote access to and improve the youth sport experience for all. Thus, the ambitious goal is somewhat to reinvent the youth sport experience and to reduce barriers and disparities to participation. The stated vision of the NYSS is that "*one day all youth will have the opportunity, motivation, and access to play sports, regardless of their race, ethnicity, sex, ability, or ZIP code.*" (See Suggested Resources and Readings.)

How did youth sports impact your current lifestyle, values, or perceptions?

connect
ACTIVITY

such as fishing, bowling, and golf, which are typically classified as lifestyle or moderate activities (step 1 in the pyramid). Examples of vigorous recreational activities include common snow activities (downhill skiing, snowboarding), water activities (surfing, wakeboarding, kayaking, canoeing), and mountain activities (hiking, mountain biking). As with sports, recreational activities can be done at different intensities. If done for a sufficient length of time, vigorous recreational activities can provide the same benefits as vigorous sports or other vigorous activities. Note that vigorous activities such as cycling, jogging, and skiing could be classified in both the vigorous recreational and vigorous aerobic activities sections. Sports can also be considered vigorous recreational activities, depending on how the individual views them.

Recreational activities have benefits beyond fitness. Recreational activities are pursued for a variety of reasons. Some common reasons for performing recreational activities include personal enjoyment, relaxation, the social experience, enjoyment of being outside, personal challenge, and improved fitness. Many people view recreation as simply time to relax and be outdoors, and find the resulting improvements in fitness to be just an additional benefit. This is a healthy attitude since activities pursued purely for enjoyment are easier to maintain than activities pursued purely for fitness.

Patterns and Trends in Physical Activity Participation

Personal interests and preferences influence participation in physical activity. Each year a number of different organizations conduct surveys to determine which activities are the most popular. Results vary based on how the questions are asked and who 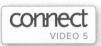 asks them. Regardless of the group doing the poll, vigorous individual activities rank high (among top 25). For example, running, aerobic exercise machines, biking, and dance aerobics are consistently in the top 10 activities. Some vigorous individual sport and recreational activities also rank among the most popular (e.g., tennis, hiking). Basketball and slow-pitch softball are among the most popular team sports, but participation is lower in other team sports. Fishing, bowling, and golf are popular but are not vigorous in nature. In many polls, walking ranks number one, but it is moderate rather than vigorous in nature, except for older people or people with health problems. Individual muscle fitness activities rank high (e.g., HIIT, mixed fitness activities, and body weight exercise), as do flexibility exercises (e.g., stretching, yoga).

Participation in physical activity varies by age group. The Physical Activity Council conducts an annual survey to evaluate trends in participation rates for different types of activities. The large, representative sample in the survey enables patterns to be compared across a variety of factors including age, ethnicity, and income. Survey results indicated that 73 percent of adults participate in physical activity but only 36 percent engage in vigorous activities. Overall participation has remained consistent over the past 5 years, but participation rates have increased in the categories of "fitness sports" and "outdoor sports" with declines evident in some other categories such as "individual sports" and "water sports."

A summary of the most recent data is provided in Figure 2 for the overall sample and for separate age segments. Overall, fitness activities are the most popular among all age groups except Gen Z (born after 2000). Outdoor sports are next, being most popular among young age groups. Individual sports also rank high, especially among younger age groups.

Team sports are less popular than other activities among adults, but they are among the most popular activities for youth (i.e., Gen Z). Racquet sports, water sports, and winter sports were the least popular general activity types, probably because of their need for special facilities and equipment, their relatively high cost, and requirements for specific weather (e.g., snow for skiing) and geographic conditions (e.g., lakes for boating).

Casual participation is different from participating on a regular basis. Some polls seek to capture the relative popularity of activities by asking participants to indicate which ones they have performed in the past year. A person who has done the activity once can check "yes" for that activity, but casual participation (once to a few times a year) does not provide the same health, wellness, and fitness benefits as regular participation.

Not surprisingly, far more people are casual exercisers than regular participants. For example, according to the Sport and Fitness Industry Association over 25 million Americans report jogging/running for exercise, but only 10 million report 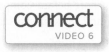 running regularly (about 6 million males and 4 million females). Distinctions in participation and regular participation are even more evident for other activities. An estimated 50 million Americans report riding their bike for recreation, but only 15 million report frequent recreational bike riding, and a still smaller segment of the population (about 2 million) participates in regular fitness bicycling. Nearly 100 million people report participating in recreational swimming; however, the number of people who report regular fitness swimming is only about 2.5 million.

Fitness trends are different than fitness fads. The ACSM's *Health and Fitness Journal* conducts annual surveys to evaluate patterns and trends in the fitness field. The reports provide useful insights about shifting interests of consumers as well as trends in fitness classes and programming. The top 10 trends in the 2020 report are summarized in Table 2.

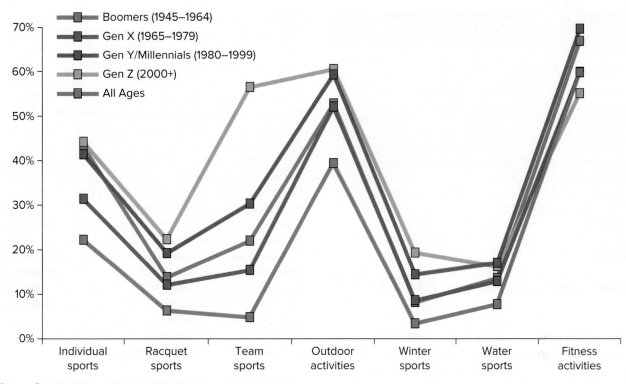

Figure 2 ▶ Patterns of physical activity by age group.

Table 2 ▶ ACSM's *Health and Fitness Journal*'s Top 10 Fitness Trends

Rank	Product/Trend	Description
1	Wearable technology	Wearable activity trackers, smartwatches, heart rate monitors, and GPS tracking devices continue to be popular for monitoring activity.
2	High-intensity interval training (HIIT)	The short bursts of activity followed by short periods of rest or recovery in HIIT allow users to maximize the intensity and efficiency of workouts.
3	Group training	Group exercise remains popular since it can help promote motivation while also providing reinforcing and supportive social networks.
4	Free weight training	The interest in mixed fitness activities and hybrid training is leading to more use of dumbells, kettlebells, and other free weight exercises.
5	Personal training	The growth in kinesiology degree programs has enhanced education and training of personal trainers and more effective use in health and fitness facilities.
6	Exercise Is Medicine (EIM)	This global health initiative that encourages physicians and other health-care providers to assess and prescribe physical activity is taking root and can impact future programming.
7	Body weight training	Body weight training builds on the popularity of "core" training and applied fitness regimens popular in CrossFit and other programs.
8	Exercise programming for older adults	The expanding geriatric population (and the increased interest among this age group) is driving innovations and options for exercise programming for older adults.
9	Health/wellness coaching	This area of coaching is distinct from personal training and is aimed at facilitating and promoting personal motivation for exercise and behavior change.
10	Educated and experienced fitness professionals	Stronger certification and credentialing programs have increased access to more qualified fitness professionals with better skills for planning and facilitating exercise.

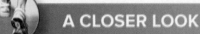

A CLOSER LOOK

23 and 1/2 Hours

Even though the benefits associated with regular physical activity are enormous, participation in exercise and physical activity still remains low. A YouTube video by Dr. Mike Evans called *23 and 1/2 Hours* presents a compelling challenge to viewers: Commit 30 minutes a day to physical activity to ensure that you get the basic health benefits that come from physical activity.

With so many powerful benefits of physical activity, why do so many people fail to put a high priority on it? Does knowing about the robust benefits make it easier for you to commit 30 minutes a day?

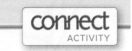

connect
ACTIVITY

When examined over time, the results also help differentiate between actual trends (generalized changes in a situation or in the way people are behaving) and fads (a temporary notion that is taken up with great enthusiasm for a brief period). The recent report indicates a continued interest in wearable technology as it has retained the number one spot over the past 4–5 years. Interest in high-intensity interval training (HIIT) has remained high (moving from third to second in the rankings). The popularity of group training (third), the incorporation of free weights into exercise routines (fourth), and the use of personal training (fifth) also reflect the current interest in mixed fitness exercises. The focus in these categories changes a bit, but they have remained in the top 10 over time. Evidence also suggests variability in interests across generations. For example, Millennials and Gen Z enthusiasts are more likely to engage in group training while Boomers are more comfortable with traditional equipment and approaches. Even though trends in fitness preferences and methods change with age (and over time), the importance of regular exercise remains constant.

Guidelines for Vigorous Physical Activity

Moderate and vigorous physical activity can be combined to meet national guidelines. National guidelines specify the total amount of activity that should be performed rather than having separate recommendations for moderate and vigorous activity. This approach helps people incorporate both moderate and vigorous activity into their lifestyle. The guidelines are based on tracking the total MET-minutes of physical activity performed. Because vigorous activity is performed at higher intensities (higher MET values), it makes a larger contribution to total activity than moderate-intensity activity performed for the same time. To determine

MET-minutes, you multiply the MET value of an activity by the number of minutes that you perform it. For example, if a person walked for 10 minutes at 4 mph (4 METs), the MET-minutes would be 40 (4 METs × 10 minutes). If the person also jogged for 20 minutes at 5 mph (8 METs), the MET-minutes for jogging would be 160 (8 METs × 20 minutes); the total MET-minutes for the day would be 200.

To meet the physical activity guidelines, a person must accumulate a minimum of 500 MET-minutes per week. These are considered to be minimal levels, and the physical activity guidelines encourage people to move toward the target of 1,000 MET-minutes per week for additional benefits. Activity should be done at least 3 days a week when the combined method is used, even though the MET-minute standard could be met with large amounts of activity performed on 1 or 2 days. MET values for a variety of moderate activities are included in the Concept on moderate physical activity. A complete list of the MET values for a variety of activities can be found online (search "Compendium of Physical Activities"). In Lab 9C you will calculate MET-minutes and learn how to combine moderate and vigorous activity to meet national goals.

Vigorous activity can present some risks, so caution is recommended. Sports medicine experts indicate that certain types of physical activities are more likely than others to result in injury. While moderate activities like walking are very safe, there are greater risks associated with performing some forms of vigorous physical activity. For example, skating or rollerblading have relatively greater risks for falls and associated injuries. Sport activities can present greater risks for concussions and various musculoskeletal injuries. Running has the greatest risk among aerobic activities, followed by cycling, high-impact dance aerobics, and step aerobics which have moderate risk for injury. Swimming and water aerobics are among those least likely to cause injuries because they do not involve impact, falling, or collision. In general, activities that require high-volume training (aerobics and jogging), collision (football, basketball, and softball), falling (biking, skating, cheerleading, and gymnastics), the use of specialized equipment that can fail (biking), and repetitive movements that stress the joints (tennis and high-impact aerobics) increase risk for injury. To minimize risks it is important to use proper safety equipment, proper performance techniques, and proper training techniques.

Vigorous physical activity is not for everyone! While some people enjoy pushing their body to the limits or appreciate the challenge of intense sporting competitions, other people may not. The key is to find activities that you enjoy and that provide meaning and value to your life since these are the activities that you are most likely to adhere to over time. Classes offered in many fitness centers often hype high-intensity training regimens that promise maximal results or that use different formats or approaches to promote interest. Examples include the CrossFit movement, boot-camp fitness classes, HIIT, and ninja-training classes. While these classes may appeal to some, they may be overly structured or too intense for others. There are many forms of vigorous activity to explore, but moderate physical activity can provide many of the benefits and with minimal risks.

Using Self-Management Skills

Becoming skillful will help you enjoy sports and recreation. Improving your skill can increase the chances that you will participate in the activity or sport for a lifetime. The following self-management strategies can help you improve your sport performance:

● *When learning a new activity, focus on the general idea of the skill first; worry about details later.* Concentrating on too many details at one time may result in **paralysis by analysis**. For example, a golfer who is told to keep the head down, the left arm straight, and the knees bent cannot possibly concentrate on all of these details at once. As a result, neither the details nor the general idea of the golf swing is performed properly.

● *Once the general idea of a skill is learned, a skill analysis of the performance may be helpful.* Watching videos of skilled performances can be helpful to learners. It can also be helpful to have a knowledgeable person pinpoint your strengths and weaknesses.

● *Avoid competition in the early stages of learning a lifetime sport or physical activity.* Beginners who compete are likely to concentrate on beating their opponent rather than on learning a skill properly. For example, in bowling, you may abandon the newly learned hook ball in favor of a straight ball to ensure hitting pins. This may help your score in the present game, but is not likely to improve bowling skills for the future.

● *To be performed well, sports skills must be overlearned.* The best way to learn a skill is to overlearn it, or practice it until it becomes habit. Frequently, games do not allow you to overlearn skills. For example, it is not effective to learn to serve during a tennis match since there may be only a few opportunities to do so. It is more productive to hit many serves (overlearn) until the general idea of the serve is well learned.

● *When unlearning an old (incorrect) skill and learning a new (correct) skill, a person's performance may get worse before it gets better.* For example, you may have learned how to score well in golf with a flawed swing. Accept that your performance may get worse initially as you try to learn better technique. As the new swing pattern is refined and over-learned, your skill will improve, as will your golf score.

● *There is no substitute for good instruction.* Getting good instruction, especially at the beginning level, will help you learn skills faster and better. Instruction will help you apply these rules and use practice more effectively.

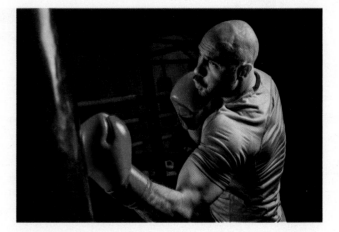

Intermittent anaerobic exercise can improve fitness and health.
Microgen/Shutterstock

Preparing a vigorous physical activity plan requires the use of multiple self-management skills. You can use the six steps in program planning outlined in the Concept on self-management to prepare a vigorous physical activity plan. Preparing a plan requires the use of a variety of self-management skills including self-assessment, goal setting, and self-monitoring. Preparing a plan also helps you manage your time—an important self-management skill. Lack of time is a common reason for not exercising. Preparing a plan helps you fit your activity into your daily schedule. (More information is provided in Strategies for Action: Lab Information.)

Choosing activities that are self-promoting can enhance confidence and fun. Self-promoting activities are activities that make you feel successful. They require relatively little skill and can be done in a way that avoids comparison with other people. They allow you to set your own standards of success and can be done individually or in small groups that are suited to your personal needs. Examples include wheelchair distance events, jogging, resistance training, swimming, bicycling, and dance exercise.

A key for long-term exercise adherence is to find exercises that you enjoy and that fit into your lifestyle. Sports are a common form of activity for younger people, but other aerobic and recreational activities have become more common among adults. This is partially because of changing interests, but also because of changing opportunities and lifestyles.

Choose effective monitors and apps for activity tracking. A variety of consumer activity monitors are available to assist in tracking the volume and intensity of exercise.

Paralysis by Analysis An overanalysis of skill behavior. This occurs when more information is supplied than a performer can use or when concentration on too many details results in interference with performance.

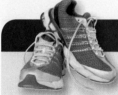

Strategies for Action: Lab Information

Understanding the factors that influence physical activity adherence will improve your chances of staying active throughout life. In Lab 9A, you will evaluate predisposing, enabling, and reinforcing factors that may help you identify the types of activity best suited to you and that enhance the chances that you will stay active over time.

Preparing a vigorous physical activity plan can help you with adherence. Lab 9B is designed to help you plan and perform a 1-week physical activity program. It helps you practice the steps in program planning and provides an opportunity to self-monitor adherence to your plan. This initial plan focuses on short-term activity goals. Future plans can focus more on long-term goals for both fitness and physical activity. If you like, you can copy the lab worksheet to make a log book for long-term self-monitoring.

Consider combining moderate and vigorous physical activity to meet activity guidelines. *Cross training* is a term used to describe the performance of a variety of activities to meet exercise goals. For example, on different days you can do a moderate activity such as walking, a vigorous aerobic activity such as jogging on a treadmill, a vigorous sport such as tennis, and a vigorous recreational activity such as mountain biking. These activities from different levels on the activity pyramid can be combined to meet activity guidelines. Lab 9C will help you learn and use this MET-minute system.

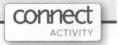

Various smartphone apps can also be used to help prompt you to stay active and to help you chart progress. The devices are designed only to provide estimates of movement, heart rate, and steps, so don't focus too much on the actual numbers. Use the information primarily to remind yourself of your goals and to track progress over time. Research is still evolving with monitors, but many people find that regular use keeps them more engaged in their exercise programs.

Suggested Resources and Readings

The websites for the following sources can be accessed by searching online for the organization, program, or title listed. Specific scientific references are available at the end of this edition of *Concepts of Fitness and Wellness.*

- Physical Activity Council. *2021 Physical Activity Council's Overview Report on U.S. Participation Report.* (pdf)
- President's Council on Sports, Fitness and Nutrition. *PCSFN Science Board Report on Youth Sports.* (pdf)
- Statista. Physical Activity–Statistics & Facts.
- U.S. Bureau of Labor Statistics. American Time Use Survey.
- U.S. Department of Health and Human Services. *Physical Activity Guidelines for Americans.*
- Thompson, Walter. (2019). "Worldwide Survey of Fitness Trends for 2020." *ACSM's Health & Fitness Journal, 23*(6), 10-18.

Lab 9A The Physical Activity Adherence Questionnaire

Name	Section	Date

Purpose: To help you understand the factors that influence physical activity adherence and to see which factors you might change to improve your chances of achieving the action or maintenance level for physical activity.

Procedures

1. The factors that predispose, enable, and reinforce adherence to physically active living are listed. Read each statement. Place an X in the circle under the most appropriate response for you: very true, somewhat true, or not true.
2. When you have answered all of the items, determine a score by summing the four numbers for each type of factor. Then sum the three scores (predisposing, enabling, reinforcing) to get your total score.
3. Record your scores in Chart 1 of the Results section (using Chart 2 to determine the ratings). Answer the questions in the Conclusions and Implications section.

	Very True	Somewhat True	Not True	
Predisposing Factors				
1. I am very knowledgeable about physical activity.	3	2	1	
2. I have a strong belief that physical activity is good for me.	3	2	1	
3. I enjoy doing regular exercise and physical activity.	3	2	1	
4. I am confident of my abilities in sports, exercise, and other physical activities.	3	2	1	
			Predisposing Score =	
Enabling Factors				
5. I possess good sports skills.	3	2	1	
6. I know how to plan my own physical activity program.	3	2	1	
7. I have a place to do physical activity near my home or work.	3	2	1	
8. I have the equipment I need to do physical activities I enjoy.	3	2	1	
			Enabling Score =	
Reinforcing Factors				
9. I have the support of my family for doing my regular physical activity.	3	2	1	
10. I have many friends who enjoy the same kinds of physical activities that I do.	3	2	1	
11. I have the support of my boss and my colleagues for participation in activity.	3	2	1	
12. I have a doctor and/or an employer who encourages me to exercise.	3	2	1	
			Reinforcing Score =	
			Total Score (Sum 3 Scores) =	

Results: Record your scores in the "Score" column. Use your score and the Physical Activity Adherence Ratings Chart to determine your ratings. Record your ratings in the "Rating" column.

Chart 1 Physical Activity Adherence Ratings

Adherence Category	Score	Rating
Predisposing		
Enabling		
Reinforcing		
Total		

Chart 2 Physical Activity Adherence Ratings Chart

Classification	Predisposing Score	Enabling Score	Reinforcing Score	Total Score
Adherence likely	11–12	11–12	11–12	33–36
Adherence possible	9–10	9–10	9–10	27–32
Adherence unlikely	<9	<9	<9	<27

Conclusions and Implications: In several sentences, discuss your ratings from this questionnaire. Also discuss the predisposing, enabling, and reinforcing factors you may need to alter in order to increase your prospects for lifetime activity.

In several sentences, discuss what type of activity you find most enjoyable (vigorous aerobics, vigorous anaerobics, vigorous recreation, or vigorous sports). Comment on *why* you enjoy the activities that you have selected.

Lab 9B Planning and Logging Participation in Vigorous Physical Activity

Name	**Section**	**Date**

Purpose: To set 1-week vigorous physical activity goals, to prepare a plan, and to self-monitor progress in your 1-week vigorous aerobics, anaerobics, sports, and recreation plan.

Procedures

1. Consider your current stage of change for vigorous activity using the questions provided. Read the five stages of change questions and place a check by the stage that best represents your current vigorous physical activity level.
2. Determine vigorous activity (aerobics, anaerobics, sports, or recreation) goals for each day of a 1-week period. In Chart 1, under the heading "Vigorous Activity Goals," record the total minutes per day that you expect to perform. Record the specific date for each day of the week in the "Date" column, and the activity or activities that you expect to perform in the "Activity" column.
3. The daily goals should be at least 20 minutes a day in the target zone for vigorous activity for at least 3 days of the week.
4. Use Chart 2 to keep track of the number of minutes of activity that you perform on each day of the 7-day period. Record the number of minutes for each bout of activity of at least 10 minutes in length performed during each day in Chart 2. Determine a total number of minutes for the day and record this total in the last column of Chart 2 and also in the last column ("Summary Performance Log") of Chart 1.
5. After completing Charts 1 and 2, answer the questions and complete the Conclusions and Implications section (use full sentences for your answers).

Determine your Stage of Change for vigorous physical activity. Check only the stage that represents your current vigorous activity level.

☐ Precontemplation. I do not meet vigorous activity guidelines and have not been thinking about starting.

☐ Contemplation. I do not do vigorous activity but have been thinking about starting.

☐ Preparation. I am planning to start doing regular vigorous activity to meet guidelines.

☐ Action. I am regularly doing vigorous activity but have been doing it only recently (less than 6 months)

☐ Maintenance. I regularly perform vigorous activity and have been doing it consistently for a while (more than 6 months).

Results

Chart 1 Vigorous Physical Activity Goals and Summary Performance Log

Select a goal for each day in a 1-week plan. Keep a log of the activities performed to determine if your goals are met (see Chart 2), and record total minutes performed in the chart below.

	Date	Vigorous Activity Goals		Summary Performance Log Total Minutes Performed/Day
		Minutes/Day	**Activity**	
Day 1				
Day 2				
Day 3				
Day 4				
Day 5				
Day 6				
Day 7				

Chart 2 Physical Activity Adherence Ratings Chart

Record the number of minutes for each bout of vigorous activities performed each day. Add the minutes in each column for the day and record a daily total (total minutes of vigorous activity per day) in the "Daily Total" column. Record your daily totals in the last column of Chart 1.

	Date	Vigorous Activity Bouts					Daily Total
		Bout 1	Bout 2	Bout 3	Bout 4	Bout 5	
Day 1							
Day 2							
Day 3							
Day 4							
Day 5							
Day 6							
Day 7							

Did you meet your vigorous activity goals for at least 3 days of the week? Yes No

Do you think that you can consistently meet your vigorous activity goals? Yes No

What activities did you perform most often when doing vigorous activity?
List the most common activities that you performed in the spaces (using a specific category).

Vigorous Aerobics   Vigorous Anaerobics   Vigorous Sports / Recreation
_____   _____   _____
_____   _____   _____
_____   _____   _____

Conclusions and Implications

Are the activities that you listed above ones that you think you will perform regularly in the future?   Yes No

Did setting goals and logging activity make you more aware of your daily vigorous physical activity patterns? Explain why or why not.

Lab 9C Combining Moderate and Vigorous Physical Activity

Name	**Section**	**Date**

Purpose: To learn about MET-minutes and how to combine moderate and vigorous physical activity to meet physical activity guidelines and goals.

Procedures

1. National guidelines recommend at least 150 minutes of moderate or 75 minutes of vigorous physical activity as the minimum amount per week. The guidelines indicate that you can combine the two forms to meet your activity goal. When combining moderate and vigorous activities, MET-minutes are used. The minimum goal for beginners is 500 MET-minutes, and 1,000 MET-minutes is the minimum goal for a reasonably fit and active person. Consider this information as you complete the rest of this lab.

2. In Chart 1 list several moderate activities and several vigorous activities for each day of one week. Next to the activities indicate the number of minutes you plan to perform each activity. Be sure to choose both moderate and vigorous activities.

3. Use the information in Chart 2 to determine a MET value for each activity or use the list of MET values found by searching the Internet for "Compendium of Physical Activities" to determine values for those not listed in Chart 2. Record the MET value in the space provided for each activity.

4. Multiply the MET values for each activity by the number of minutes you plan to perform each activity to determine MET-minutes for each activity.

5. Total the MET-minute columns for both moderate and vigorous activities to be performed during the week.

6. Answer the questions in the Conclusions and Implications section.

Results

Chart 1 Moderate and Vigorous Activity Plan for One Week

Day	Date	Moderate Activity				Vigorous Activity			
		Activity	Min	METs	MET-min	Activity	Min	METs	MET-min
1									
2									
3									
4									
5									
6									
7									
Totals									

Total MET-mins = Moderate MET-mins + Vigorous MET-mins =

Did you meet the 500 MET-minute recommendation for beginners? (Yes) (No)

Did you meet the 1,000 MET-minute recommendation for more active people? (Yes) (No)

Which is your weekly activity plan most likely to include?

☐ Moderate activity only

☐ Vigorous activity only

☐ Both moderate and vigorous activity

Chart 2 MET Values for Selected Moderate and Vigorous Physical Activities

Moderate Activities	METs	Vigorous Activities	METs
Bowling	3.0	Shoveling Snow	6.0
Vacuuming/Mopping	3.0	Walking (4.5 mph)	6.3
Walking (3 mph)	3.0	Aerobic Dance	6.5
Child Care	3.5	Bricklaying	7.0
Golf (riding)	3.5	Cross-Country Skiing (leisure)	7.0
Biking (10 mph flat)	4.0	Soccer (leisure)	7.0
Fishing (moving, not stationary)	4.0	Basketball (game)	8.0
Raking Leaves	4.0	Biking (12–17 mph)	8.0
Table Tennis	4.0	Hiking Terrain (pack)	8.0
Volleyball (non-comp.)	4.0	Jogging (5 mph)	8.0
Working as Waiter/Waitress	4.0	Tennis (singles)	8.0
Ballroom Dance (social)	4.5	Volleyball (games)	8.0
Basketball (shooting)	4.5	Digging Ditches	8.5
Mowing Lawn (power)	4.5	Step Aerobics	8.5
Painting	4.5	Cross-Country Skiing (fast, 5–7 mph)	9.0
Tennis (doubles)	5.0	Swimming Laps (varies with strokes)	9.0
Walking (4 mph)	5.0	Jogging (6 mph)	10.0
Construction	5.5	Racquetball (games)	10.0
Farming	5.5	Soccer (competitive)	10.0
Golf (walking)	5.5	Running (11.5 mph)	11.5
Softball (games)	5.5	Handball (games)	12.0
Swimming (leisure)	5.5		

Note: MET values are based on the Compendium of Physical Activities Tracking Guide (available at http://prevention.sph.sc.edu/tools/docs/documents_compendium.pdf).

Conclusions and Implications: In the space provided below discuss the MET-minute method of combining activities to meet goals. Do you think that this method will be useful to you? Explain why or why not.

Muscle Fitness and Resistance Exercise

LEARNING OBJECTIVES

After completing the study of this Concept, you will be able to:

▶ Identify and explain the factors that influence strength, muscular endurance, and power.

▶ List the health benefits of muscle fitness and resistance exercise.

▶ Describe the types of progressive resistance exercise (PRE) and their advantages and disadvantages, including some basic exercises for each type of PRE.

▶ Describe different types of PRE equipment and the advantages and disadvantages of each.

▶ Determine the amount of exercise necessary to improve muscle fitness and explain the FIT formulas for the different types of PRE.

▶ Describe how to design PRE programs for optimal effectiveness.

▶ Evaluate facts and fallacies about PRE and the risks of performance-enhancing drugs, supplements, and steroids.

▶ Describe several self-assessments for muscle fitness, understand the self-assessments that help you identify personal needs, and plan (and self-monitor) a personal PRE program.

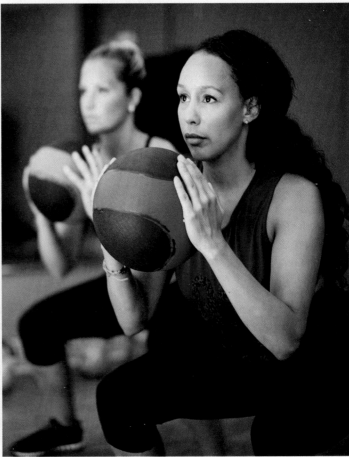

Progressive resistance exercise promotes muscle fitness that permits efficient and effective movement, contributes to ease and economy of muscular effort, promotes successful performance, and lowers susceptibility to some types of injuries, musculoskeletal problems, and illnesses.

SG Hirst/Getty Images

Why It Matters!

Muscle fitness provides a number of benefits for both health and wellness. Like other dimensions of fitness, the key to building and sustaining good muscle fitness is regular exercise. Current guidelines call for resistance exercise at least 2 days a week, but specific training plans and prescriptions depend on whether your primary goals are to improve strength, muscular endurance, or power, or for general conditioning. The varying quality of fitness information on the Internet has led many people to have misconceptions about progressive resistance exercise. This Concept covers the scientific basis and health benefits of muscle fitness as well as principles, guidelines, and specific exercises that can help you establish an appropriate muscle fitness program.

Factors Influencing Muscle Fitness

Muscle fitness is a multidimensional construct. The three components of muscle fitness (strength, muscular endurance, and power) each reflect different capacities of human movement. Strength is the amount of force you can produce with a single maximal effort of 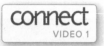 a muscle group. Muscular endurance is the capacity of the skeletal muscles, or group of muscles, to continue contracting over a long period of time. Muscle power is the ability to exhibit strength quickly and it depends on the combination of strength and speed. Power is associated with enhanced sports performance and has historically been considered a skill-related component of fitness. However, it is now considered to be a health-related component because of its link to bone health and other health factors.

Skeletal muscle tissue has unique properties that are important to muscle fitness. The three types of muscle tissue—smooth, cardiac, and skeletal—have different structures and functions. Smooth muscle tissue consists of long, spindle-shaped fibers, with each fiber containing only one nucleus. The smooth muscle fibers are located in the walls of the esophagus, stomach, and intestines, where they contract involuntarily to move food and waste products through the digestive tract. Cardiac muscle tissue is also involuntary and, as its name implies, is found only in the heart. These fibers contract in response to demands on the cardiovascular system. The heart muscle contracts at a slow, steady rate at rest but contracts more frequently and forcefully during physical activity. Skeletal muscle tissues consist of long, cylindrical, multinucleated fibers. They provide the force needed to move the skeletal system and can be controlled voluntarily.

Muscle fiber types influence adaptations to training and muscle fitness performance. There are three distinct types of muscle fibers: slow-twitch (Type I), fast-twitch (Type IIb), and intermediate (Type IIa). Each responds and adapts differently to muscle fitness activities. Therefore, muscle fitness is influenced directly by fiber type distribution and the extent to which fibers have adapted as a result of training.

The slow-twitch fibers are generally red in color (due to good blood flow) and are well suited to produce energy with aerobic metabolism. Slow-twitch fibers generate less tension but are more resistant to fatigue. Endurance training leads to adaptations in the slow-twitch fibers that allow them to produce energy more efficiently and to better resist fatigue. Fast-twitch fibers are generally white in color and are well suited to produce energy with anaerobic processes. They generate greater tension than slow-twitch fibers, but they fatigue more quickly. These fibers are particularly well suited to fast, high-force activities that require strength and power, such as explosive weight-lifting movements, sprinting, and jumping. Resistance exercise enhances strength primarily by increasing the size (muscle **hypertrophy**) of fast-twitch fibers, but cellular adaptations also take place to enhance various metabolic properties. Intermediate fibers have biochemical and physiological properties that are between those of the slow-twitch and fast-twitch fibers. A distinct property of these intermediate fibers is that they are highly adaptable, depending on the type of training that is performed.

The relative amount of fast- and slow-twitch fibers can influence performance and adaptations to training. An applied example of fiber types is evident in the different coloration of meat in chickens compared to ducks. The chicken is heavy and must exert a powerful force to fly a few feet up to a perch. Thus, flying muscles in chickens tend to be white (fast-twitch). In contrast, a wild duck that flies for hundreds of miles has dark meat (slow-twitch fibers) in the flying muscles for better endurance. Humans have a mix of fast- and slow-twitch fibers, but each person might inherit a certain predisposition to one type or another. The mix of fibers can influence potential to adapt to different types of training. Muscle fitness activities generally lead to improved fitness and performance primarily through changes in fast-twitch fibers, while aerobic fitness activities lead to adaptations in slow-twitch fibers.

Leverage is an important mechanical principle that influences muscle fitness. The body uses a system of levers to produce movement. Muscles are connected to bones via tendons, and some muscles (referred to as "primary movers") cross over a particular joint to produce movement. When a muscle contracts, it physically shortens and pulls the two bones connected by the joint together to produce movement. Figure 1 shows the two heads of the biceps muscle inserting on the forearm. When the muscle contracts, the forearm is pulled up toward the upper arm (elbow flexion).

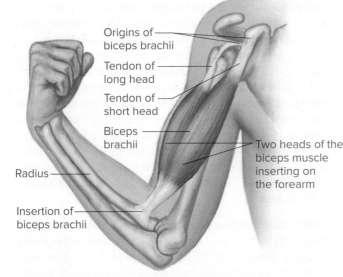

Figure 1 ▶ Muscles contract (shorten) to produce movement.

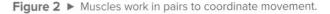

When the thigh muscles (quadriceps) contract to extend the knee they are the agonist (hamstrings are the antagonist)

When the muscles on the back of thigh (hamstrings) flex the knee they are the agonist (quadriceps are the antagonist)

Figure 2 ▶ Muscles work in pairs to coordinate movement.

The muscle on the opposite side (triceps) relaxes or lengthens to allow the movement.

Figure 2 shows a related image of knee flexion and extension to show the distinctions between **agonist muscles** and **antagonist muscles** that work together to coordinate movement.

A person with long arms and legs has a mechanical advantage in most movements, since the force that is exerted can act over a longer distance. Although it is not possible to change the length of your limbs, it is possible to learn to use your muscles more effectively. The ability of elite golfers to hit a golf ball 350 yards, for example, is due primarily to the ability to generate torque and power rather than due to strength.

Genetics, sex, and age affect muscle fitness performance.
Each person inherits a certain proportion of muscle fiber types in his or her skeletal muscle. This allocation influences the potential a person has for muscle fitness activities. Regardless of genetics, all people can 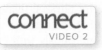 improve their strength and muscular endurance with proper training. Females generally are smaller than males, have smaller amounts of the anabolic hormone testosterone, and, therefore, have less muscle mass than males. Because of this, females typically have 60–85 percent of the absolute strength of males. However, when expressed relative to lean body mass, females have similar relative strength as males. For example, a 150-pound female who lifts 150 pounds has relative strength equivalent to that of a 250-pound male who lifts 250 pounds, even though absolute strength is lower. Sex differences between males and females for both absolute and relative power are similar to those for strength. Absolute muscular endurance tends to be greater for males, but the

difference again is negated if relative muscular endurance is considered.

Measures of **relative muscle fitness** are typically better indicators of performance since they take into account differences in size and muscle mass. However, for some activities, **absolute muscle fitness** may be more important. Maximum strength and power are usually reached in the 20s and typically decline with age. However, after age 30, people who are physically inactive can lose as much as 3–5 percent of their muscle mass per decade, a phenomenon known as **sarcopenia**. Muscular endurance also typically declines as people grow

Hypertrophy Increase in the size of muscles as a result of strength training; increase in bulk.

Agonist Muscles Muscle or muscle group that contracts to cause movement during an isotonic exercise.

Antagonist Muscles Muscle or muscle group on the opposite side of the limb from the agonist muscles.

Relative Muscle Fitness Muscular performance (strength, endurance, or power) adjusted for body size.

Absolute Muscle Fitness A maximum performance for strength (e.g., number of pounds lifted at one time), muscular endurance (e.g., number of times a specific weight can be lifted), or power (e.g., maximum distance in putting the shot).

Sarcopenia An age-related decline in muscle mass that is due, in part, to declines in physical activity.

older, but the decrease is less dramatic for muscular endurance than for strength and power.

The components of muscle fitness are interrelated. Most activities rely on various combinations of strength and muscular endurance; thus, it is important to have sufficient amounts of both. Training protocols are specific for each, but a person who trains for strength will develop some endurance and a person who trains for endurance will develop some strength. Power is sometimes referred to as "explosive strength" because it is the product of both strength and speed. Strength contributes to power, but specific training is necessary for building power.

While not a component of muscle fitness, cardiorespiratory endurance is conceptually related to muscular endurance. Both are necessary for performing exercise for extended periods of time. Cardiorespiratory endurance depends primarily on the efficiency of the circulatory and respiratory systems, while muscular endurance depends primarily on the efficiency of the local skeletal muscles.

Health Benefits of Muscle Fitness Activities

Good muscle fitness and regular muscle fitness activities contribute to the prevention of chronic diseases and early death. Muscle fitness (often described as the functional outcome of muscular strength, muscular endurance, and power) enhances the functionality of the skeletal system, the cardiovascular system, and the metabolic system. The current *Physical Activity Guidelines for Americans* (as well as the World Health Organization's *Global Recommendations on Physical Activity for Health*) emphasizes the importance of regular muscle fitness activities for optimal health. The guidelines call for adults to perform **muscle fitness activities** at least two times a week (in addition to regular aerobic activity). Following are some of the established health benefits associated with muscle fitness activities and good muscle fitness:

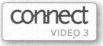

- Lower risk of all-cause mortality
- Fewer heart attacks; a better heart disease risk profile
- Lower incidence of high blood pressure (hypertension)
- Reduced risk of some cancers
- Healthier blood lipid profile
- Better insulin sensitivity and improved blood glucose
- Reduced risk of metabolic syndrome
- Better body composition (i.e., less body fat and more lean muscle)
- Greater bone mass and less risk of osteoporosis
- Lower risk for osteoarthritis and musculoskeletal disorders

Good muscle fitness and regular muscle fitness activities contribute to weight control. The primary determinant of daily energy expenditure is lean body mass since it influences your overall basal metabolic rate. Gradual increases in body fatness with age are attributable (in large part) to declines in muscle mass and corresponding declines in metabolism. Regular muscle fitness activities can preserve muscle mass and contribute to improved weight control. For each pound of muscle gained, a person can burn approximately 35–50 calories more per day. Physical activity has been shown to be critical for maintaining weight loss and a recent longitudinal study confirmed that muscle fitness exercise is especially important for controlling excess abdominal body fatness.

Good muscle fitness and regular muscle fitness activities help maintain the ability to function effectively in daily life. Muscle fitness allows work to be done more easily. With good muscle fitness, you have the energy needed to perform daily tasks efficiently and effectively and the reserve energy to enjoy leisure time. Regular muscle fitness activities are particularly important for older adults since it helps prevent the loss of muscle mass that occurs with age. Adults that perform muscle fitness activities can delay the effects of sarcopenia, improve their mobility, and maintain independence, delaying premature aging.

Regular muscle fitness activities are important for both prevention and treatment of injuries and chronic conditions. As muscle balance is important in reducing the risk for injury, resistance training should build both agonist and antagonist muscles. For example, if you do resistance exercise to build the quadriceps muscles (front of the thigh), you should also exercise the hamstring muscles (back of the thigh). In this instance, the quadriceps are the agonist (muscle being used), and the hamstrings are the antagonist. If the quadriceps become too strong relative to the antagonist hamstring muscles, the risk for injury increases (see Figure 2).

Muscle fitness exercise provides the cornerstone for effective physical therapy and is prescribed for injury rehabilitation and recovery after a variety of musculoskeletal surgeries. Individuals with cancer and other chronic conditions have also been shown to benefit in different ways from muscle fitness exercise. For example, breast cancer survivors report fewer symptoms after performing muscle fitness activities.

Good muscle fitness is associated with good posture and reduced risk for back problems. When muscles in specific body regions are weak or underdeveloped, poor posture can result. Lack of fitness of the abdominal and low back muscles is particularly related to poor posture and potential back problems. Muscle fitness of the core (e.g., abdominal, paraspinal [back], and gluteal muscles) also influences posture and may reduce the risk of injuries and back problems. (Review the Concept on body mechanics for more comprehensive information on posture and back care.)

Table 1 ▶ Advantages and Disadvantages of Isotonic, Isometric, Plyometric, and Isokinetic Exercises

	Advantages	Disadvantages
Isotonic	• Can effectively mimic movements used in sport skills • Enhance dynamic coordination • Challenge muscles through full range of motion	• Do not offer equal resistance at all joint angles • May require equipment or machines
Isometric	• Can be done anywhere • Require only low-cost/little equipment • Can rehabilitate an immobilized joint	• Build strength at only one position • Cause less muscle hypertrophy • Are a poor link or transfer to sport skills
Plyometric	• Build power that is especially useful in sports • Typically do not require expensive equipment • Facilitate bone development when used appropriately	• Can be risky for the untrained • Require good knowledge of training technique to be safe • Require good strength for safe and effective use
Isokinetic	• Offer equal resistance at all joint angles • Are beneficial for rehabilitation and evaluation • Are safe and less likely to promote soreness	• Require specialized equipment • Cannot replicate natural acceleration found in sports • Are more complicated to use and cannot work all muscle groups

Good muscle fitness and regular muscle fitness activities are associated with wellness and quality of life. Recent research has documented a number of wellness and mental health benefits associated with resistance exercise including increased vigor, improved cognition, improved mood states, reduced depression, reduced anxiety, and reduced fatigue. A recent meta-analysis concluded that regular resistance exercise was associated with reduced anxiety symptoms among both healthy participants and participants with a physical or mental illness. Another systematic review specifically examined the psychological benefits of strength exercise in people who are overweight. The results showed small but consistent benefits in a variety of psychological outcome measures with effects comparable to or sometimes stronger than those found in aerobic and diet interventions. Thus (similar to aerobic exercise), resistance exercise can increase healthspan (years of quality of life) as well as lifespan. (See the HELP feature to further explore this topic.)

Progressive Resistance Exercise

Progressive resistance exercise is the principal method of improving muscle fitness. Exercise that gradually and systematically increases overload to the muscles is called **progressive resistance exercise (PRE)**. *Weight training* and *progressive resistance training (PRT)* are often used as synonyms for *PRE*, but they should not be confused with the various competitive events related to resistance exercise. Weight lifting is a competitive sport that involves two lifts: the snatch and the clean and jerk. Powerlifting, also a competitive sport, includes three lifts: the bench press, the squat, and the dead lift. Bodybuilding is a competition in which participants are judged on the size and **definition** of their muscles. Participants in these competitive events rely on highly specialized

forms of PRE to optimize their training. Individuals interested in general muscular fitness also rely on PRE but do not need to follow the same routines or regimens to achieve good results. Others may engage in muscle fitness activities for reasons other than to improve fitness.

There are different types of PRE, and each has its advantages and disadvantages. The main types of PRE are isotonic, isometric, plyometric, and isokinetic. All use overload progressively to build muscle fitness, each in a unique way. The advantages and disadvantages of each type are summarized in Table 1.

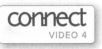

- **Isotonic** exercises are the most common type of PRE. They include calisthenics (body weight exercise), resistance machine exercises, free weight exercises, and exercises using other types of resistance such as exercise bands. The defining feature of isotonic exercise is that the muscle shortens and lengthens to cause movement. Isotonic exercise allows for the use of resistance through a full range of joint motion and provides an effective stimulus for muscle development.

Muscle Fitness Activities Higher-intensity resistance activities that contribute to improved muscle strength, muscle endurance, and power. (See step 4 of the physical activity pyramid.)

Progressive Resistance Exercise (PRE) The type of physical activity done with the intent of improving muscle fitness.

Definition The detailed external appearance of a muscle.

Isotonic Type of muscle contraction in which the muscle changes length, either shortening (concentrically) or lengthening (eccentrically).

Resistance Exercise Boosts Confidence and Mental Health

It's clear that resistance exercise provides numerous benefits for physical health, but there is increasing evidence documenting the benefits of resistance exercise on mental health. Although the mechanisms for mental health benefits are not well established, regular participation can help promote a positive cycling of mood and confidence. The gains in muscle fitness from resistance exercise are thought to directly contribute to the increased confidence and enhanced mood which, in turn, tend to spur on continued participation.

Are you more inclined to be motivated by the physical benefits of resistance exercise or by the mental benefits? Why?

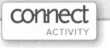

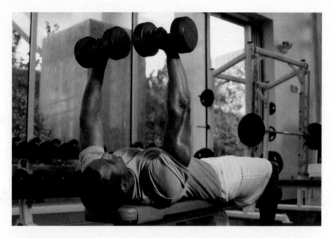

Progressive resistance exercises are used in programs designed to build muscle fitness.
©Fuse/Corbis/Getty Images

When performing isotonic exercise, both **concentric contractions** (shortening) and **eccentric contractions** (lengthening) are important. For example, in a standard biceps curl, the biceps contract concentrically to lift the weight and then eccentrically to lower the weight back down to the starting position. Many people emphasize only the lifting (concentric) phase, but isotonic exercises are most effective when weights are lowered in a slow and controlled manner. Depending on the resistance used, isotonic exercises can build both **dynamic strength** and **dynamic muscular endurance**. *Dynamic* refers to movement, so strength and muscular endurance that cause movement are referred to as dynamic.

- **Isometric** exercises are those in which no movement takes place while a force is exerted against an immovable object. When properly done, isometric exercise can build **static strength** or **static muscular endurance**. However, isometric exercises are not emphasized in PRE programs because the gains are evident only at the angle of the joint used in the exercise.

- **Plyometric** exercises are a form of isotonic exercises that involves a stretch-shortening cycle: an active prestretch (eccentric phase) followed by a fast powerful contraction (concentric phase). An example is landing following a jump (eccentric phase) and then jumping again (concentric phase). More aggressive forms include "depth jumping," such as jumping up off a box to landing (eccentric phase) and then jumping back on top of the box (concentric phase). The loading or eccentric phase stretches the muscle before it contracts, allowing the muscle to contract with greater force. Less aggressive forms include activities such as repetitive hopping, sequential jumping, jumping

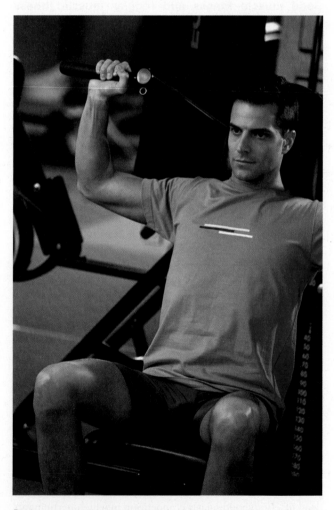

Resistance exercise can promote lean body mass and contribute to a healthy appearance.
Tom Grill/Corbis/Getty Images

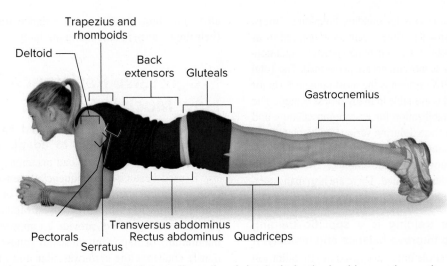

Trapezius and
rhomboids

Deltoid

Back
extensors   Gluteals

Gastrocnemius

Pectorals

Serratus

Transversus abdominus
Rectus abdominus   Quadriceps

Figure 3 ▶ The plank is a core exercise that strengthens the abdominals, back, shoulders, and a number of other stabilizing muscles of the core.
Mark Ahn Creative Services

rope, and medicine ball throws. Plyometrics build power (explosive strength). A foundation in strength is necessary prior to performing plyometric exercises.

- **Isokinetic** exercises are isotonic-concentric muscle contractions performed on machines that keep the velocity of the movement constant through the full range of motion. Isokinetic machines essentially match the resistance to the effort of the performer, permitting maximal tension to be exerted throughout the range of motion. Isokinetic exercises are effective, but they are typically found only in sport training or rehabilitation settings.

Core training uses a variety of resistance training methods to build the core muscles of the body. **Core training** is not a specific type of resistance training such as isokinetics, isometrics, or plyometrics. It can be done with a variety of methods. However, specific types of exercises are used to more effectively engage the core musculature. Inadequate development of these muscles has been shown to be a risk factor for back pain, so it is important to incorporate specialized core exercises into a resistance training program.

The plank is one of the most common isometric core training exercises as it effectively activates a number of stabilizing core muscles. In the front plank, a person holds a horizontal push-up position, bearing the body weight on the forearms, elbows, and toes. The plank strengthens primarily the abdominals, back, and shoulders, but a variety of stabilizing muscles are engaged to resist the pull of gravity and keep the body horizontal (see Figure 3). Many variations of the plank exist, and they can be modified to fit different fitness levels.

Functional fitness training focuses on improving movements used in real life. Interest in functional fitness has increased dramatically in recent years, and it is now widely promoted in both fitness centers and rehabilitation facilities. The ACSM recommends the use of neuromotor

exercises designed to improve motor skills, balance, coordination, gait, and agility for the maintenance and improvement of functional fitness. Balance tends to deteriorate with age, partly due to corresponding declines in muscle strength, range of motion, and a reduced ability to coordinate muscle movements. Therefore, neuromuscular exercise and functional fitness are especially important for older individuals.

Concentric Contractions Isotonic muscle contractions in which the muscle gets shorter as it contracts, such as when a joint is bent and two body parts move closer together.

Eccentric Contractions Isotonic muscle contractions in which the muscle gets longer as it contracts—that is, when a weight is gradually lowered and the contracting muscle gets longer as it gives up tension. Eccentric contractions are also called *negative exercise.*

Dynamic Strength A muscle's ability to exert force that results in movement. It is typically measured isotonically.

Dynamic Muscular Endurance A muscle's ability to contract and relax repeatedly. This is usually measured by the number of times (repetitions) you can perform a body movement in a given period. It is also called *isotonic endurance.*

Isometric Type of muscle contraction in which the muscle remains the same length. Also known as *static contraction.*

Static Strength A muscle's ability to exert a force without changing length; also called *isometric strength.*

Static Muscular Endurance A muscle's ability to remain contracted for a long period. This is usually measured by the length of time you can hold a body position.

Plyometrics A training technique used to develop explosive power. It consists of isotonic-concentric muscle contractions performed after a prestretch or an eccentric contraction of a muscle.

Isokinetic Isotonic-concentric exercises done with a machine that regulates movement velocity and resistance.

Core Training A specialized training regimen designed to improve the strength and functionality of core muscles.

There are multiple methods for building functional fitness, but one approach common in fitness centers is referred to as "suspension training," which uses a cabling system to intentionally destabilize the body as movements are performed. The Total Resistance Exercise (TRX) system is the most popular form for suspension training and is available in many fitness centers. The concept is that the destabilization forces core musculature and joint stabilizers to be activated during various multi-joint movements. Research has supported the contention that TRX increases muscle activation and joint stability, but long-term benefits have not been demonstrated. There are also many alternative approaches to building functional fitness.

Functional balance training is a specific training method designed to improve balance and mobility. It is beneficial to older people but is also used in rehabilitation and in specialized training regimens for sports. This type of training is typically conducted with specialized devices, such as exercise balls (Swiss balls), BOSU platforms, and balance boards. Because these devices challenge you to remain balanced, they recruit muscles that are not typically worked in most strength training regimens. Core fitness exercises are also important for functional balance training because of their importance in stabilizing the body.

Progressive Resistance Exercise: How Much Is Enough?

Progressive overload is needed to challenge the musculoskeletal system to adapt. The foundational principle of PRE is the overload principle. The word *progressive* is used because the frequency, intensity, and length of time of muscle overload are gradually, or progressively, increased as muscle fitness increases. Moderate and vigorous physical activity do not provide an appropriate stimulus for maintaining or improving muscular fitness because they primarily challenge the cardiovascular and respiratory system. Thus, muscle fitness activities are placed as a separate step in the physical activity pyramid (see Figure 4). The activities at this level are primarily anaerobic activities that challenge the muscular and skeletal systems to work at maximal or near maximal levels. Over time, the body adapts to enable gains in muscular strength, muscular endurance, and power.

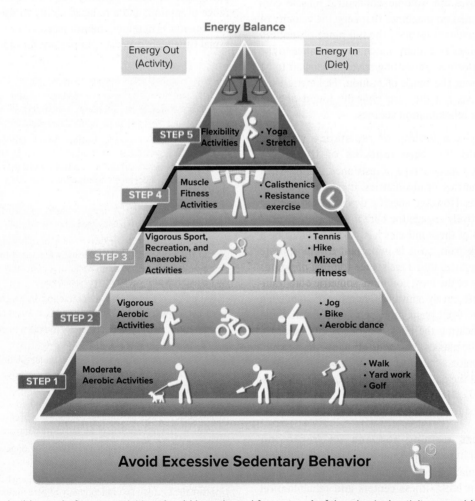

Figure 4 ▶ To build muscle fitness, activities should be selected from step 4 of the physical activity pyramid.

Table 2 ▶ Threshold of Training and Fitness Target Zones for Different Components of Muscular Fitness

	Threshold of Training	Fitness Target Zones
Muscular Strength Training		
Frequency	2 days a week for each muscle group	2–3 days a week for each muscle group
Intensity*	40–60% of 1RM	60 to 85% of 1RM
Time (sets and repetitions)	1–2 sets of 8–12 reps	2–4 sets of 8–12 reps
Muscular Endurance Training		
Frequency	2 days a week for each muscle group	2–3 days a week for each muscle group
Intensity*	<50% of 1RM	50% of 1RM
Time (sets and repetitions)	1–2 sets of 15–25 reps	2–4 sets of 15–25 reps
General Muscle Fitness Training (combined strength and muscular endurance)		
Frequency	2 days a week for each muscle group	2–3 days a week for each muscle group
Intensity*	40–60% of 1RM	60 to 85% of 1RM
Time	1 set of 8–12 reps	1–3 sets of 8–12 reps
Power Training (plyometrics are recommended only for those with a sufficient base of fitness)**		
Frequency	2 days a week	2–3 days a week
Intensity*	Body weight	Body weight or with load
Time	1 set of jumps or movements	1–3 sets of jumps or movements

*Recommendations are for typical exercisers. Beginners or older individuals may benefit from loads of even 40–60 percent of 1RM for strength and muscular endurance. Advanced lifters may need to use higher intensities and with different formats.

**Plyometrics is an effective way to build power, but it is recommended only for those with a sufficient base level of fitness. Body weight may be sufficient for most people but intensity can be increased with added weight or medicine balls (see Concept 12 for more details). Exercises may include depth jumps or bounding calisthenics.

There is a FIT formula for each type of PRE. The FIT formula varies for each type of isotonic PRE, depending on the expected benefit. Days of exercise per week are used to determine frequency (F). Intensity (I) is determined using a percentage of your **1 repetition maximum (1RM)** for isotonic and isokinetic exercises and percentage of maximum exertion for isometric exercises (see Lab 10A). Time (T) is determined by the number of repetitions and sets (groups of repetitions) of an exercise. Table 2 illustrates the FIT formulas for PRE designed primarily to build different components of muscle fitness (strength, muscular endurance, general muscle fitness, and power). Most people will benefit from the general muscle fitness regimen, but customized programs may be needed for more specific goals.

The recommended frequency of PRE depends on personal fitness goals. As illustrated in Table 2, the recommended frequency of exercise for muscle fitness varies based on the expected outcomes. For beginners and older people, 2–3 days per week is recommended. For most everyone else, 3 days per week is recommended. The ACSM recommends 48 hours of rest between exercise sessions to provide appropriate time for recovery. The great proportion of potential strength gains can be accomplished with 2 days of training per week. Exercise done on a third day results in additional increases, but the amount of gain is relatively small, compared with gains resulting from 2 days of training per week. For people interested in health benefits rather than performance benefits, 2 days a week saves time and may result in greater adherence to a strength training program. For people interested in performance benefits, more frequent training may be warranted (4–6 days a week). Rotating exercises so that certain muscles are exercised on one day and other

1 Repetition Maximum (1RM) The maximum amount of resistance you can move a given number of times—for example, 1RM = maximum weight lifted one time; 6RM = maximum weight lifted six times.

muscles are exercised the next allows for more frequent training. For example, upper body exercises can be performed on alternating days so that each can be performed 2-3 days per week.

The optimal intensity of PRE depends on the relative importance of strength and endurance. The amount of resistance (intensity of exercise) used in a PRE program is based on a percentage of your 1 repetition maximum (1RM)—the maximum amount of resistance you can move (or weight you can lift) one time. The 1RM value provides an indicator of your maximum strength, but desired levels of resistance are determined using percentages of the 1RM value. The specific prescription depends on the program goals (see Table 2). For strength, the percentages typically vary 60-80 percent of the 1RM value depending on experience and fitness level. For older adults, the percentage of 1RM is less (40-50 percent). For muscular endurance, the recommended percentage is 50 percent of 1RM for most adults, with slightly lower ranges recommended for older adults (40-50 percent).

The total amount of time for PRE sessions is quantified by sets and repetitions. For cardiorespiratory endurance exercise, the recommendations for time (T) refers to minutes but, with PRE, the T refers to sets and repetitions. Each set should be performed to muscle fatigue, but not to muscle failure as this can result in increased injury risk and muscle soreness that reduces adherence to regular training.

The recommended number of repetitions varies with the type of PRE. The stimulus for strength is high-level exertion, so the goal is to select a load that can be lifted a maximum of 8-12 times. A total of 1-3 sets are recommended with at least 2-3 minutes between sets. For muscular endurance the stimulus is more related to volume, so the focus should be on lighter weights that can be lifted 15-25 times. A total of 2-4 sets are recommended with rest intervals of approximately 1 minute. Individuals interested in general muscle fitness can select weights that allow an intermediate range of reps (10-18). Advanced lifters may need to select higher intensities and perform more sets to provide a stimulus that continues challenging the muscles.

The graph in Figure 5 illustrates the relationship between strength and muscular endurance. Training that requires high resistance and low repetitions (top bar) results in the least gain in endurance but the greatest gain in strength. Training with moderate resistance and moderate repetitions (second bar) results in moderate gains in both strength and endurance. Training that requires a high number of repetitions and

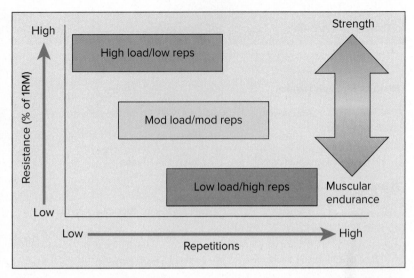

Figure 5 ▶ Comparison of muscular endurance with muscle strength by different repetitions and resistance.

a relatively low resistance (third bar) results in small gains in strength but large increases in muscular endurance.

The FIT formula for power varies based on the type of exercise and the abilities of the person performing it. Even though power is viewed as a dimension of health-related fitness, achieving power requires a good foundation of strength. This is because power reflects both the force and speed of movement. Beginners should build strength before trying to improve power. Following the FIT formula for strength (see Table 2) for 6 weeks would provide a sound foundation of strength.

Once a foundation of strength is achieved, more specific power training can be used as part of an overall program. When using body weight refer to Table 2. When using other forms of resistance (e.g., free weights or pulleys), the ACSM recommends 1 to 6 sets using 30-60% of 1RM for upper body exercises and 0-60% of 1RM for lower body exercises. Higher percentages are used to increase the force component of the power equation and light to moderate loading are performed at an explosive velocity to enhance the speed component of power. Multi-set routines are often used to enable training in both strength and speed.

A training technique that is specifically designed to improve power is plyometric exercise. This technique takes advantage of a quick prestretch prior to a movement to increase power. By repeatedly doing these movements in training, it is possible to provide a greater stimulus to the muscles and improve the body's ability to perform power movements over time. Examples of plyometric drills for leg power are hopping drills or depth jumps. During these exercises, the leg muscles lengthen in an eccentric contraction to absorb the force of the drop and then follow immediately with a strong concentric contraction to complete the next jump or stride. The

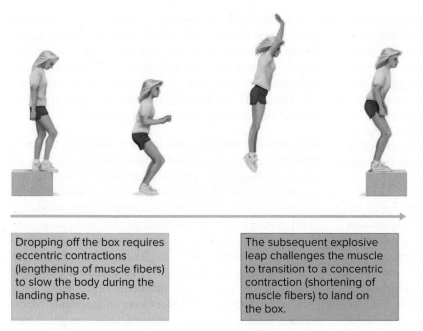

Dropping off the box requires eccentric contractions (lengthening of muscle fibers) to slow the body during the landing phase.

The subsequent explosive leap challenges the muscle to transition to a concentric contraction (shortening of muscle fibers) to land on the box.

Figure 6 ▶ Plyometric exercise—a technique for developing power.

prestretch of the muscle during landing adds an elastic recoil that provides extra force to the push-off (see Figure 6). A push-up that thrusts the hands and arms off the floor is an example of the same principle applied to upper body exercise. A medicine ball throw provides another good option to build power in the upper body.

Muscle Fitness Activities and Equipment

Free weights are the most commonly used equipment for resistance exercise. Free weight equipment consists of weights that are typically loaded onto a barbell or a dumbbell. They have often been considered to be the domain of serious weight lifters, but now they are widely used by more casual fitness enthusiasts. Based on 3-year-trend data from the Sports and Fitness Industry Association (SFIA), use of free weight equipment has increased by 5–15 percent while use of machines has decreased by 2–5 percent. Factors that contribute to the popularity of free weights are their versatility, the ability to change weight in gradual increments, and the ability to modify exercises for specific muscles or movements (see Table 3). Because free weights require balance and technique, they may be more difficult for beginners to use.

Resistance training machines offer many advantages for overall conditioning. Resistance training machines can be effective in developing strength and muscular endurance if used properly. They can save time because, unlike free weights, the resistance can be changed easily and quickly. They may be safer because you are less likely to drop weights.

Table 3 ▶ Advantages (+) and Disadvantages (−) of Free Weights and Machine Weights

		Free Weights		Machine Weights
Isolation of Major Muscle Groups	−/+	Movements require balance and coordination; more muscles are used for stabilization.	+/−	Body stabilizes during lift, allowing isolation, but muscle imbalances can develop.
Applications to Real-Life Situations	+	Movements can be developed to be truer to real life.	−	Movements are determined by the paths allowed on the machine.
Risk for Injury	−	There is more possibility for injury because weights can fall or drop on toes.	+	They are safer because weights cannot fall on participants.
Need for Assistance	−	Spotters are needed for safety with some lifts.	+	No spotters are required.
Time Requirement		More time is needed to change weights.	+	It is easy and quick to change weights or resistance.
Number of Available Exercises	+	Unlimited number of exercises is possible.	−	Exercise options are determined by the machine.
Cost	+	They are less expensive, but good (durable) weights are still somewhat expensive.	−	They are expensive; access to a club is usually needed.
Space Requirement	+/−	Equipment can be moved, but loose weights may clutter areas.	−/+	Machines are stationary but take up large spaces.

A disadvantage is that the kinds of exercises that can be done on these machines are more limited than free weight exercises. They also may not promote optimal balance in muscular development, since a stronger muscle can often make up for a weaker muscle in the completion of a lift. Some machines have mechanisms that provide variable, or accommodating, resistance. These features allow the machine to provide a more appropriate resistance across the full range of motion. New lines of equipment allow the arms and legs to work more independently and enable the exercises to better simulate free living movements.

Circuit resistance training (CRT) is an effective way to build muscular endurance as well as cardiorespiratory endurance. Circuit resistance training (CRT) is a mixed fitness activity that combines several different activities in a workout. CRT consists of the performance of high repetitions of an exercise with low to moderate resistance, progressing from one station to another, performing a different exercise at each station. The stations are usually placed in a circle to facilitate movement. CRT typically uses about 15–25 reps against a resistance that is 30–50 percent of 1RM for 45 seconds. Fifteen seconds of rest is provided while changing stations. Approximately 10 exercise stations are used, and the participant repeats the circuit two to three times (sets). Because of the short rest periods, significant cardiovascular benefits have been reported in addition to muscular endurance gains.

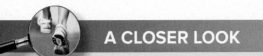

A CLOSER LOOK

CrossFit Controversy

Mixed fitness activities are popular; however, the approaches used in some programs have been controversial. CrossFit is a company that uses high-intensity mixed fitness training conducted in its specially designed and franchised gyms. Although CrossFit has maintained a steady following in the fitness industry, its overall popularity has declined considerably over time. Some people value the forced accountability, the inherent challenge, and the support provided in CrossFit programs. However, the pressures and "cultish" atmosphere are also what drive many people away. Experts have continued to express concerns that CrossFit may push people too hard and increase risk of injury. Advocates have argued that consumers have a choice regarding physical activity and that the media highlights isolated negative events.

Do you think you need a high-pressure environment and high-intensity activities to stay fit or do you prefer a more relaxed environment for your workouts?

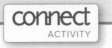

CRT strategies are commonly used in new hybridized group fitness classes aimed at building both muscular fitness and aerobic fitness. They are also incorporated into mixed fitness regimens and high-intensity interval training (HIIT) regimens to provide more of a functional, whole-body workout. Thus, CRT can be broadly viewed as a method of integrating resistance exercise with aerobic exercise.

A variety of resistance devices are available to aid in plyometric and functional fitness training. To improve functional fitness, it is important to mimic movements that occur in real life. The TRX cable system mentioned earlier leverages gravity and body position to change resistance. However, there are simple alternatives that can be done using elastic bands. Kettlebells are also commonly used for functional fitness training. While kettlebells are not really different from a traditional dumbbell, the handles make them more versatile for more dynamic, functional fitness movements. Other simple resistance devices used in functional fitness training include weighted "medicine balls," weighted bars (e.g., Bodybar), and sand/water bag resistance cords. The same equipment can be used in plyometric training for power.

Body weight exercises are popular alternatives to traditional exercise equipment. While equipment can facilitate some aspects of training, there is also a movement toward greater reliance on bodyweight exercises. Examples of common bodyweight exercises include squats, push-ups, sit-ups, and pull-ups, but there are many other variations, including many options with elastic tubing. Bodyweight training naturally engages muscles of the core, forcing the deep muscles to stabilize the trunk in neutral alignment while utilizing the superficial muscles to power movement of the arms and legs. Many advocates appreciate the simplicity of bodyweight exercises, especially since many exercises can be done at home (see Technology Update).

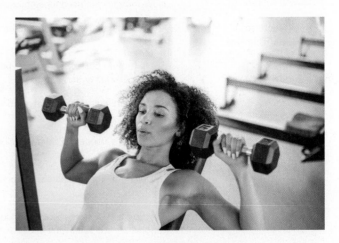

Good technique using slow and controlled movements help to optimize gains from resistance exercise.
vitapix/E+/Getty Images

Online Resistance Training Options

Resistance training has historically been conducted in gyms since most people don't have access to their own equipment. However, there are now many options for interactive online training routines and fitness programming that can be done at home, spurred in part by gyms being closed in response to the COVID-19 pandemic. *Mirror* by Lululemon is one example of a home workout system that uses an interactive computer monitor that looks like a regular mirror hung on the wall. The monitor offers a variety of workouts (both live and interactive and prerecorded) that you can "mirror" as the exercises are demonstrated. The company obé fitness also provides online muscle fitness classes similar to the popular Peloton program for bicycling.

Would you consider online muscle fitness workouts to help you stay fit?

connect
ACTIVITY

Principles of Muscle Fitness Training

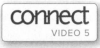

Apply the overload principle to determine appropriate workloads. For the body to adapt and improve, the muscles and systems of the body must be challenged. As noted earlier, the concept behind PRE is that the frequency, intensity, and duration of lifts are progressively increased to maintain an effective stimulus as the muscle fitness improves. When the overload principle is followed, the muscles are progressively challenged and the body adapts with structural and metabolic improvements that lead to increases in strength and endurance. Progress may be hard to detect, and this may contribute to the many misconceptions about resistance training. Table 4 summarizes some common myths and fallacies about resistance exercise (e.g., "no pain, no gain") and explains what really happens with correctly planned resistance exercise.

Apply the principle of progression to adapt and change the program. An effective PRE program should build progressively over time as your fitness level improves.

Table 4 ▶ Fallacies and Facts about Resistance Training

Fallacies	Facts
Resistance training will make you muscle-bound and cause you to lose flexibility.	Normal resistance training will not reduce flexibility if exercises are done through the full range of motion and with proper technique. Powerlifters who do highly specific movements have been shown to have poorer flexibility than other weight lifters.
Females will become masculine-looking if they gain strength.	Females will not become masculine-looking from resistance exercise. Females have less testosterone and do not bulk up from resistance training to the same extent as males. Females and males can make similar relative gains in strength and hypertrophy from a resistance training program, however. The greater percentage of fat in most females prevents the muscle definition possible in males and camouflages the increase in bulk.
Strength training makes you move more slowly and look uncoordinated.	Strength training, if done properly, can enhance sport-specific strength and increase power. There are no effects on coordination from having high levels of muscular fitness.
No pain, no gain.	It is not true that you have to get to the point of soreness to benefit from resistance exercise. It may be helpful to strive until you can't do a final repetition, but you should definitely stop before it is painful. Slight tightness in the muscles is common 1–2 days following exercise but is not necessary for adaptations.
Soreness occurs because lactic acid builds up in the muscles.	Lactic acid is produced during muscular work but is converted back into other substrates within 30 minutes after exercising. Soreness is due to microscopic tears or damage in the muscle fibers, but this damage is repaired as the body builds the muscle. Excessive soreness occurs if you violate the law of progression and do too much too soon.
Strength training can build cardiorespiratory endurance and flexibility.	Resistance exercise can increase heart rate, but this is due primarily to a pressure overload rather than a volume overload on the heart that occurs from endurance (aerobic) exercise. Gains in muscle mass do cause an increase in resting metabolism that can aid in controlling body fatness.
Strength training is beneficial only for young adults.	Studies have shown that people in their 80s and 90s can benefit from resistance exercise and improve their strength and endurance. Most experts would agree that resistance exercise increases in importance with age rather than decreases.

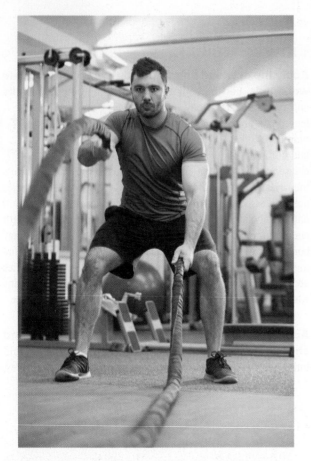

A variety of training methods can be used to improve functional fitness.
Shutterstock

Many beginning resistance trainers experience soreness after the first few days of training. The reason for the soreness is that the principle of progression has been violated. Soreness can occur with even modest amounts of training if the volume of training is considerably more than normal. In the first few days or weeks of training, the primary adaptations in the muscle are due to motor learning factors rather than to muscle growth. Because these adaptations occur no matter how much weight is used, start your program slowly with light weights. After these adaptations occur and the rate of improvement slows down, the intensity and volume of training can increase to achieve proper overload.

The most common progression used in resistance training is the double progressive system, so called because this system periodically adjusts both the resistance and the number of repetitions of the exercise performed. For example, if you are training for strength, you may begin with three repetitions in one set. As the repetitions become easy, additional repetitions are added. When you have progressed to eight repetitions, increase the resistance and decrease the

repetitions in each set back to three and begin the progression again.

Apply the principle of specificity to get specific results. The adaptations resulting from exercise are specific to the type and intensity of exercise performed. If you are not training for a specific task, but merely wish to develop muscle fitness for daily living, a general fitness program (or a functional fitness program) will provide good, overall benefits. However, specific training is needed if you have specific goals. Factors that can be varied in your program are the type of muscle contraction (isometric or isotonic), the speed or cadence of the movement, and the amount of resistance being moved. For example, if you want strength in the elbow extensor muscles (e.g., triceps) so that you can more easily lift heavy boxes onto a shelf, you can train using isotonic contractions, at a relatively slow speed, with a relatively high resistance. If you want muscle fitness of the fingers to grip a heavy bowling ball, much of your training should be done isometrically using the fingers the same way you normally hold the ball. If you are training for a skill that requires explosive power, such as in throwing, striking, kicking, or jumping, your strength exercises should be done with less resistance and greater speed. If you are training for a skill that uses both concentric and eccentric contractions, you should perform exercises using these characteristics (e.g., plyometrics).

Apply the principles of dose-response and reversibility to understand adaptations. The body is an amazing and unique machine since it adapts to make exercise easier on itself. The nature of the adaptations depends on the type and amount of activity performed as well as on the presence of a regular stimulus or challenge. Compromise is sometimes needed depending on the relative importance of different facets of fitness. Too much endurance training can cause a loss of strength and power because of the modification of different muscle fibers. Strength and power athletes need some endurance training, but not too much, just as endurance athletes need some strength and power training, but not too much.

Apply the principle of diminishing returns for program efficiency. To get optimal strength gains from progressive resistance training, several sets of exercise repetitions should be performed. However, research indicates that considerable fitness (and health benefits) can be achieved with a single set. The first set produces approximately 50 percent of the available gain, with successive sets yielding smaller incremental benefits. A single set is recommended for beginners, but two or more are recommended for most people (see Table 2). For those interested in high-level performance, extra benefits from additional sets may be worth the effort. However, for many people this may not be the case.

Apply the principle of rest and recovery to avoid overtraining. Rest is an important part of the body's adaptation to exercise. The frequency guidelines proposed in Table 2 are based on the need for rest following vigorous resistance training exercise. For most people, 3 days of resistance training provides an appropriate amount of overload and rest. If PRE is done more often than this, injuries and overtraining are more likely.

While often not appreciated, an adequate rest period between workouts ensures that there is appropriate time for cellular adaptations to occur. The repeated repetitions in a PRE workout create some minor damage to the outer layers of the contracting muscle fibers. With adequate rest, these muscle fibers rebuild and become stronger. The cycle of catabolic and anabolic processes is critical for effective adaptation to PRE. The ACSM recommends about 48 hours between workouts for the same muscle groups (about three workouts a week).

Apply the principle of individuality to adjust training to meet personal goals. The general guidelines for muscular fitness must be adapted to meet personal needs and goals. Advanced lifters may need to train more than 3 days a week to optimize gains, but it is also important to vary the muscle groups and provide adequate rest between workouts. Serious strength training athletes also employ principles of *periodization* to ensure a proper balance between training and rest. In a periodization plan, the volume and intensity of training are altered to impose different challenges while still keeping the body rested. (See the Concept on advanced training principles.)

Risks with Muscle Supplements

Steroids and related analogs present significant and permanent health risks. The use of **anabolic steroids** in sports has received considerable media attention over the years. The harmful effects of use are well documented, but it is important to continue to emphasize that they are illegal and extremely dangerous. Steroid use directly increases risk for heart disease, liver disease, and early death. It leads to a variety of negative psychological outcomes (e.g., hostility, violence, depression, mood swings, apathy, and addiction) and undesirable body changes such as hair loss, acne, breast enlargement (males), and breast reduction (females). Perhaps more salient to young adults is the fact that steroids lead to adverse sexual/reproductive effects in both males (e.g., testicular atrophy, impotence, and sterility) and females (e.g., uterine atrophy, menstrual irregularities, and sterility).

Synthetic "designer" steroids, such as tetrahydrogestrinone (THG), have the same properties (and risks) of other anabolic steroids. Other steroid analogs such as androstenedione (andro) have been used by athletes to get around regulations and testing of steroids. Andro is a precursor of naturally occurring testosterone and estrogen so it was harder to detect supplementation. Early studies suggested that andro did not lead to increases in testosterone levels; but later evidence documented that andro produced anabolic effects at the high doses used by athletes and it also has the same health risks as conventional steroids. It has been banned by the FDA.

Many athletes have been caught using human growth hormone (HGH) or synthetic analogs to improve performance. As a main effect is increasing bone strength, athletes have believed this would protect them from some of the bone injuries that occur among steroid users. However, evidence has also documented compounded health risks. The use of steroids and analogs presents major health risks and remain illegal.

Supplements touting muscle-building effects are marketed without documentation of safety or efficacy. A number of other dietary supplements are marketed (either legally or illegally) to capitalize on interest in muscular development and sports performance. Contrary to popular belief, they are typically ineffective or dangerous (often both). Although the Food and Drug Administration (FDA) helps protect against fraud and quackery in the supplement industry, the current legislation makes it easy for supplement manufacturers to market and sell products without documenting the safety or efficacy of the ingredients. Reports of adverse effects eventually accumulate with sufficient enough frequency to allow the FDA to take action. An example is with a muscle-building supplement containing a compound called DMAA (dimethylamylamine). The FDA received multiple reports of illness and death following usage and released warnings about supplements containing DMAA. The use of DMAA is known to raise blood pressure and lead to cardiovascular problems such as shortness of breath, arrhythmias, tightening in the chest, and heart attack, as well as seizures and other neurological and psychological conditions. The FDA has since informed manufacturers that they must stop selling products with DMAA; however, companies often ignore the warnings or switch to other ingredients with similarly untested effects (see In the News).

Supplements containing creatine may be safe but have limited effectiveness. Creatine is a nutrient involved in the production of energy during short-term, high-intensity exercise, such as resistance exercise. The body produces creatine naturally from foods containing protein, but some athletes take creatine supplements to increase the amounts available in the muscle. The concept behind supplementation

Anabolic Steroids Synthetic hormones similar to the male sex hormone testosterone. They function androgenically to stimulate male characteristics and anabolically to increase muscle mass, weight, bone maturation, and virility.

is that additional creatine intake enhances energy production and therefore increases the body's ability to maintain force and delay fatigue. Some studies have shown improvements in athletic performance with creatine, but reviews indicate that it may only help athletes who are already well trained. Studies have demonstrated performance-enhancing effects of creatine on muscle strength, but the benefits are due to the ability to work the muscles harder during an exercise session, not to the supplement itself. At present, creatine usage hasn't been linked to any major health problems, but the long-term effects are unknown.

Guidelines for Safe and Effective PRE

Beginners should emphasize lighter weights and progress their program gradually. When beginning a resistance training program, start with light weights so that you can learn proper technique and avoid soreness and injury. Most of the adaptations that occur in the first few months of a program are due to improvements in the body's ability to recruit muscle fibers to contract effectively and efficiently. These neural adaptations occur in response to the movement itself and not the weight that is used. Therefore, beginning lifters can achieve significant benefits from lighter weights. As experience and fitness levels improve, use heavier loads and more challenging sets to continually challenge the muscles.

Use proper technique to reduce the risks for injury and to isolate the intended muscles. An important consideration in resistance exercise is to complete all lifts through the full range of motion using only the intended muscle groups. A common cause of poor technique is using too heavy of a weight. If you have to jerk the weight up or use momentum to lift the weight, it is too heavy. Using heavier weights will provide a greater stimulus to your muscles only if your muscles are actually doing the work. Therefore, it is best to use a weight that you can control safely. By lifting through the full range of motion, you increase the effectiveness of the exercise and maintain good flexibility. Some safety tips are presented in Table 5.

Perform lifts in a slow, controlled manner to enhance both effectiveness and safety. Lifting at a slow cadence provides a greater stimulus to the muscles and increases strength gains. A good recommendation is to take 2 seconds on the lifting phase (concentric) and 3–4 seconds on the lowering (eccentric) phase.

Provide sufficient time to rest during and between workouts. The body needs time to rest in order to allow beneficial adaptations to occur. Choose an exercise sequence that alternates muscle groups so muscles have a chance to

Table 5 ▶ How to Prevent Injury
• Warm up 10 minutes before the workout and stay warm.
• Do not hold your breath while lifting. This may cause blackout or hernia.
• Avoid hyperventilation before lifting a weight.
• Avoid dangerous or high-risk exercises.
• Progress slowly.
• Use good shoes with good traction.
• Avoid arching the back. Keep the pelvis in normal alignment.
• Keep the weight close to the body.
• Do not lift from a stoop (bent over with back rounded).
• When lifting from the floor, do not let the hips come up before the upper body.
• For bent-over rowing, lay your head on a table and bend the knees, or use one-arm rowing and support the trunk with your free hand.
• Stay in a squat as short a time as possible and do not do a full squat.
• Be sure collars on free weights are tight.
• Use a moderately slow, continuous, controlled movement and hold the final position a few seconds.
• Overload but don't overwhelm! A program that is too intense can cause injuries.
• Do not allow the weights to drop or bang.
• Do not train without medical supervision if you have a hernia, high blood pressure, a fever, an infection, recent surgery, heart disease, or back problems.
• Use chalk or a towel to keep your hands dry when handling weights.

rest before another set. Lifting every other day or alternating muscle groups (if lifting more than 3–4 days per week) provides rest for the muscles.

Include exercises to build muscle fitness of all muscle groups. A common mistake made by many beginning lifters is to perform only a few different exercises or to emphasize a few body parts. Training the biceps without working the triceps, for example, can lead to muscle imbalances that can compromise flexibility and increase risks for injury. In some cases, training must be increased in certain areas to compensate for stronger antagonist muscle groups. Many sprinters, for example, pull their hamstrings because the quadriceps are so overdeveloped

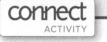

connect
ACTIVITY

that they overpower the hamstrings. The recommended ratio of quadriceps to hamstring strength is 60:40.

Customize your training program to fit your specific needs. Athletes should train muscles the way they will be used in their skill, using similar patterns, range of motion, and speed (the principle of specificity). If you wish to develop a particular group of muscles, remember that the muscle group can be worked harder when isolated than when worked in combination with other muscle groups. However, a good guideline is to choose exercises that build muscle fitness in the major muscle groups of the body. For more information, consult the supplemental Tables at the end of the Concept. Table 6 provides eight basic exercises for free weights. Table 7 presents eight basic exercises for resistance machines. Table 8 shows calisthenic exercises that can serve as alternatives for resistance training. Table 9 includes eight core strength exercises, and Table 10 shows specific options for trunk muscle fitness. Since good muscular fitness in the abdominals is important, it is recommended that some abdominal or core training be performed as part of any program.

It is important to understand your limitations and establish reasonable expectations for your training. Many people get inspired to exercise based on goals to be slimmer or to look good for a special occasion. Appropriately designed muscle fitness activities can improve muscle fitness but will not lead to meeting these personal goals without corresponding reductions in body fatness. If your goals are mostly focused on improving your figure or physique, the most appropriate base program would be of the muscular endurance type. High-repetition, low-resistance exercise is suitable for this because it usually brings about some strengthening and higher volume would expend more calories. Muscle fitness activities do not spot-reduce fat, but they do speed up metabolism which can contribute to weight loss. Including aerobic activity or using CRT approaches may offer advantages since they contribute to both weight loss and muscle fitness.

Using Self-Management Skills

Practicing self-assessments for muscle fitness can help you determine your strengths and weaknesses. Simple screening tools may help determine if you have sufficient muscular fitness for good health. A long-term study of firefighters found that those able to complete 40 push-ups had significantly lower rates of cardiovascular disease than those that could only do 10. Similar studies have documented that grip strength is predictive of chronic disease and early death risk, cognitive disorders, and risk for hospitalization in older adults. The ability to do push-ups or to have a good grip are not specifically important, but the results suggests that these assessments may serve as a simple proxy or screening tool for evaluating functional capacity. The assessments in Lab 10A and 10B allow you to try several different field tests of muscle fitness. The results can help you determine if you have sufficient muscular strength and endurance for good health.

Preparing a muscle fitness exercise plan requires the use of multiple self-management skills. Preparing a plan requires the use of self-assessment skills, goal setting skills, and self-monitoring skills. Following a plan also requires self-management skills, skills in overcoming barriers, and relapse-prevention skills. The planning labs inLabs 10C and 10D help you plan muscle fitness exercises and then monitor your progress in adhering to your plan. It isn't important that you stick with this specific plan, but the practice in setting up and following a plan can build confidence and skills for the future.

Strategies for Action: Lab Information

An important step in taking action for developing and maintaining muscle fitness is assessing your current status. A 1RM test of isotonic strength is described in the Lab Resource Materials: Muscle Fitness Tests. This test allows you to determine absolute and relative strength for the arms and legs. In addition, the 1RM values can be used to help you select the appropriate resistance for your muscle fitness training program. A grip strength test of isometric strength is also provided in the Lab Resource Materials for Lab 10A.

Three tests of muscular endurance and two tests of power are described in the Lab Resource Materials for Lab 10B. It is

recommended that you perform the assessments for strength, muscular endurance, and power before you begin your progressive resistance training program. Periodically reevaluate your muscle fitness using these assessments.

Keeping records of progress will help you adhere to a PRE program. Labs 10C and 10D provide activity logging sheets to help you keep records of your progress as you regularly perform PRE to build and maintain good muscle fitness. (A guide to the major muscle groups is presented in the Lab Resource Materials at the end of this Concept.)

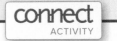

Suggested Resources and Readings

The websites for the following sources can be accessed by searching online for the organization, program, or title listed. Specific scientific references are available at the end of this edition of *Concepts of Fitness and Wellness*.

- Alvar, B. A, Sell, K., & Deuster, P. A. (eds.). (2017). *NSCA's Essentials of Tactical Strength and Conditioning.* Champaign, IL: Human Kinetics.
- American College of Sports Medicine. (2013). *Resistance Training for Health and Fitness.* (pdf)
- American College of Sports Medicine. (2022). *ACSM's Guidelines for Exercise Testing and Prescription* (11th ed.). Philadelphia: Wolters Kluwer.
- American College of Sports Medicine Position Stand. (2009). Progression Models in Resistance Training for Healthy Adults.
- Jacobs, P. (ed.). (2018). *NSCA's Essentials of Training Special Populations.* Champaign, IL: Human Kinetics.
- Kravitz, L. R. (2019). Developing a Lifelong Resistance Training Program. *ACSM's Health & Fitness Journal, 23*(1), 9–15.
- National Strength and Conditioning Association. (2016). *Exercise Technique Manual for Resistance Training* (3rd ed.). Champaign, IL: Human Kinetics.
- Performance Health. Thera-band Academy: Exercises.
- Schwecherl, L. (2020, November 24). "50 Exercises for a Bodyweight Workout You Can Do Anywhere." *The Active Times.*
- U.S. Food and Drug Administration. DMBA in Dietary Supplements.
- U.S. Food and Drug Administration. MedWatch: The FDA Safety Information and Adverse Event Reporting Program.
- World Health Organization (2020, January). *Global Recommendations on Physical Activity for Health.* (pdf)

Lab Resource Materials: Muscles of the Body (anterior view)

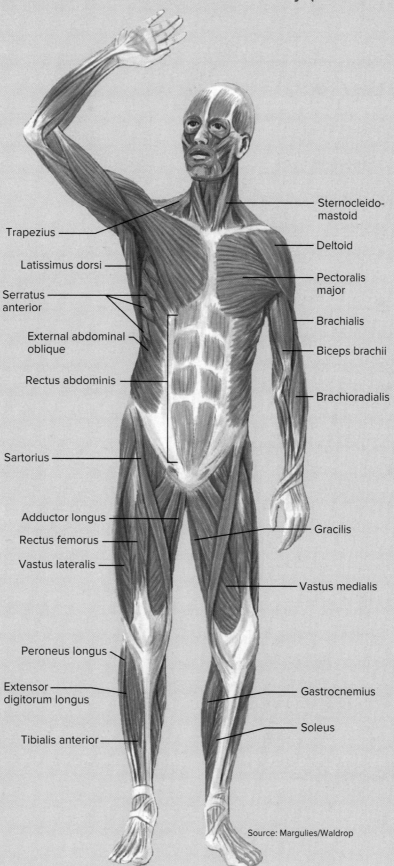

Trapezius

Latissimus dorsi

Serratus anterior

External abdominal oblique

Rectus abdominis

Sartorius

Adductor longus

Rectus femorus

Vastus lateralis

Peroneus longus

Extensor digitorum longus

Tibialis anterior

Sternocleido-mastoid

Deltoid

Pectoralis major

Brachialis

Biceps brachii

Brachioradialis

Gracilis

Vastus medialis

Gastrocnemius

Soleus

Source: Margulies/Waldrop

173

Lab Resource Materials: Muscles of the Body (posterior view)

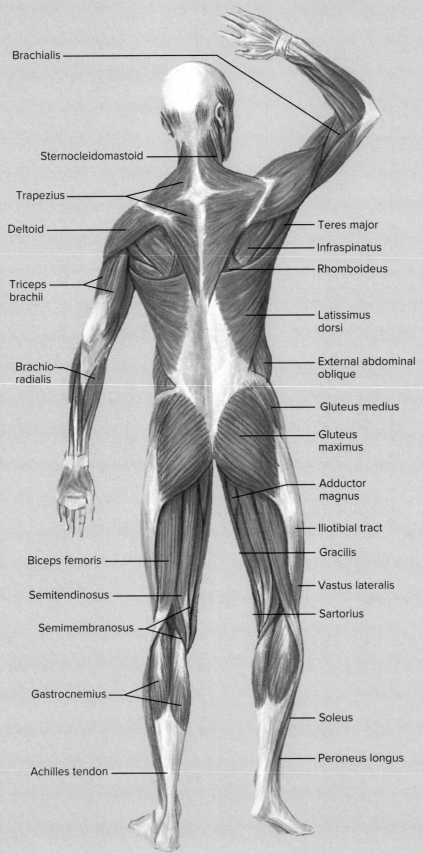

Brachialis

Sternocleidomastoid

Trapezius

Deltoid

Triceps brachii

Brachioradialis

Teres major

Infraspinatus

Rhomboideus

Latissimus dorsi

External abdominal oblique

Gluteus medius

Gluteus maximus

Adductor magnus

Iliotibial tract

Gracilis

Vastus lateralis

Sartorius

Biceps femoris

Semitendinosus

Semimembranosus

Gastrocnemius

Soleus

Peroneus longus

Achilles tendon

Source: Margulies/Waldrop

Lab Resource Materials: Muscle Fitness Tests

Evaluating Isotonic Strength: 1RM

1. Use a weight machine for the leg press and seated arm press (or bench press) for the evaluation.
2. Estimate how much weight you can lift 2 or 3 times. Be conservative; it is better to start with too little weight than too much. If you lift the weight more than 10 times, the procedure should be done again on another day when you are rested.
3. Using correct form, perform a leg press with the weight you have chosen. Perform as many times as you can up to 10.
4. Use Chart 1 to determine your 1RM for the leg press. Find the weight used in the left-hand column and then find the number of repetitions you performed across the top of the chart.
5. Your 1RM score is the value where the weight row and the repetitions column intersect.
6. Repeat this procedure for the seated arm press.
7. Record your 1RM scores for the leg press and seated arm press in the Results section.
8. Next, divide your 1RM scores by your body weight in pounds to get a "strength per pound of body weight" (str/lb/body wt.) score for each of the two exercises.
9. Finally, determine your strength rating for your upper body strength (arm press) and lower body (leg press) using Chart 2.

Chart 1 Predicted 1RM Based on Reps-to-Fatigue

Wt.	1	2	3	4	5	6	7	8	9	10	Wt.	1	2	3	4	5	6	7	8	9	10
30	30	31	32	33	34	35	36	37	38	39	170	170	175	180	185	191	197	204	211	219	227
35	35	37	38	39	40	41	42	43	44	45	175	175	180	185	191	197	203	210	217	225	233
40	40	41	42	44	46	47	49	50	51	53	180	180	185	191	196	202	209	216	223	231	240
45	45	46	48	49	51	52	54	56	58	60	185	185	190	196	202	208	215	222	230	238	247
50	50	51	53	55	56	58	60	62	64	67	190	190	195	201	207	214	221	228	236	244	253
55	55	57	58	60	62	64	66	68	71	73	195	195	201	206	213	219	226	234	242	251	260
60	60	62	64	65	67	70	72	74	77	80	200	200	206	212	218	225	232	240	248	257	267
65	65	67	69	71	73	75	78	81	84	87	205	205	211	217	224	231	238	246	254	264	273
70	70	72	74	76	79	81	84	87	90	93	210	210	216	222	229	236	244	252	261	270	280
75	75	77	79	82	84	87	90	93	96	100	215	215	221	228	235	242	250	258	267	276	287
80	80	82	85	87	90	93	96	99	103	107	220	220	226	233	240	247	255	264	273	283	293
85	85	87	90	93	96	99	102	106	109	113	225	225	231	238	245	253	261	270	279	289	300
90	90	93	95	98	101	105	108	112	116	120	230	230	237	244	251	259	267	276	286	296	307
95	95	98	101	104	107	110	114	118	122	127	235	235	242	249	256	264	273	282	292	302	313
100	100	103	106	109	112	116	120	124	129	133	240	240	247	254	262	270	279	288	298	309	320
105	105	108	111	115	118	122	126	130	135	140	245	245	252	259	267	276	285	294	304	315	327
110	110	113	116	120	124	128	132	137	141	147	250	250	257	265	273	281	290	300	310	321	333
115	115	118	122	125	129	134	138	143	148	153	255	256	262	270	278	287	296	306	317	328	340
120	120	123	127	131	135	139	144	149	154	160	260	260	267	275	284	292	302	312	323	334	347
125	125	129	132	136	141	145	150	155	161	167	265	265	273	281	289	298	308	318	329	341	353
130	130	134	138	142	146	151	156	161	167	173	270	270	278	286	295	304	314	324	335	347	360
135	135	139	143	147	152	157	162	168	174	180	275	275	283	291	300	309	319	330	341	354	367
140	140	144	148	153	157	163	168	174	180	187	280	280	288	296	305	315	325	336	348	360	373
145	145	149	154	158	163	168	174	180	186	193	285	285	293	302	311	321	331	342	354	366	380
150	150	154	159	164	169	174	180	186	193	200	290	290	298	307	316	326	337	348	360	373	387
155	155	159	164	169	174	180	186	192	199	207	295	295	303	312	322	332	343	354	366	379	393
160	160	165	169	175	180	186	192	199	206	213	300	300	309	318	327	337	348	360	372	386	400
165	165	170	175	180	186	192	198	205	212	220	305	305	314	323	333	343	354	366	379	392	407

Source: JOPERD.

Chart 2 Fitness Classification for Relative Strength in Males and Females (1RM/Body Weight)

Age:	Leg Press			Arm Press		
	30 or Less	31–50	51+	30 or Less	31–50	51+
Ratings for Males						
High-performance zone	2.06+	1.81+	1.61+	1.26+	1.01+	0.86+
Good fitness zone	1.96–2.05	1.66–1.80	1.51–1.60	1.11–1.25	0.91–1.00	0.76– 0.85
Marginal fitness zone	1.76–1.95	1.51–1.65	1.41–1.50	0.96–1.10	0.86– 0.90	0.66– 0.75
Low fitness zone	1.75 or less	1.50 or less	1.40 or less	0.95 or less	0.85 or less	0.65 or less
Ratings for Females						
High-performance zone	1.61+	1.36+	1.16+	0.76+	0.61+	0.51+
Good fitness zone	1.46–1.60	1.21–1.35	1.06–1.15	0.66– 0.75	0.56– 0.60	0.46– 0.50
Marginal fitness zone	1.31–1.45	1.11–1.20	0.96–1.05	0.56– 0.65	0.51– 0.55	0.41– 0.45
Low fitness zone	1.30 or less	1.10 or less	0.95 or less	0.55 or less	0.50 or less	0.40 or less

Evaluating Isometric Strength

Test: Grip Strength

Adjust a hand dynamometer to fit your hand size. Squeeze it as hard as possible. You may bend or straighten the arm, but do not touch the body with your hand, elbow, or arm. Perform with both right and left hands. *Note:* When not being tested, perform the basic eight isometric strength exercises, or squeeze and indent a new tennis ball (after completing the dynamometer test).

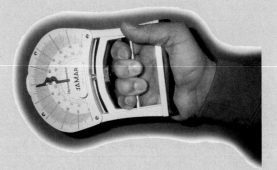

©Charles B. Corbin

Evaluating Muscular Endurance

Test: Curl-Up (Dynamic)

Sit on a mat or carpet with your legs bent more than 90 degrees so your feet remain flat on the floor (about halfway between 90 degrees and straight). Make two tape marks 4½ inches apart or lay a 4½-inch strip of paper on the floor. Lie with your arms extended at your sides, palms down and the fingers extended so that your fingertips touch one tape mark (or one side of the paper strip). Keeping your heels in contact with the floor, curl the head and shoulders forward until your fingers reach 4½ inches (second piece of tape or other side of strip). Lower slowly to beginning position. Repeat one curl-up every 3 seconds. Continue until you are unable to keep the pace of one curl-up every 3 seconds. Two partners may be helpful. One stands on the paper strip (to prevent movement); the second ensures that the head returns to the floor after each repetition.

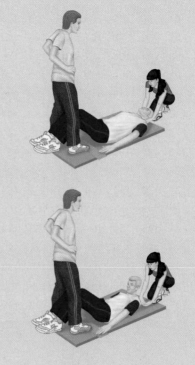

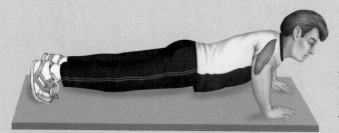

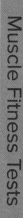

Test: Ninety-Degree Push-Up (Dynamic)

Support the body in a push-up position from the toes. The hands should be just outside the shoulders, the back and legs straight, and toes tucked under. Lower the body until the upper arm is parallel to the floor or the elbow is bent at 90 degrees. The rhythm should be approximately 1 push-up every 3 seconds. Repeat as many times as possible up to 35.

Test: Flexed-Arm Support (Static)

Females: Support the body in a push-up position from the knees. The hands should be outside the shoulders, the back and legs straight. Lower the body until the upper arm is parallel to the floor or the elbow is flexed at 90 degrees.

Males: Use the same procedure as for women except support the push-up position from the toes instead of the knees. (Same position as for 90-degree push-up.) Hold the 90-degree position as long as possible, up to 35 seconds.

Evaluating Power

Test: Vertical Jump

Hold a piece of chalk so that its end is even with your fingertips. Stand with both feet on the floor and your side to the wall; reach and mark as high as possible. Mark the height of your standing reach with the chalk. Jump upward with both feet as high as possible. Swing arms upward and make a chalk mark on the wall at the peak of your jump. Measure the distance between the reaching height and the jumping height. Your score is the best of three jumps. *Note:* You may use a vertical jump measuring device if available.

Test: Medicine Ball Throw

Place a sturdy chair against a wall. Sit with your back firmly against the back of the chair. Hold a 14-pound medicine ball against your chest with both hands. Keeping your back against the chair, throw (push) the ball as far as possible. Your score is the distance from the spot where the ball landed (nearest edge of ball landing) to the wall.

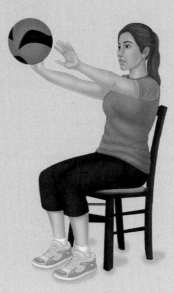

Chart 3 Isometric Strength Rating Scale (Pounds)

Classification	Left Grip	Right Grip	Total Score
Ratings for Males			
High-performance zone	125+	135+	260+
Good fitness zone	100–124	110–134	210–259
Marginal fitness zone	90–99	95–109	185–209
Low fitness zone	<90	<95	<185
Ratings for Females			
High-performance zone	75+	85+	160+
Good fitness zone	60–74	70–84	130–159
Marginal fitness zone	45–59	50–69	95–129
Low fitness zone	<45	<50	<95

Note: Suitable for use by young adults between 18 and 30 years of age. After 30, an adjustment of 0.5–1 percent per year is appropriate because some loss of muscle tissue typically occurs as you grow older.

Chart 4 Isometric Strength Rating Scale (Pounds)

Age:	17–26		27–39		40–49		50–59		60+	
Classification	Curl-Ups	Push-Ups	Curl-Ups	Push-Ups	Curl-Ups	Push-Ups	Curl-Ups	Push-Ups	Curl-Ups	Push-Ups
Ratings for Males										
High-performance zone	35+	29+	34+	27+	33+	26+	32+	24+	31+	22+
Good fitness zone	24–34	20–28	23–33	18–26	22–32	17–25	21–31	15–23	20–30	13–21
Marginal fitness zone	15–23	16–19	14–22	15–17	13–21	14–16	12–20	12–14	11–19	10–12
Low fitness zone	<15	<16	<14	<15	<13	<14	<12	<12	<11	<10
Ratings for Females										
High-performance zone	25+	17+	24+	16+	23+	15+	22+	14+	21+	13+
Good fitness zone	18–24	12–16	17–23	11–15	16–22	10–14	15–21	9–13	14–20	8–12
Marginal fitness zone	10–17	8–11	9–16	7–10	8–15	6–9	7–14	5–8	6–13	4–7
Low fitness zone	<10	<8	<9	<7	<8	<6	<7	<5	<6	<4

Chart 5 Rating Scale for Static Endurance (Flexed-Arm Support)

Classification	Score in Seconds
High-performance zone	30+
Good fitness zone	20–29
Marginal fitness zone	10–19
Low fitness zone	<10

Chart 6 Rating Scale for Power

Classification	Vertical Jump (inches)		Medicine Ball Throw (inches)	
	Males	Females	Males	Females
High-performance zone	22.5+	15+	186+	121+
Good fitness zone	17.5–22.4	12.5–14.9	171–185	111–120
Marginal fitness zone	15.5–17.4	10.5–11.4	156–170	101–110
Low fitness zone	<15.5	<10.5	155 or less	100 or less

Note: Metric conversions are in Appendix A.

1. Bench Press

This exercise develops the chest (pectoral) and triceps muscles. Lie supine on bench with knees bent and feet flat on bench or flat on floor in stride position. Grasp bar at shoulder level. Push bar up until arms are straight. Return and repeat. Do not arch lower back. *Note:* Feet may be placed on floor if lower back can be kept flattened. Do not put feet on the bench if it is unstable.

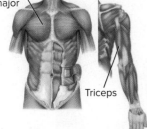

Pectoralis major

Triceps

3. Biceps Curl

This exercise develops the muscles of the upper front part of the arms (biceps). Stand erect with back against a wall, palms forward, bar touching thighs. Spread feet in comfortable position. Tighten abdominals and back muscles. Do not lock knees. Move bar to chin, keeping body straight and elbows near the sides. Lower bar to original position. Do not allow back to arch. Repeat. Spotters are usually not needed. *Variations:* Use dumbbell and sit on end of bench with feet in stride position; work one arm at a time. Or use dumbbell with the palm down or thumb up to emphasize other muscles.

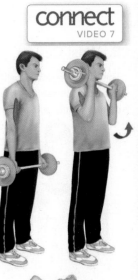

Biceps

2. Overhead (Military) Press

This exercise develops the muscles of the shoulders and arms. Sit erect, bend elbows, palms facing forward at chest level with hands spread (slightly more than shoulder width). Have bar touching chest; spread feet (comfortable distance). Tighten your abdominal and back muscles. Move bar to overhead position (arms straight). Lower bar to chest position. Repeat. *Caution:* Keep arms perpendicular and do not allow weight to move backward or wrists to bend backward. Spotters are needed.

Deltoid

4. Triceps Curl

This exercise develops the muscles on the back of the upper arms (triceps). Sit erect, elbows and palms facing up, bar resting behind neck on shoulders, hands near center of bar, feet spread. Tighten abdominal and back muscles. Keep upper arms stationary. Raise weight overhead, return bar to original position. Repeat. *Variation:* Substitute dumbbells (one in each hand, or one held in both hands, or one in one hand at a time).

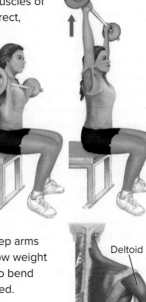

Triceps

Table 6   The Basic Eight for Free Weights

Table 6

5. Wrist Curl

This exercise develops the muscles of the fingers, wrist, and forearms. Sit astride a bench with the back of one forearm on the bench, wrist and hand hanging over the edge. Hold a dumbbell in the fingers of that hand with the palm facing forward. To develop the flexors, lift the weight by curling the fingers then the wrist through a full range of motion. Slowly lower and repeat. To strengthen the extensors, start with the palm down. Lift the weight by extending the wrist through a full range of motion. Slowly lower and repeat. *Variation:* Both wrists may be exercised at the same time by substituting a barbell in place of the dumbbell.

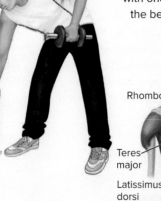

Wrist flexors

7. Half Squat

This exercise develops the muscles of the thighs and buttocks. Stand erect, feet shoulder-width apart and turned out 45 degrees. Rest bar behind neck on shoulders. Spread hands in a comfortable position. Begin squat by first moving hips backward, keeping back straight, eyes ahead. By moving first at the hips and then bending knees, shins will remain vertical. Bend knees to approximately 90 degrees. Pause; then stand. Repeat. Spotters are needed. *Variation:* Substitute dumbbell in each hand at sides.

Gluteus maximus
Rectus femoris
Biceps femoris, long head
Vastus lateralis
Semi-membranosus

6. Dumbbell Rowing

This exercise develops the muscles of the upper back. It is best performed with the aid of a bench or chair for support. Grab a dumbbell with one hand and place opposite hand on the bench to support the trunk. Slowly lift the weight up until the elbow is parallel with the back. Lower the weight and repeat to complete the set. Switch hands and repeat with the opposite arm. *Variation:* The exercise can also be performed with one leg kneeling on the bench.

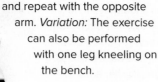

Rhomboids
Teres major
Latissimus dorsi

8. Lunge

This exercise develops the thigh and gluteal muscles. Place a barbell (with or without weight) behind your head and support with hands placed slightly wider than shoulder-width apart. In a slow and controlled motion, take a step forward and allow the leading leg to drop so that it is nearly parallel with the ground. The lower part of the leg should be nearly vertical and the back should be maintained in an upright posture. Take stride with opposite leg to return to standing posture. Repeat with other leg, remaining stationary or moving slowly in a straight line with alternating steps.

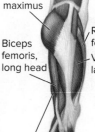

Rectus femoris
Vastus lateralis
Gluteus maximus

The Basic Eight for Resistance Machine Exercises   Table 7

Table 7

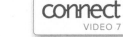

1. Chest Press

This exercise develops the chest (pectoral) and tricep muscles. Position seat height so that arm handles are directly in front of chest. Position backrest so that hands are at a comfortable distance away from the chest. Push handles forward to full extension and return to starting position in a slow and controlled manner. Repeat. *Note:* Machine may have a foot lever to help position, raise, and lower the weight.

Pectoralis major

Triceps

2. Overhead Press

This exercise develops the muscles of the shoulders and arms. Position seat so that arm handles are slightly above shoulder height. Grasp handles with palms facing away and push lever up until arms are fully extended. Return to starting position and repeat. *Note:* Some machines may have an incline press.

Deltoid

3. Biceps Curl

This exercise develops the elbow flexor muscles on the front of the arm, primarily the biceps. Adjust seat height so that arms are fully supported by pad when extended. Grasp handles palms up. While keeping the back straight, flex the elbow through the full range of motion.

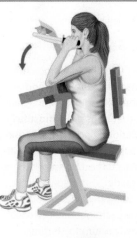

Biceps

4. Triceps Press

This exercise develops the extensor muscles on the back of the arm, primarily the triceps. Adjust seat height so that arm handles are slightly above shoulder height. Grasp handles with thumbs toward body. While keeping the back straight, extend arms fully until wrist contacts the support pad (arms straight). Return to starting position and repeat.

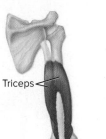

Triceps

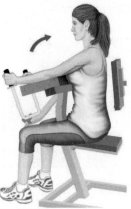

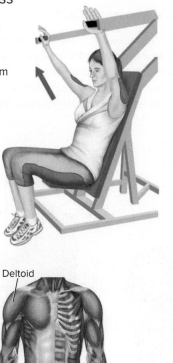

Table 7

Table 7   The Basic Eight for Resistance Machine Exercises

5. Lat Pull-Down

This exercise primarily develops the latissimus dorsi, but the biceps, chest, and other back muscles may also be developed. Sit on the floor. Adjust seat height so that hands can just grasp bar when arms are fully extended. Grasp bar with palms facing away from you and hands shoulder-width (or wider) apart. Pull bar down to chest and return. Repeat.

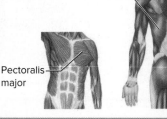

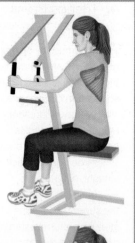

Middle trapezius
Latissimus dorsi
Rhomboid minor
Teres major
Pectoralis major

7. Knee Extension

This exercise develops the thigh (quadriceps) muscles. Sit on end of bench with ankles hooked under padded bar. Grasp edge of table. Extend knees. Return and repeat. *Alternative:* Leg press (similar to half squat). *Note:* The knee extension exercise isolates the quadriceps but places greater stress on the structures of the knee than the leg press or half squat.

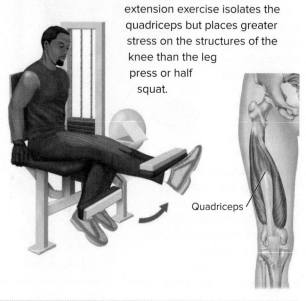

Quadriceps

6. Seated Rowing

This exercise develops the muscles of the back and shoulder. Adjust the machine so that arms are almost fully extended and parallel to the ground. Grasp handgrip with palms turned down and hands shoulder-width apart. While keeping the back straight, pull levers straight back to chest. Slowly return to starting position and repeat.

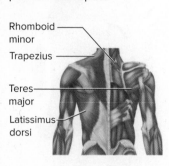

Rhomboid minor
Trapezius
Teres major
Latissimus dorsi

8. Hamstring Curl

This exercise develops the hamstrings (muscles on back of thigh) and other knee flexors. Sit on bench with legs over padded bar, pads contracting lower leg or calf just above the ankles. Grasp handles or edge of seat. Bend knees as far as possible. Return slowly and repeat.

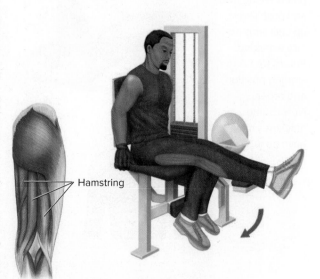

Hamstring

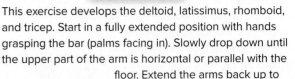

1. Push-Ups

This exercise develops the muscles of the arms, shoulders, and chest. Lie on the floor, face down with hands under shoulders. Keep body straight from the knees to the top of the head. Push up until the arms are straight. Slowly lower chest to floor. Repeat. *Variation:* If this exercise is too difficult, modify by performing on bent knees.

Variation: Start from the up position and lower until the arm is bent at 90 degrees; then push up until arms are extended. *Caution:* Do not arch back.

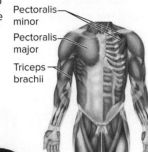

Pectoralis minor
Pectoralis major
Triceps brachii

2. Modified Pull-Ups

This exercise develops the muscles of the arms and shoulders. Hang (palms forward and shoulder-width apart) from a low bar (may be placed across two chairs), heels on floor, with the body straight from feet to head. Bracing the feet against a partner or fixed object is helpful. Pull up, keeping the body straight; touch the chest to the bar; then lower to the starting position. Repeat. *Note:* This exercise becomes more difficult as the angle of the body approaches horizontal and easier as it approaches the vertical. *Variations:* Perform so that the feet do not touch the floor (full pull-up). Or, perform with palms turned up. When palms are turned away from the face, pull-ups tend to use all the elbow flexors. With palms facing the body, the biceps are emphasized more.

Trapezius
Rhomboids
Deltoid
Teres major
Latissimus dorsi

3. Dips

This exercise develops the deltoid, latissimus, rhomboid, and tricep. Start in a fully extended position with hands grasping the bar (palms facing in). Slowly drop down until the upper part of the arm is horizontal or parallel with the floor. Extend the arms back up to the starting position and repeat. *Note:* Many gyms have a dip/pull-up machine with accommodating resistance that provides a variable amount of assistance to help you complete the exercise.

Rhomboid major
Deltoid
Triceps
Latissimus dorsi

4. Crunch (Curl-Up)

This exercise develops the upper abdominal muscles. Lie on the floor with the knees bent and the arms extended or crossed with hands on shoulders or palms on ears. If desired, legs may rest on bench to increase difficulty. For less resistance, place hands at side of body (do not put hands behind head or neck). For more resistance, move hands higher. Curl up until the shoulder blades leave floor; then roll down to the starting position. Repeat. *Note:* Twisting the trunk on the curl-up develops the oblique abdominals.

Internal abdominal oblique
External abdominal oblique
Rectus abdominis

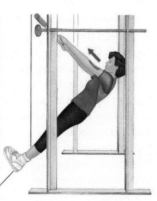

183

Table 8

Table 8   The Basic Eight for Calisthenics

5. Trunk Lift

This exercise develops the muscles of the upper back and corrects round shoulders. Lie face down with hands clasped behind the neck. Pull the shoulder blades together, raising the elbows off the floor. Slowly raise the head and chest off the floor by arching the upper back. Return to the starting position; repeat. For less resistance, hands may be placed under thighs. *Caution:* Do not arch the lower back. Lift only until the sternum (breastbone) clears the floor. *Variations:* Arms down at sides (easiest), hands by head, arms extended (hardest).

Back extensors

7. Step-Ups

This exercise develops the muscles of the thighs and buttocks. Stand facing an 8- to 15-inch-high box or stair. Step up, straightening knee. Keep back straight. Slowly lower opposite foot back to the floor by bending the knee. Repeat. *Variation:* Hold onto dumbbells for greater resistance.

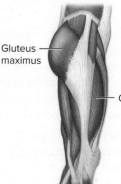

Gluteus maximus

Quadriceps

6. Side Leg Raises

These exercises develop the muscles of the outer and inner thigh. Lie on your side. With knee pointing forward, slowly raise and lower the top leg. Next, bend the top leg and cross it in front of bottom leg for support. Raise and lower the bottom leg. *Variation:* Ankle weights may be added for greater resistance.

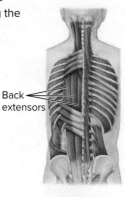

Pectineus

Adductor brevis

Adductor longus

Gracilis

Adductor magnus

Gluteus medius

Tensor fasciae latae

8. Lunge Walk

This exercise develops the muscles of the legs and hips. Stand tall, feet together. Take a step forward with the right foot, touching the left knee to the floor. The knees should be bent only to a 90-degree angle. Rise and step forward with the opposite leg, repeating. *Variation:* Dumbbells may be held in the hands for greater resistance.

Gluteus maximus

Rectus femoris

Vastus lateralis

Biceps femoris, long head

Semimembranosus

Biceps femoris, short head

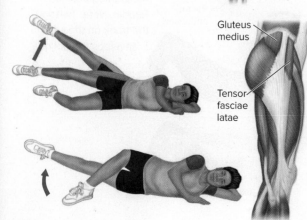

Table 9

Exercises for Abdominal Muscle Fitness   Table 9

1. Crunch

This exercise develops the upper abdominal muscles. Lie on the floor with the knees bent and the arms extended or crossed with hands on shoulders or palms on ears. If desired, legs may rest on bench to increase difficulty. For less resistance, place hands at side of body (do not put hands behind neck). For more resistance, move hands higher. Curl up until shoulder blades leave floor; then roll down to the starting position. Repeat. *Note:* Twisting the trunk on the curl-up develops the oblique abdominals.

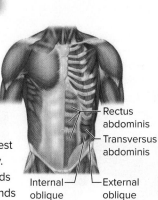

Rectus abdominis

Transversus abdominis

Internal oblique (cut)

External oblique (cut)

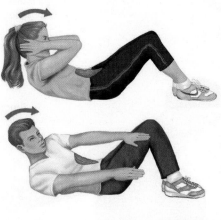

2. Reverse Curl

This exercise develops the lower abdominal muscles. Lie on the floor. Bend the knees, place the feet flat on the floor, and place arms at sides. Lift the knees to the chest, raising the hips off the floor. Do not let the knees go past the shoulders. Return to the starting position. Repeat.

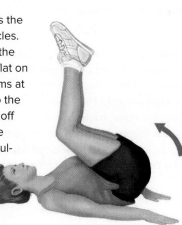

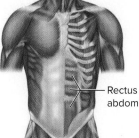

Rectus abdominis

3. Crunch with Twist (on Bench)

This exercise strengthens the oblique abdominals and helps prevent or correct lumbar lordosis, abdominal ptosis, and backache. Lie on your back with your feet on a bench, knees bent at 90 degrees. Arms may be extended or on shoulders or hand on ears (the most difficult). Same as crunch except twist the upper trunk so the right shoulder is higher than the left. Reach toward the left knee with the right elbow. Hold. Return and repeat to the opposite side.

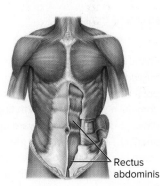

Internal oblique

External oblique

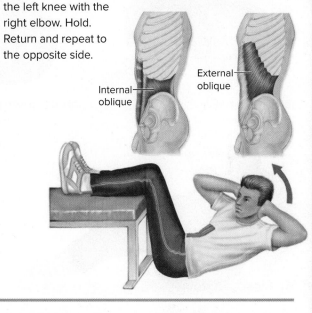

4. Sitting Tucks

This exercise strengthens the lower abdominals, increases their endurance, improves posture, and prevents backache. (This is an advanced exercise and is not recommended for people who have back pain.) Sit on floor with feet raised, arms extended for balance. Alternately bend and extend legs without letting back or feet touch floor.

Rectus abdominis

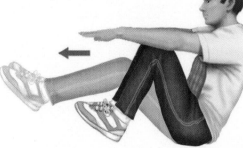

Table 10 Exercises for Trunk Muscle Fitness

Table 10

1. Dynamic Trunk Exercises

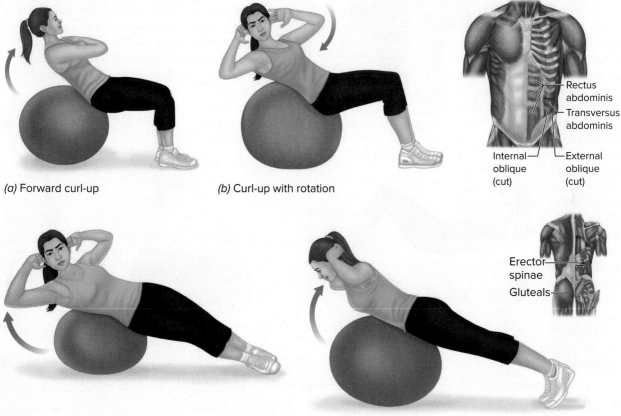

(a) Forward curl-up

(b) Curl-up with rotation

Rectus abdominis

Transversus abdominis

Internal oblique (cut)

External oblique (cut)

(c) Lateral trunk raise

(d) Trunk extension raise

Erector spinae

Gluteals

These exercises strengthen the abdominal and back muscles by moving the trunk through a small arc of motion: *(a)* The *forward curl-up* targets the rectus abdominis. Sit on large ball with hands crossed over chest. Recline backward to the point where feet just begin to lose grip on floor. Curl forward. Repeat. *(b)* The *curl-up with rotation* targets the oblique abdominal muscles. Begin with fingertips by ears and trunk reclined approximately 45 degrees. Curl forward with rotation by drawing one shoulder toward opposite knee. Recline back. Curl forward again, rotating trunk in the opposite diagonal. Repeat. *(c)* The *lateral trunk raise* also targets the oblique muscles. Lie side-bent over ball with fingertips by ears. Straighten spine by raising head and shoulders upward. Repeat. *(d)* The *trunk extension raise* targets the back extensor muscles. Lie flexed on stomach over ball with fingertips by ears. Straighten spine by raising head and chest upward, away from ball. Repeat.

Lab 10A Evaluating Muscle Strength: 1RM and Grip Strength

Name	**Section**	**Date**

Purpose: To evaluate your muscle strength using 1RM and to determine the best amount of resistance to use for various strength exercises.

Procedures: 1RM is the maximum amount of resistance you can lift for a specific exercise. Testing yourself to determine how much you can lift only one time using traditional methods can be fatiguing and even dangerous. The procedure you will perform here allows you to estimate 1RM based on the number of times you can lift a weight that is less than 1RM.

Evaluating Strength Using Estimated 1RM

1. Use a resistance machine for the leg press and arm or bench press for the evaluation part of this lab.
2. Estimate how much weight you can lift 2 or 3 times. Be conservative; it is better to start with too little weight than too much. If you lift a weight more than 10 times, the procedure should be done again on another day when you are rested.
3. Using correct form, perform a leg press with the weight you have chosen. Perform as many times as you can up to 10.
4. Use Chart 1 in Lab Resource Materials to determine your 1RM for the leg press. Find the weight used in the left-hand column and then find the number of repetitions you performed across the top of the chart.
5. Your 1RM score is the value where the weight row and the repetitions column intersect.
6. Repeat this procedure for the arm or bench press using the same technique.
7. Record your 1RM scores for the leg press and bench press in the Results section.
8. Next divide your 1RM scores by your body weight in pounds to get a "strength per pound of body weight" (1RM/body weight) score for each of the two exercises.
9. Determine your strength rating for your upper body strength (arm press) and lower body (leg press) using Chart 2 in Lab Resource Materials. Record in the Results section. If time allows, assess 1RM for other exercises you choose to perform (see Lab 10C).
10. If a grip dynamometer is available, determine your right-hand and left-hand grip strength using the procedures in Lab Resource Materials. Use Chart 3 in Lab Resource Materials to rate your grip (isometric).

Results

Arm press: Wt. selected ____ Reps ____ Estimated 1RM ____

(or bench press) (Chart 1, *Lab Resource Materials, page* 175)

Strength per lb body weight ____ Rating ____

(1RM ÷ body weight) (Chart 2, *Lab Resource Materials, page* 176)

Leg press: Wt. selected ____ Reps ____ Estimated 1RM ____

(Chart 1, *Lab Resource Materials, page* 175)

Strength per lb body weight ____ Rating ____

(1RM ÷ body weight) (Chart 2, *Lab Resource Materials, page* 176)

Grip strength: Right grip score ____ Right grip rating ____

Left grip score ____ Left grip rating ____

Total score ____ Total rating ____

(Chart 3, *Lab Resource Materials, page* 178)

Seated Press (Arm Press)

This test can be performed using a seated press (see image) or using a bench press machine. When using the seated press, position the seat height so that arm handles are directly in front of the chest. Position backrest so that hands are at comfortable distance away from the chest. Push handles forward to full extension and return to starting position in a slow and controlled manner. Repeat. *Note:* Machine may have a foot lever to help position, raise, and lower the weight.

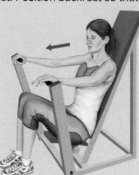

Leg Press

To perform this test, use a leg press machine. Typically, the beginning position is with the knees bent at right angles with the feet placed on the press machine pedals or a foot platform. Extend the legs and return to beginning position. Do not lock the knees when the legs are straightened. Typically, handles are provided. Grasp the handles with the hands when performing this test.

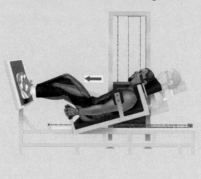

Conclusions and Implications: In several sentences, discuss your current strength, whether you believe it is adequate for good health, and whether you think that your "strength per pound of body weight" scores are representative of your true strength.

Lab 10B Evaluating Muscular Endurance and Power

Name	**Section**	**Date**

Purpose: To evaluate dynamic muscular endurance, static muscular endurance, and power.

Procedures

1. Perform the curl-up, push-up, flexed-arm support, vertical jump, and medicine ball throw tests described in the Lab Resource Materials.
2. Record your test scores in the Results section. Determine and record your rating in Chart 1, based on Charts 4, 5, and 6 in the Lab Resource Materials.

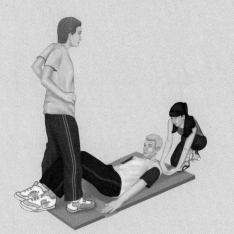

1. Curl-up (dynamic muscular endurance)

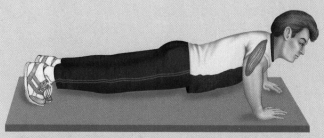

2. Ninety-degree push-up (dynamic muscular endurance)

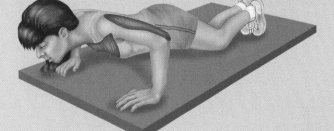

3. Flexed-arm support (static muscular endurance): females in knee position and males in full support position

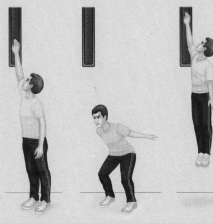

4. Vertical jump (power)

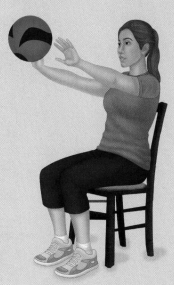

5. Medicine ball throw (power)

Results

Record your scores.

Curl-up [   ]   Push-up [   ]   Flexed-arm support (seconds) [   ]

Vertical jump [   ]   Medicine ball throw [   ]

Check your ratings in Chart 1.

Chart 1 Rating Scale

	Curl-Up	Push-Up	Flexed-Arm Support	Vertical Jump	Medicine Ball Throw
High	○	○	○	○	○
Good	○	○	○	○	○
Marginal	○	○	○	○	○
Poor	○	○	○	○	○

Conclusions and Implications: In several sentences, discuss your current levels of muscular endurance and power. Indicate whether you think you are fit enough to meet your health, work, and leisure-time needs.

Lab 10C Planning and Logging Muscle Fitness Exercises: Free Weights or Resistance Machines

Name	**Section**	**Date**

Purpose: To set lifestyle goals for muscle fitness exercise, to prepare a muscle fitness exercise plan, and to self-monitor progress for the 1- to 2-week plan.

Procedures

1. Using Chart 1, provide some background information about your experience with resistance exercise, your goals, and your plans for incorporating these exercises into your normal exercise routine.
2. Using Chart 2, select at least eight muscle fitness exercises as directed. Perform the exercises for 3 days over a 1- to 2-week period. Be sure to plan your exercise program so that it fits with the goals you described in Chart 1. If you are just starting out, it is best to start with light weights and more repetitions (e.g., 12–15). For best results, take the log with you during your workout, so that you can remember the weights, reps, and sets you performed.
3. Complete the Results section and then answer the questions in the Conclusions and Implications section.

Chart 1 Muscle Fitness Survey

1. Determine your current stage for resistance exercise. Check only the stage that represents your current activity level.

   ⚪ Precontemplation. I do not meet resistance exercise guidelines and have not been thinking about starting.

   ⚪ Contemplation. I do not do resistance exercises but have been thinking about starting.

   ⚪ Preparation. I am planning to start doing regular resistance exercises to meet guidelines.

   ⚪ Action. I do resistance exercises, but am inconsisent or have only recently started being consistent (less than 6 months).

   ⚪ Maintenance. I regularly meet guidelines for resistance exercises and have been doing it for more than 6 months.

2. What are your primary goals for resistance exercise?

   ⚪ General conditioning   ⚪ Improved appearance   ⚪ Other_____

   ⚪ Sports training   ⚪ Avoidance of back pain

Chart 2 Muscle Fitness Exercise Log

Check (√) the exercises you plan to perform in the first column. Choose eight exercises from free weight, machine, or a combination of the two types of exercises. Record the weight (resistance), number of reps, and number of sets you plan to perform. Perform the exercises for 3 days over a period of 1–2 weeks. Write the date (month/day) in the day column for the date you performed the exercise. You may do upper body and lower body exercises on different dates.

Exercises	Exercise Plan			Day 1 _____ (date)			Day 2 _____ (date)			Day 3 _____ (date)		
	Wt.	Reps	Sets	Wt.	Reps	Sets	Wt.	Reps	Sets	Wt.	Reps	Sets
Free Weight Exercises (Table 6, pages 179–180)												
☐ 1. Bench press												
☐ 2. Overhead (military) press												
☐ 3. Biceps curl												
☐ 4. Triceps curl												
☐ 5. Wrist curl												
☐ 6. Dumbbell rowing												
☐ 7. Half squat												
☐ 8. Lunge												
Machine Exercises (Table 7, pages 181–182)												
☐ 1. Chest press												
☐ 2. Overhead press												
☐ 3. Biceps curl												
☐ 4. Triceps press												
☐ 5. Lat pull-down												
☐ 6. Seated rowing												
☐ 7. Knee extension												
☐ 8. Hamstring curl												

Results

Were you able to do your basic eight exercises at least 2 days in the week?   Yes ◯   No ◯

Conclusions and Implications: Do you feel that you will use muscle fitness exercises as part of your regular lifetime physical activity plan, either now or in the future? In the box, indicate what modifications you would make in your program in the future.

connect
ACTIVITY

Lab 10D Planning and Logging Muscle Fitness Exercises: Calisthenics, Core Exercises, or Plyometrics

Name	Section	Date

Purpose: To set lifestyle goals for muscle fitness exercises that can easily be performed at home, to prepare a muscle fitness exercise plan, and to self-monitor progress for a 1-week plan.

Procedures

1. Using Chart 1, provide some background information about your experience with calisthenic, core exercise, or plyometrics, and your plans for incorporating these exercises into your normal exercise routine.
2. Using Chart 2, select at least eight calisthenics or core exercises as directed. Perform the exercises for 2 or 3 days. Record the reps and sets performed on each day.
3. Complete the Results section and then answer the questions in the Conclusions and Implications section.

Chart 1 Muscle Fitness Survey

1. What is your level of experience with calisthenic, core, and plyometric exercises? Check a box for each of the three types of exercise.

	Inexperienced	Somewhat Experienced	Very Experienced
Calisthenic Exercises			
Core Exercises			
Plyometric Exercises			

2. What are your primary reasons for doing calisthenic or core exercise?

- ⭘ General conditioning
- ⭘ Improved appearance
- ⭘ Sports training
- ⭘ Avoidance of back pain

Chart 2 Muscle Fitness Exercise Log

Check (√) the exercises you plan to perform in the first column. Choose eight exercises from the calisthenic, core, and plyometric sections. Record the number of reps and number of sets you plan to perform. Perform the exercises for 3 days over a period of 1–2 weeks. Write the date (month/day) in the day column for the date you performed the exercise. You may do upper body and lower body exercises on different dates.

Exercises	Exercise Plan		Day 1 _____ (date)		Day 2 _____ (date)		Day 3 _____ (date)	
	Reps	Sets	Reps	Sets	Reps	Sets	Reps	Sets
Calisthenic Exercises (Table 8, pages 183–184)								
☐ 1. Push-ups								
☐ 2. Modified pull-ups								
☐ 3. Dips								
☐ 4. Crunch (curl-up)								
☐ 5. Trunk lift								
☐ 6. Side leg raises								
☐ 7. Step-ups								
☐ 8. Lunge walk								
Abdominal and Trunk Exercises (Tables 9 and 10, pages 185–186)								
☐ 1. Crunch (curl-up)								
☐ 2. Reverse curl								
☐ 3. Crunch with twist (on bench)								
☐ 4. Sitting tucks								
☐ 5. Forward curl-up								
☐ 6. Curl-up with rotation								
☐ 7. Lateral trunk raise								
☐ 8. Trunk extension raise								
Plyometric Exercises (See Figure 6 for a sample of Depth Jumps, page 165)								
☐ 1. Rope jumping or hopping								
☐ 2. Medicine Ball (chest pass) Exercise								
☐ 3. Box or Depth Jumps (advanced)								

Results

Were you able to do your planned exercises at least 2 days in the week?   Yes ◯   No ◯

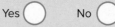

Conclusions and Implications: Do you feel that you will use these muscle fitness exercises as part of your regular lifetime physical activity plan, either now or in the future? Discuss the exercises you feel benefited you and the ones that did not. What modifications would you make in your program for it to work better for you?

Flexibility and Stretching Activities

LEARNING OBJECTIVES

After completing the study of this Concept, you will be able to:

▶ Identify and explain several misconceptions about flexibility.

▶ List the health benefits of flexibility and stretching.

▶ Describe the various methods of stretching and their advantages and disadvantages.

▶ Determine the amount of exercise necessary to improve flexibility, explain the FIT formulas for the different types of stretching, and describe factors in the "do and don't list for stretching."

▶ Describe a variety of flexibility-based activities for improving flexibility.

▶ Identify some of the guidelines for safe and effective stretching.

▶ Describe several self-assessments for flexibility, select the self-assessments that help you identify personal needs, and plan (and self-monitor) a personal flexibility exercise program.

Regular stretching exercises promote flexibility, a component of fitness that permits freedom of movement, contributes to ease and economy of muscular effort, allows for successful performance in certain activities, and provides less susceptibility to some types of injuries or musculoskeletal problems.

Tom Grill/Corbis/Getty Images

Why It Matters!

Flexibility is an important component of functional fitness, but there are many misconceptions about how it contributes to health and how it can be enhanced. It is important to first understand the difference between *stretching* (the principal type of exercise used to build flexibility) and *flexibility* (a component of fitness resulting from stretching). It is also important to distinguish between stretching exercises for building flexibility as part of your workout and stretching as a warm-up. Finally, it is important to understand how much flexibility is needed (some is clearly needed to perform efficiently and effectively in daily life, but excessive flexibility is not desirable). This Concept will clarify the distinctions between flexibility and stretching and provide guidelines for safe and effective ways to include various flexibility-based activities into your program.

Factors Influencing Flexibility

The range of motion in a joint or joints is a reflection of the flexibility at that joint. Clinically, the **range of motion (ROM)** of a joint is the extent *and* direction of movement that is possible. The extent of movement is described by the arc through which a joint moves. It is typically measured in degrees using a tool called a goniometer. The direction of movement at a specific joint is determined by the shapes of the bony surfaces that are in contact. Certain types of joints allow for greater movement than others. In fact, flexibility is highly joint specific. An individual may demonstrate optimal flexibility in one region of the body but not in others. For example, a person may have good enough flexibility of the spine, hips, and legs to reach down and perform a toe touch, but may be unable to clasp both hands behind the back due to stiffness of the shoulder joints.

Medical professionals use a specific vocabulary to describe the movement of joints. Figure 1 illustrates some of these movement terms as they relate to hip, knee, or ankle motion. Similar terms are applied in describing movement of the spine and upper body. Note that the same terms (such as *flexion/extension*) can be applied to different joints, while other terms (such as *dorsiflexion/plantar flexion*) are unique to a specific joint like the ankle.

The shape, size, and orientation of a joint greatly influence the amount of motion available. The circular surface of the ball-and-socket joint of the hip, for example, allows for considerable mobility, including movement to the side (adduction and abduction), forward and backward (flexion and extension), and in and out (internal and external rotation). The hinge joint of the knee is more restrictive and limits movement to primarily forward and backward (flexion and extension). Motion at other joints, such

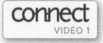

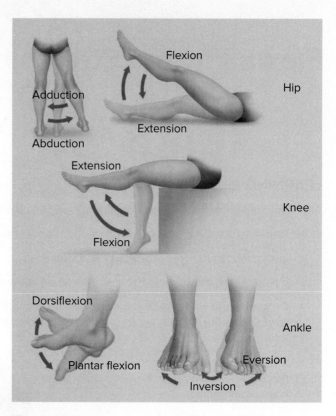

Figure 1 ▶ Ranges of joint motion.

as the ankle, involves the combined movements of numerous bony surfaces. A hinge-type portion permits the up-and-down motion of the foot (dorsiflexion and plantar flexion), while a separate planar-type joint allows the side-to-side motion (inversion and eversion) of the foot. A basic understanding of this terminology is important in understanding principles of flexibility and stretching.

Flexibility is influenced by the extensibility of soft tissues such as muscles, tendons, and ligaments. Soft tissues are made up of a number of substances, including fibers called collagen and elastin. These structural building blocks influence the degree of extensibility of tissues such as **ligaments**, **tendons**, and muscles. Tissues with a greater proportion of collagen fibers tend to be stiffer while those with more elastin tend to bend and stretch more readily. Ligaments contain a greater proportion of collagen, and this enhances their function in providing rigidity and stability to a joint and their role in restricting excessive joint motion. Damage to ligaments from repeated sprains can lead to excessive joint **laxity** and increased risk for injuries. Tendons contain a greater proportion of elastin than ligaments, but muscles contain even more contributing to the relatively high degree of elasticity. Together, the muscles and tendons are referred to as a **muscle-tendon unit (MTU)** and, due to their connection, they are both stretched together. However, the terms *muscles* or *tissues* will generally be used instead of *MTU* for ease of interpretation.

Viscoelastic properties of muscles have an influence on flexibility. The short-term gains in range of motion immediately following stretching can be attributed, in large part, to viscoelastic properties of the muscle. During a sustained stretch, the viscous (fluid-like) and elastic properties of the muscle allow it to slowly increase in length with less effort. Repeated stretching bouts promote further gains in length (creep) and reduced tension in the muscle (stretch-relaxation). These properties of creep and stretch-relaxation partially explain why a static stretch feels easier the longer it is held. However, these viscoelastic influences on flexibility are relatively short-lived, lasting from just a few seconds up to 2 hours in duration.

Viscoelasticity is also rate-dependent. Rapid, bouncing stretches tend to increase muscle tension more than a slow, steady stretch, and this limits the overall extent of elongation. A slower, static stretch avoids this effect and produces more elongation of the muscle. These viscoelastic properties of muscle tissue influence guidelines about the most effective dose (frequency, intensity, time) and type of stretch used to improve flexibility. (Specific guidelines will be covered later in this Concept.)

Short-term changes in muscle flexibility differ from long-term changes. The effectiveness of a flexibility program is largely assessed by its ability to improve ROM. Significant short-term gains in ROM can be achieved by a single (acute) bout of stretching, but a regular, long-term (chronic) stretching program will lead to more sustained gains in flexibility. Research on flexibility suggests that the resulting gains in motion immediately following stretching are due as much to sensory changes in the nervous system as they are to increased muscle length or changes in muscle **stiffness**. Thus, the acute changes in flexibility that occur following a stretch are due to both the viscoelastic properties of muscles and the nervous system's regulation of **stretch tolerance**. Stretch tolerance is the nervous system's way of allowing a person to stretch further toward end range of motion with less perception of pain. Stretch tolerance varies among individuals and can be enhanced by flexibility training.

In contrast to short-term changes, the mechanisms influencing long-term changes in flexibility are considered to be more complex and are not as well understood. Long-term gains in ROM that occur after weeks of participating in a stretching program are believed to be the result of repeated cycles of increased stretch tolerance and changes in muscle length. Increased muscle length is believed to occur when sarcomeres, the building blocks of the muscle fiber, are added to the muscle fiber.

Certain types of muscles are more prone to tightness than others. A number of muscles in the body have a predictable tendency toward tightness. Clinicians refer to these muscles as "tonic" or "postural" muscles because of their tendency to tighten or shorten. Structurally, these muscles tend to be composed of a higher proportion of slow-twitch (Type I) muscle fibers, which tend to be less elastic (stiffer) than fast-twitch (Type II) fibers. Another characteristic of these postural muscles is that they tend to cross more than one joint. Examples include the upper trapezius, the muscles at the base of the skull, the pectorals, hip flexors, back extensors, hamstrings, adductors, and calf muscles. These muscles typically benefit the most from stretching and therefore are often targeted by common stretching exercises. (Specific exercises for these muscle groups are provided at the end of this Concept.)

Static flexibility is different from dynamic flexibility. The flexibility of a joint differs under static versus dynamic conditions. Static flexibility is the maximum range a joint can achieve under stationary conditions, and it is limited by the structural (viscous and elastic) properties of the muscles. An example of static flexibility would be the amount of hamstring flexibility needed to perform the sit-and-reach test, touching fingertips to toes. Dynamic flexibility is the maximum range a joint can achieve under active conditions, and it is influenced by both structural characteristics and neural factors. Dynamic flexibility refers to the ability of the body to move during functional, real-life movements. An example of dynamic flexibility would be the amount of hamstring flexibility needed to clear a track hurdle with the lead leg during a race. Although good static flexibility is necessary for good dynamic flexibility, it does not ensure it. (Techniques for both static and dynamic stretching are discussed later in the Concept.)

Flexibility is influenced by temperature. Muscle and joint temperature directly influence flexibility, with warm muscles being more flexible than cold ones. The higher temperature improves the extensibility of collagen within the joint capsules, muscles, and tendons. Heat also facilitates relaxation by altering the nervous system's response to stretch, making the body less sensitive to the stretch reflex. Thus, a warm shower or heating pad used prior to stretching can help improve flexibility. While the application of an external source of heat has the potential to improve muscle flexibility, an active warm-up is considered to be the most effective method in raising internal temperature of the muscle. In order to prepare the body for exercise or an athletic event, an active warm-up is recommended. Some people specifically

---

Range of Motion (ROM) The full motion possible in a joint or series of joints.

Ligaments Bands of tissue that connect bones. Unlike muscles and tendons, overstretching ligaments is not desirable.

Tendons Fibrous bands of tissue that connect muscles to bones and facilitate movement of a joint.

Laxity Motion in a joint outside the normal plane for that joint, due to loose ligaments.

Muscle-Tendon Unit (MTU) The functional union of a skeletal muscle and its associated tendon. Strengthening and stretching affect both elements of the MTU.

Stiffness Elasticity in the MTU; measured by force needed to stretch.

Stretch Tolerance Greater degree of stretch before onset of pain.

prefer to exercise in warm conditions, possibly because it helps them feel more limber. For example, weight lifters typically prefer to train in a warmer gym.

Flexibility varies considerably across the lifespan. Flexibility is generally high in children but declines during adolescence because of the rapid changes in growth—essentially, the bones grow faster than the soft tissues, leading to tightness. In early adulthood, the muscles and tendons catch up to the skeletal system, allowing flexibility to improve (with peaks generally occurring in the mid- to late 20s). With increasing age, range of motion tends to decline, but this is due to both age-dependent (biologic) changes as well as to modifiable lifestyle factors (e.g., sedentary behavior). The intrinsic factors influencing reduced flexibility with age include a loss of elasticity and water content in soft tissues, reduced size of muscle fibers, age-related cross-linkages within the collagen fibers, and more restricted movement of joints. Over the span of their working lives, adults typically lose 3–4 inches of lower back and leg flexibility as measured by the common sit-and-reach test. Likewise, hip and shoulder ROM have been noted to decrease by approximately 6 degrees per decade in females and males aged 55–86 years old, with the most significant decline noted after age 70.

Decreased flexibility throughout the lifespan has implications for health-related quality of life. For example, reduced leg range of motion can alter gait mechanics and increase risk for falls while reduced flexibility of the spine can increase risk of neck or back pain. Reduced flexibility may also have an impact on functional independence. For instance, reduced joint ROM may adversely affect the ability to perform simple tasks such as bending over to tie shoes or reaching into an overhead cupboard. While loss of flexibility is considered to be a natural part of the aging process, research studies have confirmed that declines in flexibility can be minimized by maintaining regular patterns of physical activity. Thus, adherence to a regular stretching program is one way to somewhat offset declines in function that occur with age.

Flexibility differences exist between males and females. Flexibility differences exist between males and females. Females tend to be more flexible than males at young ages, but the differences are less apparent among adults. The greater flexibility of females is generally attributed to anatomical differences (e.g., wider hips) and hormonal influences.

Genetic factors can explain some individual variability in flexibility. Joint **hypermobility** is sometimes referred to as joint laxity. The term *hypermobility* refers to joints that stretch further than normally expected because of increased elasticity in the connective tissues, including ligaments, muscles, and tendons. In some families, the trait for hypermobile joints is passed from generation to generation. Hypermobile joints are one feature of inherited conditions such as Ehlers-Danlos, Down, and Marfan syndromes. Studies show that people with

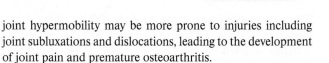

Technology Update

Take-a-Break Reminders

Sedentary office jobs that require sitting at a desk all day can take a toll on both our body and our mind. The recent shift to home-based jobs has created additional challenges by restricting our movement and forcing us to spend even more time online. To avoid computer eye strain and negative outcomes from sitting, it is important to take periodic breaks. While this seems simple, evidence suggests that people need reminders to take small breaks in their day. Programs such as StretchClock.com provide prompts through your computer. A number of other apps such as Stretchly, Stretch Reminder, Unhook, and Microbreak provide reminders to break up sitting time or to take stretch breaks.

Would this type of behavioral prompt help you remember to get up and move periodically? Why or why not?

connect
ACTIVITY

joint hypermobility may be more prone to injuries including joint subluxations and dislocations, leading to the development of joint pain and premature osteoarthritis.

Flexibility, Injuries, and Rehabilitation

Reduced flexibility may contribute to injuries in some individuals. Established risk factors for activity-related injuries include overall level of fitness, previous history of injuries, level of experience, and the type and intensity of activity performed. Reduced flexibility has been commonly viewed as a potential cause of injuries during exercise, but research is not clear on the subject. Some studies have reported significant correlations between flexibility deficits and specific types of injuries. For example, reduced hip and ankle range of motion has been associated with falls in older adults. Similarly, tight hamstring and quadriceps muscles have been associated with knee injuries in soccer players, and tight calf muscles have been associated with leg injuries during basic training in army recruits. However, a number of other studies have not revealed associations between muscle tightness and injury rates.

The emerging consensus is that a combination of fitness-related factors contribute to overall risk of injury risk, including flexibility, strength, power, agility, and balance. Comprehensive injury prevention programs (IPPs) are now used to help decrease risks of injuries among athletes, firefighters, and military personnel. In addition to flexibility training, these programs include other forms of exercises to improve muscle strength, balance, proprioception, and agility. The combination of exercises and movement skills in these programs depends on the needs of the activities. While results can't be attributed directly to flexibility, research has shown promising results from structured IPPs for reducing risks of some injuries.

Excessive flexibility may contribute to injuries in some individuals with hypermobility. Hypermobility is a condition diagnosed by specific clinical findings. Those with increased ligamentous laxity are often believed to be at risk for injury through overstraining their muscles or joints. For example, studies have documented higher injuries in ballet dancers with excessive flexibility and higher risk of ankle sprains in soldiers with hypermobility disorders. Yet not all persons with excessive flexibility suffer from injuries. Despite excessive joint laxity, it appears that people can learn to control their movements and posture in order to protect joints from harm. Clearly, too little or too much flexibility can increase risk of injury, but it doesn't fully predict its occurrence.

Stretching is used to assist in injury rehabilitation and to prevent future injuries. Physical therapists and athletic trainers frequently prescribe **stretching exercises** to help patients regain normal range of motion or function after injury. Stretching also helps promote healing by improving the alignment of collagen fibers. Muscle strains and ligamentous sprains are typically responsive to appropriately prescribed stretching exercise. Stretching also helps alleviate joint stiffness, a common problem following surgeries of the shoulder, knee, and ankle as well as following use of casts or walking boots. In each case, gentle stretching and range of motion exercises are used to stimulate the healing process and add strength to the healing tissues. Prior to stretching, tissues are warmed up through the use of active exercise, massage techniques, or modalities such as moist heat or ultrasound. Stretching is followed by exercises to increase strength within the newly gained range of motion and neuromuscular activities to restore functional movement patterns. However, once prescribed, the effectiveness of rehabilitation is directly dependent on the willingness of the individual to perform the recommended stretching exercises on their own. The strongest predictor of injury is a prior history of injury, so proper rehabilitation is critical to decrease risks in the future.

Stretching can help with treatment of musculoskeletal pain. Stretching is often one component of a larger treatment plan for addressing low back and neck pain. Because it is rarely used as the sole treatment approach, it is difficult to isolate its effectiveness from other treatments commonly provided. However, stretching has been shown to be as effective as strengthening or massage in the treatment of chronic neck pain. Additionally, movement-based activities such as tai chi have been shown to facilitate movement and reduce low back pain.

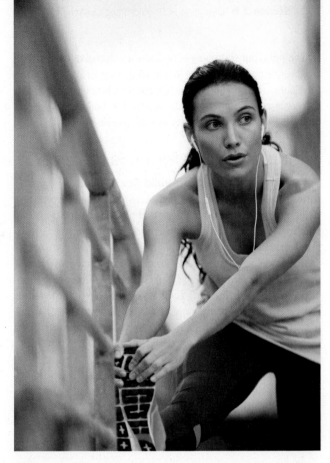

Stretching is most effective following a workout after your body is warmed up.
Sam Edwards/Getty Images

Stretching may help relieve muscle cramps and pain associated with myofascial trigger points. Many people experience some form of muscle cramping during or following exercise. A muscle spasm or cramp may result for various reasons, including overexertion, dehydration, and heat stress. Stretching can often help relieve mild cramps. It also contributes to reducing pain associated with **myofascial trigger points.** Trigger points are characterized by localized areas of taut bands within skeletal muscle that have a nodular texture. They can produce a radiating pain in specific regions of the body when touched. Trigger points can be caused by trauma, but may occur after overuse or from prolonged spasm in the muscles. Physical therapists and clinicians may use needling, massage, and the application of direct pressure over trigger points to help

Hypermobility Looseness or slackness in the joint and of the muscles and ligaments (soft tissue) surrounding the joint.

Stretching Exercise A structured flexibility activity that is intended to maintain or improve range or motion of a specific joint.

Myofascial Trigger Points Tight bands or knots in a muscle or fascia (a sheath of connective tissue that binds muscles and other tissues together). Trigger points often refer pain to another area of the body.

relieve pain, but stretching is typically recommended as part of the overall treatment plan. While stretching helps with some forms of cramps and pain, it is less effective for relieving nonspecific areas of soft tissue tenderness in the body (often called tender points) or delayed onset muscle soreness.

Flexibility: How Much Is Enough?

A variety of activities can build flexibility and improve functional fitness. The Physical Activity Pyramid depicts the different types of physical activity that produce health, wellness, and fitness benefits. Flexibility activities are referenced as a separate level since they have unique benefits. Normal daily activities, and even other activities from the physical activity pyramid, do relatively little to develop flexibility. For this reason, it is important to include flexibility activities from step 5 of the pyramid to build flexibility (see Figure 2). Stretching exercise is the primary way to improve flexibility, but a number of other activities and movement disciplines also build flexibility.

Flexibility is joint specific, so the needed amount of flexibility varies by joint. Norms are available for the amount of flexibility for males and females of different ages,

but it is not clear how much is needed for health. For example, there is little scientific evidence to indicate that a person who can reach 2 inches beyond the toes on a sit-and-reach test is less fit (or less healthy) than a person who can reach 8 inches past the toes. The standards presented in the Lab Resource Materials are based on the best available evidence.

Too much flexibility (hyperflexibility) in a joint may increase susceptibility to injury. While an appropriate amount of flexibility is beneficial, too much flexibility can actually compromise the integrity of the joint and make it less stable and prone to injury. Most muscles and tendons can lengthen and return to their normal length after appropriate stretching. However, short, tight muscles and tendons can be easily overstretched (i.e., strained). Even more likely to be injured are the ligaments that connect bone to bone. Ligaments and the joint capsule lack the elasticity and tensile strength of the muscles and tendons. When involuntarily overstretched, they may remain in a lengthened state or become ruptured (i.e., sprained). If this occurs multiple times, the joint loses stability and is susceptible to repeated dislocation, repeated sprains, and excessive wear and tear of the joint surface. This is particularly true of weight-bearing joints, such as the hip, knee,

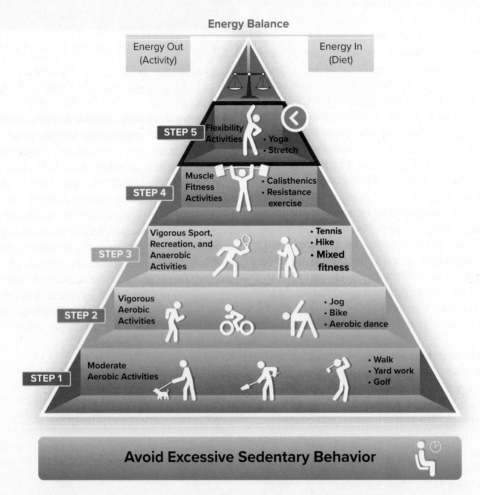

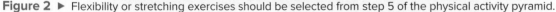

Figure 2 ▶ Flexibility or stretching exercises should be selected from step 5 of the physical activity pyramid.

and ankle. Appropriate stretching techniques can increase flexibility without leading to hyperflexibility.

Flexibility contributes to improvements in functional fitness. Good range of joint motion (flexibility) is necessary to participate in some sports and recreational activities; however, it is also important for a variety of normal daily tasks (e.g., reaching and bending). As

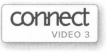

we age, flexibility becomes increasingly important for maintaining function and independence including ease with basic tasks such as standing up from a low chair or bending over to pick up an item from the floor. Properly performed stretching exercise has been shown to improve flexibility in people of all ages and is a key contributor to a broader construct of **functional fitness**, which also incorporates core strength, balance, and agility.

A number of research studies have demonstrated improved functional outcomes in older adults following a stretching program, including improved scores on sit-to-stand time, and walking speed. However, few research studies have directly examined the relationship between older adults' flexibility (ROM) and performance of activities of daily living (ADLs). Therefore, more evidence is needed before recommendations can be made about the role of flexibility exercises in improving daily functioning. Flexibility plays a key role in functional fitness along with core strength, balance, and agility.

Flexibility is critical for achieving and maintaining optimal posture. Poor posture typically develops over time due to lifestyle choices and/or poor habits. For example, people who sit a lot may develop tightness of the hip flexors. Weight lifters who follow a specific training regimen may develop tightness of the pectoral and biceps muscles. Over time, poor posture can result in muscle imbalance where muscles on one side of a joint become short and "overactive" while muscles on the opposite side become long and "underactive." The positions tend to become reinforced over time through

neural programming. Flexibility is critical for improving posture, but it is also important to strengthen the long and underactive muscles and to improve overall body awareness. Additional details are provided in the Concept on Body Mechanics and Care of the Back.

Flexibility can improve performance. Many sports require good flexibility for optimal performance. Dancers, gymnasts, and divers stretch extensively to meet the unique flexibility demands of their activities. Baseball catchers and those who play first base are well aware of the benefits of flexibility when stretching to reach a ball while still staying in contact with the base. The same is true for many other sports, such as soccer, tennis, and swimming.

Flexibility is also important for daily life activities, especially for older people. For example, range of motion in the neck is important for safe driving, and the ability to bend forward to pick up objects also requires flexibility. As already noted, those who train future firefighters and military personnel recognize the need for flexibility as part of readiness programs. People who work in other professions such as plumber, painter, and construction worker also need to stretch and reach to perform the demands of their jobs.

Stretching Methods

Static stretching is the most commonly used method of stretching. Static stretching is done slowly and held for a period of several seconds. This type of stretch is relatively safe if performed properly. For best results, stretching should be performed when the body is warm, after exercise, or as a separate routine. There is ample evidence that static stretching can have a temporary negative effect on performance in certain athletes requiring speed and power. Strength and power have been shown to decrease by 4–30 percent following brief stretching, with effects lasting up to an hour. For this reason, static stretching is not recommended immediately prior to athletic competitions involving power, strength, and speed activities.

Static stretches can be performed with **active assistance** or with **passive assistance**. When active assistance is used, the opposing muscle group is contracted to produce a reflex relaxation (**reciprocal inhibition**) in the muscle being stretched. This enables the muscle to be more easily stretched. For example, when doing a calf stretch exercise, the muscles on the front of

Functional Fitness The ability to perform activities of daily life.

Active Assistance An assist to stretch from an active contraction of the opposing (antagonist) muscle.

Passive Assistance Stretch imposed on a muscle with the assistance of a force other than the opposing muscle.

Reciprocal Inhibition Reflex relaxation in stretched muscle during contraction of the antagonist.

Contrasting Three Methods of Stretching

I. Static Stretch

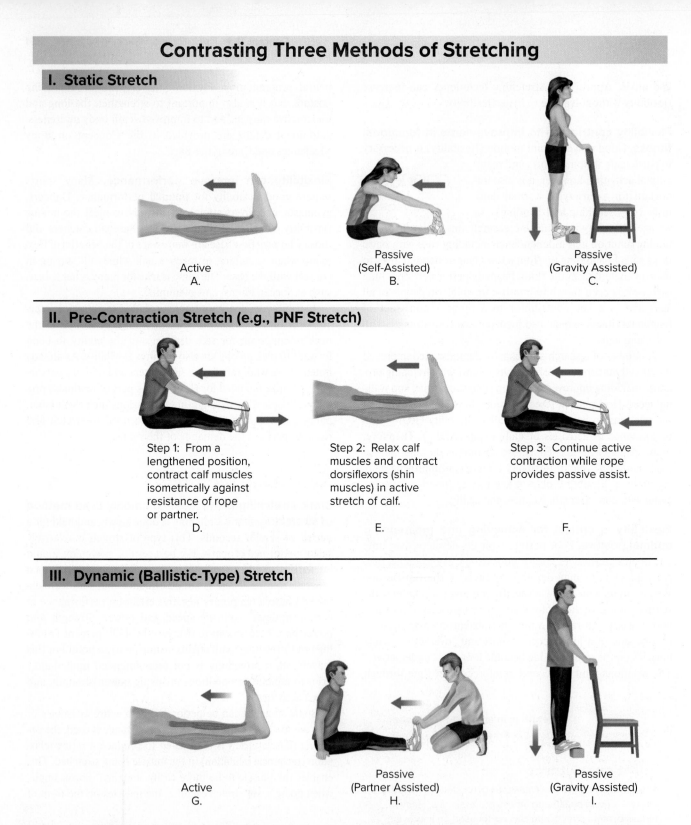

Active
A.

Passive
(Self-Assisted)
B.

Passive
(Gravity Assisted)
C.

II. Pre-Contraction Stretch (e.g., PNF Stretch)

Step 1: From a lengthened position, contract calf muscles isometrically against resistance of rope or partner.
D.

Step 2: Relax calf muscles and contract dorsiflexors (shin muscles) in active stretch of calf.
E.

Step 3: Continue active contraction while rope provides passive assist.
F.

III. Dynamic (Ballistic-Type) Stretch

Active
G.

Passive
(Partner Assisted)
H.

Passive
(Gravity Assisted)
I.

Figure 3 ▶ Examples of static, pre-contraction, and dynamic stretches of the calf muscles (gastrocnemius and soleus). Muscles shown in dark pink are the muscles being contracted. Muscles shown in light pink are those being stretched.

the shin can be contracted to assist in the stretch of the muscles of the calf (see Figure 3A). However, a limitation of this method is that it is difficult to produce adequate overload by simply contracting the opposing muscles. With passive assistance, an outside force or gravity helps put the muscle on stretch. In the calf stretch example, passive assistance can be provided by using the hands to pull the foot forward in a sitting stretch (Figure 3B), or with the aid of gravity in a standing stretch (Figure 3C). This type of stretch does not create the relaxation in the muscle associated with active assisted stretch.

An unrelaxed muscle cannot be stretched as far, and injury may happen. Therefore, it is best to combine the active assistance with a passive assistance when performing a static stretch. This gives the advantage of a relaxed muscle and a sufficient force to provide an overload to stretch it. A good way to begin static stretching exercises is to stretch until tension is first felt, back off slightly and hold the position several seconds, and then gradually stretch a little farther, back off, and hold. Decrease the stretch slowly after the hold.

Specific stretching techniques can enhance gains in flexibility. Proprioceptive neuromuscular facilitation (PNF) stretching utilizes techniques to stimulate muscles to contract more strongly (and relax more fully) in order to enhance the effectiveness of stretching. The contract-relax-antagonist-contract (CRAC) technique is the most popular. CRAC PNF involves three specific steps: (1) Move the limb so the muscle to be stretched (agonist) is initially elongated, and then contract it isometrically (at 20–75 percent maximum voluntary contraction) for several seconds (against an immovable object or the resistance of a partner); (2) relax the muscle; and (3) immediately statically stretch the muscle with the active assistance of the antagonist muscle and passive assist from a partner or gravity. Figures 3D, 3E, and 3F provide an illustration of how this technique is applied to the calf stretch. Research shows that this and other types of PNF stretch are more effective than a simple static stretch.

Dynamic stretching can be safe and effective if performed properly. There are two types of dynamic stretching: active and ballistic. *Active stretching* refers to the gradual controlled movement of body parts through a joint's normal range of motion, with the motion repeated a number of times. Stretches may involve 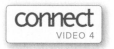 arm or leg swings of increasing reach or increasing speed. These types of stretches are often incorporated into the warm-up phase of many sport activities as well as functional fitness programs. Compared to static stretching, dynamic techniques have been shown to be equally effective at improving flexibility without impairing measures of athletic performance immediately following their use. The second type of dynamic stretch is *ballistic stretching*. Ballistic techniques involve rapid, alternating movements or bouncing at end range of motion. Due to their speed, they can increase muscle tension and increase the risk of muscle strain. Therefore, ballistic-type stretches are primarily used in sport-specific warm-ups rather than recommended for the general population. Examples of dynamic (ballistic-type) stretching are provided in Figures 3G, 3H, and 3I.

Specific FIT guidelines are established for safe and effective stretching. The guidelines from the American College of Sports Medicine (ACSM) indicate that stretching can be done using static stretches (active or passive),

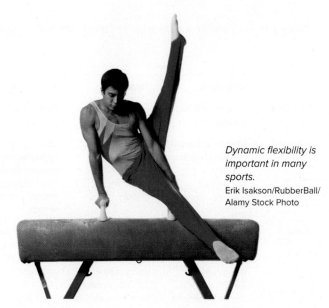

Dynamic flexibility is important in many sports.
Erik Isakson/RubberBall/ Alamy Stock Photo

pre-contraction stretches, and dynamic stretches. The recommended threshold and target zones for safe and effective stretching are provided in Table 1. The threshold of training refers to the minimum amount of stretching required to make gains and/or maintain a level of flexibility. Target zone refers to the overload needed to make significant gains in flexibility or to progress one's level of flexibility following a plateau.

Stretching exercises should be performed 2–3 times per week but daily is most effective (frequency). Some stretching is better than none, but gains are greater if performed at least three times a week (ideally daily). A recent review determined that the frequency of stretching is more important than the total time or volume of stretching; thus, building a habit of regular stretching is best for improving flexibility.

The evidence is also clear that stretching is most effective when the muscles are warm. Performing a general or dynamic warm-up activity prior to stretching can increase internal muscle temperature and the extensibility of soft tissues, allowing for a more effective stretch. Since some people do not want to interrupt their workout in the middle, they prefer to stretch at the end. Stretching at the end of the workout serves a dual purpose: building flexibility and cooling down. It is, however, appropriate to stretch at any time in the workout after the muscles have been active and are warm. If you prefer to include it at the beginning of a workout, ease into the stretching gradually after a light warm-up.

> **Proprioceptive Neuromuscular Facilitation (PNF)** A stretching technique that incorporates muscle contraction prior to stretch.

Table 1 ▶ FIT Formula for Stretching—Thresholds and Target Zones

	Static		Dynamic		PNF (CRAC)	
	Threshold	**Target**	**Threshold**	**Target**	**Threshold**	**Target**
Frequency	At least 2–3 days a week	2–7 days a week	At least 2–3 days a week	2–7 days a week	At least 2–3 days a week	2–7 days a week
Intensity	Stretch to the point of feeling tightness or slight discomfort.	Add passive assistance. Avoid over-stretching or pain.	Use a gentle swing (active) or bounce (ballistic) to stretch slightly beyond normal length.	Use same formula as for dynamic threshold.	Use an active 3- to 6-second contraction prior to an assisted stretch and stretch to point of tightness.	Use a 6-second contraction prior to an assisted stretch to point of tightness.
Time	For each exercise, stretch for total of 60 seconds using reps of 10–30 seconds. Rest 30 seconds between reps.	For each exercise, stretch for total of 90 seconds using reps of 10–30 seconds. Rest 30 seconds between reps.	Perform 1 set with 30 continuous seconds of motion.	Perform 1–3 sets with 30 consecutive seconds of motion. Rest 1 minute between sets.	For each exercise, stretch for total of 60 seconds using reps of 10–30 seconds. Rest 30 seconds between reps.	For each exercise, stretch for total of 90 seconds using reps of 10–30 seconds. Rest 30 seconds between reps.
Application	General population as well as rehab from injuries.		Sports and functional fitness.		Rehab from injuries and goal of increased ROM.	

To increase the length of a muscle, stretch it more than its normal length but do not overstretch it (intensity). The best evidence suggests that muscles should be stretched to about 10 percent beyond their normal length to bring about an improvement in flexibility. A more practical indicator of the intensity of stretching is to stretch just to the point of tension or slight discomfort. A small overload stimulus is needed in order to increase flexibility. Exercises that do not cause an overload will not increase flexibility. Once adequate flexibility has been achieved, range of motion is best maintained by regular stretching to the desired point of elongation.

To increase flexibility, stretch and hold muscles for a total of 90 seconds using several repetitions of 10–30 seconds (time). ACSM guidelines suggest that to get the most benefit for the least effort, stretches should be maintained for 10-30 seconds and with the total time for several repetitions equaling 90 seconds (See Table 1). Holding the stretch for a sustained period is important in overcoming the **stretch reflex** and to enhance the viscoelastic properties of the muscle and tendon. Repeating the stretch several times is also important, as the muscle will elongate further with each repetition (up to a point) based on the viscoelastic properties. When the muscle is first stretched, neural factors resist the stretch but the reflex contraction subsides, allowing the muscle to be stretched more easily. Repeating the stretch several times is important to gradually increase the overload and promote adaptations. Figure 4 shows the typical responses to a stretched muscle during a series of stretches. Tension in a muscle decreases as the stretch is held over time, with most of the decrease occurring during the first 15-30 seconds. The multicolor curves in the figure illustrate that each successive stretch further reduces tension in the muscle, allowing greater stretch. For most people, three repetitions of 30 seconds (total of 90 seconds) are most efficient. In older adults, stretching for longer duration (e.g. 30-60 seconds) may be more beneficial.

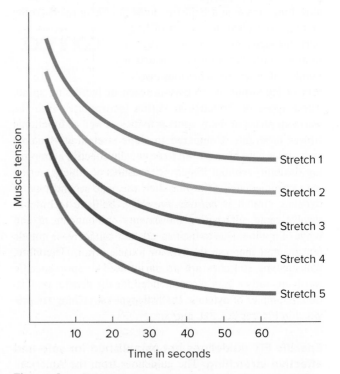

Figure 4 ▶ Typical responses to a stretched muscle during a series of stretches.

Popular Flexibility Activities

Flexibility activities continue to be popular among fitness enthusiasts. The acceptance and popularity of flexibility activities such as yoga, tai chi, and Pilates have remained high. This has been attributed, in part, to increased acceptance of these activities by medical professionals. For example, clinicians now more routinely refer patients to evidence-based programs for arthritis and fall prevention that utilize these activities. This also explains why "specialized training for older adults" has consistently ranked as a top 10 fitness trend. And as people turned to more home-based fitness during the COVID-19 pandemic, practicing yoga increased even more. The following sections provide distinctions among these similar activities.

Tai chi is a relaxing and contemplative martial art with established health benefits. Tai chi (often translated as Chinese shadow boxing) involves the execution of slow, flowing movements called "forms." Tai chi has been shown to improve a wide variety of health outcomes including improved flexibility, improved balance, improved lower leg strength, improved immune capacity, increased bone density, reduced fall risk among older adults, improved cardiovascular function, reduced stress, reduced pain from arthritis, and improved quality of life. For older people, the improved muscle fitness translates into joint protection and stability as well as improved functional fitness. Younger participants can benefit as well.

Yoga is a popular and diverse mind–body movement discipline. *Yoga* is an umbrella term that refers to a number of yoga traditions. The foundation for most yoga traditions is hatha yoga, which incorporates a variety of asanas (postures). Iyengar yoga is another popular variation. It uses similar asanas as hatha yoga but uses props and cushions to enhance the movements. Emphasis is placed on balance through coordinated breathing and precise body alignment.

The popularity of yoga continues to grow, encompassing numerous yoga forms from gentle and meditative to challenging and sweaty. Although yoga practices are thousands of years old, they are continually reinvented and refreshed, helping them retain popularity with people of diverse ages and interests. While yoga is commonly assumed to be a safe and healthy form of exercise, it is important to remember that, like any other form of exercise, there is potential for injury. Some extreme forms of yoga use contraindicated poses or movements that are potentially harmful to beginning exercisers. Care should be used when performing movements that require unnatural movements of the body or high stress loads placed on small joints. Props such as blocks and straps can be used to ease poses and make yoga gentler on the joints. Likewise, participants of Bikram ("hot") yoga should be aware of symptoms of heat intolerance and avoid overexertion.

Yoga is believed to contribute to a number of health benefits including improvements in flexibility, strength, balance,

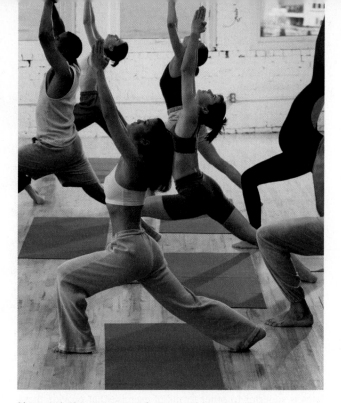

Yoga and other movement classes involving stretching are increasingly popular.
Ryan McVay/Getty Images

stress management, cardiovascular health, and pain management (see In the News). A number of studies support these benefits while others suggest that some claims may be exaggerated. A number of high-quality research studies have provided evidence that yoga has a beneficial effect on improved cardiovascular health markers. Additional research studies have documented benefits on pain reduction and improved function in those with low back pain. More studies are needed to better understand the health-related effects of yoga, to differentiate the effects of varying yoga forms, and to compare the effectiveness of yoga to other exercise interventions.

Pilates is a therapeutic regimen that combines strength training with body awareness and flexibility. Pilates differs from yoga in its emphasis on core strengthening and the absence of an overt spiritual or meditative component. Created in the 1920s as more of a therapeutic program, Pilates has now been adapted for use in fitness centers and recreation programs. Research has supported the utility of Pilates for building flexibility, muscle strength, trunk endurance, and cardiorespiratory endurance, as well as enhancing physical function and reducing pain and disability. Studies examining the relationship between Pilates and flexibility have found benefits related to a number of case-specific issues, including improved iliotibial band and hamstring flexibility in dancers,

Stretch Reflex A reflexive contraction (shortening) of a muscle that occurs when sensory neurons in the MTU perceive a stretch of a muscle. The reflex subsides gradually, allowing the muscle to be stretched beyond resting length.

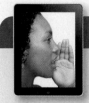

In the News

Yoga as a Complementary Health Approach

Yoga has been around for thousands of years, but research studies have now been able to formally evaluate the health benefits. The National Center for Complementary and Integrative Health (a division of the National Institutes of Health) has identified yoga as a top 10 complementary health approach. A survey conducted by the National Center for Health Statistics examined Americans' use of alternative or complementary medicine approaches, and yoga was among the strongest trends. Yoga was also on the list of prominent trends in the most recent ACSM fitness trend report. Experts attribute the wide appeal of yoga to the diversity of disciplines and applications. The positive impacts on health and mental well-being likely also keep people engaged once they try it.

What factors do you think explain the increased popularity of yoga?

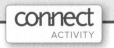

improved shoulder range of motion (ROM) in breast cancer survivors, and gains in chest excursion and trunk ROM in adolescents with scoliosis. While effective, it is not clear that Pilates is superior to other forms of exercise that provide these same health benefits. Thus, Pilates is a good option for many people, but it is just one of many routes to improved fitness and better health. It is important to also check for credentials of instructors to ensure effective programming.

Guidelines for Improving Flexibility

Build in time for specific flexibility exercises. Many people presume that a stretch warm-up counts as a flexibility workout. People who choose to do a stretch warm-up do it to prepare for their workout. Stretching exercises done to build flexibility, as described in this Concept, are performed intentionally as a stand-alone workout or as part of a complete workout. Although similar exercises can be used in both the stretch warm-up and the flexibility workout, each has a different purpose. Both should be preceded by a general or dynamic warm-up.

The consensus is that stretching exercise is most effective when the body is already warmed up. For this reason, some people prefer to perform their stretching routine at the end of a workout when muscles are warm. Others prefer to perform their flexibility workout at a time when they can concentrate specifically on building flexibility. In either case, sufficient time should be allowed to ensure that the exercises are done correctly. The guidelines in Table 2 will help you gain the most benefit from your stretching exercises.

Apply the principle of specificity to improve flexibility. Flexibility is joint specific and so is stretching. No single exercise can produce total flexibility. For example, stretching

Table 2 ▶ Do and Don't List for Stretching

Do	Don't
Do warm muscles before you attempt to stretch them.	Don't stretch to the point of pain. Remember, you want to stretch muscles, not joints.
Do stretch with care if you have osteoporosis or arthritis.	Don't use ballistic stretches if you have osteoporosis or arthritis.
Do use static or PNF stretching rather than ballistic stretching if you are a beginner.	Don't perform ballistic stretches with passive assistance unless you are under the supervision of an expert.
Do stretch weak or recently injured muscles with care.	Don't ballistically stretch weak or recently injured muscles.
Do use great care in applying passive assistance to a partner; go slowly and ask for feedback.	Don't overstretch a muscle after it has been immobilized for a long period of time (such as in a sling or cast).
Do perform stretching exercises for each muscle group and at each joint where flexibility is desired.	Don't bounce muscles through excessive range of motion. Begin ballistic stretching with gentle movements and gradually increase intensity.
Do make certain the body is in good alignment when stretching.	Don't stretch swollen joints without professional supervision.
Do stretch the smaller muscle groups of the arms and legs first; then progress to the larger muscle groups of the trunk and hips.	Don't stretch several muscles at one time until you have stretched individual muscles. For example, stretch muscles at the ankle, then the knee, then the ankle and knee simultaneously.

tight hamstrings can increase the length of these muscles but will not lengthen the muscles in other areas of the body. For total flexibility, it is important to stretch each of the major muscle groups. However, performing additional exercises for joints with limited flexibility may be needed. Exercises should be based on specific needs, conducted through a full range of normal motion and be focused on a functional goal.

Follow the principles of progression to safely build flexibility over time. Flexibility activities and stretching are low-impact activities, and they are generally very safe to perform. However, it is important to build up slowly and allow time for your body to adapt. Experts in yoga and tai chi may make some movements look easy, but it takes considerable training to develop the skills and flexibility needed to hold certain positions. Some movements may also increase risk for injuries if you aren't properly conditioned. Therefore, it is important to build up slowly by following the principle of progression.

Select exercises that promote flexibility in all areas of the body. For total-body flexibility, 8–10 stretching exercises for the major muscle groups of the body are recommended. Table 3 (See end of Concept) describes some of the most effective exercises for a basic flexibility routine. Individual

stretching needs may vary, but the most common areas to target are the trunk, legs, and arms. A variety of stretches for these areas are described in Tables 3, 4, and 5. Most are designed for static stretching, but the pectoral stretch and back-saver hamstring stretch use PNF techniques.

Using Self-Management Skills

Preparing a flexibility exercise plan requires the use of multiple self-management skills. You can use the six steps in program planning outlined in the Concept on Self-Management Skills for Health Behavior Change to prepare a flexibility exercise plan. Preparing a plan requires the use of a variety of self-management skills including self-assessment, goal setting, and self-monitoring. Preparing a plan also gives

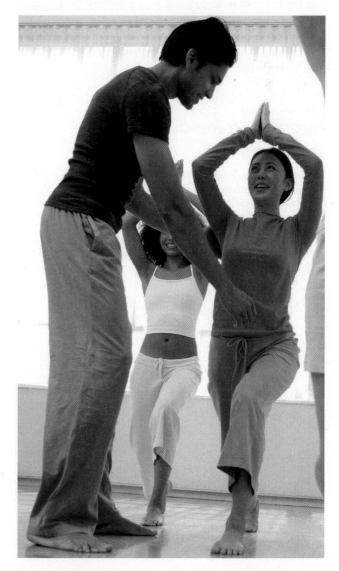

To get the most out of yoga, tai chi, and Pilates classes, find a qualified instructor.
Comstock/Stockbyte/Getty Images

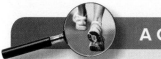

A CLOSER LOOK

Massage Rollers

Massage rollers are specialized devices used to massage sore muscles, alleviate muscle soreness, and improve flexibility. Use of massage rollers is referred to as "foam rolling" (FR) and is considered a form of self-directed deep soft tissue massage. The targeted musculature is essentially rolled and compressed utilizing an FR device. Massage roller devices come in a variety of sizes, shapes, and textures including the foam roll, massage stick, and massage ball. It can be conducted as a warm-up activity before exercise (pre-rolling) as well as a recovery strategy following exercise (post-rolling). Research on the purported benefits of roller devices is limited, but recent studies have demonstrated improvements in range of motion and reduced severity and incidence of delayed onset muscle soreness after their use. Scientists don't fully understand the mechanisms by which rollers work but believe the rollers help by reducing pain thresholds, influencing the central nervous system's modulation of pain, and possibly altering local circulation.

Do you think foam rollers can provide benefits for your stretching program?

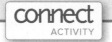

connect
ACTIVITY

you a chance to practice using these skills. (More information is provided in Strategies for Action: Lab Information.)

Apply consumer skills to ensure you receive good instruction. The popularity of flexibility exercise has led to an increasing array of classes, videos, and on-demand links available for yoga, Pilates, tai chi, and ballet-inspired barre exercises. Be sure to check the credentials of instructors providing these courses.

Apply performance skills by developing better mind–body awareness. Effective stretching requires careful attention to signals from your body. As described, gains in flexibility are influenced by body perceptions and complex stretch reflexes. By paying attention to flexibility and tension in your muscles, you can gain mind–body awareness. Familiarity with your body's capabilities will also help determine safe limits for stretching. Some yoga positions, for example, may be contraindicated exercises that could increase risk for injury in some individuals. For safety, exercises should always be performed within the safe limits, and only you can know how far is too far.

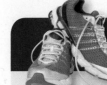

Strategies for Action: Lab Information

An important step for developing and maintaining flexibility is assessing your current status. There are dozens of tests for flexibility. Four tests that assess range of motion in the major joints of the body, that require little equipment, and that can be easily administered are presented in the Lab Resource Materials in this Concept. In Lab 11A you will get an opportunity to try these self-assessments. Perform these assessments before you begin your regular stretching program and use these assessments to reevaluate your flexibility periodically.

Keeping records of progress will help you adhere to a stretching program. A stretching exercise log is provided in Lab 11B to help you keep records of your progress as you regularly perform stretching exercises to build and maintain good flexibility.

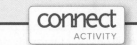

Suggested Resources and Readings

The websites for the following sources can be accessed by searching online for the organization, program, or title listed. Specific scientific references are available at the end of this edition of *Concepts of Fitness and Wellness*.

- American College of Sports Medicine. (2021). *ACSM's Guidelines for Exercise Testing and Prescription* (11th ed.). Philadelphia: Wolters Kluwer, Chapter 5.
- Davis, N. (2020, April 23). "Why Functional Fitness Is Important for Everyone." *Healthline*.
- Lindberg, S. (2018, June 18). "Stretching: 9 Benefits, Plus Safety Tips and How to Start." *Healthline*.
- National Center for Complementary and Integrative Health. (2020). *Yoga for Health*. (pdf)
- National Center for Complementary and Integrative Health. Yoga: What You Need to Know.
- Nyman, S. (2020, February 14). "Tai Chi Health Benefits? What the Research Says." *The Conversation*.

The Basic Eight for Trunk Stretching Exercises   Table 3

1. Upper Trapezius/Neck Stretch

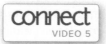

This exercise stretches the muscles on the back and sides of the neck. To stretch the right trapezius, place left hand on top of your head. Gently look down toward your left underarm, tucking your chin toward your chest. Let the weight of your arm gently draw your head forward. Hold. Repeat to the opposite side. *Variations:* The stretch may be modified to stretch the muscles on the front and sides of the neck. Start from the stretch position described. Tip your left ear near your left shoulder. Turn your head slightly and look up toward the ceiling, lifting your chin 2–3 inches. Hold.

Trapezius

2. Chin Tuck

This exercise stretches the muscles at the base of the skull and reduces headache symptoms. Sit up straight, with chest lifted and shoulders back. Gently tuck in the chin by making a slight motion of nodding "yes." Imagine a string attached to the back of your head, which is pulling your head upward, like a puppet. As your chin draws inward, attempt to lengthen the back of your neck. Hold.

Longissimus capitis
Splenius capitis
Semispinalis capitis
Semispinalis cervicis

3. Pectoral Stretch

This exercise stretches the chest muscles (pectorals).

1. Stand erect in doorway, with arms raised 45 degrees, elbows bent, hands grasping the doorjamb, and feet in front-stride position. Press out on door frame, contracting your arm muscles maximally for 6 seconds. Relax and shift weight forward on legs. Lean into doorway, so that the muscles on the front of your shoulder joint and chest are gently stretched. Do not overstretch. Hold.
2. Repeat with your arms raised 90 degrees.
3. Repeat with your arms raised 135 degrees. This exercise is useful to prevent or correct round shoulders and sunken chest.

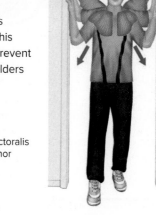

Pectoralis major
Pectoralis minor

4. Lateral Trunk Stretch

This exercise stretches the trunk lateral flexors. Stand with feet shoulder width apart. Stretch left arm overhead to right. Bend to right at waist, reaching as far to right as possible with left arm. Hold. Do not let trunk rotate or lower back arch. Repeat on opposite side.

Trunk lateral flexors

Table 3

Table 3

Table 3 The Basic Eight for Trunk Stretching Exercises

5. Leg Hug

This exercise stretches the hip and back extensor muscles. Lie on your back. Bend one leg and grasp your thigh under the knee. Hug it to your chest. Keep the other leg straight and on the floor. Hold. Repeat with the opposite leg.

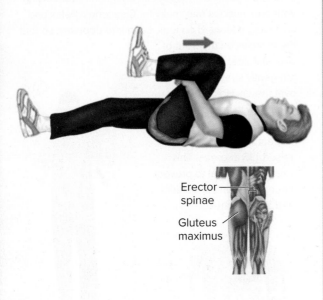

Erector spinae

Gluteus maximus

7. Trunk Twist

This exercise stretches the trunk muscles and the muscles on the outside of the hip. Sit with your right leg extended, left leg bent and crossed over the right knee. Place your right arm on the left side of the left leg and push against that leg while turning the trunk as far as possible to the left. Place the left hand on the floor behind the buttocks. Stretch and hold. Reverse position and repeat on the opposite side.

Erector spinae

Gluteals

6. Cobra and Child's Pose

This exercise stretches the back and hips. Begin on stomach with legs extended behind you. Place hands on floor directly under shoulders and fingertips pointed forward. Press tops of feet and thighs into floor. Gently raise head and chest from the ground, straightening the elbows. Hold 30 seconds. Relax. Keeping hands on the ground, sit back toward heels, rounding out low back and lowering forehead toward the floor. Hold for 30 seconds.

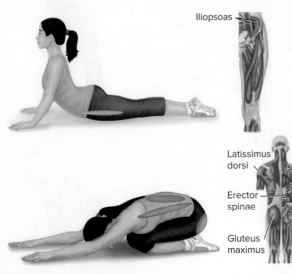

Iliopsoas

Latissimus dorsi

Erector spinae

Gluteus maximus

8. Spine Twist

This exercise stretches the trunk rotators and lateral rotators of the thighs. Start in hook-lying position, arms extended at shoulder level. Cross your left knee over the right. Drop both knees toward the floor on the left side of your body. Keep your arms and shoulders on the floor while moving your legs. Stretch and hold. Reverse leg position and lower your knees to right.

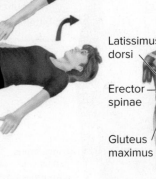

Latissimus dorsi

Erector spinae

Gluteus maximus

The Basic Eight for Leg Stretching Exercises Table 4

Table 4

1. Calf Stretch

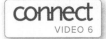

This exercise stretches the calf muscles and Achilles tendon. Face a wall with your feet 2 or 3 feet away. Step forward on your left foot to allow both hands to touch the wall. Keep the heel of your right foot on the ground, toe turned in slightly, knee straight, and buttocks tucked in. Lean forward by bending your front knee and arms and allowing your head to move nearer the wall. Hold. *Variation:* Repeat, bending your right knee, keeping your heel on floor. Stretch and hold. Repeat with the other leg.

Gastrocnemius

3. Back-Saver Hamstring Stretch

This exercise stretches the hamstrings and calf muscles and helps prevent or correct backache caused in part by short hamstrings. Sit on the floor with the feet against the wall or an immovable object. Bend left knee and bring foot close to buttocks. Clasp hands behind back. Contract the muscles on the back of the upper leg (hamstrings) by pressing the heel downward toward the floor. Hold, relax. Bend forward from hips, keeping lower back as straight as possible. Let bent knee rotate outward so trunk can move forward. Lean forward keeping back flat; hold and repeat on each leg.

Hamstrings

2. Shin Stretch

This exercise relieves shin muscle soreness by stretching the muscles on the front of the shin. Kneel on both knees, turn to the right, and press down and stretch your right ankle with your right hand. Move your pelvis forward. Hold. Repeat on the opposite side. Except when they are sore, most people need to strengthen rather than stretch these muscles.

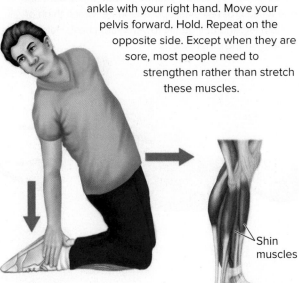

Shin muscles

4. Hip and Thigh Stretch

This exercise stretches the hip (iliopsoas) and thigh muscles (quadriceps) and is useful for people with lordosis and back problems. Kneel on the floor with your left leg behind you and the knee touching the floor. Place your right leg out in front with the right knee directly above your right ankle. If necessary, place your hands on floor for balance.

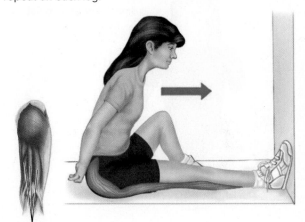

1. Tilt the pelvis backward by tucking in the abdomen and flattening the back.
2. Then shift the weight forward until a stretch is felt on the front of the left thigh. Hold. Repeat on the opposite side.
   Caution: Do not bend your front knee more than 90 degrees.

Iliopsoas

Quadriceps

Table 4

Table 4 The Basic Eight for Leg Stretching Exercises

5. Groin Stretch

This exercise stretches the muscles on the inside of the thighs. Sit with the soles of your feet together; place your hands on your knees or ankles and lean your forearms against your knees; resist (contract) by attempting to raise your knees. Hold. Relax and press the knees toward the floor as far as possible. Hold. This exercise is useful for pregnant women and anyone whose thighs tend to rotate inward, causing backache, knock-knees, and flat feet.

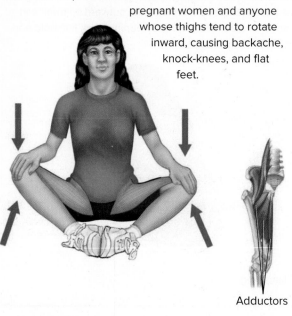

Adductors

6. Lateral Thigh and Hip Stretch

This exercise stretches the muscles and connective tissue on the outside of the legs (tensor fascia lata and iliotibial band). Stand with your left side to the wall, left arm extended and palm of your hand flat on the wall for support. Cross the left leg behind the right leg and turn the toes of both feet out slightly. Bend your left knee slightly and shift your pelvis toward the wall (left) as your trunk bends toward the right. Adjust until tension is felt down the outside of the left hip and thigh. Stretch and hold. Repeat on the other side.

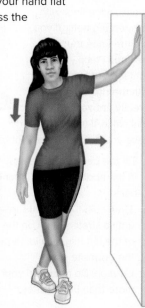

Iliotibial band

7. Inner Thigh Stretch

This exercise stretches the muscles of the inner thigh. Stand with feet spread wider than shoulder-width apart. Shift weight onto the right foot and bend the right knee slightly. Straighten left knee and raise toes of left foot off the floor. Lean forward slightly from the waist, keeping back straight/shoulders back. Shift weight back over the right foot by moving hips diagonally away from the left foot. Hold. Repeat in the opposite direction.

Adductors

8. Deep Buttock Stretch

This exercise stretches the deep buttock muscles, such as the piriformis. Lie on your back with knees bent and one ankle crossed over opposite knee. Grasp thigh of bottom leg and pull gently toward your chest. Hold. Repeat on the other side.

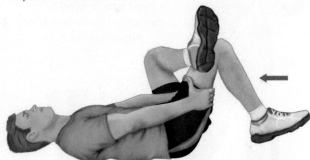

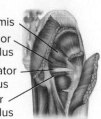

Piriformis
Superior gemellus
Obturator internus
Inferior gemellus

The Basic Four for Arm Stretching Exercises Table 5

Table 5

1. Forearm Stretch

This exercise stretches the muscles on the front and back sides of the lower arm. It is particularly useful in relieving stress from excessive keyboarding activity. Hold your right arm straight out in front, with your palm facing down. Use your left hand to gently stretch the fingertips of your right hand toward the floor. Hold. Turn your right arm over with your palm facing up. Use your left hand to gently stretch the fingertips of your right hand toward the floor. Hold. Repeat on the opposite side.

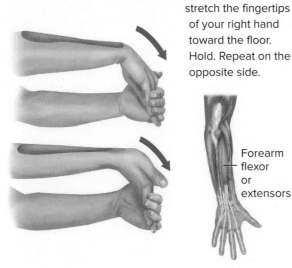

Forearm flexor or extensors

3. Overhead Arm Stretch

This exercise stretches the triceps and latissimus dorsi muscles. Stretch your arms up overhead. Grasp your right elbow with your left hand. Pull your right elbow back behind your head. Hold. Repeat on opposite side.

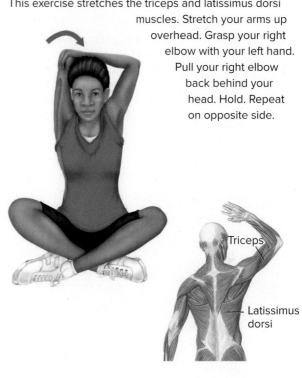

Triceps

Latissimus dorsi

2. Back Scratcher

This exercise stretches the muscles on the front of the shoulder. Stand straight with back of left hand held flat against back. With right hand, throw one end of a towel over right shoulder from front to back. Grab end of towel with left hand. Pull down gently on the towel with right hand, raising left arm in back as high as is comfortable. Hold. Repeat to opposite side.

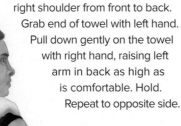

Pectoralis
Deltoid

4. Arm Hug Stretch

This exercise stretches the shoulder muscles (lateral rotators and posterior deltoid). Hold onto right arm above the elbow with left hand and gently pull arm across chest.

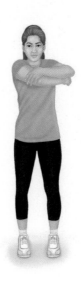

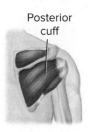

Posterior cuff

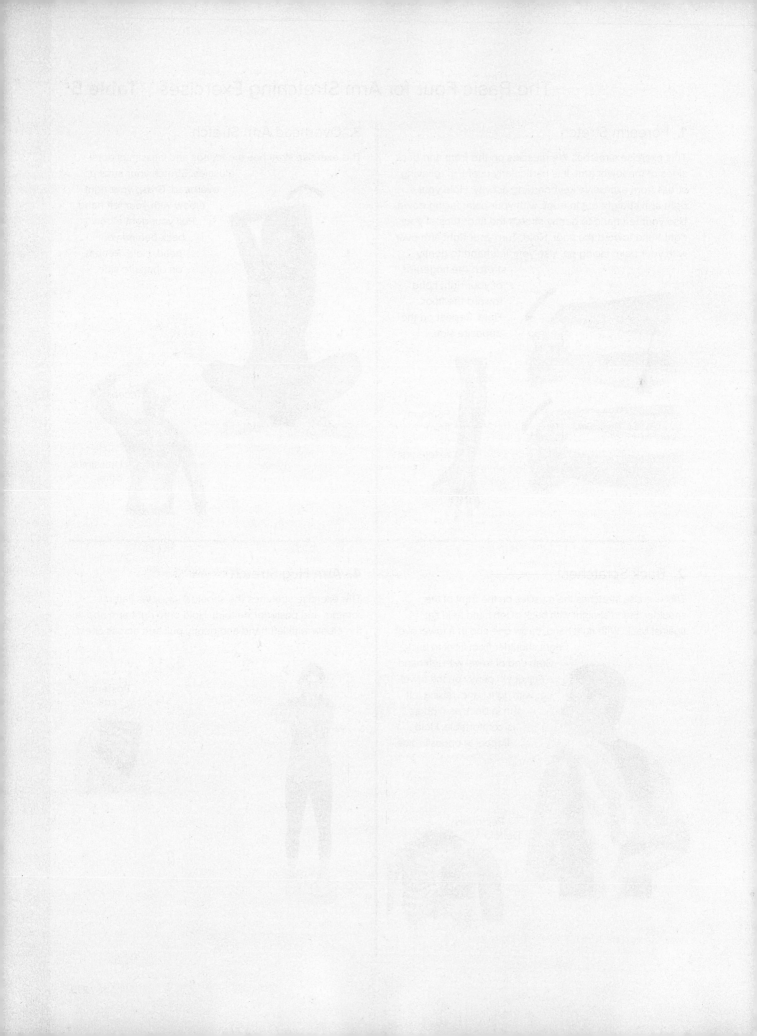

Lab Resource Materials: Flexibility Tests

Directions: To test the flexibility of all joints is impractical. These tests are for frequently tight muscle groups that can limit joint flexibility. Follow the instructions carefully. Determine your flexibility using Chart 1.

1. Test: Modified Sit-and-Reach (Flexibility Test of Hamstrings)

   a. Remove shoes and sit on the floor. Place the sole of the foot of the extended leg flat against a box or bench. Bend opposite knee and place the head, back, and hips against a wall with a 90-degree angle at the hips.

   b. Place one hand over the other and slowly reach forward as far as you can with arms fully extended. Keep head and back in contact with the wall. A partner will slide the end of the measuring stick on the bench until it touches the fingertips.

   c. With the measuring stick fixed in the new position, reach forward as far as possible, allowing head and trunk to move away from the wall. Perform three times, holding the position on the third reach for at least 2 seconds while the partner records the distance fingertips slide forward on the ruler. Keep the knee of the extended leg straight (see illustration).

   d. Repeat the test a second time and average the scores of the two trials.

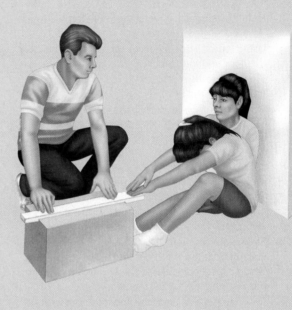

2. Test: Shoulder Flexibility (Zipper Test)

   a. Raise your right arm overhead, bend your elbow, and reach down across your back as far as possible.

   b. At the same time, extend your left arm down and behind your back, bend your elbow up across your back, and try to cross your fingers over those of your right hand as shown in the accompanying illustration.

   c. Measure the distance between fingertips to the nearest half-inch. If your fingers overlap, score as a plus. If they fail to meet, score as a minus. Score as a zero if your fingertips just touch.

   d. Repeat with your arms crossed in the opposite direction (left arm up). Most people will find that they are more flexible on one side than the other.

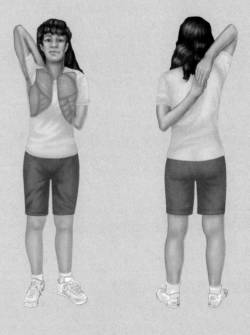

3. Test: Hamstring and Hip Flexor Flexibility

   a. Lie on your back on the floor beside a wall.

   b. Slowly lift one leg off the floor. Keep the other leg flat on the floor.

   c. Keep both legs straight.

   d. Continue to lift the leg until either leg begins to bend or the lower leg begins to lift off the floor.

   e. Place a yardstick against the wall and underneath the lifted leg.

   f. Hold the yardstick against the wall after the leg is lowered.

   g. Using a protractor, measure the angle created by the floor and the yardstick. The greater the angle, the better your score.

   h. Repeat with the other leg.

   Note: For ease of testing, you may want to draw angles on a piece of posterboard, as illustrated. If you have goniometers, you may be taught to use them instead.

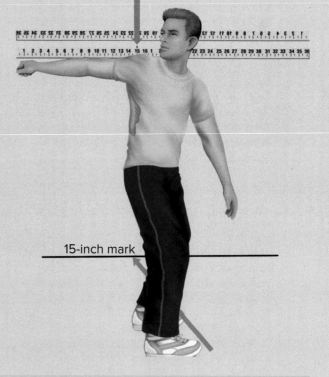

15-inch mark

15-inch mark

4. Test: Trunk Rotation

   a. Tape two yardsticks to the wall at shoulder height, one right side up and the other upside down. Position yardsticks directly over one another.

   b. Stand with your left shoulder an arm's length (fist closed) from the wall. Toes should be on the line, which is perpendicular to the wall and even with the 15-inch mark on the yardstick.

   c. Drop the left arm and raise the right arm to the side, palm down, fist closed.

   d. Without moving your feet, rotate the trunk to the right as far as possible, reaching along the yardstick, and hold it 2 seconds. Do not move the feet or bend the trunk. Your knees may bend slightly.

   e. A partner will read the distance reached to the nearest half-inch. Record your score. Repeat two times and average your two scores.

   f. Next, perform the test facing the opposite direction. Rotate to the left. For this test, you will use the second yardstick (upside down) so that, the greater the rotation, the higher the score. If you have only one yardstick, turn it right side up for the first test and upside down for the second test.

Chart 1 Flexibility Rating Scale for Tests 1–4

Classification	Males					Females				
	Test 1	Test 2		Test 3	Test 4	Test 1	Test 2		Test 3	Test 4
		Right Up	Left Up				Right Up	Left Up		
High-performance zone*	16+	5+	4+	111+	20+	17+	6+	5+	111+	20.5+
Good fitness zone	13–15	1–4	1–3	80–110	16–19.5	14–16	2–5	2–4	80–110	17–20
Marginal fitness zone	10–12	0	0	60–79	13.5–15.5	11–13	1	1	60–79	14.5–16.5
Low fitness zone	<9	<0	<0	<60	<13.5	<10	<1	<1	<60	<14.5

*Though performers need good flexibility, hypermobility may increase injury risk.

Lab 11A Evaluating Flexibility

Name		Section	Date

Purpose: To evaluate your flexibility in several joints.

Procedures

1. Take the flexibility tests outlined in the Lab Resource Materials.
2. Record your scores in the Results section.
3. Use Chart 1 in the Lab Resource Materials to determine your ratings on the self-assessments; then place an X over the circle for the appropriate rating.

Results

Flexibility Scores and Ratings

Record Scores			Record Ratings			
			High Performance	Good Fitness	Marginal	Low
Modified sit-and-reach						
Test 1	Left		○	○	○	○
	Right		○	○	○	○
Zipper						
Test 2	Left		○	○	○	○
	Right		○	○	○	○
Hamstring/hip flexor						
Test 3	Left		○	○	○	○
	Right		○	○	○	○
Trunk rotation						
Test 4	Left		○	○	○	○
	Right		○	○	○	○

Do any of these muscle groups need stretching? Check yes or no for each muscle group.

	Yes	No
Back of the thighs and knees (hamstrings)	◯	◯
Calf muscles	◯	◯
Lower back (lumbar region)	◯	◯
Front of right shoulder	◯	◯
Back of right shoulder	◯	◯
Front of left shoulder	◯	◯
Back of left shoulder	◯	◯
Most of the body	◯	◯
Trunk muscles	◯	◯

Conclusions and Implications: In several sentences, discuss your current flexibility and your flexibility needs for the future. Include comments about your current state of flexibility, need for improvement in specific areas, and special flexibility needs for sports or other special activities.

Lab 11B Planning and Logging Stretching Exercises

Name	**Section**	**Date**

Purpose: To set 1-week lifestyle goals for stretching exercises, to prepare a stretching for flexibility plan, and to self-monitor progress in your 1-week plan.

Procedures

1. Using Chart 1, provide some background information about your experience with stretching exercise, your goals, and your plans for incorporating these exercises into your normal exercise routine.
2. Using Chart 2, select at least 8–10 flexibility exercises as directed. Perform the exercises for 3–6 days over a 1-week period. Be sure to plan your exercise program so that it fits with the goals you described in Chart 1. For best results, take the log with you during your workout, so that you can record the exercises you performed.
3. Answer the questions in the Results and Conclusions and Implications sections.

Chart 1 Stretching Exercise Survey

1. Determine your current stage for flexibility exercise. Check only the stage that represents your current activity level.

   ○ Precontemplation. I do not meet flexibility exercise guidelines and have not been thinking about starting.

   ○ Contemplation. I do not meet flexibility exercise guidelines but have been thinking about starting.

   ○ Preparation. I am planning to start doing regular flexibility exercises to meet guidelines.

   ○ Action. I do flexibility exercises, but I am not as regular as I should be.

   ○ Maintenance. I regularly meet guidelines for flexibility exercises.

2. What are your primary goals for flexibility exercise?

   ○ General conditioning

   ○ Sports improvement (specify sport: _____)

   ○ Health benefits

3. Are you currently involved in a regular stretching program?

   ○ Yes

   ○ No

Results

	Yes	No
Did you do eight exercises at least 3 days in the week?	○	○
Did you notice any changes in flexibility?	○	○

Chart 2 Stretching Exercise Log

Check (√) the exercises you plan to perform in the first column. Choose 8–10 or more exercises from the three lists (trunk, leg, and arm). Be sure to include at least two exercises from each of the three lists. Perform the exercises for 3–6 days over the 1-week period. Write the date (month/day) in the day column for the date you performed the exercise.

Exercises	Day 1	Day 2	Day 3	Day 4	Day 5	Day 6	Day 7
Trunk Stretching Exercises (Table 3, pages 209–210)							
☐ 1 Upper trapezius/neck stretch							
☐ 2 Chin tuck							
☐ 3 Pectoral stretch							
☐ 4 Lateral trunk stretch							
☐ 5 Leg hug							
☐ 6 Cobra and child's pose							
☐ 7 Trunk twist							
☐ 8 Spine twist							
Leg Stretching Exercises (Table 4, pages 211–212)							
☐ 1 Calf stretch							
☐ 2 Shin stretch							
☐ 3 Back-saver hamstring stretch							
☐ 4 Hip and thigh stretch							
☐ 5 Groin stretch							
☐ 6 Lateral thigh and hip stretch							
☐ 7 Inner thigh stretch							
☐ 8 Deep buttock stretch							
Arm Stretching Exercises (Table 5, page 213)							
☐ 1 Forearm stretch							
☐ 2 Back scratcher							
☐ 3 Overhead arm stretch							
☐ 4 Arm hug stretch							

Conclusions and Implications: Do you think you will use stretching exercises as part of your regular physical activity plan, either now or in the future? What modifications would you make in your program in the future?

Advanced Fitness Training

LEARNING OBJECTIVES

After completing the study of this Concept, you will be able to:

► Describe characteristics and training necessary for high-level performance.

► Identify the unique training considerations for cardiorespiratory endurance, speed, muscular strength, muscular endurance, power, functional fitness, and flexibility.

► Explain how principles of periodization are used to optimize training effectiveness.

► Describe types of ergogenic aids and how they may or may not work to improve performance.

► Evaluate your personal skill-related fitness.

► Identify and self-assess overtraining symptoms.

Specialized forms of training are needed to optimize adaptations to exercise and for enhancing performance in sports.

Why It Matters!

Sports, competitive events, and recreational activities provide opportunities for individuals to explore the limits of their ability and to challenge themselves. Some enjoy competitive aerobic activities, such as running, cycling, swimming, and triathlons. Others enjoy the challenges associated with competitive resistance training activities, such as powerlifting and bodybuilding. The pursuit of high-level performance requires training that is well beyond what is needed for good health and well-being, but many find these endeavors to be very compelling. This Concept will provide insights into the approaches used to train for high-level performance. While the focus is on sports, high-level performance is also a requirement for some types of work, such as fire safety, military service, and police work.

High-Level Performance and Training Characteristics

High-level performance requires health-related and skill-related fitness and the specific motor skills necessary for the performance. Improving performance requires more specific training than the type needed to improve health. **Training** (regular physical activity) builds health-related fitness that enhances both health and high-level performance (see Figure 1). High-level performance is not necessary for all people, only for those who need exceptional performances. A distance runner needs exceptional cardiorespiratory endurance and muscular endurance, a lineman in football needs exceptional strength, and a gymnast needs exceptional flexibility.

Exceptional performance also requires high-level skill-related physical fitness and good physical and motor skills. It is important to understand that skill-related fitness and skills are not the same thing. Skill-related fitness components are abilities that help you learn skills faster and better, thus the arrow in Figure 1 from skill-related fitness to skills. Skills, on the other hand, are things such as throwing, kicking, catching, and hitting a ball. Practice enhances

skills. Practicing the specific skills of a sport or a job can help improve performance, but specific levels of skill-related fitness that influence skills are less amenable to change.

High-level performance requires more focused and structured training. The amount of effort and training required to excel in sports, competitive athletics, or work requiring high-level performance is greater than the amount needed for good health and wellness. Because adaptations to exercise are specific to the type of activity that is performed, training must also be matched to the specific needs of a given activity. Athletes learn to optimize training by carefully planning workouts that maximize adaptations and performance gains. While all principles are important, several are particularly important for high-level training, including overload, progression, specificity, individuality, and rest/recovery.

Success in endurance sports requires optimal performance of multiple systems. A report of the National Academy of Medicine (NAM; formerly the Institute of Medicine) recommends the use of the term **cardiorespiratory endurance** to describe one's ability to persist in sustained bouts of physical activity. **Aerobic capacity** is a term that describes a lab measure of one's ability to effectively use multiple systems to deliver and use oxygen during vigorous exercise. However, cardiorespiratory endurance reflects one's ability to sustain performance in real-life conditions. For the reasons described, the term *cardiorespiratory endurance* is used in this edition to describe how body systems work together to enhance endurance performance.

Endurance athletes such as distance runners, cyclists, and triathletes focus training on building aerobic capacity because it is essential to performing cardiorespiratory endurance bouts of high intensity for long periods of time. Adaptations from vigorous **aerobic exercise** increase aerobic capacity by enhancing the body's ability to supply oxygen to the muscles as well as their ability to use it. Slow-twitch muscle fibers are most suited for aerobic exercise, and these fibers adapt most to aerobic training. Activities and events that require sustained, high-intensity aerobic exercise place special demands on the slow-twitch fibers and require a high level of aerobic capacity.

Cardiorespiratory endurance is important for all athletes, but success in many sports also requires speed, strength, and power. The sprinting, jumping, and powerful movements needed in most competitive sports are good examples. Strength competitions and sprint events in running, bicycling, and swimming also require short bursts of high-intensity activity. These activities use more energy than can be provided with aerobic metabolism. Anaerobic processes (i.e., processes that do not require oxygen) provide the additional energy needs, but a by-product of these processes (**lactic acid**) eventually causes the muscles to fatigue. See the Concept on Vigorous Aerobic, Anaerobic, Sport, and Recreational Activities to understand the differences between aerobic and **anaerobic exercise**.

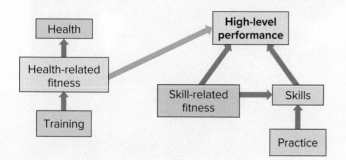

Figure 1 ▶ Factors influencing high-level performance.

Understanding how your body responds and adapts to exercise is important for advanced training. During any bout of exercise, the body initially attempts to meet energy demands with the aerobic metabolism. This is most evident with changes in ventilation and heart rate. However, as intensity increases, the body can no longer supply enough oxygen to sustain performance. There is a limited supply of high-energy fuel that the body can use to keep going, but when this fuel is used up, you cannot continue to perform. After exercise, your body starts to recover and replenish these energy stores. You keep breathing hard during recovery because the body needs to take in extra oxygen to rebuild the stores of the high-energy fuel used in anaerobic exercise. This is sometimes called **oxygen debt**. The body essentially "borrows" oxygen that it cannot provide when it is using high-energy fuel during anaerobic exercise. It then "pays back the debt" by supplying extra oxygen after the anaerobic exercise. The active recovery phase helps break down lactic acid and return the body to its normal resting state. The notion of "borrowing" oxygen during anaerobic exercise and paying the oxygen debt later can be likened to using a credit card to borrow money that is paid back later.

Athletes involved in anaerobic activities typically perform specialized forms of anaerobic exercise to help improve their **anaerobic capacity**, often reported to in fitness magazines as an **anaerobic threshold**. This ability is different than aerobic capacity and refers to the body's ability to produce energy anaerobically (without oxygen) and to tolerate higher levels of lactic acid. Using the credit card analogy mentioned, anaerobic capacity can be equated to the increase in available credit that is provided to customers who demonstrate they can pay their credit card bills. With training, the body can increase capacity for anaerobic physical activity and this can contribute to improved performance. Fast-twitch muscle fibers are used primarily during intense anaerobic activity, and these fibers are more likely to adapt and respond to anaerobic exercise. Most sports require

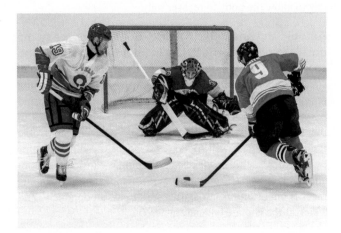

Performance in most sports requires good levels of fitness (health-related and skill-related) as well as practice to improve skills.
Simonkr/Getty Images

A CLOSER LOOK

"Heads Up" Concussion Awareness

The tragic stories about the long-term consequences of concussions have raised many concerns by medical and public health professionals. Great strides have been made in recent years with formalized regulations now in place in professional, collegiate, secondary school, and recreational sports. These efforts are focused on improving screening, testing, and rehabilitation to minimize long-term consequences. However, less attention has been placed on prevention. The CDC's comprehensive campaign "Heads Up" has helped promote awareness and education about concussions and head injuries in sports. Evidence has supported the benefits from these and other campaigns, but there are still questions about whether sports like football and hockey put athletes at too great of risk for head injuries.

Do campaigns such as "Heads Up" do enough or are other measures needed to reduce the prevalence of head injuries and concussions in sports?

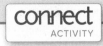
connect
ACTIVITY

a combination of aerobic and anaerobic capacity, so it is important to conduct training that is most specific to the needs of a given activity.

Training Physical activity performed by people interested in high-level performance (e.g., athletes, people in specialized jobs).

Cardiorespiratory Endurance The ability to perform whole-body aerobic exercise at a moderate to high intensity for extended periods of time.

Aerobic Capacity A measure of the ability of the heart and lungs to get oxygen to the muscles. Typically expressed as the maximum amount of oxygen that can be consumed in one minute of high intensity aerobic activity.

Aerobic Exercise A structured and intentional form of aerobic physical activity intended to maintain or improve cardiorespiratory fitness.

Lactic Acid Substance that results from the process of supplying energy during anaerobic exercise; a cause of muscle fatigue.

Anaerobic Exercise A structured and intentional form of exercise characterized by repeated, short bouts of high-intensity physical activity intended to maintain or improve cardiorespiratory and muscular fitness.

Oxygen Debt The oxygen consumed following anaerobic exercise that is used to rebuild the supply of high-energy fuel.

Anaerobic Capacity The ability to perform repeated anaerobic activity. It reflects the maximum amount of high energy fuel (ATP) that can be resynthesized during maximal exercise; is often reported as an anaerobic threshold.

Anaerobic Threshold The intensity of physical activity where the rate of lactic acid production exceeds the body's ability to break it down. It is determined as an inflection in blood lactate during a progressive exercise test.

Genetics can influence a person's potential for high-level performance. We inherit a unique genetic profile that predisposes us to success in different sports and activities. A higher percentage of slow-twitch muscle fibers allows a person to adapt most effectively to aerobic exercise, while a higher percentage of fast-twitch muscle fibers enhance adaptations from and performance in anaerobic exercise. Heredity also influences the dimensions of skill-related fitness, such as balance, coordination, and reaction time, that enhance development of motor skills. The most successful performers are those who inherit good potential for health- and skill-related fitness, who train to improve their health-related fitness, and who do extensive practice to improve the skills needed for the activity or sport.

Training for Cardiorespiratory Endurance

Specific forms of training are needed to optimize cardiorespiratory endurance. Speed and endurance are at opposite ends of the performance continuum. Speed events in running are as short as 100 meters, while endurance events, such as a marathon, last 26 miles. These are just two events, but they effectively capture extremes of human performance. The world record holder for the 100m achieved a top speed of 27.8 mph in the middle of the sprint. The world record for the marathon is now under 2 hours and this required an average speed of over 13.1 mph (an average of 4:35 per mile). Both performances are incredible accomplishments, but they required very different forms of training and very different physiological adaptations. Middle-distance events, such as the mile run, fall between these extremes and present unique challenges, since it is important for athletes to have both speed and endurance. While these examples both involve running, the types of training needed for these events are very different.

Involvement in regular physical activity will lead to increases in cardiorespiratory endurance in most people, but improvements are harder to achieve once a good level of fitness has been attained (the principle of diminishing returns). To continue to improve performance, athletes need to perform more specific forms of training. The same training principles and parameters apply, but endurance athletes need to exercise more frequently, at higher intensities, and for longer lengths of time than individuals seeking general levels of fitness. Supplemental training to improve technique and efficiency are also used to enhance performance. For example, very different skills, techniques, and abilities are required for excellence in running, swimming, cycling, or cross-country skiing.

Long-slow distance training is important for building cardiorespiratory endurance. Extended periods of aerobic exercise are needed to achieve high-level endurance performance. Athletes generally refer to this type of training as **long-slow distance (LSD) training**. Emphasis is placed on the overall duration or length of the exercise session rather than on speed. The reason for this is that specific adaptations take place

within the muscles when used for long periods of time. These adaptations improve the muscles' ability to take up and use the oxygen in the bloodstream. Adaptations within the muscle cell also improve the body's ability to produce energy from fat stores. Long-slow distance training involves performances longer than the event for which you are performing but at a slower pace. For example, a mile runner will regularly perform 6- to 7-mile runs (at 50–60 percent of racing pace) to improve aerobic conditioning, even though the event is much shorter. A marathoner may perform runs of 20 miles or more to achieve even higher levels of endurance. Although this 20-mile distance is shorter than the marathon race distance, research suggests that ample adaptations occur from this volume of exercise. Excess mileage in this case may just wear down the body. Long-slow distance training should be performed once every 1–2 weeks, and a rest day is recommended on the subsequent day to allow the body to recover fully.

Aerobic and anaerobic capacity both contribute to the ability to perform effectively in intermittent sports and recreational activities. Sports such as tennis, basketball, and soccer and recreational activities such as downhill skiing require intermittent periods of sustained aerobic activity and bursts of vigorous anaerobic activity. Therefore, athletes in these sports must also perform both aerobic and anaerobic training to perform well and to resist fatigue. Even participants in activities such as long-distance running can benefit from anaerobic training, especially if performance times or winning races is important. A fast start, a sprint past an opponent, and a kick at the end are typically anaerobic.

Interval training can be effective in building both aerobic and anaerobic capacity. High-level performance requires high-level training. **Interval training** is an advanced

Table 1 ▶ Work and Rest Bouts for Different Types of Interval-Training Workouts

Type of Interval	Short-Length Intervals			Long-Length Intervals		
	Intensity	Duration	Frequency	Intensity	Duration	Frequency
Aerobic (50–70% MaxHR)	50–70%	2- to 3-minute bouts with 10–15 seconds rest	Perform 7–8 with rest; repeat after 3–4 minutes (recovery)	50–60%	15–20 minutes	Perform full bout; repeat after 3–4 minutes (recovery)
Aerobic/Anaerobic (70–90% MaxHR)	75–85%	1- to 2-minute bouts with 30–60 seconds rest	Perform 5–6 with rest; repeat after 5–6 minutes (recovery)	70–75%	6–8 minutes	Perform full bout; repeat after 5–6 minutes (recovery)
Anaerobic (85–95% MaxHR)	90–95%	10- to 15-second bouts with 15–120 seconds rest	Perform 3–4 with rest; repeat after 7–8 minutes (recovery)	85–90%	30–60 seconds with 60–240 seconds rest	Perform 10–12 with rest; repeat after 7–8 minutes (recovery)

training technique that helps athletes optimize the effectiveness of their training. The premise behind interval training is that by providing periodic rest you can increase the overall intensity of the exercise session and provide a greater stimulus to the body. Interval training can be performed in different ways to achieve different training goals. It can be done at lower intensities to improve aerobic metabolism or at extremely high intensities to enhance anaerobic capacity. Interval training can be done using a series of shorter intervals that are strung together after short rests or with fewer, but longer, bouts. Examples of interval training options are summarized:

- *Aerobic intervals improve the efficiency of the aerobic metabolism.* The goal of aerobic intervals is to provide a sustained challenge to the cardiorespiratory system. The intensity should be challenging (but manageable) since the goal is to train the aerobic system to function efficiently over an extended period of time. In general, the pace would be similar to (or slightly slower than) the pace used for a 30- to 40-minute continuous event (about 50–70 percent of maximum heart rate). The body adapts to the pace and becomes better at providing oxygen to the muscles and clearing lactic acid that accumulates during the bout. Aerobic interval training can be done using a series of short 2- to 3-minute intervals (with short 10- to 15-second rests). Alternately, it can be done as a pace workout using a longer continuous bout lasting 15–20 minutes. Advanced athletes may repeat the workout after a short recovery period to further enhance the training stimulus.

- *Aerobic/anaerobic intervals help improve maximal aerobic capacity.* To improve aerobic capacity ($\dot{V}O_2$ max) it is necessary to push the body to perform near your aerobic capacity for an extended period of time (4–6 minutes is a good target). A person's aerobic capacity is reached at intensities above the anaerobic threshold, so this requires a fairly high intensity (typically about 70–85 percent maximum heart rate). For runners, a series of repeated mile runs at

a faster than normal training pace provides a good challenge to the aerobic system. However, a series of quarter-mile repeats can also achieve the same goal as long as the total time at a high intensity is similar. In this case, the rest intervals for the set must be short enough to allow only partial recovery between intervals. The adaptations here are based on sustaining a high intensity for the 4- to 6-minute period so full recovery is desirable between sets. Similar workouts can be devised for other sports.

- *Anaerobic intervals help improve anaerobic capacity.* This is typically accomplished with a series of high-intensity bouts of activity at 85–95 percent of maximum heart rate. In response to this training, the body improves its ability to produce energy anaerobically and to tolerate anaerobic by-products such as lactic acid. A series of 4–5 short bouts of activity that are 10–15 seconds long at maximum speed provide a good stimulus (e.g., 100-yard dash). Work-to-rest ratios may range from 1:1 to 1:10 depending on the individual's fitness and the goal of the training. Longer intervals (30–60 seconds) at a slightly slower speed (85–90 percent of maximum heart rate) with more extended rest breaks (60–240 seconds) can also be effective.

The purpose of the training session should dictate the intensity, duration, and rest periods with interval training. Examples of aerobic, aerobic/anaerobic, and anaerobic intervals are provided in Table 1. A highly fit person may use shorter rests and repeat the interval session multiple times in a given workout.

Long-Slow Distance (LSD) Training Training technique used by marathon runners and other endurance performers that emphasizes slow, sustained exercise rather than speed.

Interval Training A training technique often used for high-level aerobic and anaerobic training that involves alternating periods of high- and low-intensity activity to maximize the quality of the workout.

Principles of interval training can be adapted for different activities. While athletes have routinely used interval training to optimize their workouts, the use of *high-intensity interval training (HIIT)* has also been promoted for use by fitness leaders in commercial fitness centers. The group structure may help some stay focused, but it can be incorporated into any exercise routine in structured or unstructured ways by including intermittent bursts of higher-intensity activity. Runners sometimes use *fartlek* training to break up their workouts. A fartlek run incorporates bursts of higher-intensity running followed by recovery periods of lower intensity. The difference from interval training is that the intermittent bursts in fartlek training are dictated by the nature of the terrain or the feelings of the moment. The term is from a Swedish word meaning "speed play," because the unstructured nature is more relaxed than interval training.

Many competitive sports involve alternating bursts of high-intensity activity followed by periods of recovery. Basketball, for example, involves intermittent sprints and jumps interspersed with periods of short recovery. Similarly, tennis involves bursts of activity separated by short recovery periods between points. To prepare for success in sports, it is important for athletes to incorporate intermittent interval–type training into their conditioning. Simulated games that require repeated sprints up and down the basketball court are a form of interval training specific to basketball players. Tennis players can also incorporate a variety of forward and lateral movements into a high-intensity agility drill to improve conditioning that specifically matches the common challenges in tennis.

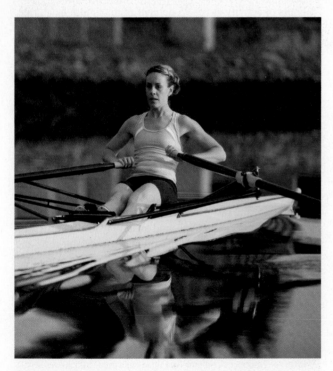

Training needs to be sport specific to improve performance.
Ty Milford/Aurora Open/Getty Images

Training for Strength, Muscular Endurance, and Power

Specific progressive resistance training programs are needed to achieve high-level muscle fitness. A basic progressive resistance program for overall good health might involve performing a single exercise for each major muscle group two or three times a week. This level of training provides a regular stimulus to maintain good **muscle fitness**. However, many people challenge themselves to achieve higher levels of fitness or muscular performance. Olympic weight-lifting competitors use free weights and compete in two exercises: the snatch and the clean and jerk. Powerlifting competitors use free weights and compete in three lifts: the bench press, squat, and dead lift. Bodybuilding competitors use several forms of resistance training and are judged on muscular hypertrophy (large muscles) and **definition of muscle**. Performers in these activities and athletes in strength-related sports need to use more advanced training methods to reach their full potential. The essential goal in high-level training is to provide the optimal stimulus so that the muscles adapt in the desired way. Because the goals are clearly different for athletes interested in strength/power, muscular hypertrophy, or muscular endurance, it is important to follow appropriate programs. The essential aspects of these different training programs are described in the sections that follow. The basic concepts are summarized in Figure 2.

Performers training for high-level strength should use multiple sets with heavier weights. The best stimulus for strength gains is repeated lifts with very heavy loads. Guidelines for intermediate lifters call for multiple sets of 6–12 reps performed using 70–80 percent of 1RM values. The load and intensity guidelines are higher for advanced lifters (1–12 reps performed using 70–100 percent 1RM) because they may need to use a higher overload to get continued improvements. Rest intervals must be long (2–3 minutes) for high-intensity strength training to allow full recovery of the muscles between sets.

Multiple-joint exercises, such as the bench press, have been found to be more effective in strength enhancement, since they allow a greater load to be lifted. The sequencing of exercises within a workout is also an important consideration for strength development. When training all major muscle groups in a workout, large muscle groups should be done before small muscle groups, and multiple-joint exercises should be done before single-joint ones.

Performers training for muscular endurance should emphasize many repetitions with lighter weights. Completing multiple sets of 10–25 repetitions is required to build endurance. Short rest periods of 1–2 minutes are recommended for high-repetition sets, and periods of less than 1 minute should be used for lower-repetition sets. This challenges the muscles to perform repeatedly and with little or

Strength/power

Load	Low	Medium	High
Reps	Low	Medium	High
Sets	Low	Medium	High
Volume	Low	Medium	High
Rest	Low	Medium	High

Hypertrophy/size

Load	Low	Medium	High
Reps	Low	Medium	High
Sets	Low	Medium	High
Volume	Low	Medium	High
Rest	Low	Medium	High

Muscular endurance

Load	Low	Medium	High
Reps	Low	Medium	High
Sets	Low	Medium	High
Volume	Low	Medium	High
Rest	Low	Medium	High

Figure 2 ► Differences in training stimulus for different resistance training programs.

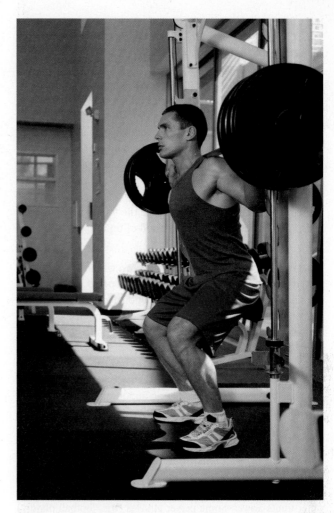

Training for high-level performance requires focus and determination.
Fuse/Corbis/Getty Images

no rest. Variation in the order in which exercises are performed is also recommended to vary the stimulus. Intermediate lifters should aim for two to four times per week, but advanced lifters may perform up to six sessions per week if appropriate variation in muscle groups is used between workouts.

Performers training for bulk and definition often use extra reps and/or sets. Bodybuilders are more interested in definition and hypertrophy than in absolute strength. Gaining both size and definition requires a balance between strength and muscular endurance training. Most bodybuilders use 3–7 sets of 10–15 repetitions, rather than the 3 sets of 3–8 repetitions recommended for most weight lifters. Sometimes definition is difficult to obtain because it is obscured by fat. It should be noted that people with the largest-looking muscles are not always the strongest. The word *tone* is often used inappropriately to explain fitness gains. (More information regarding the misuse of the word *tone* is provided in the Concept on Making Informed Consumer Choices.)

Cardiorespiratory endurance training can limit adaptations from strength or power training. The body adapts to the type of training that is performed. If too much endurance training is performed, the body tries to adapt to the needs of aerobic activity, and this makes it more difficult to gain muscle mass or achieve maximal increases in strength. The effect would be an issue only for competitive strength or power athletes and should not deter people from getting the important health benefits associated with moderate amounts of aerobic activity. Regular aerobic activity is considered essential for bodybuilders to help them reduce unwanted body fat.

Muscle Fitness A generalized term that reflects the ability of the musculoskeletal system to perform strength, endurance, or power activities.

Definition of Muscle The detailed external appearance of a muscle.

Training for Speed and Power

Speed is important for optimal performance in many sports. Speed is categorized as a dimension of skill-related fitness since it is more directly related to performance than to health (see the introductory Concept on healthy lifestyles). Speed can be improved with training, but trainability is more dependent on genetics than other dimensions of fitness such as cardiorespiratory endurance. Individuals with greater percentages of fast-twitch muscle fibers will tend to adapt more readily to sprint training since these fibers are specialized for anaerobic energy production. Training for speed resembles protocols for strength training since the focus is on maximal exertion or force over a short period of time.

Power reflects the rate at which force can be applied, and it depends on both strength and speed. Some experts consider power to be the most functional mode in which all human motion occurs. Power is exceptionally important in sport activities such as hitting a baseball, blocking in football, putting the shot, and throwing the discus. Power is also essential for good vertical jumping—a movement critical for basketball and many other sports. While power is emphasized in sports training, it is also now viewed as an important attribute for successful aging. A typical progressive resistance exercise program will build sufficient power for normal activities of daily living; however, people interested in high-level performance should consider using additional exercises that specifically develop power. To increase power, you must do more work in the same time or the same work in less time. Increasing one without the other limits power. Some power athletes (e.g., football players) might benefit by achieving less strength and more speed.

Training for power requires highly specific training. If you need power for an activity in which you are required to move heavy weights, then you need to develop *strength-related power* by working against heavy resistance at slower speeds. If you need to move light objects at great speed, such as in throwing a ball, you need to develop *speed-related power* by training at high speeds with relatively low resistance. There are trade-offs between speed- and strength-related power training because the heavier the resistance, the slower the movement. Therefore, the focus of training should be on the primary need for the specific sport or activity.

Performers who need explosive power to perform a specific task or event should use training that closely resembles that movement. Jumpers, for example, should jump as a part of their training programs in order to learn correct timing and mechanics. If they use machines, it is better to use the leg press than a knee extension machine because the press more nearly resembles the leg action of the jump. In general, power training with weights should be done with light loads (30%–60% of 1 RM) and with an intentional fast velocity. Aim for 3 to 6 repetitions.

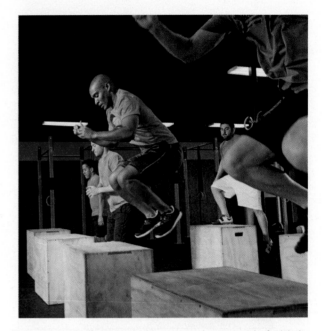

Plyometrics are effective at building power, but pose risks for injuries due to the intensity and the settings where it might be performed.
Erik Isakson/Blend Images LLC

Plyometrics refer to a specific type of training that is well suited for power development. Plyometric exercises can be customized to help build power for specific performance skills, but typically involve explosive bounding and jumping movements. The eccentric landing phase in the movement is important since it allows the exercise to be maximally loaded and challenged in a dynamic, sport-specific way. However, the eccentric muscle contractions can lead to muscular soreness, so it is important to ease into this type of training to give your body time to adapt. It is also important to have good flexibility before beginning a plyometrics program. Table 2 lists safety guidelines for plyometrics.

Table 2 ▶ Safety Guidelines for Plyometrics
• Progression should be gradual to avoid extreme muscle soreness.
• Adequate strength should be developed prior to plyometric training. (As a general rule, you should be able to do a half squat with one-and-a-half times your body weight.)
• Obstacles used for jumping-over should be padded to reduce risks for injuries. The landing surface should be semi-resilient, dry, and unobstructed.
• Shoes should have good lateral stability, be cushioned with an arch support, and have a nonslip sole.
• The training should be preceded by a general and specific warm-up. Don't perform at the end of a workout if fatigued.
• Beginners should aim to perform 3 or 4 drills (2–3 sets and 10–15 reps per set) with rest between each one. Perform no more than twice per week.

Source: Adapted from Brittenham.

Training for Functional Fitness and Flexibility

Functional fitness training builds skill-related fitness dimensions such as balance, coordination, and agility as well as muscle fitness and flexibility. Functional fitness training (also called neuromotor training) refers to specific efforts to improve the integration of the body's motor (muscle) system with the neural (sensory) system. This integration can improve the body's ability to perform real-life activities such as bending, squatting, lunging, kicking, climbing, reaching, or lifting.

Functional fitness training can be conducted in a variety of ways, but athletes often use task-specific or sport-specific training regimens such as squatting, tossing a ball against a rebounder, performing a "grapevine" movement, or running through agility ladders. Resistance needed for building strength comes from the weight of the moving body part(s) or the movement of devices such as kettlebells, medicine balls, or elastic cords. These devices are swung, tossed, caught, stretched, or pulled to provide added resistance to the workout. The ideal dosage (intensity, repetitions, and sets) has not been determined but would likely depend on the type of functional fitness exercise being performed.

Functional balance training is a specific type of functional fitness training that can promote better body control. Functional balance training involves the execution of skilled movements that improve **proprioception** and promote balance. The unique aspect of this form of training is that exercises typically require movement and stabilization force production at the same time. In other words, one part of the body is in motion while another is stabilized. These actions train the body's many somatic sensory organs to respond and adjust to different postures and positions—thereby improving balance. Functional balance training is frequently performed with exercise balls, balance boards, or BOSU trainers (see the Concept on muscle fitness). It is important to start slowly with easy movements and work up to more challenging positions and movements. This type of training is not recommended for people who have had recent orthopedic injuries, or individuals who have degenerative joint disease or knee instability.

Dynamic stretching provides some advantages for athletes preparing for competition. While static stretching is often recommended for general applications, athletes often need to perform more active (dynamic) stretching to prepare for activity. More dynamic forms of stretching (including ballistic stretching) are considered appropriate for high-level performers because many of the motions of the activities in which they perform require dynamic movements. Although ballistic stretching movements have an associated risk, athletes are trained to tolerate them, and the risk is not as significant. The ballistic movements also better prepare an athlete for the dynamic nature of activities during competition.

> **Plyometrics** A training technique used to develop explosive power. It consists of isotonic–concentric muscle contractions performed after a prestretch or an eccentric contraction of a muscle.
>
> **Proprioception** Awareness of body movements and orientation of the body in space; often used synonymously with *kinesthesis*.

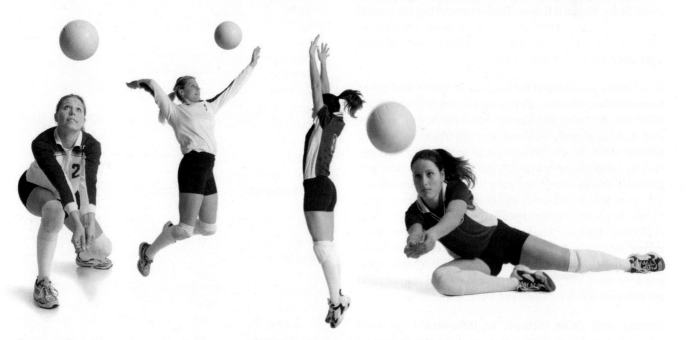

Sport-specific training and warm-ups help prepare athletes for the unique demands of their sport.
lfet: Alan Bailey/Rubberball/Getty Images; middle: Alan Bailey/Rubberball/Photodisc/Getty Images right: Alan Bailey/Rubberball/Getty Images

Dynamic stretching may provide other advantages for athletes. Static stretching may impair performance if done right before a competition. The reason for this is that the neuro-muscular system somewhat fights the stretch with an inhibitory response. The muscles become less responsive and stay weakened for up to 30 minutes after stretching, and this is certainly not beneficial for performance. Dynamic forms of stretching that stretch muscles while moving avoid this problem. Dynamic stretching is thought to enhance performance since muscles receive more of a stimulation response rather than an inhibition. Examples of ballistic stretches for sport-related activities include practice swings with a baseball bat, a golf club, or a tennis racquet. In each case, start by swinging backward and forward rhythmically and continuously. Gradually increase the speed and vigor of the swing until it approaches the speed used in the actual movement.

Training for High-Level Performance: Skill-Related Fitness and Skill

Good skill-related fitness is needed for success in many sports. There are five primary dimensions of skill-related fitness: agility, coordination, balance, reaction time, and speed. Having these attributes can make it easier to learn the necessary skills for many competitive sports. Balance and reaction time are critical for hitting a baseball, considered by many to be the toughest skill in sports. Similarly, agility and coordination may help one master advanced dribbling skills for sports such as basketball or soccer. Because skill-related fitness can enhance performance in sports, it is often called **motor fitness** or **sports fitness**. Table 3 summarizes the general skill-related fitness requirements of 44 sport activities. In Lab 12A you will evaluate your skill-related fitness and learn what activities you are most suited for.

Good skills are needed for success in sports and other competitive activities. Skill-related fitness helps you learn skills, but possessing the specific skills of an activity is probably more important. Skill refers to the ability to perform specific tasks. Sports examples include throwing, kicking, striking (as in hitting a baseball), and jumping. A person with good skill-related fitness may learn skills more easily and ultimately be able to achieve a higher level of skills than other people, but with practice anyone can learn skills. High-level performers typically must practice more often than recreational athletes and typically require more coaching on the specific skills of their chosen activity. Feedback from coaches, peers, or video analyses can help improve skill learning and performance if it is provided and utilized appropriately.

Fitness and skills interact to influence high-level performance. The ability to play games or sports is determined by combined abilities in separate skill-related components along

Table 3 ▶ Skill-Related Requirements of Sports and Other Activities

Activity	Balance	Coordination	Reaction Time	Agility	Power	Speed
Archery	***	****	*	*	*	*
Backpacking	**	**	*	**	**	*
Badminton	**	****	***	***	**	***
Baseball/softball	***	****	****	***	****	***
Basketball	***	****	****	****	****	***
Bicycling	****	**	**	*	**	**
Bowling	***	****	*	**	**	**
Canoeing	***	***	**	*	***	*
Circuit training	**	**	*	**	***	**
Dance, aerobic	**	****	**	***	*	*
Dance, ballet	****	****	**	****	***	
Dance, disco	**	***	**	****	*	**
Dance, modern	****	****	**	****	***	*
Dance, social	**	***	**	***	*	**
Fencing	***	****	****	***	***	****
Fitness calisthenics	**	**	*	***	**	*
Football	***	***	****	****	****	****
Golf (walking)	**	****	*	**	***	*
Gymnastics	****	****	***	****	****	**
Handball	**	****	***	****	***	***
Hiking	**	**	*	**	*	*
Horseback riding	***	***	**	***	*	*
Interval training	**	**	*	*	*	**
Jogging	**	**	*	*	*	*
Judo	***	****	****	****	****	****
Karate	***	****	****	****	****	****
Mountain climbing	****	****	**	***	***	*
Pool/billiards	**	***	*	**	**	*
Racquetball	**	****	***	****	**	***
Rope jumping	**	***	**	***	**	*
Rowing, crew	**	****	*	***	****	**
Sailing	***	***	***	***	*	*
Skating	****	***	**	***	**	***
Skiing, cross-country	**	****	*	***	****	**
Skiing, downhill	****	****	***	****	***	*
Soccer	**	****	***	****	***	***
Surfing	****	****	***	****	***	*
Swimming (laps)	**	***	*	***	**	*
Table tennis	**	***	****	**	**	**
Tennis	**	****	****	***	***	***
Volleyball	**	****	****	***	**	**
Walking	**	**	*	*	*	*
Waterskiing	***	***	*	***	**	*
Weight training	**	**	*	*	**	*

* = minimal needed; **** = a lot needed.

In the News

Youth Sports: When Is It Too Much?

Youth sports are an institution in contemporary society, if not a rite of passage. There are many potentially desirable outcomes from youth sports, but many experts question the excessive structure and pressure that it imposes on young children. Parents are left with the challenge of deciding whether the advantages of sports outweigh the limitations. While intentions may be good, many parents also find it hard to know how hard to push in trying to help or motivate their child. It is common for many talented young athletes to burn out or lose interest if faced with too much pressure. A 2017 *Time* magazine cover story "How Kids' Sports Became a $15 Billion Industry" exposed the personal, financial, and time commitments families have been devoting to youth sports. (See link in Suggested Resources and Readings.)

Are the pressures and demands of contemporary youth sports too high? Were you involved in sports as a youth? If so, did your experiences have a positive or negative influence on you?

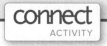

with a number of intangible factors. Following are key points about skill-related fitness:

- *Exceptional performers tend to be outstanding in more than one dimension of skill-related fitness.* Though people possess skill-related fitness in varying degrees, great athletes are likely to be above average in most, if not all, aspects.

- *Excellence in one skill-related fitness dimension may compensate for a lack in another.* For example, a tennis player may use good coordination to compensate for lack of speed.

- *Excellence in skill-related fitness may compensate for a lack of health-related fitness when playing sports and games.* Health-related fitness potential tends to decline with age, but experience and good skill-related fitness can help sustain high performance.

High-Level Performance Training

The quality of training is clearly more important than the quantity. A characteristic of high-level performance training is the need to continually challenge the body (overload principle). Involvement in regular physical activity will lead to improvements in fitness for most people, but they are harder to achieve once a good level of fitness has been attained (the principle of diminishing returns). It takes considerably more training to improve fitness than it does to maintain fitness.

To maximize performance, perform more specific types of workouts that provide a greater challenge to the body. Serious athletes may exercise 6 or 7 days a week, but easier workouts are generally done after harder and more intense workouts. The hard workouts are generally very specific and are designed to challenge the body in different ways. The easier workouts provide time to recover while building other dimensions of fitness. Quality is clearly more important than quantity.

Overtraining is a common problem among athletes. Most Americans suffer from hypokinetic conditions resulting from too little activity. Athletes, on the other hand, often push themselves too hard and do not allow adequate time for rest, making them susceptible to a variety of hyperkinetic conditions, such as *overload syndrome*. This condition is characterized by fatigue, irritability, and sleep problems, as well as an increased risk for injuries. Performance can decline sharply in an overtrained status, causing athletes to train even harder and become even more overtrained. Athletes should pay close attention to possible symptoms of overtraining and back off their training if they notice increased fatigue, lethargy, or unexpected decreases in their performance. Lab 12B helps you identify some symptoms of overtraining.

A slightly elevated morning heart rate (four or five beats more than normal values) is a useful physical indicator of overtraining. The body has had to work too hard to recover from the exercise and isn't in its normal resting mode. To use this indicator, regularly monitor your resting heart rate before getting out of bed in the morning. Another indicator that is increasingly used by elite endurance athletes is compressed or reduced "heart rate variability." A lower beat-to-beat variability indicates fatigue or overtraining, since it reflects sympathetic dominance over the normally dominant parasympathetic system that exists during more rested states. Newer heart rate monitors provide an indicator of heart rate variability.

Rest and a history of regular exercise are both important for reducing the risks for overuse injuries. Adequate rest helps the body recover from the stress of vigorous training—it promotes the physiological adaptations that improve performance and reduces the likelihood of developing overuse injuries.

Motor Fitness Skill-related physical fitness. Also called *sports fitness.*

Sports Fitness Skill-related physical fitness. Also called *motor fitness.*

A history of regular exercise is also important for reducing risks for injury. Research conducted by the military has determined that recruits with a history of regular exercise were less likely to get injured during basic training than recruits without this experience. This suggests that regular exercise can build up the strength and integrity of bones and joints and reduce the risk for injury. While experienced athletes may have less risk for injuries, they often push themselves too hard and develop overuse injuries or other conditions. Listening to your body and getting rest are important for decreasing risk of overtraining.

Periodization of training may help prevent overtraining. Athletes must plan carefully to reach peak performance at the right time and to avoid overtraining and injuries. **Periodization** is an advanced training principle that involves manipulating repetition, resistance, and exercise selection so there are periodic peaks and valleys during the training program. The peaks are needed to challenge the body, and the valleys allow the body to recover and adapt fully.

A training program is usually divided into a series of cycles that allow the intensity and volume to change in a systematic way. A hypothetical periodization cycle is depicted in Figure 3. Note that the overall training program (one macrocycle) is made up of three mesocycles that are each made up of three microcycles. The intensity increases gradually in each microcycle to provide a progressive training stimulus. Also note that the volume increases somewhat in opposition to the intensity with volume actually decreasing at the higher-intensity phases. The overall training stimulus increases throughout the mesocycle. Rest is a critical point of an effective periodization program as the body needs time to recover from (and adapt to) the challenging training stimulus. The intensity and volume drop to lower levels at the start of each microcycle with larger drops after each mesocycle. Periodization training is usually focused on preparing a person for a competition and, as the competition gets closer, the athlete typically begins a **tapering** plan to ensure a full recovery prior to the event. The tapering plan typically involves reductions in both intensity and volume of training to help facilitate recovery. Following a periodization plan helps an athlete optimize the effectiveness of training while also decreasing the risk of overtraining.

Athletes should be aware of various psychological disorders related to overtraining. Compulsive physical activity, often referred to as activity neurosis or exercise addiction, can be considered a hyperkinetic condition. People with activity neurosis become irrationally concerned about their exercise regimen. They may exercise more than

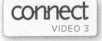

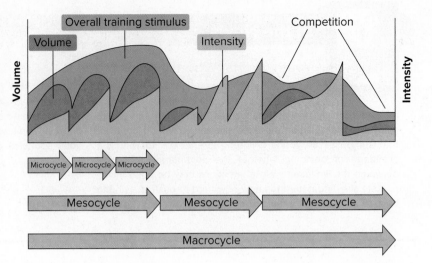

Figure 3 ▶ Conceptual pattern of cycles within a periodized training program.

once a day, rarely take a day off, or feel the need to exercise even when ill or injured. One condition related to activity neurosis is an obsession with having an attractive body (body neurosis). Among females, it is usually associated with an extreme desire to be thin, whereas among males it is more often associated with an extreme desire to be muscular. This excessive desire to be fit or thin can negatively affect other aspects of life, threaten personal relationships, and cause extreme stress.

Performance Trends and Ergogenic Aids

Many athletes look to ergogenic aids as an additional way to improve performance. Athletes are always looking for a competitive edge. In addition to pursuing rigorous training programs, many athletes look for alternative ways to improve their performance. Substances, strategies, and treatments designed to improve physical performance beyond the effects of normal training are collectively referred to as **ergogenic aids**. People interested in improving their appearance (including those with body neurosis) also abuse products they think will enhance their appearance. Ergogenic aids can be classified as mechanical, psychological, and physiological. Each category will be discussed in the subsequent sections.

Mechanical ergogenics may improve efficiency and performance. Mechanical ergogenic aids consist of equipment or devices that aid performance. Examples include oversized tennis racquets, more flexible poles for pole vaulting, spring-loaded ice skates (klap skates), Lycra body suits for reducing drag in swimming, carbon fiber bike frames to increase stiffness and force transmission in biking, and ultralight performance running shoes. The major innovations tend to spark controversy since the technology seems to provide an unfair advantage. However, sports seem to evolve and

Technology Update

Shoe Technology and the 2-Hour Marathon

The Kenyan runner Eliud Kipchoge recently made history by being the first person to run a marathon in under 2 hours. The achievement is remarkable since the 2-hour barrier had been considered to be almost at the realm of human limits. Innovations in running shoes, such as the Nike Vaporfly NEXT%, have been contributing to lower marathon times of high-performing runners for a number of years. Features in the Nike Alphafly model that Kipchoge used in his record run likely provided some additional advantages. The Nike shoes feature a carbon fiber plate, a springy foam midsole, and small air-filled sacs that act like a suspension system. The shoes essentially provide a rebound effect that improves efficiency. Time will tell whether this technology will be used more broadly or whether it may be banned.

Is the impact of technology in sports just "part of the game" or does it make competition less fair?

connect
ACTIVITY

adapt just as athletes do, and soon the new technology becomes more standardized (see Technology Update). While mechanical ergogenic aids may help maximize performance, the advantages are probably noticeable only for highly elite athletes. For example, a recreational athlete may not play any better with an expensive tennis racquet or new golf clubs. Expert players, on the other hand, can appreciate subtle differences in equipment and may benefit. Athletes, however, should continue to focus on improving fitness and practicing skills, since these will have bigger impacts on performance.

Psychological ergogenics may improve motivation and concentration and reduce anxiety during competitive activities. Many competitive activities require extreme levels of concentration, motivation, and focus. Athletes who can maintain a mental edge during an event are at a clear advantage over athletes who cannot. Competitive anxiety can impair performance, and psychological ergogenics can help reduce anxiety before and during an event. Psychological ergogenics include mental imagery, hypnosis, performance modeling, and established skill routines, to name but a few.

Physiological ergogenics are designed to improve performance by enhancing various biochemical and physiological processes in the body. Physiological ergogenics are primarily nutritional supplements thought to have a positive effect on various metabolic processes. Because the supplement industry is largely unregulated, many products are developed and marketed with little or no research to

document their effects. Producers of these products prey on an athlete's lack of knowledge and concern over performance.

Products with little or no evidence of benefits often have questionable safety. For example, protein supplements are unregulated products for which evidence of effectiveness is lacking. Many strength athletes continue to believe that extra protein in the diet can contribute to strength and muscle mass gains, despite the fact that this has been clearly refuted in the scientific literature. The aggressive marketing and propaganda in many muscle-related fitness publications convince many people to buy and try unproven supplements. Do not be swayed by ads and unsubstantiated claims. Physiological ergogenics with established performance benefits are described.

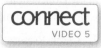

- *Fluid replacement beverages and energy bars.* Fluid replacement beverages, such as Gatorade, Exceed, and Powerade, contain carbohydrates needed for endurance exercise. People exercising for more than an hour can benefit from these supplements, and research shows that they can replace fluid lost in sweat at the same or a faster rate than water. Energy bars (e.g., Power Bars and Clif Bars), energy gels (e.g., GU), or energy chews (e.g., Clif Shot Blocks) also provide valuable energy for extended endurance exercise.

- *Creatine.* The body produces creatine naturally from foods containing protein, but some athletes take creatine supplements (usually a powder dissolved in a liquid) to increase the amounts available in the muscle. Some studies have shown improvements in performance and anaerobic capacity, but recent reviews indicate that the supplement may be effective only for athletes who are already well trained. Products containing creatine do not work by themselves; instead, they only help athletes maximize their training or performance during an event. Effects are not evident unless training is performed while taking the supplements.

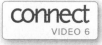

Using Self-Management Skills

Use appropriate self-planning skills to take responsibility for your own training program. Coaches handle these tasks for many competitive athletes, but recreational athletes typically have to plan their own program. Although you can contract with a personal trainer to help you, the principles and guidelines described in this Concept (and throughout this

Periodization A planned sequence of training designed to optimize adaptations and minimize overtraining.

Tapering A reduction in training volume and intensity prior to competition to elicit peak performance.

Ergogenic Aids Substances, strategies, and treatments intended to improve performance in sports or competitive athletics.

edition) provide a strong foundation for effective training. To plan your own program, use the self-planning skills described in the Concept on Self-Management Skills for Health Behavior Change. Brief summaries are:

1. **Clarify Reasons:** High-level training requires a strong personal commitment, so consider your motives to build your drive.

2. **Identify Needs:** Critically evaluate your fitness needs using the various self-assessments in this edition or consider more specialized assessments conducted through exercise labs or fitness facilities.

3. **Set Personal Goals:** Use SMART goal principles to set specific, measurable, attainable, realistic, and timely goals. Also, put your goals in writing since a goal really isn't a "goal" unless it is written down.

4. **Select Program Components:** The type of program needs to be designed to specifically help you make progress toward your goals. Training usually needs to be more specifically planned and intentional. Because the training is likely higher intensity, it is important to get adequate rest. Consider periodized training to adhere to principles of progression.

5. **Write Out Your Plan:** A written plan provides the needed structure to help you stick with your training program and to stay focused on your goals. Modifications will likely be needed along the way, so you should expect to revisit and adjust the plan as needed.

6. **Evaluate Progress:** Periodic evaluation is a key step to ensure that your program is on the right track. Athletes need to carefully monitor their progress to determine how to adjust their training.

Use good consumer skills to avoid being a victim of fraud and quackery. The strong interest in training and improved performance makes athletes a primary target for companies selling fraudulent fitness and performance supplements. Many athletes search online for information or visit "nutrition" stores to try to learn how to improve their performance. Unfortunately, there are few (if any) policies that regulate what is communicated in print or online sources. Many companies take small "truths" about fitness or health and then misuse them or apply them incorrectly. The consumer can be hooked by the apparent logic and the company cashes in on the sale. Companies are also not required to document that their products are safe or effective. Therefore, consumers waste millions of dollars a year on fraudulent products that have little or no benefit (and may even be harmful). Caveat emptor (buyer beware)! (See the Concept on Making Informed Consumer Choices for more information.)

Strategies for Action: Lab Information

Select activities that match your abilities. People differ in many factors, including skills and abilities that influence sports and athletic performance. You may be well suited to some sports but not to others. Behavioral scientists have also determined that perceptions of competence are important predictors of long-term exercise adherence. To give yourself the best chance of being successful in sports (and exercise involvement), choose activities that are well matched to your abilities. The assessments in Lab 12A provide a way to get a basic sense of which skill-related fitness dimensions you are stronger in

and which ones you are weaker in. Referring to Table 3 can help you determine the sports and activities that best match your individual abilities. These are just conceptual assessments, so the best way to assess your potential in a specific activity is to give it a try.

Get adequate rest and listen to your body. Many athletes make the mistake of training too hard and don't include enough time for rest. Without rest, the body does not have sufficient time to make the needed adaptations, and overtraining syndrome can result. Lab 12B helps you learn how to monitor for signs of overtraining.

connect
ACTIVITY

Suggested Resources and Readings

The websites for the following sources can be accessed by searching online for the organization, program, or title listed. Specific scientific references are available at the end of this edition of *Concepts of Fitness and Wellness*.

- American College of Sports Medicine. *Progression Models in Resistance Training for Healthy Adults.* (pdf)
- Bompa, T. O. (2021). *Periodization of Strength Training for Sports.* Champaign, IL: Human Kinetics.
- Burgess, M. (2020, February 5). "Nike Has Finally Revealed the Secrets of Its 1:59 Marathon Shoe." *Wired.*
- Gregory, S. (2017, August 24). "How Kids' Sports Became a $15 Billion Industry." *Time.*
- Laursen, P., & Buchheit, M. (eds.). (2019). *Science and Application of High-Intensity Interval Training.* Champaign, IL: Human Kinetics.
- McGuigan, M. (2017). *Monitoring Training and Performance in Athletes.* Champaign, IL: Human Kinetics.
- Simpson, R. (2020, March 30). "Exercise, Immunity, and the COVID Pandemic." American College of Sports Medicine.
- Topend Sports. Anaerobic Capacity Fitness Tests.

Design Element: (*magnifying glass*): Siede Preis/Getty Images; (*runners shoes*): Maridav/Getty Images; (*tablet*): McGraw Hill; (*woman*): GlobalStock/Getty Images; (*blue sports shoes*): chictype/Getty Images; (*smartphone*): Alexey Boldin/Shutterstock; (*Why It Matters*): MHHE

Lab Resource Materials: Skill-Related Physical Fitness

Important Note: Because skill-related physical fitness does not relate to good health, the rating charts used in this section differ from those used for health-related fitness. The rating charts that follow can be used to compare your scores with those of other people. You *do not* need exceptional scores on skill-related fitness to be able to enjoy sports and other types of physical activity; however, it is necessary for high-level performance.

Evaluating Skill-Related Physical Fitness

I. Evaluating Agility: The Illinois Agility Run An agility course using four chairs 10 feet apart and a 30-foot running area will be set up as depicted in this illustration. The test is performed as follows:

1. Lie prone with your hands by your shoulders and your head at the starting line. On the signal to begin, get on your feet and run the course as fast as possible.

2. Your score is the time required to complete the course. Check your rating in Chart 1.

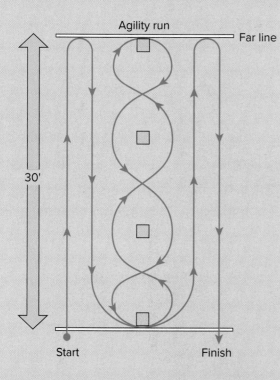

Agility run

Far line

30'

Start   Finish

II. Evaluating Balance: The Bass Test of Dynamic Balance
Eleven circles (9½ inches in diameter) are drawn on the floor as shown in the illustration. The test is performed as follows:

1. Stand on the right foot in circle X. *Leap* forward to circle 1, then circle 2 through 10, alternating feet with each leap.

2. The feet must leave the floor on each leap and the heel may not touch. Only the ball of the foot and toes may land on the floor.

3. Remain in each circle for 5 seconds before leaping to the next circle. If you lose balance, reestablish position and count for 5 seconds

4. The score is 50, plus the number of seconds taken to complete the test, minus the number of errors.

5. For every error, deduct 3 points each. Errors include touching the heel, moving the supporting foot, touching outside a circle, and touching any body part other than the supporting foot to the floor. See Chart 2 to check your rating.

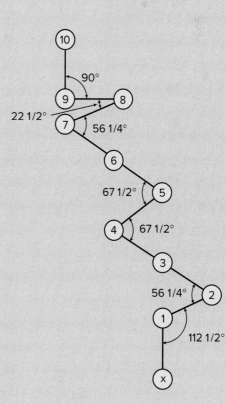

Chart 1 Agility Rating Scale

Classification	Male	Female
Excellent	15.8 or faster	17.4 or faster
Very good	16.7–15.9	18.6–17.5
Good	18.6–16.8	22.3–18.7
Fair	18.8–18.7	23.4–22.4
Poor	18.9 or slower	23.5 or slower

Source: Adams et al.

Chart 2 Balance Rating Scale

Rating	Score
Excellent	90–100
Very good	80–89
Good	70–79
Fair	60–69
Poor	50–59

Chart 3 Coordination Rating Scale

Classification	Male	Female
Excellent	14–15	13–15
Very good	11–13	10–12
Good	5–10	4–9
Fair	3–4	2–3
Poor	0–2	0–1

III. Evaluating Coordination: The Stick Test of Coordination

The stick test of coordination requires you to juggle three wooden sticks. The sticks are used to perform a half flip and a full flip, as shown in the illustrations.

1. *Half flip.* Hold two 24-inch (12 inches in diameter) dowel rods, one in each hand. Support a third rod of the same size across the other two. Toss the supported rod in the air so that it makes a half turn. Catch the thrown rod with the two held rods.

2. *Full flip.* Perform the preceding task, letting the supported rod turn a full flip.

The test is performed as follows:

1. Practice the half flip and full flip several times before taking the test.

2. When you are ready, attempt a half flip five times. Score 1 point for each successful attempt.

3. When you are ready, attempt the full flip five times. Score 2 points for each successful attempt. Check your rating in Chart 3.

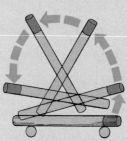

Half flip

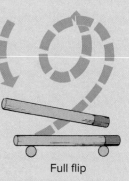

Full flip

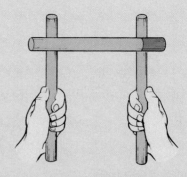

Hand position

IV. Evaluating Reaction Time: The Stick Drop Test To perform the stick drop test of reaction time, you will need a yardstick, a table, a chair, and a partner to help with the test. To perform the test, follow this procedure:

1. Sit in the chair next to the table so that your elbow and lower arm rest on the table comfortably. The heel of your hand should rest on the table so that only your fingers and thumb extend beyond the edge of the table.

2. Your partner holds a yardstick at the top, allowing it to dangle between your thumb and fingers.

3. The yardstick should be held so that the 24-inch mark is even with your thumb and index finger. No part of your hand should touch the yardstick.

4. Without warning, your partner will drop the stick, and you will catch it with your thumb and index finger.

5. Your score is the number of inches read on the yardstick just above the thumb and index finger after you catch the yardstick.

6. Try the test three times. Your partner should be careful not to drop the stick at predictable time intervals, so that you cannot guess when it will be dropped. It is important that you react only to the dropping of the stick.

7. Use the middle of your three scores (e.g., if your scores are 21, 18, and 19, your middle score is 19). The higher your score, the faster your reaction time. Check your rating in Chart 4.

Chart 4 Reaction Time Rating Scale

Classification	Score
Excellent	More than 21″
Very good	19″–21″
Good	16″–18¾″
Fair	13″–15¾″
Poor	Below 13″

Note: Metric conversions for this chart appear in Appendix A.

V. Evaluating Speed: The 3-Second Run To perform the running test of speed, it will be necessary to have a specially marked running course, a stopwatch, a whistle, and a partner to help you with the test. To perform the test, follow this procedure:

1. Mark a running course on a hard surface so that there is a starting line and a series of nine additional lines, each 2 yards apart, the first marked at a distance 10 yards from the starting line.

2. From a distance 1 or 2 yards behind the starting line, begin to run as fast as you can. As you cross the starting line, your partner starts a stopwatch.

3. Run as fast as you can until you hear the whistle, which your partner will blow exactly 3 seconds after the stopwatch is started. Your partner marks your location at the time the whistle was blown.

4. Your score is the distance you covered in 3 seconds. You may practice the test and take more than one trial if time allows. Use the better of your distances on the last two trials as your score. Check your rating in Chart 5.

Chart 5 Speed Rating Scale

Classification	Male	Female
Excellent	24–26 yards	22–26 yards
Very good	22–23 yards	20–21 yards
Good	18–21 yards	16–19 yards
Fair	16–17 yards	14–15 yards
Poor	Less than 16 yards	Less than 14 yards

Note: Metric conversions for this chart appear in Appendix A.

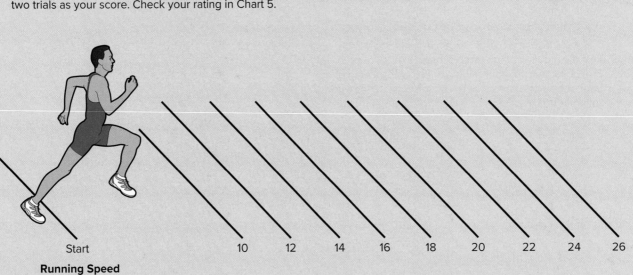

Start   10   12   14   16   18   20   22   24   26

Running Speed

Lab 12A Evaluating Skill-Related Physical Fitness

connect
ACTIVITY

Name	Section	Date

Purpose: To help you evaluate your own skill-related fitness, including agility, balance, coordination, power, speed, and reaction time; this information may be of value in helping you decide which sports match your skill-related fitness abilities.

Procedures

1. Read the directions for each of the skill-related fitness tests presented in the Lab Resource Materials.
2. Take as many of the tests as possible, given the time and equipment available.
3. Be sure to warm up before and to cool down after the tests.
4. It is all right to practice the tests before trying them. However, you should decide ahead of time which trial you will use to test your skill-related fitness.
5. After completing the tests, write your scores in the appropriate places in the Results section.
6. Determine your rating for each of the tests from the rating charts in the Lab Resource Materials.

Results

Place a check in the circle for each of the tests you completed.

Agility (Illinois run) ○

Balance (Bass test) ○

Coordination (stick test) ○

Reaction time (stick drop test) ○

Speed (3-second run) ○

Record your scores and ratings in the following spaces.

	Score	Rating	
Agility			(Chart 1)
Balance			(Chart 2)
Coordination			(Chart 3)
Reaction time			(Chart 4)
Speed			(Chart 5)

Conclusions and Implications: In two or three paragraphs, discuss the results of your skill-related fitness tests. Comment on the areas in which you did well or did not do well, the meaning of these findings, and the implications of the results, with specific reference to the activities you will perform in the future.

Lab 12B Identifying Symptoms of Overtraining

Name	**Section**	**Date**

Purpose: To help you identify the symptoms of overtraining.

Procedures

1. Answer the questions concerning overtraining syndrome in the Results section. If you are in training, rate yourself; if not, evaluate a person you know who is in training. As an alternative, you may evaluate a person who was formerly in training (and who experienced symptoms) or evaluate yourself when you were in training (if you trained for performance in the past).
2. Use Chart 1 to rate the person (yourself or another person) who is (or was) in training.
3. Use Chart 2 to identify some strategies you can try to treat or prevent overtraining syndrome.
4. Answer the questions in the Conclusions and Implications section.

Results

Answer "Yes" (place a check in the circle) to any of the questions relating to overtraining symptoms you (or the person you are evaluating) experienced.

◯ 1. Has performance decreased dramatically in the last week or two?

◯ 2. Is there evidence of depression?

◯ 3. Is there evidence of atypical anger?

◯ 4. Is there evidence of atypical anxiety?

◯ 5. Is there evidence of general fatigue that is not typical?

◯ 6. Is there general lack of vigor or loss of energy?

◯ 7. Have sleeping patterns changed (inability to sleep well)?

◯ 8. Is there evidence of heaviness of the arms and/or legs?

◯ 9. Is there evidence of loss of appetite?

◯ 10. Is there a lack of interest in training?

Chart 1 Ratings for Overtraining Syndrome

Number of "Yes" Answers	Rating
9–10	Overtraining syndrome is very likely present. Seek help.
6–8	Person is at risk for overtraining syndrome if it is not already present. Seek help to prevent additional symptoms.
3–5	Some signs of overtraining syndrome are present. Consider methods of preventing further symptoms.
0–2	Overtraining syndrome is not present, but attention should be paid to any symptoms that do exist.

Conclusions and Implications

Chart 2 lists some of the strategies that may help eliminate or prevent overtraining syndrome. Check the strategies that you think would be (or would have been) most useful to the person you evaluated.

Chart 2 Strategies for Treating or Preventing Overtraining Syndrome

○ 1. Consider a break from training.

○ 2. Taper the program to help reduce symptoms.

○ 3. Seek help to redesign the training program.

○ 4. Alter your diet.

○ 5. Evaluate other stressors that may be producing symptoms.

○ 6. Reset performance goals.

○ 7. Talk to someone about problems.

○ 8. Have a medical checkup to be sure there is no medical problem.

○ 9. If you have a coach, consider a talk with him or her.

○ 10. Add fluids to help prevent performance problems from dehydration.

Discuss overtraining syndrome in general. Elaborate on one or two of the strategies in Chart 2 that you think would be (or would have been) most effective in treating or preventing overtraining syndrome for the person you evaluated.

Body Composition and Health

LEARNING OBJECTIVES

After completing the study of this Concept, you will be able to:

▶ Understand and interpret body composition measures.

▶ Describe common methods of assessing body composition.

▶ List health risks associated with overfatness.

▶ List health risks associated with excessively low body fatness.

▶ Identify and describe the origins of body fatness.

▶ Explain the relationship between physical activity and body composition and apply the FIT formula for achieving and maintaining a healthy body composition.

▶ Evaluate your body composition using several self-assessments and identify personal needs, set goals, and create a plan for achieving and maintaining a healthy body composition.

▶ Self-assess your daily energy expenditure.

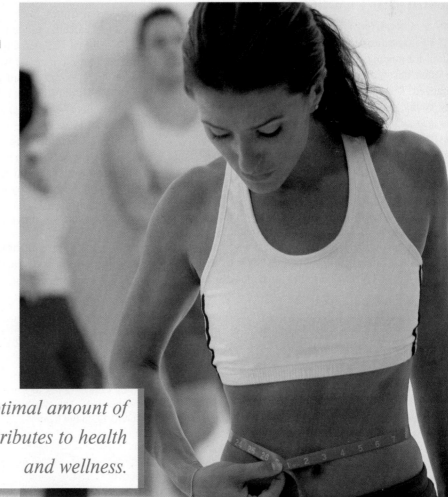

Possessing an optimal amount of body fat contributes to health and wellness.

Comstock/Getty Images

Maintaining a healthy body composition can be challenging in our contemporary society. This Concept provides information about how to assess and interpret your body composition status using several indicators. It also provides information about the causes and consequences of obesity to provide a foundation for effective weight management practices. Having knowledge about factors influencing body composition can help you set appropriate goals and not put excessive pressure on yourself to look a certain way or to achieve a certain weight. Having a good understanding of these factors can also help you develop lifestyles that are more conducive to establishing and maintaining a healthy weight. Numerous studies have demonstrated that fitness is more important than fatness as far as overall health is concerned. Therefore, instead of focusing on weight, the more important goal is to adopt an active and healthy lifestyle.

Understanding Obesity

Obesity **is a clinical term that simply means "excess body fat."** The classifications of "overweight" and "obesity" are important for guiding clinical care but, unfortunately, the words are often misused and individuals may be inappropriately stigmatized. There is growing sensitivity in society related to diversity, equity, and inclusion (DEI) issues and these considerations also apply to obesity. This edition endorses (and encourages) the movement to "person-first language" when explaining issues related to obesity by putting the person before the diagnosis (e.g., "a person with obesity").

Obesity continues to be a major public health challenge. The rapid increases in obesity rates in society have been referred to as an "epidemic." An epidemic is technically defined as "an outbreak of disease that spreads quickly and affects many individuals at the same time." While obesity is not contagious like COVID-19 or other infectious diseases,

it has exhibited epidemic-like characteristics as the prevalence began increasing. For example, 30 years ago almost no states in the United States had an obesity rate higher than 20 percent, but now only 1 state (Colorado) has a prevalence of less than 25 percent. Approximately half of the states have rates that exceed 30 percent, and 24 percent (12 out of 50 states) have rates above 35 percent. Some evidence suggested that increases in obesity rates were starting to level off; however, these figures reflect increases over those from a few years ago. Projections by researchers in Harvard's School of Public Health indicate that obesity rates could reach 50 percent by 2030. These projections were made before the COVID-19 pandemic which has already contributed to weight gain for many Americans (see In the News).

Obesity is influenced by genetics, culture, and environmental factors. As described in the Concept on lifelong determinants, a variety of factors influence health and fitness, and many are not within our control. Obesity is known to be strongly linked to genetics, but a hereditary predisposition can be compounded by social, cultural, and environmental factors. There are clear regional patterns in obesity in the United States, with the highest prevalence in the Midwest (34 percent) and South (33 percent) and the lowest in the Northeast (29 percent) and the West (27 percent). Prevalence tends to increase with age and varies considerably across ethnic groups. Recent estimates reveal higher prevalence in non-Hispanic Black adults (40 percent), followed by Hispanic adults (34 percent) and non-Hispanic white adults (30 percent). However, the drivers of obesity are most directly tied to the underlying social determinants of health. For example, the prevalence of obesity is higher among those without a college education and those with lower incomes. There are also disparities by urbanicity, with higher rates in rural areas than urban ones. Additional information on the causes of obesity is provided in a later section.

Obesity has major impacts on personal health and well-being. Excess body fat is associated with greater risks for many medical conditions, including high blood pressure,

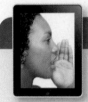

In the News

Quarantine 15

The "freshman 15" is an expression used to describe the weight gain that often happens to students during their first year in college. Research has verified that first-year college students do gain weight, though the average gain is closer to 6–9 pounds. This has been attributed to stress as well as aspects of the social and physical environments. The isolation, stress, and lifestyle changes

caused by COVID-19 led to similar amounts of weight gain in adults nationwide. This has been called the "quarantine 15" or the "COVID 19" in the media.

Did social isolation due to COVID-19 make it harder for you to manage your weight? What have you learned from the experience?

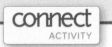
connect
ACTIVITY

diabetes, heart disease, and cancer. However, the implications of obesity on overall health status were also evident throughout the COVID-19 pandemic. People with obesity were at least twice as likely to end up in the hospital if they contracted COVID-19, and they were 50 percent more likely to die than people of a healthy weight. Individuals with overweight or obesity were less able to battle COVID-19 due to impaired function in a number of body systems (immune, cardiovascular, respiratory, and metabolic). Clinicians referred to the challenges of treating COVID-19 as a "pandemic laying on top of an ongoing epidemic" (i.e., obesity).

A prominent study in the journal *Circulation* documented that COVID-19-related risks from obesity were more pronounced in younger individuals. Another study documented an increased prevalence of various cancers among Millennials (individuals born 1981 to 1996). Thus, obesity presents risks for all ages and not just for older individuals. The health risks of obesity are explained in a later section to help you understand personal implications.

Obesity is classified as a disease. While obesity is linked to preventable behaviors of healthy eating and physical activity, it is officially recognized by the American Medical Association (AMA) as a disease. The designation was controversial since some felt that it allowed individuals to justify unhealthy lifestyle or dietary practices rather than accepting personal responsibility for their condition. However, the decision has brought increased attention to the problem and has impacted how obesity is treated by the medical community. The labeling of obesity as a disease also changed policies related to insurance coverage. For example, it led to the passage of the Patient Access to Evidence-Based Obesity Services resolution by the AMA that has helped improve patient access to evidence-based obesity treatments. Despite progress, the obesity epidemic continues to have financial consequences and places considerable burdens on the health-care system. A CDC web page devoted to obesity sums up the issue very concisely: "Obesity is common, serious, and costly."

Weight shaming contributes to negative outcomes and experiences. The continued pressure on individuals with overweight or obesity to change, to diet, or to lose weight can backfire. Clinicians are often blamed for weight shaming when they press patients too hard about their weight. However, weight shaming can come from many sources. It can come directly through verbal references to a person's weight status or their failure to lose weight. It can also occur as small micro-aggressions that a person experiences from work or social interactions that subtly draw attention to his or her weight. Weight shaming doesn't help a person's weight control efforts, and it has also been linked to depression, anxiety, low self-esteem, and eating disorders. In addition to being unfair, evidence suggests that weight discrimination and bias cause considerable harm (see the HELP feature).

HELP Health is available to Everyone for a Lifetime, and it's Personal

Weight Discrimination

Individuals with excess weight or obesity may be susceptible to forms of bias, prejudice, and discrimination. Bias and prejudice can be subtle or overt, but they contribute to unfair labeling, exclusion, victimization, and rejection. *Weight discrimination* is distinct from stigmatization and refers to unequal or unfair treatment because of weight status. For example, a person with obesity may be passed over for a job or a promotion because of his or her weight status. The increased emphasis on social justice issues in society provides hope for addressing inequities associated with weight discrimination.

Have you perceived or been a victim of weight discrimination? What can you do to contribute to ending this inequity?

connect ACTIVITY

Body Composition Indicators and Standards

Body composition is a component of health-related fitness. Body composition is different from other dimensions of health-related physical fitness in that it is not a performance measure. Cardiorespiratory endurance, strength, power, muscular endurance, and flexibility are typically assessed using movement or performance, while body composition is considered to be an anthropometric measure. Body composition is an important determinant of metabolic fitness and also impacts the health and performance of many organs and body systems. This is why it is categorized as an important dimension of health-related fitness. Labs 13A and 13B provide opportunities for you to assess your body composition using appropriate standards.

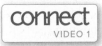

connect VIDEO 1

Standards have been established for healthy levels of body fatness. Fat has important functions in the body, and it is distributed naturally into different tissues and storage depots. The indicator of **percent body fat** is typically used to reflect the overall fat content of the body. This indicator takes into account differences in body size and allows recommendations to be made for healthy levels of body fatness.

A certain minimal amount of fat is needed to allow the body to function. This level of **essential fat** is necessary for

Percent Body Fat The percentage of total body weight that is composed of fat.

Essential Fat The minimum amount of fat in the body necessary to maintain healthful living.

Body fatness (percent body fat)		Too low	Borderline	Good fitness	Marginal	At risk
	Male	5 or less	6–9	10–20	21–25	26+
	Female:	10 or less	11–16	17–28	29–35	36+

Body Mass Index (kg/m²)		Too low	Borderline	Good fitness	Overweight	Obesity
	Male	12 or less	13–18.4	18.5–24.9	25–30	30+
	Female:	12 or less	13–18.4	18.5–24.9	25–30	30+

Figure 1 ▶ Health-related standards for body fatness (percent body fat) and Body Mass Index.

temperature regulation, shock absorption, and the regulation of essential body nutrients, including vitamins A, D, E, and K. The exact amount of fat considered essential to normal body functioning has been debated, but most experts agree that males should possess no less than 5 percent and females no less than 10 percent. For females, an exceptionally low body fat percentage (**underfat**) is of special concern, particularly when associated with overtraining, low calorie intake, competitive stress, and poor diet. **Amenorrhea** may occur, placing the female at risk for bone loss (osteoporosis) and other health problems. A body fat level below 10 percent is one of the criteria often used by clinicians for diagnosing eating disorders, such as anorexia nervosa.

Figure 1 shows the health-related standards for body composition (percent body fat) for both males and females. Because individuals differ in their response to low fatness, a borderline range is provided above the essential fat (too low) zone. Values in this zone are not necessarily considered to be healthy, but some individuals may seek to have lower body fat levels to enhance performance in certain sports. Fat that is stored above essential fat levels is classified as **nonessential fat.** Just as percent body fat should not drop too low, it should not get too high. The healthy range for body fatness in males is between 10 and 20 percent, while the healthy range for females is between 17 and 28 percent. These levels are associated with good metabolic fitness, good health, and wellness. The marginal zone includes levels that are above the healthy fitness zone but not quite into the range used to reflect obesity. The term *obesity* often carries negative connotations and stereotypes but, as mentioned previously, it is important to understand that it is a clinical term that simply means excessively high body fat.

Health standards have been established for the Body Mass Index. The **Body Mass Index (BMI)** is a commonly used indicator of **overweight** and obesity in our society but is often misunderstood. The measure of BMI is basically an indicator of your weight relative to your height. It does not provide an indicator of body fatness, although BMI values tend to correlate with body fatness in most people. Because

of this association, it is widely used in clinical settings and as a general indicator of body composition.

The accepted international standards for defining overweight and obesity are the same for both males and females. BMI values over 25 are used to define overweight, and values over 30 are used to define obesity (see Figure 1). These values are widely used and accepted for general population surveillance but may not be useful for certain individuals. People with high levels of muscle fitness or large muscle mass will often be categorized as overweight or obese using the standard BMI criteria. This is because muscle weighs more than fat. The BMI values are based solely on a person's weight relative to his or her height, so it cannot detect differences in muscle and fat in the body. However, BMI is still a useful indicator for most people.

Because BMI is a frequently used measure, you should know how to calculate and interpret your BMI and your "healthy weight range." Mathematically, BMI is calculated with the following formula: BMI = weight (kg)/(height [m] × height [m]). Instructions for calculating BMI, including the nonmetric formula and rating charts, are provided in the Lab Resource Materials later in this Concept. There are also many BMI calculators on the Internet that make it easy to calculate.

Methods Used to Assess Body Composition

Methods of body composition assessment vary in accuracy and practicality. Your body is made up of water, fat, protein, carbohydrate, and various vitamins and minerals. However, assessments of body composition typically focus on the relative amount of fat in the body. A number of techniques have been developed to assess body composition. They vary in terms of practicality and accuracy, so it is important to understand the limitations of each method. Even established techniques have potential for error. The most common methods are summarized in this section.

connect
VIDEO 2

Dual-energy X-ray absorptiometry (DXA) has emerged as the accepted "gold standard" measure of body composition. The DXA technique uses the attenuation of two energy sources to estimate the density of the body. A specific advantage of DXA is that it can provide whole-body measurements of body fatness as well as amounts stored in different parts of the body. An additional advantage is that it provides estimates of bone density. For the procedure, the person lies on a table and the machine scans up along the body. While some radiation exposure is necessary with the procedure, it is quite minimal compared with X-ray and other diagnostic scans. Because the machine is expensive, this procedure is found only in medical centers and well-equipped research laboratories. The DXA (also called DEXA) procedure provides a highly accurate measure of body composition for research and a criterion measure that has been used to validate other, more practical measures of body composition.

Underwater weighing and Bod Pod are two highly accurate methods. Underwater weighing is another excellent method of assessing body fatness. Before the development of DXA it was considered to be the "gold standard" method of assessment. In this technique, a person is weighed in air and underwater, and the difference in weight is used to assess the levels of body fatness. People with a lot of muscle, bone, and other lean tissue sink like a rock in water because muscle and other lean tissue are dense. Fat is less dense, so people with more fat tend to float in a water environment. A limitation of this method is that participants must exhale all their air while submerged in order to obtain an accurate reading. Additional error from the estimations of residual lung volumes also tends to reduce the accuracy of this approach.

A device called the Bod Pod uses the same principles as underwater weighing but relies on air displacement to assess body composition. The Bod Pod tends to overestimate body fat percentage in thinner participants and underestimate body fat percentage in heavier participants (compared to DXA). Discrepancies are smaller in normal-weight individuals.

Skinfold measurements are a practical method of assessing body fatness. About one-half of the body's fat is located around the various body organs and in the muscles. The other half of the body's fat is located just under the skin, or in skinfolds (Figure 2). A skinfold is two thicknesses of skin and the amount of fat that lies just under the skin. By measuring skinfold thicknesses of various sites around the body, it is possible to estimate total body fatness (Figure 3). Skinfold measurements are often used because they are relatively easy to do. They are not nearly as costly as underwater weighing and other methods that require expensive equipment. Research-quality skinfold calipers cost more than $100, but consumer models are available for $10 to $20.

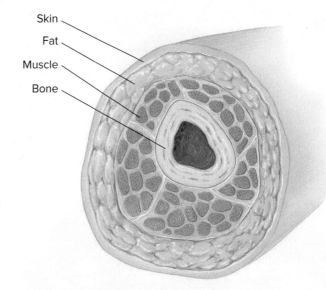

Figure 2 ▶ Location of body fat.

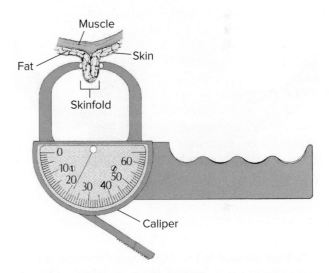

Figure 3 ▶ Measuring skinfold thickness with calipers.

In general, the more skinfolds measured, the more accurate the fatness estimate. However, measurements with two or three skinfolds have been shown to be reasonably accurate and can be done in a relatively short period. Two skinfold

Underfat Too little of the body weight composed of fat.

Amenorrhea Absent or infrequent menstruation.

Nonessential Fat Extra fat or fat reserves stored in the body.

Body Mass Index (BMI) A measure of body composition using a height–weight formula. High BMI values have been related to increased disease risk.

Overweight A clinical term that implies higher than normal levels of body fat and potential risk for development of obesity.

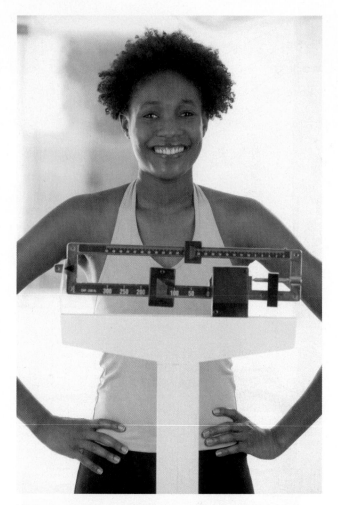

Monitoring weight can be helpful, but measures of body fatness provide a better indication of body composition.
JGI/Blend Images LLC

techniques are used in Lab 13A. You are encouraged to try both to see how they compare. While you might not have access to calipers in the future, it is important to understand the concept behind the assessment.

Bioelectric impedance analysis has become a practical alternative for body fatness assessment. Bioelectric impedance analysis (BIA) ranks quite favorably for accuracy and has overall rankings similar to those of skinfold measurement techniques. The test can be performed quickly and is more effective for people high in body fatness (a limitation of skinfolds). The technique is based on measuring resistance to current flow. Electrodes are placed on the body, and low doses of current are passed through the skin. Because muscle has greater water content than fat, it is a better conductor and has less resistance to current. The overall amount of resistance and body size are used to predict body fatness. The results depend heavily on hydration status, so do not test after exercising or immediately after eating or drinking. Accuracy is

also affected by the quality of the equipment. Portable BIA scales are available that allow you to simply stand on metal plates to get an estimate of body fatness. These devices are easier to use and are now widely available to consumers. They provide a reasonable estimate but are less accurate than research-grade devices.

Health Risks Associated with Obesity

Obesity contributes directly and indirectly to a number of major health problems. The presence of excess body fat impairs the function of most systems of the body (e.g., the cardiovascular system, the pulmonary system, the skeletal system, the reproductive system, the immune system, and the metabolic system). For example, obesity contributes to a respiratory condition called hypoventilation syndrome which, in turn, contributes to respiratory failure and death (such as happened with many people with COVID-19). Obesity increases risks for a variety of other chronic diseases, including cardiovascular disease and diabetes. It also increases risks for 13 different types of cancer, contributing to approximately 40 percent of all cancer diagnoses. The overall negative impact of excess body fat on the various body systems is summarized in Figure 4.

Obesity contributes to early death but even greater losses in quality of life. A number of studies have sought to predict the impact of obesity on life expectancy. Results indicate that obesity may cut 8–10 years from life, but the absolute impact varies by the severity of the condition as well as by many other social, demographic, lifestyle, and health factors. Public health experts suggest that efforts to estimate risk of mortality are not of much value. They contend that the clear evidence of increased mortality fails to capture the real damage that obesity causes across a lifetime. New statistical models have focused on computing "healthy years lost" rather than total years lost. This distinction is consistent with the shift from the notion of "lifespan" to one of "healthspan."

Physical activity and physical fitness provide protection from the health risks of obesity. A common misconception is that if you are thin, you are fit and healthy, and that if you are overweight, you are unfit and unhealthy. Numerous studies have demonstrated that it is possible to be fit while still being overweight. In fact, the findings consistently show that active people who have a high BMI are at less risk than inactive people with normal BMI levels (see Figure 5). Even high levels of body fatness may not increase disease risk if a person has good metabolic fitness as indicated by healthy blood fat levels, normal blood pressure, and normal blood sugar levels. For this reason, it is important to consider your cardiorespiratory endurance and

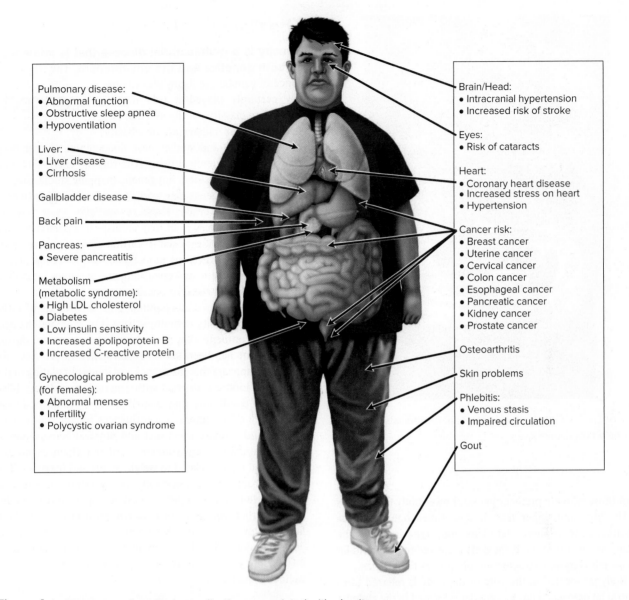

Pulmonary disease:
• Abnormal function
• Obstructive sleep apnea
• Hypoventilation

Liver:
• Liver disease
• Cirrhosis

Gallbladder disease

Back pain

Pancreas:
• Severe pancreatitis

Metabolism
(metabolic syndrome):
• High LDL cholesterol
• Diabetes
• Low insulin sensitivity
• Increased apolipoprotein B
• Increased C-reactive protein

Gynecological problems
(for females):
• Abnormal menses
• Infertility
• Polycystic ovarian syndrome

Brain/Head:
• Intracranial hypertension
• Increased risk of stroke

Eyes:
• Risk of cataracts

Heart:
• Coronary heart disease
• Increased stress on heart
• Hypertension

Cancer risk:
• Breast cancer
• Uterine cancer
• Cervical cancer
• Colon cancer
• Esophageal cancer
• Pancreatic cancer
• Kidney cancer
• Prostate cancer

Osteoarthritis

Skin problems

Phlebitis:
• Venous stasis
• Impaired circulation

Gout

Figure 4 ▶ Diseases and medical complications associated with obesity.

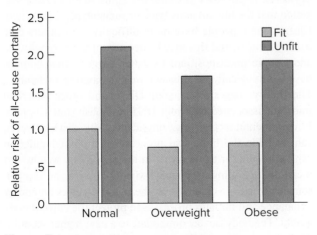

Figure 5 ▶ Risks of fatness versus fitness.

Source: Lee, C. D., et al.

metabolic fitness levels before drawing conclusions about the effects of high body weight or high body fat levels on health and wellness. This information also documents the importance of focusing on adopting and maintaining a habit of regular physical activity.

Excessive abdominal fat and excessive fat of the upper body can increase the risk for various diseases. The location of body fat can influence the health risks associated with obesity. Fat in the upper part of the body is sometimes referred to as "Northern Hemisphere" fat, and a body type high in this type of fat is called the "apple" shape. Upper body fat is also referred to as android fat because it is more characteristic of males than females. Postmenopausal females typically have a higher amount of upper body fat

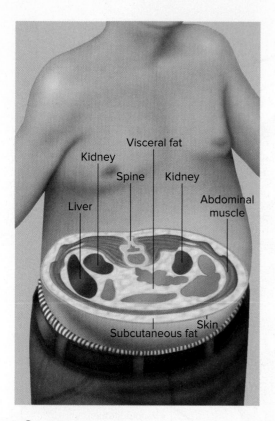

Figure 6 ▶ Visceral, or abdominal, fat is associated with increased disease risk.

than those who are premenopausal. Lower body fat, such as in the hips and upper legs, is sometimes referred to as "Southern Hemisphere" fat. This body type is called the "pear" shape. Lower body fat is also referred to as gynoid fat because it is more characteristic of females than males.

Body fat located in the core of the body is referred to as central fat or visceral fat. Visceral fat is located in the abdominal cavity (see Figure 6), as opposed to subcutaneous fat, which is located just under the skin. Though subcutaneous fat (skinfold measures) can be used to estimate body fatness, it is not a good indicator of central fatness. Your waist size is a useful indicator of visceral fat distribution. It can be used alone, in combination with BMI, in combination with your birth assigned sex and height, and/or in combination with hip size (waist-to-hip ratio) to determine health risk (see the Lab Resource Materials). Visceral fat is considered more harmful than other forms and is associated with high blood fat levels as well as other metabolic problems. It is also associated with high incidence of heart attack, stroke, chest pain, breast cancer, and early death.

A number of studies have documented that aerobic physical activity and muscle fitness activities promote preferential loss of abdominal body fat. This metabolic benefit is likely a key reason why physical activity improves health and provides protection against the risks of obesity.

The Causes of Obesity

Obesity is a multifactorial disease that is influenced by both genetics and the environment. The strong evidence of genetic predisposition to obesity certainly played a role in the decision to classify obesity as a disease. There is clear clustering of obesity

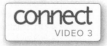

within families, and studies have documented similar body composition in identical twins. The role of genetic factors is still not well understood, but genetic mapping studies suggest that a number of genes may work in combination to influence susceptibility to obesity. These *susceptibility genes* may not lead directly to obesity but may predispose a person to overweight or obesity if exposed to certain environmental conditions. Thus, the prevailing model guiding obesity research is that complex genetic and environmental variables interact to increase potential risks for obesity.

It is important to understand that the "environment" influences risk for obesity in multiple ways. For example, the neonatal environment that the child is exposed to during development has been shown to influence future risks for obesity. It appears that hormones and lipids circulating in the maternal blood can interact with genetic factors to establish metabolic conditions that contribute to elevated body fat. The family environment also influences weight status since parents and siblings affect diet and physical activity habits. The social/cultural environment further influences norms, values, and beliefs related to weight status and lifestyles. The built environment (e.g., sidewalks, parks, safe play areas) also plays a role in access to active lifestyle opportunities. As discussed earlier, you may not have control over most of these factors; however, you do have control over your own lifestyle decisions as an adult. Lifestyles are the most important factor influencing your weight status as well as your overall health, wellness, and fitness.

Body weight is regulated and maintained through complex regulatory processes. Some scholars have suggested that the human body type, or **somatotype,** is inherited. Clearly, some people have more difficulty than others controlling fatness, and this may be because of their somatotype and genetic predisposition. Evidence suggests that humans have a biologically established weight baseline (**set-point**). The theory suggests that your DNA, and other inherited traits not associated with your DNA, establish your set-point. Environmental factors (e.g., physical activity, diet), however, can override the biological processes. Set-point regulation can be helpful for those trying to maintain body weight, but it can be frustrating for people trying to lose weight. If a person slowly tries to cut calories, the body perceives an energy imbalance and initiates processes to protect the current body weight. The body can accommodate to a new, higher set-point if weight gain takes place over time, but there is greater resistance to adopting a lower set-point. Many people lose weight, only to see the weight come back months later. One of the reasons physical activity is so critical for weight maintenance is that it may help in resetting a person's set-point.

Changes in basal metabolic rate can be the cause of obesity. Your **basal metabolic rate (BMR)** is the largest component of total daily energy expenditure. BMR is typically expressed in the number of **calories** needed to maintain your body functions under resting conditions. When resting, your body expends calories because your heart is pumping and other body organs are working. Processing the food you eat also expends calories. People with more lean tissue have a higher BMR than those with less lean tissue and greater amounts of body fat. People who are physically active will also have a higher BMR on days they exercise, contributing to long-term weight control.

During childhood and adolescence, BMR is high to support growth and development. This is why teenagers can typically eat more without gaining weight. However, when a person reaches full growth, the BMR decreases and is determined primarily by the amount of muscle mass a person has. Regular physical activity throughout life helps keep the muscle mass higher, which helps maintain a higher BMR. Evidence suggests that regular exercise can contribute in other ways to increasing BMR. For example, BMR can stay elevated for up to 10 hours following a bout of vigorous physical activity. This boost in BMR helps burn extra calories during the day.

"Creeping obesity" is a problem as you grow older. With age, people tend to become less active, causing declines

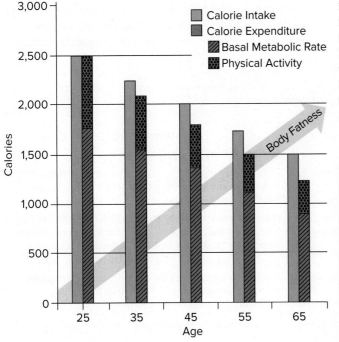

Figure 7 ▶ Creeping obesity.

Technology Update

Is Technology the Problem or the Solution?

Advances in technology have changed the way we work, socialize, and recreate. While it has improved many facets of our life, it may also be the key driver in the relatively recent rise in obesity in our society. Research has convincingly documented associations between television viewing and the risk of obesity. Research has also demonstrated associations between sedentary behavior and obesity. However, it is difficult to confirm that the underlying cause of obesity is exposure to "technology." The 30-year progression in the obesity epidemic largely parallels the evolution of computer and phone technology, which makes the causation seem probable. However, research and technology have provided advances that support positive lifestyle changes and have improved medical and pharmaceutical options.

Do you see technology as part of the problem or can it be part of the solution to tackling the obesity epidemic?

connect ACTIVITY

in BMR. Caloric intake does seem to decrease somewhat with age, but the decrease does not adequately compensate for the decreases in BMR and activity levels. For this reason, body fat increases gradually with age for the typical person (see Figure 7). This increase in fatness over time is commonly referred to as "creeping obesity" because the increase in fatness is gradual. For a typical person, creeping obesity can result in a gain of 1/2 to 1 pound per year. People who stay active can keep muscle mass high and delay changes in BMR. For those who are not active, it is suggested that caloric intake decrease by 3 percent each decade after 25 so that by age 65 caloric intake is at least 10 percent less than it was at age 25. The decrease in caloric intake for active people need not be as great.

Somatotype A term that refers to a person's body type. One simple somatotopic classification system emphasizes three body types: ectomorph (linear), mesomorph (muscular), and endomorph (round).

Set-Point A theoretical concept that describes the way the body protects current weight and resists change.

Basal Metabolic Rate (BMR) The minimal number of calories needed to perform your body's most basic (basal) functions (typically expressed and assessed as resting metabolic rate).

Calories Units of energy supplied by food; the quantity of heat necessary to raise the temperature of a kilogram of water 1°C (actually, a kilocalorie, but usually called a calorie for weight control purposes).

Treatment and Prevention of Overweight and Obesity

Current treatment guidelines for obesity emphasize lifestyle behavior change. The labeling of obesity as a disease led to refinements in the clinical treatment of obesity. There is now wide consensus that lifestyle approaches emphasizing dietary change and physical activity are the most effective treatment of obesity. A joint statement by the American Heart Association, American College of Cardiology, and the Obesity Society has helped promote screening and referral to obesity prevention programs. The adoption of screening and counseling strategies by clinicians is still relatively low (approximately 30–40 percent), but progress has been made with referrals to evidence-based programs in community settings. For example, most states have networks in place to offer a standardized Diabetes Prevention Program (DPP) in community settings to help reduce further risks for diabetes, heart disease, and stroke. Lifestyle interventions like DPP typically include guidance on dietary change, physical activity, and behavioral skills training and are delivered by trained interventionists (e.g., dietitians, psychologists, exercise specialists, and health coaches).

A combination of regular physical activity and dietary restriction is the most effective means of losing body fat. Weight control is based on principles of **caloric balance** (a balance between energy intake and energy expenditure). For optimal results, all weight loss programs should combine a lower energy intake with an enhanced energy expenditure to create a larger caloric deficit. Table 1 presents thresholds of training and target zones for body fat reduction, including information for both physical activity and diet. A general guideline is to try to lose no more than 1 to 2 pounds a week. Because a pound of fat contains 3,500 calories (see note in Table 1), this requires a caloric deficit of approximately 500 calories per day. (See the Concept on the Principles of Effective Weight Control for details.)

Physical activity burns calories but also helps maintain lean body mass. National activity guidelines recommend a minimum of 30 minutes of moderate to vigorous activity a day or 150 minutes per week, but these guidelines are based on needs for health and not weight control. More time is often needed either to maintain weight over time or to lose weight. The ACSM guidelines suggest that it may be necessary to work progressively up to 200 to 300 minutes a week to expend enough calories to lose weight. One study found that females who maintained weight across the lifespan average approximately 60 minutes of activity per day. Table 2 shows calories expended in various activities to help promote understanding of how many calories are burned over time.

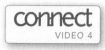

Physical activity provides advantages for weight maintenance and improved body composition. As discussed in other Concepts, there are limitations associated with trying to lose weight only with changes in **diet**. Weight loss from dieting can come from both fat and muscle. The rate of weight loss also tends to slow because the metabolism slows down when calories are cut. When physical activity and diet are both used in a weight loss program, the same amount of weight may be lost but more of it is from fat. Physical activity also helps maintain resting metabolic rate at a higher level. This can contribute to further weight loss or facilitate weight maintenance. Individuals who want to increase lean body mass need to increase caloric intake while carefully increasing the intensity and duration of exercise (mainly muscular activity).

Table 1 ▶ Threshold of Training and Target Zones for Body Fat Reduction

	Threshold of Training*		Target Zones*	
	Physical Activity	**Diet**	**Physical Activity**	**Diet**
Frequency	Daily activity is best for weight loss and long-term weight control.	Adopt a healthy daily eating pattern.	Daily activity is best for weight loss and long-term weight control.	Adopt a healthy daily eating pattern.
Intensity	Moderate-intensity activity is best since it can be done comfortably for a longer time.	Aim to cut 250 calories per day from normal intake.	Moderate-intensity activity is best since it can be done comfortably for a longer time.	Aim to cut 500 calories per day. Larger cuts can lead to larger weight loss but are hard to sustain.
	Aim for at least 30 minutes a day to expend a reasonable number of calories.	Eating smaller but regular meals is best.	Aim for 60 minutes a day (or more) to maximize daily caloric expenditure.	Eating smaller but regular meals is best.

Note: A gram of fat is 9 calories; thus, a pound is equal to 4,086 calories (9 cal/g × 454 g/pound). However, fat in the body is 10 percent water and contains some protein and minerals that reduce the effective caloric equivalent to 3,500 calories (the accepted standard).

*It is best to combine exercise and diet to achieve the 3,500-calorie imbalance necessary to lose a pound of fat. Using both exercise and diet in the target zone is most effective.

Table 2 ▶ Calories Expended per Hour in Various Physical Activities (Performed at a Recreational Level)*

Activity	Calories Used per Hour				
	100 lb (46 kg)	120 lb (55 kg)	150 lb (68 kg)	180 lb (82 kg)	200 lb (91 kg)
Archery	180	204	240	276	300
Backpacking (40-lb. pack)	307	348	410	472	513
Badminton	255	289	340	391	425
Baseball	210	238	280	322	350
Basketball (half-court)	225	255	300	345	375
Bicycling (10 mph)	182	218	273	327	364
Bowling	136	164	205	245	273
Canoeing	227	273	341	409	455
Circuit training	247	280	330	380	413
Dance, aerobics	315	357	420	483	525
Dance, ballet (choreographed)	240	300	360	432	480
Dance, modern (choreographed)	240	300	360	432	480
Dance, social	205	245	307	368	409
Fencing	225	255	300	345	375
Fitness calisthenics	232	263	310	357	388
Football	225	255	300	345	375
Golf (walking)	250	300	375	450	500
Gymnastics	232	263	310	357	388
Handball	450	510	600	690	750
Hiking	225	255	300	345	375
Horseback riding	182	218	273	327	364
Interval training	487	552	650	748	833
Jogging (5 1/2 mph)	487	552	650	748	833
Judo/karate	232	263	310	357	388
Mountain climbing	450	510	600	690	750
Pool/billiards	97	110	130	150	163
Racquetball/paddleball	450	510	600	690	750
Rope jumping (continuous)	525	595	700	805	875
Rowing, crew	615	697	820	943	1025
Running (10 mph)	625	765	900	1035	1125
Sailing (pleasure)	135	153	180	207	225
Skating, ice	262	297	350	403	438
Skating, roller/inline	262	297	350	403	438
Skiing, cross-country	318	382	477	573	636
Skiing, downhill	450	510	600	690	750
Soccer	405	459	540	621	775
Softball (fast-pitch)	210	238	280	322	350
Softball (slow-pitch)	217	246	290	334	363
Surfing	416	467	550	633	684
Swimming (fast laps)	420	530	630	768	846
Swimming (slow laps)	273	327	409	491	545
Table tennis	182	218	273	327	364
Tennis	315	357	420	483	525
Volleyball	262	297	350	403	483
Walking	173	207	259	311	346
Waterskiing	306	390	468	564	636
Weight training	352	399	470	541	558

*Locate your weight to determine the calories expended per hour in each of the activities shown in the table based on recreational involvement. More vigorous activity, as occurs in competitive athletics, may result in greater caloric expenditures.
Source: Corbin and Lindsey.

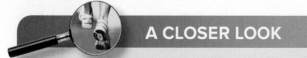

A CLOSER LOOK

What Happened to Body Positivity?

Body positivity refers to the idea that all body shapes and sizes are acceptable. The body positivity movement has had an interesting evolution. As a social movement, it helped challenge assumptions about beauty and empowered individuals to be more accepting of their bodies, regardless of size or shape. The movement was popularized through movies, music, and social media and spawned wholesale changes in fashion and marketing. While the principles of the body positivity movement are sound, the structure and new forms of social and personal pressure have led some to become disillusioned. Some have become frustrated by how the movement has been taken over by commercial industry as a new marketing strategy. Others find that it doesn't address or acknowledge the reasons why people struggle to accept their bodies in the first place. The terms *body neutrality* and *body acceptance* are now being promoted as alternatives.

Do you support the general notions of body positivity or is it a standard that can't be attained?

connect
ACTIVITY

Body Image and Eating Disorders

Body image issues contribute to compromised health and wellness. The social pressures related to body weight and attractiveness may contribute to disordered eating in some individuals. Evidence suggests that body image issues and fear of obesity

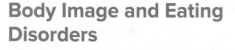
connect
VIDEO 5

can occur early in life while children are in elementary school, but other pressures accrue over time. A variety of eating disorders have been documented, including extreme restriction of food intake, binged eating, or periods of binge-ing and purging. While most common in high-achievement-oriented young females, these conditions affect virtually all segments of the population, including males. It is important to note that patterns of *disordered eating* are not the same as clinically diagnosed eating disorders. However, people who adopt disordered eating tend to have a greater chance of developing an eating disorder. The body positivity move-ment helped promote changes in social norms related to body image, but evidence suggests that it has led to different forms of pressure and continued focus on one's body (see A Closer Look).

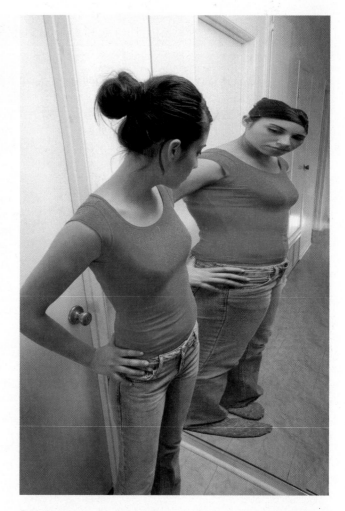

Body image disorders can influence self-esteem and wellness.
Ted Foxx/Alamy Stock Photo

Anorexia nervosa is the most severe eating disorder. Anorexia nervosa is characterized by extreme food restric-tion as a result of a pursuit for excessive leanness. Indi-viduals with anorexia nervosa typically have highly inaccurate perceptions of their bodies and often see them-selves as "too fat" even when they are excessively thin. They restrict food intake to promote more weight loss, but they are typically undernourished. If untreated, anorexia is life-threatening. People who are anorexic may exercise compulsively (about 25 percent) or use laxatives to pre-vent the digestion of food in an attempt to "stay thin." In-dividuals with signs or symptoms of this disorder should obtain medical and psychological help immediately, as the consequences are severe.

Binge eating disorder is the most common eating disorder. Binge eating disorder (BED) is characterized by periods of eating large quantities of food in a short amount of time, often in isolation. Individuals may eat very rapidly until they are uncomfortably full and feel out of control and powerless to stop eating. It is by far the most common eating disorder with rates estimated to be three times as high as the rates for anorexia and bulimia combined (approximately 3.5 percent of females and 2 percent of males). Clinically diagnosed BED involves recurrent episodes of binge eating at least once a week for 3 months. Treatments are shown to be effective for reversing this condition.

Bulimia is an eating disorder characterized by bingeing and purging. Bulimia involves a distorted body image and an obsessive desire to lose weight or to be thin. However, the pressure and stress can contribute to binge eating, followed by guilt, depression, and self-induced vomiting, purging, or fasting. A person with bulimia might binge after a relatively long period of dieting and consume excessive amounts of junk foods containing empty calories. Another form of bulimia is bingeing on one day and severely restricting calorie intake on the next. The consequences of bulimia include serious mental, gastrointestinal, and dental problems. Individuals who are bulimic may or may not be anorexic, but disordered eating patterns can become habitual and hard to change. Purging disorder is a related condition that may involve purging but without the bingeing. It may be hard to identify a person at risk for bulimia or purging disorder, as he or she may be lean, normal weight, overweight, or obese.

Muscle dysmorphia is a body image disorder that mainly affects males. Muscle dysmorphia is a body dysmorphic disorder in which an individual becomes preoccupied with the idea that his or her body is not sufficiently lean and/or muscular. It has been referred to as "reverse anorexia" since it relates to the delusional belief that one's own body is too small even when it is normal or even exceptionally large. Both athletes and non-athletes can experience this condition. Those with muscle dysmorphia may be more inclined to use performance-enhancing drugs, to exercise while sick, or to have an eating disorder. Additional risks include depression and social isolation.

Athletes are susceptible to eating disorders and health risks from low body fatness. *Anorexia athletica* is a body image disorder related to participation in sports and activities emphasizing body leanness. Studies show that participants in sports such as gymnastics, wrestling, and bodybuilding and activities such as ballet and cheerleading are at greater risk of developing anorexia athletica. This disorder has many of the symptoms of anorexia nervosa, but not of the same severity. In some cases, anorexia athletica leads to anorexia nervosa. Surveys of college athletes reveal tendencies toward disordered eating, but it also manifests as excessive exercise as a way to try to continue to lose weight.

Female athletes that are excessively lean are at specific risk of a condition known as the *female athlete triad*. This condition refers to the presence of three related and linked symptoms that affect some female athletes (eating disorders/low energy availability, amenorrhea, and decreased bone mineral density). The conditions are linked because low body fat levels lead to the amenorrhea. The alterations in menstrual cycles lead to low levels of estrogen, which subsequently lead to the reduced bone density and risk for osteoporosis.

Using Self-Management Skills

Self-assessments of body weight can be helpful if done correctly. Many people chronically check their weight on scales, but this is not a good indicator of body composition. Your weight can vary from day to day and even hour to hour, based solely on your level of hydration. Short-term changes in weight are often due to water loss or gain, yet many people erroneously attribute the weight changes to their diet, a pill they have taken, or the exercise they recently performed. There is some evidence that monitoring weight daily can help normal-weight people from gaining weight. However, for people trying to lose weight, monitoring weight less frequently (maybe once a week) is more useful. When you do weigh yourself, weigh at the same time of day, preferably early in the morning, because it reduces the chances that your weight variation will be a result of body water changes. Of course, it is best to use body composition assessments in addition to those based on body weight.

Self-assessments of body composition should be used and interpreted carefully. Estimates of body composition provide meaningful information about body fatness, but the limitations of the measures need to be considered. Estimates from even the best techniques may be off by as much as 2–3 percent. The formulas used to determine body fatness from skinfolds and other procedures are also based on typical body types and nonrepresentative samples. Thus, the estimation errors may be larger for some people than others. View the values as estimates and not as absolute indicators of body fatness. Using the same measuring device each time you assess your body composition is also recommended. This reduces measurement error and allows you to track your progress over time.

Caloric Balance Consuming calories in amounts equal to the number of calories expended.

Diet The usual food and drink for a person or an animal.

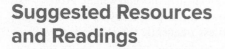

Strategies for Action: Lab Information

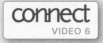

Doing several self-assessments can help you make informed decisions about body composition. In Labs 13A and 13B you will take various body composition self-assessments. It is important that you take all of the measurements and consider all of the information before making final decisions about your body composition. Each self-assessment technique has strengths and weaknesses to be aware of when you make personal decisions. The importance you place on one particular measure may be different from the importance another person places on that measure. You are a unique individual and should use information that is more relevant for you personally. If doing a self-assessment around other people makes you self-conscious, do the measurement in private. If the measurement requires the assistance of another person, choose a person you trust and feel comfortable with.

Understanding the factors that contribute to energy expenditure can help you determine the number of calories you expend each day. In Lab 13C you will learn how to estimate your basal metabolic rate (BMR) so you can know how much energy you typically expend when you are resting. Use this information together with the information about the energy you expend in activities to help you balance the calories you consume with the calories you expend each day. You will also log the activities you perform in a day and learn how to estimate your total daily energy expenditure.

Suggested Resources and Readings

The websites for the following sources can be accessed by searching online for the organization, program, or title listed. Specific scientific references are available at the end of this edition of *Concepts of Fitness and Wellness*.

- Centers for Disease Control and Prevention. (2020). Adult Obesity Facts.
- Centers for Disease Control and Prevention. (2020). Adult Obesity Prevalence Maps.
- Centers for Disease Control and Prevention. (2020). Obesity, Race/Ethnicity, and COVID-19.
- familydoctor.org. Female Athlete Triad.
- Garrison, J. (2019, December 19). "Nearly Half of US Residents to Be 'Obese' in 2030, 1 in 4 to Have 'Severe Obesity,' Study Says." *USA Today*.
- Gunnars, K. (2019, February 27). "The Harmful Effects of Fat Shaming." *Healthline*.
- Medscape. (2018, July 5). Is Obesity a Disease or a Choice?
- Molina, B. (2019, February 6). "Obesity-Related Cancers up Among Millennials, Study Says." *USA Today*.
- National Eating Disorders Association. Helpline.
- Obesity Medicine Association.
- The Obesity Society. Obesity & COVID-19.
- Trust for America's Health. (2020). *State of Obesity 2020: Better Policies for a Healthier America*. (pdf)
- World Health Organization. (2020, April 1). Obesity and Overweight.

Lab Resource Materials: Evaluating Body Fat

General Information about Skinfold Measurements

It is important to use a consistent procedure for "drawing up" or "pinching up" a skinfold and making the measurement with the calipers. The following procedures should be used for each skinfold site.

1. Lay the calipers down on a nearby table. Use the thumbs and index fingers of both hands to draw up a skinfold, or layer of skin and fat. The fingers and thumbs of the two hands should be about 1 inch apart, or 1/2 inch on each side of the location where the measurement is to be made.

2. The skinfolds are normally drawn up in a vertical line rather than a horizontal line. However, if the skin naturally aligns itself less than vertical, the measurement should be done on the natural line of the skinfold, rather than on the vertical.

3. Do not pinch the skinfold too hard. Draw it up so that your thumbs and fingers are not compressing the skinfold.

4. Once the skinfold is drawn up, let go with your right hand and pick up the calipers. Open the jaws of the calipers and place them over the location of the skinfold to be measured and 1/2 inch from your left index finger and thumb. Allow the tips, or jaw faces, of the calipers to close on the skinfold at a level about where the skin would be normally.

5. Let the reading on the calipers settle for 2–3 seconds; then note the thickness of the skinfold in millimeters.

6. Three measurements should be taken at each location. Use the middle of the three values to determine your measurement. For example, if you had values of 10, 11, and 9, your measurement for that location would be 10. If the three measures vary by more than 3 millimeters from the lowest to the highest, you may want to take additional measurements.

Skinfold Measurement Methods

You will be exposed to two methods of using skinfolds. The first method (based on the FitnessGram method) uses the same sites for males and females and was originally developed for use with schoolchildren but has since been modified for adults. The second method (Jackson-Pollock) is the most widely used method. It uses different sites for males and females and considers your age in estimating your body fat percentage. You are encouraged to try both methods.

Calculating Fatness from Skinfolds (FitnessGram Method)

1. Sum the three skinfolds (triceps, abdominal, and calf) for males and females. Use horizontal abdominal measure.

2. Use the skinfold sum and the appropriate column (males or females) to determine your percent fat using Chart 1. Locate your sum of skinfold in the left column at the top of the chart. Your estimated body fat percentage is located where the values intersect.

3. Use the Standards for Body Fatness (Chart 2) to determine your fatness rating.

FitnessGram Locations (Males and Females)

Triceps

Make a mark on the back of the right arm, one-half the distance between the tip of the shoulder and the tip of the elbow. Make the measurement at this location.

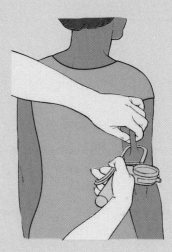

Abdominal

Make a mark on the skin approximately 1 inch to the right of the navel. Unlike the Jackson-Pollock method (done vertically), make a horizontal measurement.

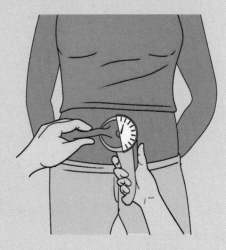

257

FitnessGram Locations *(continued)*

Calf Skinfold

Make a mark on the inside of the calf of the right leg at the level of the largest calf size (girth). Place the foot on a chair or other elevation so that the knee is kept at approximately 90 degrees. Make a vertical measurement at the mark.

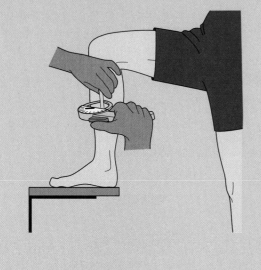

Self-Measured Triceps Skinfold

This measurement is made on the left arm so that the calipers can easily be read. Hold the arm straight at shoulder height. Make a fist with the thumb faced upward. Place the fist against a wall. With the right hand, place the calipers over the skinfold as it "hangs freely" on the back of the tricep (halfway from the tip of the shoulder to the elbow).

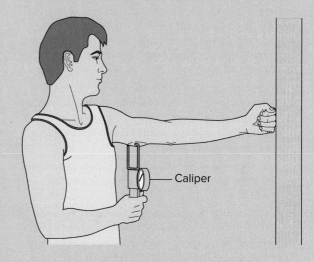

Caliper

Chart 1 Percent Fat for Sum of Triceps, Abdominal, and Calf Skinfolds (FitnessGram)

Males		Females	
Sum of Skinfolds (mm)	Percent Fat	Sum of Skinfolds (mm)	Percent Fat
8–10	3.2	23–25	16.8
11–13	4.1	26–28	17.7
14–16	5.0	29–31	18.5
17–19	6.0	32–34	19.4
20–22	6.9	35–37	20.2
23–25	7.8	38–40	21.0
26–28	8.7	41–43	21.9
29–31	9.7	44–46	22.7
32–34	10.6	47–49	23.5
35–37	11.5	50–52	24.4
38–40	12.5	53–55	25.2
41–43	13.4	56–58	26.1
44–46	14.3	59–61	26.9
47–49	15.2	62–64	27.7
50–52	16.2	65–67	28.6

Males		Females	
Sum of Skinfolds (mm)	Percent Fat	Sum of Skinfolds (mm)	Percent Fat
53–55	17.1	68–70	29.4
56–58	18.0	71–73	30.2
59–61	18.9	74–76	31.1
62–64	19.9	77–79	31.9
65–67	20.8	80–82	32.7
68–70	21.7	83–85	33.6
71–73	22.6	86–88	34.4
74–76	23.6	89–91	35.5
77–79	24.5	92–94	36.1
80–82	25.4	95–97	36.9
83–85	26.4	98–100	37.8
86–88	27.3	101–103	38.6
89–91	28.2	104–106	39.4
92–94	29.1	107–109	40.3
95–97	30.1	110–112	41.1
98–100	31.0	113–115	42.0
101–103	31.9	116–118	42.8
104–106	32.8	119–121	43.6
107–109	33.8	122–124	44.5
110–112	34.7	125–127	45.3
113–115	35.6	128–130	46.1
116–118	36.6	131–133	47.0
119–121	37.5	134–136	47.8
122–124	38.4	137–139	48.7
125–127	39.3	140–142	49.5

Chart 2 Standards for Body Fatness (Percent Body Fat)

	Too Low	Borderline	(Healthy) Good Fitness	Marginal	(At Risk) Overfat
	Below Essential Fat Levels	Unhealthy for Many People	Optimal for Good Health	Associated with Some Health Problems	Unhealthy
Males	<5%	6–9%	10–20%	21–25%	>25%
Females	<10%	11–16%	17–28%	29–35%	>35%

Calculating Fatness from Skinfolds (Jackson-Pollock Method)

1. Sum three skinfolds (tricep, iliac crest, and thigh for females; chest, abdominal [vertical], and thigh for males).

2. Use the skinfold sum and your age to determine your percent fat using Chart 3 for females and Chart 4 for men. Locate your sum of skinfold in the left column and your age at the top of the chart. Your estimated body fat percentage is located where the values intersect.

3. Use the Standards for Body Fatness (Chart 2) to determine your fatness rating.

Jackson-Pollock Locations (Females)

Triceps

Same as FitnessGram (see previous instructions).

Iliac crest

Make a mark at the top front of the iliac crest. This skinfold is taken diagonally because of the natural line of the skin.

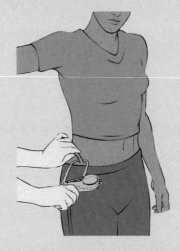

Thigh

Make a mark on the front of the thigh midway between the hip and the knee. Make the measurement vertically at this location.

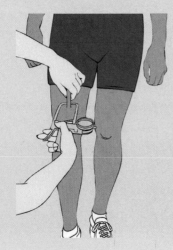

Jackson-Pollock Locations (Males)

Chest

Make a mark above and to the right of the right nipple (one-half the distance from the midline of the side and the nipple). The measurement at this location is often done on the diagonal because of the natural line of the skin.

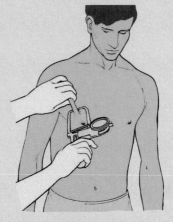

Abdominal

Make a mark on the skin approximately 1 inch to the right of the FitnessGram method.

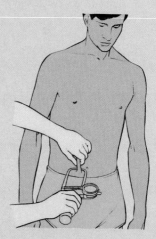

Thigh

Same as for females.

Note: Research has identified other methods that can also be used to calculate body fatness using skinfold measurements. See:

- Ball, S., Altena, T., & Swan, P. (2004). Accuracy of anthropometry compared to dual energy x-ray absorptiometry: A new generalizable equation for men. *European Journal of Clinical Nutrition,* 58, 1525–1531.

- Ball, S., Swan, P. D., & DeSimone, R. (2004). Comparison of anthropometry compared to dual energy x-ray absorptiometry: A new generalizable equation for women. *Research Quarterly for Exercise and Sports,* 75, 248–258.

Chart 3 Percent Fat for Females (Jackson-Pollock: Sum of Triceps, Iliac Crest, and Thigh Skinfolds)

Sum of Skinfolds (mm)	Age to the Last Year								
	22 and Under	23 to 27	28 to 32	33 to 37	38 to 42	43 to 47	48 to 52	53 to 57	Over 57
23–25	9.7	9.9	10.2	10.4	10.7	10.9	11.2	11.4	11.7
26–28	11.0	11.2	11.5	11.7	12.0	12.3	12.5	12.7	13.0
29–31	12.3	12.5	12.8	13.0	13.3	13.5	13.8	14.0	14.3
32–34	13.6	13.8	14.0	14.3	14.5	14.8	15.0	15.3	15.5
35–37	14.8	15.0	15.3	15.5	15.8	16.0	16.3	16.5	16.8
38–40	16.0	16.3	16.5	16.7	17.0	17.2	17.5	17.7	18.0
41–43	17.2	17.4	17.7	17.9	18.2	18.4	18.7	18.9	19.2
44–46	18.3	18.6	18.8	19.1	19.3	19.6	19.8	20.1	20.3
47–49	19.5	19.7	20.0	20.2	20.5	20.7	21.0	21.2	21.5
50–52	20.6	20.8	21.1	21.3	21.6	21.8	22.1	22.3	22.6
53–55	21.7	21.9	22.1	22.4	22.6	22.9	23.1	23.4	23.6
56–58	22.7	23.0	23.2	23.4	23.7	23.9	24.2	24.4	24.7
59–61	23.7	24.0	24.2	24.5	24.7	25.0	25.2	25.5	25.7
62–64	24.7	25.0	25.2	25.5	25.7	26.0	26.2	26.4	26.7
65–67	25.7	25.9	26.2	26.4	26.7	26.9	27.2	27.4	27.7
68–70	26.6	26.9	27.1	27.4	27.6	27.9	28.1	28.4	28.6
71–73	27.5	27.8	28.0	28.3	28.5	28.8	28.0	29.3	29.5
74–76	28.4	28.7	28.9	29.2	29.4	29.7	29.9	30.2	30.4
77–79	29.3	29.5	29.8	30.0	30.3	30.5	30.8	31.0	31.3
80–82	30.1	30.4	30.6	30.9	31.1	31.4	31.6	31.9	32.1
83–85	30.9	31.2	31.4	31.7	31.9	32.2	32.4	32.7	32.9
86–88	31.7	32.0	32.2	32.5	32.7	32.9	33.2	33.4	33.7
89–91	32.5	32.7	33.0	33.2	33.5	33.7	33.9	34.2	34.4
92–94	33.2	33.4	33.7	33.9	34.2	34.4	34.7	34.9	35.2
95–97	33.9	34.1	34.4	34.6	34.9	35.1	35.4	35.6	35.9
98–100	34.6	34.8	35.1	35.3	35.5	35.8	36.0	36.3	36.5
101–103	35.3	35.4	35.7	35.9	36.2	36.4	36.7	36.9	37.2
104–106	35.8	36.1	36.3	36.6	36.8	37.1	37.3	37.5	37.8
107–109	36.4	36.7	36.9	37.1	37.4	37.6	37.9	38.1	38.4
110–112	37.0	37.2	37.5	37.7	38.0	38.2	38.5	38.7	38.9
113–115	37.5	37.8	38.0	38.2	38.5	38.7	39.0	39.2	39.5
116–118	38.0	38.3	38.5	38.8	39.0	39.3	39.5	39.7	40.0
119–121	38.5	38.7	39.0	39.2	39.5	39.7	40.0	40.2	40.5
122–124	39.0	39.2	39.4	39.7	39.9	40.2	40.4	40.7	40.9
125–127	39.4	39.6	39.9	40.1	40.4	40.6	40.9	41.1	41.4
128–130	39.8	40.0	40.3	40.5	40.8	41.0	41.3	41.5	41.8

Note: Percent fat calculated by the formula by Siri. Percent fat = ([4.95/BD]–4.5) × 100, where BD = body density.

Source: Baumgartner and Jackson (1999). *Evaluation in Physical Education and Exercise Science.* Dubuque, IA: W.C. Brown Publishers.

Chart 4 Percent Fat for Males (Jackson-Pollock: Sum of Thigh, Chest, and Abdominal Skinfolds)

Sum of Skinfolds (mm)	Age to the Last Year								
	22 and Under	23 to 27	28 to 32	33 to 37	38 to 42	43 to 47	48 to 52	53 to 57	Over 57
8–10	1.3	1.8	2.3	2.9	3.4	3.9	4.5	5.0	5.5
11–13	2.2	2.8	3.3	3.9	4.4	4.9	5.5	6.0	6.5
14–16	3.2	3.8	4.3	4.8	5.4	5.9	6.4	7.0	7.5
17–19	4.2	4.7	5.3	5.8	6.3	6.9	7.4	8.0	8.5
20–22	5.1	5.7	6.2	6.8	7.3	7.9	8.4	8.9	9.5
23–25	6.1	6.6	7.2	7.7	8.3	8.8	9.4	9.9	10.5
26–28	7.0	7.6	8.1	8.7	9.2	9.8	10.3	10.9	11.4
29–31	8.0	8.5	9.1	9.6	10.2	10.7	11.3	11.8	12.4
32–34	8.9	9.4	10.0	10.5	11.1	11.6	12.2	12.8	13.3
35–37	9.8	10.4	10.9	11.5	12.0	12.6	13.1	13.7	14.3
38–40	10.7	11.3	11.8	12.4	12.9	13.5	14.1	14.6	15.2
41–43	11.6	12.2	12.7	13.3	13.8	14.4	15.0	15.5	16.1
44–46	12.5	13.1	13.6	14.2	14.7	15.3	15.9	16.4	17.0
47–49	13.4	13.9	14.5	15.1	15.6	16.2	16.8	17.3	17.9
50–52	14.3	14.8	15.4	15.9	16.5	17.1	17.6	18.1	18.8
53–55	15.1	15.7	16.2	16.8	17.4	17.9	18.5	18.2	19.7
56–58	16.0	16.5	17.1	17.7	18.2	18.8	19.4	20.0	20.5
59–61	16.9	17.4	17.9	18.5	19.1	19.7	20.2	20.8	21.4
62–64	17.6	18.2	18.8	19.4	19.9	20.5	21.1	21.7	22.2
65–67	18.5	19.0	19.6	20.2	20.8	21.3	21.9	22.5	23.1
68–70	19.3	19.9	20.4	21.0	21.6	22.2	22.7	23.3	23.9
71–73	20.1	20.7	21.2	21.8	22.4	23.0	23.6	24.1	24.7
74–76	20.9	21.5	22.0	22.6	23.2	23.8	24.4	25.0	25.5
77–79	21.7	22.2	22.8	23.4	24.0	24.6	25.2	25.8	26.3
80–82	22.4	23.0	23.6	24.2	24.8	25.4	25.9	26.5	27.1
83–85	23.2	23.8	24.4	25.0	25.5	26.1	26.7	27.3	27.9
86–88	24.0	24.5	25.1	25.5	26.3	26.9	27.5	28.1	28.7
89–91	24.7	25.3	25.9	25.7	27.1	27.6	28.2	28.8	29.4
92–94	25.4	26.0	26.6	27.2	27.8	28.4	29.0	29.6	30.2
95–97	26.1	26.7	27.3	27.9	28.5	29.1	29.7	30.3	30.9
98–100	26.9	27.4	28.0	28.6	29.2	29.8	30.4	31.0	31.6
101–103	27.5	28.1	28.7	29.3	29.9	30.5	31.1	31.7	32.3
104–106	28.2	28.8	29.4	30.0	30.6	31.2	31.8	32.4	33.0
107–109	28.9	29.5	30.1	30.7	31.3	31.9	32.5	33.1	33.7
110–112	29.6	30.2	30.8	31.4	32.0	32.6	33.2	33.8	34.4
113–115	30.2	30.8	31.4	32.0	32.6	33.2	33.8	34.5	35.1
116–118	30.9	31.5	32.1	32.7	33.3	33.9	34.5	35.1	35.7
119–121	31.5	32.1	32.7	33.3	33.9	34.5	35.1	35.7	36.4
122–124	32.1	32.7	33.3	33.9	34.5	35.1	35.8	36.4	37.0
125–127	32.7	33.3	33.9	34.5	35.1	35.8	36.4	37.0	37.6

Note: Percent fat calculated by the formula by Siri. Percent fat = $([4.95/BD] - 4.5) \times 100$, where BD = body density.
Source: Baumgartner and Jackson (1999). *Evaluation in Physical Education and Exercise Science.* Dubuque, IA: W.C. Brown Publishers.

Calculating Fatness from Self-Measured Skinfolds

1. Sum three skinfolds (tricep, iliac crest, and thigh for women; chest, abdominal [vertical], and thigh for men).

2. Use the skinfold sum and your age to determine your percent fat using Chart 3 for females and Chart 4 for males. Locate your sum of skinfold in the left column and your age at the top of the chart. Your estimated body fat percentage is located where the values intersect.

Height–Weight Measurements

1. *Height*—Measure your height in inches or centimeters. Take the measurement without shoes, but add 2.5 centimeters, or 1 inch, to measurements, as the charts include heel height.

2. *Weight*—Measure your weight in pounds or kilograms without clothes. Add 3 pounds, or 1.4 kilograms, because the charts include the weight of clothes. If weight must be taken with clothes on, wear indoor clothing that weighs 3 pounds, or 1.4 kilograms.

3. Determine your frame size using the elbow breadth. The measurement is most accurate when done with a broad-based sliding caliper. However, it can be done using skinfold calipers or can be estimated with a metric ruler. The right arm is measured when it is elevated with the elbow bent at 90 degrees and the upper arm horizontal. The back of the hand should face the person making the measurement. Using the calipers, measure the distance between the epicondyles of the humerus (inside and outside bony points of the elbow). Measure to the nearest millimeter (1/10 centimeter). If a caliper is not available, place the thumb and the index finger of the left hand on the epicondyles of the humerus and measure the distance between the fingers with a metric ruler. Use your height and elbow breadth in centimeters to determine your frame size (Chart 5); you need not repeat this procedure each time you use a height and weight chart.

Chart 5 Frame Size Determined from Elbow Breadth (mm)

Height	Elbow Breadth (mm)		
	Small Frame	Medium Frame	Large Frame
Males			
5'2 ½" or less	<64	64–72	>72
5'3"–5'6 ½"	<67	67–74	>74
5'7"–5'10 ½"	<69	69–76	>76
5'11"–6'2 ½"	<71	71–78	>78
6'3" or more	<74	74–81	>81
Females			
4'10 ½" or less	<56	56–64	>64
4'11"–5'2 ½"	<58	58–65	>65
5'3"–5'6 ½"	<59	59–66	>66
5'7"–5'10 ½"	<61	61–68	>69
5'11" or more	<62	62–69	>69

Note: *Height* is given including 1-inch heels.
Source: Metropolitan Life Insurance Company.

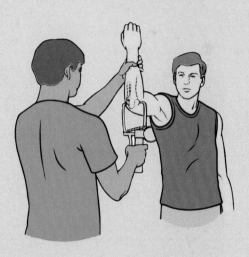

Evaluating Body Fat

4. Use Chart 6 to determine your healthy weight range. The new healthy weight range charts do not account for frame size. However, you may want to consider frame size when determining a personal weight within the healthy weight range. People with a larger frame size typically can carry more weight within the range than can those with a smaller frame size.

Body Mass Index (BMI)

Use the steps listed or use Chart 7 to calculate your BMI.

1. Divide your weight in pounds by 2.2 to determine your weight in kilograms.

2. Multiply your height in inches by 0.0254 to determine your height in meters.

3. Square your height in meters (multiply your height in meters by your height in meters).

4. Divide your weight in kilograms from step 1 by your height in meters squared from step 3.

5. If you use these steps to determine your BMI, use the Rating Scale for Body Mass Index (Chart 8) to obtain a rating for your BMI.

Chart 6 Healthy Weight Ranges for Adult Females and Males

Height			Height		
Feet	Inches	Pounds	Feet	Inches	Pounds
4	10	91–119	5	9	129–169
4	11	94–124	5	10	132–174
5	0	97–128	5	11	136–179
5	1	101–132	6	0	140–184
5	2	104–137	6	1	144–189
5	3	107–141	6	2	148–195
5	4	111–146	6	3	152–200
5	5	114–150	6	4	156–205
5	6	118–155	6	5	160–211
5	7	121–160	6	6	164–216
5	8	125–164			

Source: U.S. Department of Agriculture and Department of Health and Human Services.

Chart 7 Body Mass Index (BMI)

Height	100	105	110	115	120	125	130	135	140	145	150	155	160	165	170	175	180	185	190	195	200	205	210	215	220	225	230	235	240	245	250
5'0"	20	21	21	22	23	24	25	26	27	28	29	30	31	32	33	34	35	36	37	38	39	40	41	42	43	44	45	46	47	48	49
5'1"	19	20	21	22	23	24	25	26	26	27	28	29	30	31	32	33	34	35	36	37	38	39	40	41	42	43	43	44	45	46	47
5'2"	18	19	20	21	22	23	24	25	26	27	27	28	29	30	31	32	33	34	35	36	37	37	38	39	40	41	42	43	44	45	46
5'3"	18	19	19	20	21	22	23	24	25	26	27	27	28	29	30	31	32	33	34	35	35	36	37	38	39	40	41	42	43	43	44
5'4"	17	18	19	20	21	21	22	23	24	25	26	27	27	28	29	30	31	32	33	33	34	35	36	37	38	39	39	40	41	42	43
5'5"	17	17	18	19	20	21	22	22	23	24	25	26	27	27	28	29	30	31	32	32	33	34	35	36	37	37	38	39	40	41	42
5'6"	16	17	18	19	19	20	21	22	23	23	24	25	26	27	27	28	29	30	31	31	32	33	34	35	36	36	37	38	39	40	40
5'7"	16	16	17	18	19	20	20	21	22	23	23	24	25	26	27	27	28	29	30	31	31	32	33	34	34	35	36	37	38	38	39
5'8"	15	16	17	17	18	19	20	21	21	22	23	24	24	25	26	27	27	28	29	30	30	31	32	33	33	34	35	36	36	37	38
5'9"	15	16	16	17	18	18	19	20	21	21	22	23	24	24	25	26	27	27	28	29	30	30	31	32	32	33	34	35	35	36	37
5'10"	14	15	16	17	17	18	19	19	20	21	22	22	23	24	24	25	26	27	27	28	29	29	30	31	32	32	33	34	34	35	36
5'11"	14	15	15	16	17	17	18	19	20	20	21	22	22	23	24	24	25	26	26	27	28	29	29	30	31	31	32	33	33	34	35
6'0"	14	14	15	16	16	17	18	18	19	20	20	21	22	22	23	24	24	25	26	26	27	28	28	29	30	31	31	32	33	33	34
6'1"	13	14	15	15	16	16	17	18	18	19	20	20	21	22	22	23	24	24	25	26	26	27	28	28	29	30	30	31	32	32	33
6'2"	13	13	14	15	15	16	17	17	18	19	19	20	21	21	22	22	23	24	24	25	26	26	27	28	28	29	30	30	31	31	32
6'3"	12	13	14	14	15	16	16	17	17	18	19	19	20	21	21	22	22	23	24	24	25	26	26	27	27	28	29	29	30	31	31
6'4"	12	13	13	14	15	15	16	16	17	18	18	19	19	20	21	21	22	23	23	24	24	25	26	26	27	27	28	29	29	30	30

Weight

☐ Low   ☐ Normal (good fitness zone)   ☐ Overweight   ☐ Obese

Chart 8 Rating Scale for Body Mass Index (BMI)

Classification	BMI
Obese (high risk)	Over 30
Overweight	25–30
Normal (good fitness zone)	18.5–24.9
Low	Less than 18.4

Note: An excessively low BMI is not desirable. Low BMI values can indicate eating disorders and other health problems.

Formula

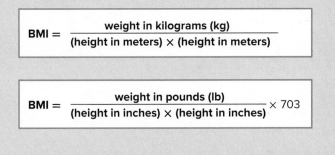

$$BMI = \frac{\text{weight in kilograms (kg)}}{(\text{height in meters}) \times (\text{height in meters})}$$

$$BMI = \frac{\text{weight in pounds (lb)}}{(\text{height in inches}) \times (\text{height in inches})} \times 703$$

Determining the Waist-to-Hip Circumference Ratio

The waist-to-hip circumference ratio is recommended as the best available index for determining risk for disease associated with fat and weight distribution. Disease and death risk are associated with abdominal and upper body fatness. When a person has high fatness and a high waist-to-hip ratio, additional risks exist. The following steps should be taken in making measurements and calculating the waist-to-hip ratio.

1. Both measurements should be done with a nonelastic tape. Make the measurements while standing with the feet together and the arms at the sides, elevated only high enough to allow the measurements. Be sure the tape is horizontal and around the entire circumference. Record scores to the nearest millimeter or 1/16th of an inch. Use the same units of measure for both circumferences (millimeters or 1/16th of an inch). The tape should be pulled snugly but not to the point of causing an indentation in the skin.

2. Waist measurement—Measure at the natural waist (smallest waist circumference). If no natural waist exists, the measurement should be made at the level of the umbilicus. Measure at the end of a normal inhale.

3. Hip measurement—Measure at the maximum circumference of the buttocks. It is recommended that you wear thin-layered clothing (such as a swimming suit or underwear) that will not add significantly to the measurement.

4. Divide the hip measurement into the waist measurement or use the waist-to-hip nomogram (Chart 9) to determine your waist-to-hip ratio.

5. Use the Waist-to-Hip Ratio Rating Scale (Chart 10) to determine your rating for the waist-to-hip ratio.

Chart 9 Waist-to-Hip Ratio Nomogram

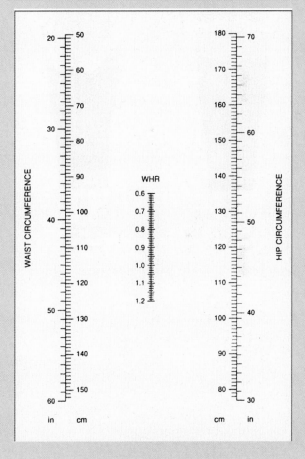

Chart 10 Waist-to-Hip Ratio Rating Scale

Classification	Male	Female
High risk	>1.0	>0.85
Moderately high risk	0.90–1.0	0.80–0.85
Lower risk	<0.90	<0.80

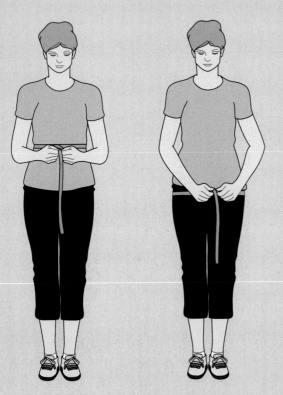

Note: Using a partner or mirror will aid you in keeping the tape horizontal.

Determining Disease Risk Based on BMI and Waist Circumference

Use Chart 11 to determine a BMI and Waist Circumference Rating. In the first column of Chart 11, locate your BMI. Locate your waist circumference in either column 2 or 3 depending on your age. Your rating is located at the point where the appropriate rows and columns intersect.

Chart 11 Waist Circumference Rating Scale

BMI	Waist Circumference (in)	
	Male	Female
High Performance	<31.5	<27.5
Good Fitness	31.5–39	27.5–35
Marginal	39.5–47	35.5–43
Low	>47	>43

Source: Adapted from ACSM.

Lab 13A Evaluating Body Composition: Skinfold Measures

Name	**Section**	**Date**

Purpose: To estimate body fatness using two skinfold procedures; to compare measures made by an expert, by a partner, and by self-measurements; to learn the strengths and weaknesses of each technique; and to use the results to establish personal standards for evaluating body composition.

General Procedures: Follow the specific procedures for the two self-assessment techniques. If possible, have one set of measurements made by an expert (instructor) for each of the two techniques. Next, work with a partner you trust. Have the partner make measurements at each site for both techniques. Finally, make self-measurements for each of the sites. If you are just learning a measurement technique, it is important to practice the skills of making the measurement. If you do measurements over time, use the same instrument (if possible) each time you measure. If your measurements vary widely, take more than one set until you get more consistent results.

  If you have had an underwater weighing, a bioelectric impedance measurement, or some other body fatness measurement done recently, record your results.

Alternative Body Fat Estimates (Other Methods)

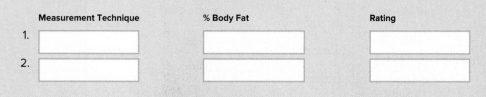

	Measurement Technique	% Body Fat	Rating
1.			
2.			

Skinfold Measurements (Jackson-Pollock Method)

Procedures for Jackson-Pollock Method

1. Read the directions for the Jackson-Pollock method measurements in the Lab Resource Materials.
2. If possible, observe a demonstration of the proper procedures for measuring skinfolds at each of the different locations before doing partner or self-measurements.
3. Make expert, partner, and self-measurements (see the Lab Resource Materials). When doing the self-measure of the triceps, use the self-measurement technique described in the Lab Resource Materials (females only).
4. Record each of the measurements in the Results section.
5. Calculate your body fatness from skinfolds by summing the appropriate skinfold values (chest, thigh, and abdominal for males; triceps, iliac crest, and thigh for females). Using your age and the sum of the appropriate skinfolds, determine your body fatness using Charts 3 and 4 in the Lab Resource Materials.
6. Rate your fatness using Chart 2 in the Lab Resource Materials.

Results for Jackson-Pollock Method

Skinfolds by an Expert (If Possible)	**Skinfolds by Partner**	**Self-Measurements**
Male	*Male*	*Male*
Chest	Chest	Chest
Thigh	Thigh	Thigh
Abdominal	Abdominal	Abdominal
Sum	Sum	Sum
% body fat	% body fat	% body fat
Rating	Rating	Rating
Female	*Female*	*Female*
Triceps	Triceps	Triceps
Iliac crest	Iliac crest	Iliac crest
Thigh	Thigh	Thigh
Sum	Sum	Sum
% body fat	% body fat	% body fat
Rating	Rating	Rating

Make a check by the statements that are true about your measurements..

☐ The person doing measurements has experience with these three skinfold measurements.

☐ Self-measurements were practiced until measurements became consistent.

☐ Results of several trials for each measure are consistent (do not vary more than 2–3 mm).

☐ You are not exceptionally low or exceptionally high in body fat.

The more checks you have, the more likely your measurements are accurate.

Skinfold Measurements (FitnessGram Method)

Procedures for FitnessGram Method

1. Read the directions for the FitnessGram measurements in the Lab Resource Materials.
2. Use the procedures as for the FitnessGram method using the triceps, abdominal, and calf sites described in the Lab Resource Materials. When doing the self-measure of the triceps, use the self-measurement technique shown earlier.
3. Calculate your body fatness from skinfolds by summing the appropriate skinfold values (same for both males and females). Using the sum of the appropriate skinfolds, determine your body fatness using Chart 1 in the Lab Resource Materials.
4. Rate your fatness using Chart 2 in the Lab Resource Materials.

Results for FitnessGram Method

Skinfolds by an Expert (If Possible)		Skinfolds by Partner		Self-Measurements	
Triceps		Triceps		Triceps	
Abdominal		Abdominal		Abdominal	
Calf		Calf		Calf	
Sum		Sum		Sum	
% body fat		% body fat		% body fat	
Rating		Rating		Rating	

Make a check by the statements that are true about your measurements.

- [ ] The person doing measurements has experience with these three skinfold measurements.
- [ ] Self-measurements were practiced until measurements became consistent.
- [ ] Results of several trials for each measure are consistent (do not vary more than 2–3 mm).
- [ ] You are not exceptionally low or exceptionally high in body fat.

The more checks you have, the more likely your measurements are accurate.

Conclusions and Implications: In the space provided, discuss your current body composition based on the two skinfold procedures and any other measures of body fatness you did. Note any discrepancies in the measurements and discuss which of the measurements you think provide the most useful information. To what extent do you think you need to alter your level of body fatness?

Lab 13B Evaluating Body Composition: Height, Weight, and Circumference Measures

Name	Section	Date

Purpose: To assess body composition using a variety of procedures, to learn the strengths and weaknesses of each technique, and to use the results to establish personal standards for evaluating body composition.

General Procedures: Follow the specific procedures for the three self-assessment techniques. If possible, work with a partner you trust to help with measurements that you have difficulty making yourself. If you are just learning a measurement technique, it is important to practice the skills of making the measurement. If you do measurements over time, use the same instrument (if possible) each time you measure. If your measurements vary widely, take more than one set until you get more consistent results. If possible, have an expert make measurements on you using these procedures.

Height and Weight Measurements

Procedures

1. Read the directions for height and weight measurements in the Lab Resource Materials.
2. Determine your healthy weight range using Chart 6 in the Lab Resource Materials. You may want to use your elbow breadth (Chart 5). People with a smaller frame size should typically weigh less than those with a larger frame size within the healthy weight range. You may need the assistance of a partner to make the elbow breadth measurement.
3. Record your scores in the Results section.

Results

Weight _____ Healthy weight range _____

Height _____

Make a check by the statements that are true about your measurements.

☐ You are confident in the accuracy of the scale you used.

☐ You are confident that the height technique is accurate.

The more checks you have, the more likely your measurements are accurate. If you are a very active person with a high amount of muscle, use this method with caution.

Body Mass Index

Procedures

1. Use the height and weight measures from above.
2. Determine your BMI score by using Chart 7 or the directions in the Lab Resource Materials. Determine your rating using Chart 8.
3. Record your score and rating in the Results section.

Results

Body Mass Index _____ Rating _____

If you are a very active person with a high amount of muscle, use this method with caution.

Waist-to-Hip Ratio

Procedures

1. Measure your waist and hip circumferences using the procedures in the Lab Resource Materials.
2. Divide your hip circumference into your waist circumference, or use Chart 9 in the Lab Resource Materials to calculate your waist-to-hip ratio.
3. Determine your rating using Chart 10 in the Lab Resource Materials.
4. Record your scores in the Results section.

Results

Waist circumference [ ]   Hip circumference [ ]   Waist-to-hip ratio [ ]   Rating [ ]

Make a check by the statements that are true about you.

☐ I am a male 5'9" or less and have a waist girth of 34 inches or more.

☐ I am a male 5'10" to 6'4" and have a waist girth of 36 inches or more.

☐ I am a male 6'5" or more and have a waist girth of 38 inches or more.

☐ I am a female 5'2" or less and have a waist girth of 29 inches or more.

☐ I am a female 5'3" to 5'10" and have a waist girth of 31 inches or more.

☐ I am a female 5'11" or more and have a waist girth of 33 inches or more.

If you checked one of the boxes, the waist-to-hip ratio is especially relevant for you.

BMI and Waist Circumference Rating

Procedures

1. Locate your BMI and waist circumference from previous Results sections in this lab.
2. Use these values to calculate your BMI and Waist Circumference Rating using Chart 11. Record the rating in the Results section.

Results

BMI and Waist Circumference Rating [ ]

Conclusions and Implications: In the space provided, discuss your results for the height, weight, and circumference procedures. Note any discrepancies in the measurements. Indicate the strengths and weaknesses of the various methods. Which of the measures do you think provided you with the most useful information? If you also did the skinfold measures (Lab 13A), discuss your body composition based on all the information you have collected (skinfolds and height, weight, and circumference measures).

Lab 13C Determining Your Daily Energy Expenditure

Name	**Section**	**Date**

Purpose: To learn how many calories you expend in a day.

Procedures

1. Estimate your basal metabolism using step 1 in the Results section in this lab. First, determine the number of minutes you sleep.
2. Monitor your activity expenditure for 1 day using Chart 1. Record the number of 5-, 15-, and 30-minute blocks of time you perform each of the different types of physical activities (e.g., if an activity lasted 20 minutes, you would use one 15-minute block and one 5-minute block). Be sure to distinguish between moderate (Mod) and vigorous (Vig) intensity in your logging. If you perform an activity that is not listed, specify the activity on the line labeled "Other" and estimate if it is moderate or vigorous. You may want to keep copies of Chart 1 for future use. One extra copy is provided at the end of this section.
3. Sum the total number of minutes of moderate and vigorous activity. Determine your calories expended during moderate and vigorous activity using steps 2 and 3.
4. Determine your nonactive minutes using step 4. This is all time that is not spent sleeping or being active.
5. Determine your calories expended in nonactive minutes using step 5.
6. Determine your calories expended in a day using step 6.

Results

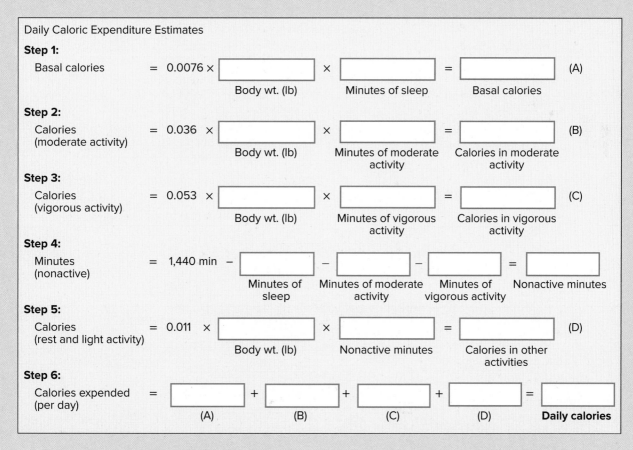

Daily Caloric Expenditure Estimates

Step 1:
Basal calories = 0.0076 × [Body wt. (lb)] × [Minutes of sleep] = [Basal calories] (A)

Step 2:
Calories (moderate activity) = 0.036 × [Body wt. (lb)] × [Minutes of moderate activity] = [Calories in moderate activity] (B)

Step 3:
Calories (vigorous activity) = 0.053 × [Body wt. (lb)] × [Minutes of vigorous activity] = [Calories in vigorous activity] (C)

Step 4:
Minutes (nonactive) = 1,440 min − [Minutes of sleep] − [Minutes of moderate activity] − [Minutes of vigorous activity] = [Nonactive minutes]

Step 5:
Calories (rest and light activity) = 0.011 × [Body wt. (lb)] × [Nonactive minutes] = [Calories in other activities] (D)

Step 6:
Calories expended (per day) = [(A)] + [(B)] + [(C)] + [(D)] = [**Daily calories**]

Answer the following questions about your daily caloric expenditure estimate.

Yes	No	
☐	☐	Were the activities you performed similar to what you normally perform each day?
☐	☐	Do you think your daily estimated caloric expenditure is an accurate estimate?
☐	☐	Do you think you expend the correct number of calories in a typical day to maintain the body composition (body fat level) that is desirable for you?

Conclusions and Implications: In several paragraphs, discuss your daily caloric expenditure. Comment on your answers to the preceding questions. In addition, comment on whether you think you should modify your daily caloric expenditure for any reason.

Chart 1

Day of Monitoring:					
Physical Activity Category		**5 Minutes**	**15 Minutes**	**30 Minutes**	**Minutes**
Lifestyle Activity		1 2 3 4 5 6	1 2 3 4 5 6	1 2 3	
Dancing (general)	Mod				
Gardening	Mod				
Home repair/maintenance	Mod				
Occupation	Mod				
Walking/hiking	Mod				
Other:	Mod				
Aerobic Activity		1 2 3 4 5 6	1 2 3 4 5 6	1 2 3	
Aerobic dance (low-impact)	Mod				
	Vig				
Aerobic machines (rowing, stair, ski)	Mod				
	Vig				
Bicycling	Mod				
	Vig				
Running	Mod				
	Vig				
Skating (roller/ice)	Mod				
	Vig				
Swimming (laps)	Mod				
	Vig				
Other:	Mod				
	Vig				
Sport/Recreation Activity		1 2 3 4 5 6	1 2 3 4 5 6	1 2 3	
Basketball	Mod				
	Vig				
Bowling/billiards	Mod				
Golf	Mod				
Martial arts (judo, karate)	Mod				
	Vig				
Racquetball/tennis	Mod				
	Vig				
Soccer/hockey	Mod				
	Vig				
Softball/baseball	Mod				
Volleyball	Mod				
	Vig				
Other:	Mod				
Flexibility Activity		1 2 3 4 5 6	1 2 3 4 5 6	1 2 3	
Stretching	Mod				
Other:	Mod				
Strengthening Activity		1 2 3 4 5 6	1 2 3 4 5 6	1 2 3	
Calisthenics (push-ups/sit-ups)	Mod				
Resistance exercise	Mod				
Other:	Mod				

Minutes of moderate activity

Minutes of vigorous activity

Total minutes of activity

Day of Monitoring:					
Physical Activity Category		**5 Minutes**	**15 Minutes**	**30 Minutes**	**Minutes**
Lifestyle Activity		1 2 3 4 5 6	1 2 3 4 5 6	1 2 3	
Dancing (general)	Mod				
Gardening	Mod				
Home repair/maintenance	Mod				
Occupation	Mod				
Walking/hiking	Mod				
Other:	Mod				
Aerobic Activity		1 2 3 4 5 6	1 2 3 4 5 6	1 2 3	
Aerobic dance (low-impact)	Mod				
	Vig				
Aerobic machines (rowing, stair, ski)	Mod				
	Vig				
Bicycling	Mod				
	Vig				
Running	Mod				
	Vig				
Skating (roller/ice)	Mod				
	Vig				
Swimming (laps)	Mod				
	Vig				
Other:	Mod				
	Vig				
Sport/Recreation Activity		1 2 3 4 5 6	1 2 3 4 5 6	1 2 3	
Basketball	Mod				
	Vig				
Bowling/billiards	Mod				
Golf	Mod				
Martial arts (judo, karate)	Mod				
	Vig				
Racquetball/tennis	Mod				
	Vig				
Soccer/hockey	Mod				
	Vig				
Softball/baseball	Mod				
Volleyball	Mod				
	Vig				
Other:	Mod				
Flexibility Activity		1 2 3 4 5 6	1 2 3 4 5 6	1 2 3	
Stretching	Mod				
Other:	Mod				
Strengthening Activity		1 2 3 4 5 6	1 2 3 4 5 6	1 2 3	
Calisthenics (push-ups/sit-ups)	Mod				
Resistance exercise	Mod				
Other:	Mod				

Minutes of moderate activity

Minutes of vigorous activity

Total minutes of activity

Nutrition and Principles of Healthy Eating

LEARNING OBJECTIVES

After completing the study of this Concept, you will be able to:

► Apply basic guidelines for healthy eating.

► List and apply dietary recommendations for carbohydrates, fats, proteins, vitamins, minerals, and water.

► Interpret and use food labels to make healthy decisions.

► Describe and incorporate sound eating practices.

► Describe and apply nutrition guidelines for active people and those interested in performance (e.g., sports).

► Analyze your diet to determine nutrient quality.

► Compare nutritional quality of various foods.

The amount and kinds of food you eat affect your health and wellness.

Rolf Bruderer/Blend Images LLC

Why It Matters!

Most people understand the importance of good nutrition for optimal health, but many still find it difficult to maintain a healthy diet. One reason for this is that foods are usually developed, marketed, and advertised for convenience and taste rather than for health or nutritional quality. Another reason is that many individuals have misconceptions about what constitutes a healthy diet. Some misconceptions are propagated by incomplete media reports, others from commercially oriented marketing efforts, and still others by confusing and often contradictory findings from nutrition research. This Concept summarizes the essential principles, guidelines, and recommendations for providing a sound foundation of nutrition knowledge. Strategies are also provided to help you adopt and maintain a healthy diet.

Guidelines and Recommendations for Healthy Eating

Good nutrition is important for both present and future health. It is well established that diets high in saturated fats, sugars, and refined carbohydrates contribute to obesity, diabetes, and many other chronic conditions. The risks of an unhealthy diet were evident during the COVID-19 pandemic. Research documented that unhealthy diets compromised adaptive immunity, contributed to greater inflammatory responses, and impaired overall defense against the virus. Dietary choices are also thought to be important for avoiding long-term consequences in those who were exposed and recovered. Nutrition influences personal health in subtle and dramatic ways, both in the short and long term.

National dietary guidelines provide a sound plan for good nutrition. National dietary guidelines have been established with the aim of promoting health and preventing disease. The first dietary guidelines were published in 1980, and federal law requires that these guidelines be updated every 5 years to incorporate new research findings. The current *Dietary Guidelines for Americans: 2020-2025* document that many of the leading chronic diseases in our society are diet-related. The report specifically identifies overweight and obesity, cardiovascular diseases (coronary artery disease, hypertension, stroke), cardiovascular disease risk factors (total blood cholesterol and high HDL), diabetes, some cancers (breast, colorectal), poor bone health (low bone density, osteoporosis), and unhealthy levels of muscle strength as diet-related health conditions. The report also emphasizes the important and complementary roles of physical activity and healthy eating to reduce chronic conditions and contribute to overall well-being.

MyPlate provides a model for adhering to dietary guidelines. Over the years, a variety of models have been used to illustrate key elements of the guidelines (see Figure 1). A common theme in the various models is that each depicts the food groups essential to a healthy diet. The first pyramid used segments of different sizes to illustrate relative amounts of food to be consumed from each food group. For example, the large segment at the bottom of the pyramid depicted carbohydrates, the largest source of calories in the diet. A refinement of the pyramid included a stairway to depict physical activity and colored bands showing the recommended proportion of the food groups. MyPlate uses a plate with four colored areas representing the different food groups (fruits, grains, vegetables, and proteins), and a glass represents the dairy food group (including solid dairy products). A key message conveyed with this image is that half of the plate should be filled with fruits and vegetables. Other countries have developed models for healthy eating as well. For example, Canada uses a rainbow and Japan uses a spinning top to depict food groups. Various organizations have developed their own models. The American Heart Association has used a modified pyramid and a heart-shaped plate to illustrate eating guidelines for heart health. The goal of all the models is to provide consumers with a conceptual way to summarize the principles of healthy eating.

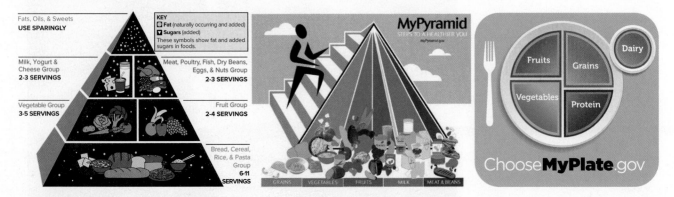

Figure 1 ▶ USDA/USDHHS models for healthy eating.

Sources: United States Department of Agriculture (USDA) and the United States Department of Health and Human Services (USDHHS).

Focus on establishing healthy eating patterns. Consistent with previous guidelines, the updated 2020–2025 guidelines emphasize the notion of "healthy dietary patterns" across the lifespan. The research underlying the guidelines documents that foods have "interactive, synergistic, and potentially cumulative relationships" and that healthy dietary patterns predict overall health status and disease risk more effectively than consumption of individual foods or nutrients. According to the Scientific Advisory report, dietary patterns associated with positive health outcomes have higher intake of vegetables, fruits, legumes, whole grains, low- or nonfat dairy, lean meat and poultry, seafood, nuts, and unsaturated vegetable oils. They are also lower in intakes of red and processed meats, sugar-sweetened foods and drinks, and refined grains. The guidelines provide tangible strategies to promote healthy eating. The main action message is to "Make Every Bite Count" and this is emphasized in four primary guidelines:

- *Follow a healthy dietary pattern at every life stage.* A healthy eating pattern should help you achieve and maintain a healthy body weight, support nutrient adequacy, and reduce the risk of chronic disease. Needs vary throughout the lifespan but by establishing patterns of healthy eating, your nutritional needs can be met throughout life. You can also contribute to broader societal changes by serving healthy food for family and friends and by advocating for healthier options.

- *Customize and enjoy nutrient-dense food and beverage choices to reflect personal preferences, cultural traditions, and budgetary considerations.* Consuming nutrient-dense foods improves the overall quality of the diet. Examples of nutrient-dense foods include vegetables, fruits, high-fiber whole grains, fat-free or low-fat milk and milk products, seafood, lean meat and poultry, eggs, soy products, nuts, seeds, and oils. Healthy foods can be prepared to suit personal preferences and on different budgets.

- *Focus on meeting food group needs with nutrient-dense foods and beverages, and stay within calorie limits.* Consuming fewer processed foods (e.g., meats, grains) and sweetened foods and drinks contributes to a healthier dietary pattern. Simple changes in beverage choices can make a big difference in overall diet quality while avoiding excess calories. Factors such as body size, activity level, and personal metabolism influence your daily energy intake needs. Most people underestimate the number of calories they eat, so it is important to learn to regulate your intake to maintain a healthy weight.

- *Limit foods and beverages higher in added sugars, saturated fat, and sodium, and limit alcoholic beverages.* Consumption of solid fats and added sugars leads to excessive intake of saturated fat and cholesterol and insufficient intake of dietary fiber and other nutrients. Smaller portions and moderation of consumption of sweets, desserts, and alcohol are good goals.

Specific Dietary Reference Intakes (DRIs) provide a target zone for healthy eating. About 45–50 nutrients in food are believed to be essential for the body's growth, maintenance, and repair. These are classified into six categories: carbohydrates (and fiber), fats, proteins, vitamins, minerals, and water. The first three provide energy, which is measured in calories. Specific dietary recommendations for each of the six nutrients are presented later in this Concept.

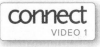

In the United States, specific nutrient requirements for good health are developed by the Food and Nutrition Board (FNB) of the National Academies of Sciences, Engineering, and Medicine. The complexity of dietary interactions has prompted the board to develop a range of indicators that collectively are referred to as **Dietary Reference Intakes (DRIs).** Each is described.

The Recommended Dietary Allowance (RDA) reflects the average daily nutrient intake that is sufficient to meet requirements for nearly all adults (97 percent). An alternative indicator called the Adequate Intake (AI) is provided as a recommendation when sufficient data aren't available to establish a firm RDA. The DRI values also include **Tolerable Upper Intake Level (UL),** which reflects the highest level of daily intake a person can consume without adverse effects on health. The guidelines make it clear that, although too little of a nutrient can be harmful to health, so can too much. The distinctions are similar to the concept of the target zone used to prescribe physical activity. The RDA or AI values are analogous to the threshold levels (minimal amount needed to meet guidelines), while the UL values represent amounts that should not be exceeded. A new DRI category is the **Chronic Disease Risk Reduction Intake (CDRRI).** It fills a need to provide better guidance on the amounts of nutrients necessary to provide health benefits. They don't replace other DRI values but are set when there is evidence to support links between intake of a specific nutrient and a chronic disease or associated risk factor. For example, CDRRI values were recently established for sodium intake based on the evidence that excessive sodium in the diet can increase blood pressure and lead to other health problems.

A "Total Diet Approach" is encouraged to achieve good nutrition. An important nutrition principle is that there are not "good" or "bad" foods, but healthy and unhealthy patterns. The phrase *Total Diet Approach* has been

Dietary Reference Intake (DRI) Appropriate amounts of nutrients in the diet (AI, RDA, and UL).

Tolerable Upper Intake Level (UL) Maximum level of a daily nutrient that will not pose a risk of adverse health effects for most people.

Chronic Disease Risk Reduction Intake (CDRRI) Nutrient intakes that are expected to reduce the risk of developing chronic disease.

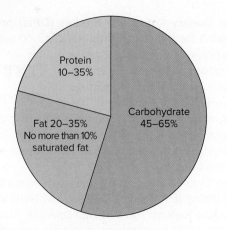

Figure 2 ▶ Dietary Reference Intake values.

used to emphasize this lifestyle approach to eating. Importantly, the word *diet* in this context should be interpreted as a pattern of eating and not something you go on (and off) to try to lose weight. The national guidelines emphasize the importance of choosing nutrient-dense foods and beverages in place of less healthy choices at every life stage. Importantly, the guidelines state that "it is never too early or too late to improve food and beverage choices to build a healthy dietary pattern."

A healthful total diet is not a rigid prescription but rather a flexible approach to eating that can be adjusted for a variety of individual tastes and preferences. This is reflected in the wide ranges in the DRI values for the macronutrients that provide energy in our diet. As shown in Figure 2, carbohydrates can contribute 45–65 percent of total calories, fat can range from 20 to 35 percent, and protein can range from 10 to 35 percent. These broad ranges allow people to make healthy but realistic choices based on their own food preferences and eating patterns.

The well-known "Mediterranean-Style" diet has been used as an example of a healthy dietary pattern. It is characterized by a higher consumption of plant-based food (e.g., fruits, vegetables, whole grains, nuts, and legumes) as well as the preferential use of healthy monounsaturated fat sources (e.g., olive oil). A prominent national study of Australian adults demonstrated that general adherence to a Mediterranean diet was associated with lower prevalence of high cholesterol and high blood pressure as well as reduced risk of cerebrovascular disease. Other studies have documented that a Mediterranean diet boosts immune function and may help reduce risks to viral infections such as COVID-19. While the Mediterranean diet is typically associated with cuisines from Italy, France, and Greece, the elements can be adopted to a variety of cooking styles. This is only one example of a healthy dietary pattern, but it illustrates how a total diet approach contributes to achieving good nutrition.

Adherence to dietary guidelines has improved in recent years, but many fail to meet them. The national nutrition survey indicates that, over the last two decades, Americans are eating better. This conclusion is based on

scores on the quality of eating index that reflects adherence to national dietary guidelines. Over the past two decades, scores (1–100) have increased slightly. The current *Dietary Guidelines* report indicates that the average American scores about 59 on the quality of eating index, indicating that there is much room for improvement. Older adults (60 and older) score the highest on the index (63) while teens (14–18) and pre-teens (9–13) score the worst, 51 and 52 respectively. Young adults (19–30) have an average index of 56 while adults (31–59) have an average index of 59.

Media influences and sociocultural factors contribute to unhealthy norms and values related to healthy eating. A recent analysis published in a prominent medical journal documented that movies tend to depict unhealthy diets and patterns that would fail to meet national dietary guidelines. While the patterns are likely akin to average American diets, the article emphasized the importance of movies and media in shaping social norms. Sociocultural factors influence many aspects of our lifestyle and especially food intake. While you don't have direct control over these factors, you can choose what you pay attention to and decide what you personally value.

Dietary Recommendations for Carbohydrates

Complex carbohydrates should be the principal source of calories in the diet. Carbohydrates have been unfairly implicated as a cause of obesity, especially by those who advocate for low-carbohydrate diets. It is true that carbohydrates cause insulin to be released and that insulin, in turn, causes the body to take up and store excess energy as fat. However, this explanation is overly simplistic and doesn't take into account differences in types of carbohydrates. Simple sugars (such as sucrose, glucose, and fructose) found in candy and soda lead to quick increases in blood sugar and tend to promote fat deposition. Complex carbohydrates (e.g., bread, pasta, rice), on the other hand, are broken down more slowly and do not cause the same effect on blood sugar. They contribute valuable nutrients and fiber in the diet and should constitute the bulk of a person's diet. Distinguishing between simple and complex carbohydrates is important, since they are processed differently and have different nutrient values.

A number of low-carb diet books have used an index known as the glycemic index (GI) as the basis for determining if foods are appropriate in the diet. Foods with a high GI value produce rapid increases in blood sugar, while foods with a low GI value produce slower increases. This may seem to be a logical way to categorize carbohydrates, but it is misleading, since it doesn't account for the amount of carbohydrates in different servings of a food. A more appropriate indicator of the effect of foods on blood sugar levels is called the glycemic load. Carrots, for example, are known to have a very high GI value, but the overall glycemic load is quite low.

The carbohydrates from most fruits and vegetables exhibit similar properties.

Despite the intuitive and logical appeal of this classification system, neither the glycemic index nor the glycemic load have been consistently associated with body weight. Diets based on low-glycemic-index diets also don't have advantages for weight loss.

Reducing consumption of dietary sugar is an important nutrition goal. People who consume high amounts of sugar also tend to consume excess calories. Foods high in sugar content also tend to be low in overall nutrient quality. Currently the average American consumes about 13 percent of daily calories from simple sugars. The current *Dietary Guidelines for Americans* recommends that no more than 10 percent of dietary calories come from simple sugars, and the World Health Organization (WHO) has a more stringent recommendation of no more than 5 percent of total calories coming from sugars. Since carbohydrates provide about 4 calories per gram, this amounts to 50 grams of sugar (about 12 teaspoons) to meet the American guideline of 10 percent and 25 grams (about 6 teaspoons) to meet the WHO guideline for a person consuming 2,000 calories (typical total calorie value on food labels). For perspective, a typical 12-ounce sweetened soft drink contains 150 calories, mostly sugar. This is why minimizing consumption of sugar-sweetened beverages is a sound dietary modification to improve your nutrition.

Increasing consumption of dietary fiber is important for overall good nutrition and health. Diets high in complex carbohydrates and **fiber** are associated with a low incidence of coronary heart disease, stroke, and some forms of cancer. Long-term studies indicate that high-fiber diets may also be associated with a lower risk for diabetes mellitus, diverticulosis, hypertension, and gallstone formation. Past guidelines distinguished soluble fiber (typically found in fruits and oat bran) from insoluble fiber (typically found in grains), but this was an oversimplification of the different types of fiber as well as how they are processed in the body. From a technical perspective, dietary fibers are defined as carbohydrate molecules that escape digestion in the small intestine and pass into the large intestine, where they are slightly or nearly completely fermented. The fermentation products actually contribute to the many physiological benefits of dietary fiber since they can be absorbed into the bloodstream.

In documenting the approaches for DRI recommendations, the FNB made distinctions between *natural fibers* in food from *functional fibers,* which are extracted, modified, or synthesized forms of fibers. However, they both contribute to total fiber intake and both provide health benefits. The functional fibers that are added to food are analogous to vitamin-fortified foods that supplement our diets to ensure that we have sufficient amounts and types of fiber in our diet.

Currently, few Americans meet the AI recommendations for dietary fiber. The average intake of dietary fiber is about 15 g/day, which is much lower than the recommended 25–35 g/day. Foods in the typical American diet contain little, if any, dietary fiber, and servings of commonly consumed grains, fruits, and vegetables contain only 1–3 g of dietary fiber. Therefore, individuals have to look for ways to ensure that they get sufficient fiber in their diet. Manufacturers are allowed to declare a food as a "good source of fiber" if it contains 10 percent of the recommended amount (2.5 g/serving) and an "excellent source of fiber" if it contains 20 percent of the recommended amount (5 g/serving). Because fiber has known health benefits, the dietary guidelines encourage consumers to select foods high in dietary fiber, such as whole-grain breads and cereals, legumes, vegetables, and fruit, whenever possible.

Fruits and vegetables are essential for good health. Fruits and vegetables are a valuable source of dietary fiber, are packed with vitamins and minerals, and contain many beneficial phytochemicals, which may have positive effects on health. The current guidelines recommend that adults eat 2½ cups of a wide variety of vegetables from all the subgroups of colors and starches a day. A major advantage of this suggestion is that it can make you feel full without eating a lot of calories. The guidelines also suggest that adults eat 2 cups of fruit a day, with half coming in the form of whole fruit. Fruit provides many essential vitamins and most are a good source of fiber as well.

The popularity of farmers' markets reflects broader interest in fresh fruits and vegetables. However, a challenge in promoting fruit and vegetable consumption is the higher relative cost. Many public health advocates have lobbied for subsidies that would help lower costs of fresh fruits and vegetables. National initiatives such as the *Fresh Food Farmacy* have sought to increase access to fruits and vegetables to individuals with lower incomes or with food insecurity.

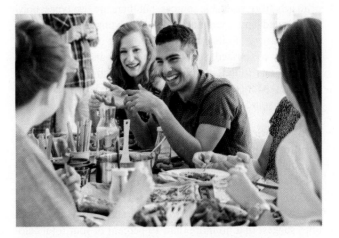

Making healthy food selections when dining out can help improve your overall nutrition and health.
Photographee.eu/Shutterstock

Fiber Indigestible bulk in foods that can be either soluble or insoluble in body fluids.

Follow the recommendations to ensure healthy amounts of carbohydrates in the diet. The following list summarizes some key dietary recommendations for carbohydrates:

- Consume a variety of fiber-rich fruits and vegetables. About 90 percent of Americans fail to meet dietary guidelines for vegetables and about 80 percent fail to meet the guideline for fruits.

- Select whole-grain foods when possible. About 40 percent of Americans fail to meet the guideline for total grains and more than 90 percent fail to meet the guideline for whole grains.

- Choose and prepare foods and beverages with little added sugars or caloric sweeteners. About 60 percent of adults (19–60) fail to meet the 10 percent guideline for simple sugars.

Dietary Recommendations for Fat

Fat is an essential nutrient and an important energy source. Humans need some fat in their diet because fats are carriers of vitamins A, D, E, and K. They are a source of essential linoleic acid, they make food taste better, and they provide a concentrated form of calories, which serve as a vital source of energy during moderate to vigorous exercise. Fats have more than twice the calories per gram as carbohydrates (9 calories per gram).

There are several types of dietary fat. **Saturated fats** come primarily from animal sources, such as red meat, dairy products, and eggs, but they are also found in some vegetable sources, such as coconut and palm oils. **Unsaturated fats** are primarily from vegetable sources, but there are two types: polyunsaturated and monounsaturated. Polyunsaturated fats include a variety of oils categorized as either omega-6 fats (e.g., safflower, cottonseed, soybean, sunflower, and corn oils), or omega-3 fats found in coldwater fish, such as salmon and mackerel. Monounsaturated fats are derived primarily from vegetable sources, including olive, peanut, and canola oil.

Consumption of saturated fat should be limited. Health recommendations related to dietary fat have changed over the years, now primarily focusing on risks from saturated fat. Excess saturated fat in the diet is known to increase the level of cholesterol in your blood, which directly increases risk of heart disease and stroke. The current dietary guidelines suggest that no more than 10 percent of your total calories should come from saturated fats. However, the American Heart Association recommends aiming for a dietary pattern that includes only 5–6 percent of calories from saturated fat (particularly if you have high blood cholesterol levels). Each gram of fat contains 9 calories, so the AHA guideline calls for about 13 grams of saturated fat per day (about 120 calories out of a daily 2,000 diet). Dietary guidelines recommend

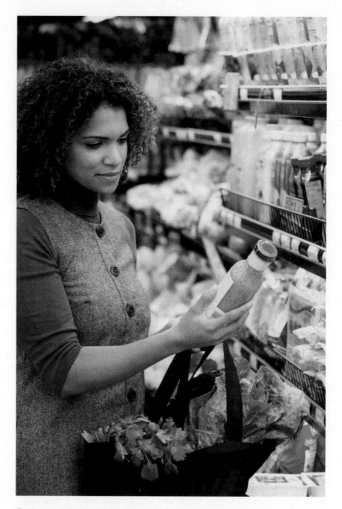

Being an informed and educated consumer can help you make healthier food choices.
Noel Hendrickson/Blend Images/Getty Images

replacing saturated fat with unsaturated fats, especially polyunsaturated fats.

Guidelines regarding consumption of cholesterol have been relaxed. Previous dietary guidelines recommended limiting consumption of cholesterol in the diet, leading consumers to carefully minimize consumption of foods high in cholesterol such as eggs. The current guidelines do not impose a specific limit on cholesterol intake; however, this does not imply that dietary cholesterol is no longer important. The technical report from the Dietary Guidelines Advisory Committee concluded that there are relatively weak relationships between consumption of dietary cholesterol and eventual levels of blood cholesterol. For example, estimates suggest that only 15 percent of circulating cholesterol is from dietary sources, with the remaining amount being manufactured by the liver as part of fat transport and metabolism. Therefore, focus has shifted to minimizing consumption of saturated fat since diets high in fat lead the liver to produce more cholesterol.

Individuals should still consume as little dietary cholesterol as possible while following a healthy eating pattern. Eggs, which were once almost forbidden in diets because of high cholesterol, are now considered to be part of a healthy eating pattern. While they have high cholesterol, they are a good source of protein and are actually low in saturated fat.

Consumption of unsaturated fats (both poly and mono) can be beneficial. Unsaturated fats are a better dietary choice than saturated fats since they are less likely to contribute to CVD, cancer, and obesity. Polyunsaturated fats (mainly omega-6 fats) can reduce total cholesterol and low-density lipoprotein (LDL) cholesterol, but they also decrease levels of high-density lipoprotein (HDL) cholesterol. They are needed in the diet, but should be minimized since they are viewed as *pro-inflammatory* for their cardiovascular effects. Avoiding fried foods and baked goods made with shortening or margarine are ways to reduce excess omega-6 fat consumption.

Omega-3 fatty acids (a special type of polyunsaturated fat found in coldwater fish) are viewed as *anti-inflammatory* and are known to help reduce the risk of cardiovascular disease. Plant source of omega-3 fatty acids (alpha-linolenic acid) found in walnuts, flaxseed, and canola oil may have similar benefits. Thus, increasing omega-3 consumption is recommended while omega-6 consumption should be minimized. Monounsaturated fats (sometimes labeled as omega-9 fats) have also been shown to decrease total cholesterol and LDL cholesterol and increase the desirable HDL cholesterol. Olive oil and canola oil are good sources.

Trans fats and hydrogenated vegetable oils should be minimized in the diet. For decades, the public has been cautioned to avoid saturated fats and foods with excessive cholesterol. Many people switched from using butter to margarine because margarine is made from vegetable oils that are unsaturated and contain no cholesterol. However, the typical hydrogenation process used to convert oils into solids produces a type of fat **(trans fats)** that was just as harmful as saturated fats, if not more so. Trans fats are known to increase LDL cholesterol and have been shown to contribute to the buildup of atherosclerotic plaque. The FDA initially enacted strong labeling laws to try to minimize consumption of trans fats, but later moved to ban food manufacturers from adding partially hydrogenated oils to foods. Trans fats still occur in some foods. Minimizing consumption of processed and high-fat foods is still a sound personal dietary habit.

Fat substitutes and nutraceuticals in food products may reduce fat consumption and lower cholesterol. For years, food scientists have sought to develop substitutes that mimic the taste and properties of fat without the negative characteristics. Olestra (often marketed as Olean) is a synthetic fat substitute that passes through the gastrointestinal system without being digested. Unfortunately, trials demonstrated that it tended to also reduce levels of beneficial fat-soluble vitamins and caused abdominal cramping. Experts recommend "replacement" over "substitution" as a better way to reduce fat content. Thus, it is more effective to make alternative food choices than to look for substitutions that allow continued consumption of specific foods.

Follow the recommendations to ensure healthy amounts of fat in the diet. The following list summarizes some key dietary recommendations for dietary fat:

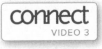

- Limit saturated fatty acid intake to less than 10 percent of total calories. More than 70 percent of adults ages 19–60 currently fail to meet the 10 percent saturated fat guideline.
- Emphasize food sources with mono- or polyunsaturated fat sources.
- Avoid trans fatty acids from processed foods (e.g., foods with hydrogenated vegetable oils).
- Consume two servings of seafood per week to provide healthy amounts of omega-3 fatty acids.

Dietary Recommendations for Proteins

Protein is the basic building block for the body, but dietary protein constitutes a relatively small amount of daily caloric intake. Proteins are often referred to as the building blocks of the body because all body cells are made of protein. More than 100 proteins are formed from 20 different **amino acids.** Eleven of these amino acids can be synthesized from other nutrients, but nine **essential amino acids** must be obtained directly from the diet. One way to identify amino acids is the *-ine* at the end of their name. For example, arginine and lysine are two of the amino acids. Only 3 of the 20 amino acids do not have the *-ine* suffix. They are aspartic acid, glutamic acid, and tryptophan.

Saturated Fats Dietary fats that are usually solid at room temperature and come primarily from animal sources.

Unsaturated Fats Monounsaturated or polyunsaturated fats that are usually liquid at room temperature and come primarily from vegetable sources.

Trans Fats Fats that result when hydrogen is added to liquid oil to make it more solid. Hydrogenation transforms unsaturated fats so that they take on the characteristics of saturated fats, as is the case for margarine and shortening.

Amino Acids The 20 basic building blocks of the body that make up proteins.

Essential Amino Acids The nine basic amino acids that the human body cannot produce and that must be obtained from food sources.

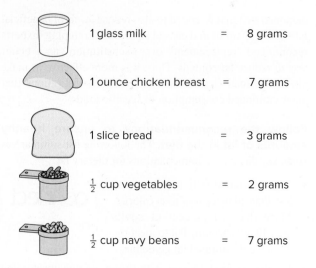

1 glass milk	=	8 grams
1 ounce chicken breast	=	7 grams
1 slice bread	=	3 grams
½ cup vegetables	=	2 grams
½ cup navy beans	=	7 grams

Figure 3 ► Protein content of various foods.
Source: Williams, M.

Certain foods, called complete proteins, contain all of the essential amino acids, along with most of the others. Examples are meat, dairy products, and fish. Incomplete proteins contain some, but not all, of the essential amino acids. Examples include beans, nuts, and rice.

Protein should account for at least 10 percent of daily calorie consumption, which can be met easily with complete (animal) or incomplete (vegetable) sources of protein. For example, a person consuming a 2,000-calorie diet should consume approximately 200 calories from protein. Protein provides 4 calories per gram, so minimum daily protein needs are as low as 50 grams per day. Figure 3 shows the relative protein content of various foods.

To provide more flexibility, dietary guidelines indicate that protein can account for as much as 35 percent of calorie intake. Experts, however, agree that there are no known benefits and some possible risks associated with consuming excess protein, particularly animal protein. High-protein diets are damaging to the kidneys, as the body must process a lot of extra nitrogen. Excessive protein intake can also lead to urinary calcium loss, which can weaken bones and lead to osteoporosis.

People who eat a variety of foods, including meat, dairy, eggs, and plants rich in protein, virtually always consume more protein than the body needs. Because of the negative consequences associated with excess intake, dietary supplements containing extra protein are not recommended for the general population.

Plant-based protein provides an alternative to meat products. Soybeans and soy-based foods are high-quality sources of protein. They may also have beneficial effects on blood pressure and cholesterol levels, possibly contributing to reductions in risk for coronary heart disease. Soy-based foods contain compounds called isoflavones, a phytoestrogen that contributes to bone health, immune function, and maintenance of menopausal health in females. Some common soy-based foods include soy milk, tofu, tempeh, and textured vegetable protein.

The popularity and acceptance of plant-based protein foods have increased dramatically in recent years. New methods have been developed to help retain more moisture in the production of plant-based proteins, which has improved the mouth-feel and taste of alternative meat products. While it may surprise people, some "veggie burgers" have more protein than beef, more omega fatty acids than salmon, more calcium than milk, and more antioxidants than blueberries. See the In the News feature for insights on the marketing and sales of plant-based meat alternatives.

Follow the recommendations to ensure healthy amounts of protein in the diet. The following list summarizes some key dietary recommendations for protein:

- As noted in Figure 2, protein should account for 10–35 percent of total calories in the diet. This guideline is designed to allow diet flexibility based on personal

In the News

Boom in Plant-Based Foods

The acceptance of plant-based foods has perhaps reached the tipping point as there have been dramatic increases in sales and consumption of plant-based foods in recent years. Interest was sparked, in part, by the promotion of the Impossible Burger in many restaurants and stores. Reports from the Good Food Institute and the Plant Based Foods Association indicate that the market for plant-based foods is almost $5 billion. The growing popularity of soy milk and alternative meat products has largely contributed. While a relatively small percentage of the population says they are vegetarian, many identify as a *flexitarian* and increasingly choose plant-based foods as part of their diet.

Have you personally noted increased marketing of plant-based foods? Have your perceptions or dietary choices been influenced by the greater societal acceptance?

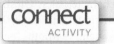

needs and interests. For most people, 10–15 percent of calories consumed as protein is adequate.

- Protein in the diet should meet the RDA of 0.8 gram per kilogram (2.2 pounds) of a person's weight (about 54 grams for a 150-pound person).

- Protein in the diet should not exceed twice the RDA (1.6 grams per kilogram of body weight). Excess protein can be harmful to the kidneys.

- Vegetarians must eat a combination of foods to ensure an adequate intake of essential amino acids. Vegans should supplement their diet with vitamin B-12.

- Dietary supplements of protein, such as tablets and powders, are not recommended.

Dietary Recommendations for Vitamins

Adequate vitamin intake is necessary for good health and wellness, but excessive vitamin intake is not necessary and can be harmful. Vitamins serve a variety of functions within the body. For example, they serve as co-enzymes for metabolism of different nutrients, contribute to the regulation of energy stores, and assist in immune function. Some vitamins (e.g., B-complex vitamins and vitamin C) are water soluble and are excreted in urine. These vitamins must be consumed on a daily basis. Other vitamins, such as A, D, E, and K, are fat soluble. These vitamins are stored over time, so daily doses of these vitamins are not necessary. Studies have supported the importance of vitamin D for reducing risks of infections, but specific roles in reducing infections or risks from SARS-CoV-2 were not conclusive. Because of reduced sun exposure, it is important to ensure sufficient vitamin D levels through dietary measures. However, excess consumption of fat-soluble vitamins should be avoided since they can actually build to toxic levels and harm cell function. The specific DRI values (minimal amounts) for some of the more important vitamins are shown in Table 1 (see page 286), along with the UL values (maximum amounts).

Some vitamins act as antioxidants, but health benefits may depend on other compounds in foods. Carotenoid-rich foods, such as carrots and sweet potatoes, contain high amounts of vitamin A and high amounts of beta-carotene. Diets high in vitamin C (e.g., citrus fruits) and vitamin E (e.g., green, leafy vegetables) are also associated with reduced risk of cancer. Vitamin E has also been associated with reduced risk of heart disease.

Vitamins A, C, and E (as well as beta-carotene) act as **antioxidants** within the body. Antioxidants are substances that are thought to inactivate free radicals (molecules that can cause cell damage and health problems). For this reason, health benefits have been attributed to antioxidant

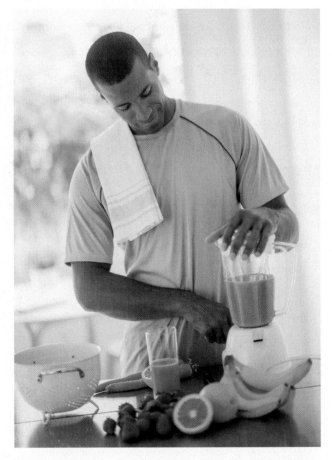

Fruits and vegetables contain vitamins as well as health-promoting phytochemicals.
Tetra Images/Shutterstock

properties. Research on vitamins is challenging since the health benefits may stem from other compounds in foods containing these vitamins (see the discussion of functional foods later in this Concept). In general, diets containing a lot of fruits and vegetables and whole grains will provide adequate intake of vitamins and other healthy food components.

Fortification of foods has been used to ensure adequate vitamin intake in the population. National policy requires many foods to be fortified. For example, milk is fortified with vitamin D, low-fat milk with vitamins A and D, and margarine with vitamin A. These foods were selected because they are common food sources for growing children. Many common grain products are fortified with folic acid because low

Antioxidants Vitamins that are thought to inactivate "activated oxygen molecules," sometimes called free radicals. Free radicals may cause cell damage that leads to diseases of various kinds. Antioxidants may inactivate the free radicals before they do their damage.

Table 1 ▶ Dietary Reference Intake (DRI), Recommended Dietary Allowance (RDA), and Tolerable Upper Intake Level (UL) for Major Nutrients

	Males	Females	UL	Function
Energy and Macronutrients				
Carbohydrates (45–65%)	130 g	130 g	ND	Energy (only source of energy for the brain)
Fat (20–35%)	ND	ND	ND	Energy, vitamin carrier
Protein (10–35%)	0.8 g/kg	0.8 g/kg	ND	Growth and maturation, tissue formation
Fiber (g/day)	38 g/day*	25 g/day*	ND	Digestion, blood profiles
B-Complex Vitamins				
Thiamin (mg/day)	1.2	1.1	ND	Co-enzyme for carbohydrates and amino acid metabolism
Riboflavin (mg/day)	1.3	1.1	ND	Co-enzyme for metabolic reactions
Niacin (mg/day)	16	14	35	Co-enzyme for metabolic reactions
Vitamin B-6 (mg/day)	1.3	1.3	100	Co-enzyme for amino acid and glycogen reactions
Folate (µg/day)	400	400	1,000	Metabolism of amino acids
Vitamin B-12 (µg/day)	2.4	2.4	ND	Co-enzyme for nucleic acid metabolism
Pantothenic acid (mg/day)	5*	5*	ND	Co-enzyme for fat metabolism
Biotin (µg/day)	30*	30*	ND	Synthesis of fat, glycogen, and amino acids
Choline (mg/day)	550*	425*	3,500	Precursor to acetylcholine
Antioxidants and Related Nutrients				
Vitamin C (mg/day)	90	75	2,000	Co-factor for reactions, antioxidant
Vitamin E (mg/day)	15	15	1,000	Undetermined, mainly antioxidant
Selenium (µg/day)	55	55	400	Defense against oxidative stress
Bone-Building Nutrients				
Calcium (mg/day)	1,000*	1,000*	2,500	Muscle contraction, nerve transmission
Phosphorus (mg/day)	700	700	3,000	Maintenance of pH, storage of energy
Magnesium (mg/day)	400–420	310–320	350	Co-factor for enzyme reactions
Vitamin D (µg/day)	5*	5*	50	Maintenance of calcium and phosphorus levels
Fluoride (mg/day)	4*	3*	10	Stimulation of new bone formation
Micronutrients and Other Trace Elements				
Vitamin K (µg/day)	120*	90*	ND	Blood clotting and bone metabolism
Vitamin A (µg/day)	900	700	3,000	Vision, immune function
Iron (mg/day)	8	18	45	Component of hemoglobin
Zinc (mg/day)	11	8	40	Component of enzymes and proteins

Notes: These values reflect the dietary needs generally for adults aged 19–50 years. Specific guidelines for other age groups are available from the Food and Nutrition Board of the National Academy of Sciences (www.nationalacademies.org; search "Food and Nutrition Board"). Values labeled with an asterisk (*) are based on Adequate Intake (AI) values rather than the RDA values; ND = not determined.

folic acid levels increase the risk for birth defects in babies. Fortification is considered essential, since more than half of all females do not consume adequate amounts of folic acid during the first months of gestation (before most even realize they are pregnant).

Vitamin supplements are not necessary for most people but may be beneficial for certain populations. Daily multiple vitamin supplements have not been shown beneficial to the general population. However, there is no current evidence to suggest that they are harmful if taken appropriately. In some cases, health professionals recommend them for specific groups. The combination of vitamin C and vitamin E proved useful as antioxidant therapy for individuals with cardiac complications of COVID-19, but these vitamins didn't have an impact on prevention. Health professionals may also recommend specific vitamin supplements for specific individuals or groups. For example, older people may need a vitamin D supplement if they get little exposure to sunlight; folic acid supplements are often recommended for pregnant females. Vitamin supplements at or below the RDA are considered safe; however, excess doses of vitamins can cause health problems. While supplementation may not be necessary for people with healthy diets, it is acceptable to take a multivitamin or mineral supplements to ensure that your needs are met. (Guidelines are presented in Table 2.)

Follow the recommendations to ensure healthy amounts of vitamins in the diet. Vitamins in the amounts equal to the RDAs should be included in the diet each day.

Table 2 ▶ Vitamin and Mineral Supplements

- Limit the use of supplements unless warranted because of a health problem or a specific lack of nutrients in the diet.

- If you decide supplementation is necessary, select a multivitamin/mineral supplement that contains micronutrients in amounts close to the recommended levels (e.g., "one-a-day"–type supplements).

- If your diet is deficient in a particular mineral (e.g., calcium or iron), it may be necessary to incorporate dietary sources or an additional mineral supplement as well, since most multivitamins do not contain the recommended daily amount of minerals.

- Choose supplements that provide between 50 and 100 percent of the AI or RDA, and avoid those that provide many times the recommended amount. The use of supplements that hype "megadoses" of vitamins and minerals can increase the risk for unwanted nutrient interactions and possible toxic effects.

- Buy supplements from a reputable company and look for products that carry a U.S. Pharmacopoeia (USP), Consumer Lab (CL), or NSP International (NSP) designation on the label.

Source: Manore.

The following guidelines will help you implement this recommendation:

- Eat a diet containing the recommended servings for carbohydrates, proteins, and fats.

- Consume extra servings of green and yellow vegetables, citrus and other fruits, and other nonanimal food sources high in fiber, vitamins, and minerals.

- People with special needs should seek medical advice before selecting supplements and should inform medical personnel as to the amounts and content of all supplements (vitamin and other).

Dietary Recommendations for Minerals

Adequate mineral intake is necessary for good health and wellness. Like vitamins, minerals have no calories and provide no energy for the body. They are important in regulating various body functions (see Table 1). A sound diet generally provides the needed amounts of most minerals, but evidence indicates that many individuals do not get recommended amounts of calcium in their diet. Calcium is important to bone, muscle, nerve, and blood development and function and has been associated with reduced risk for heart disease. Adequate intake (~2,000 mg/day) is particularly important for pregnant females, postmenopausal females, and people over 65 years of age. Consuming a calcium-rich diet is recommended, but calcium supplementation may be important for those not consuming enough in their diet.

Another mineral that merits additional attention is iron since it plays a critical role in carrying oxygen within the blood. Iron levels in blood are routinely checked by physicians to check for anemia. Increased attention has recently been paid to zinc since it is important for the development of immune cells. The use of zinc supplements and lozenges is common for fighting off colds and respiratory illnesses. Studies have found that they can help reduce the duration of a cold by about a day, but specific effects on COVID-19 are not known. Other important minerals are phosphorus, which builds teeth and bones; sodium, which regulates water in the body; and potassium, which is necessary for proper muscle function.

Reducing salt in the diet can reduce health risks. Salt is common in many processed food products, and most Americans consume way too much. Most meals at fast food chains provide more than a full day's allotment of salt. Therefore, major public health efforts have focused on encouraging manufacturers to reduce salt content in processed and fast foods. It is noteworthy that the FNB established specific health guidelines for sodium using the new CDRRI categorization in the DRIs. Salt intake increases the risk for hypertension, which is a major risk factor for heart disease and stroke. Many people have assumed that salt consumption is not a problem if you are not hypertensive, but this is not the case. Recent studies have shown that sodium intake increases risk of stroke independent of the presence of hypertension. Therefore, reducing salt consumption is important for everyone. Among American adults ages 19–60, 97 percent of males and 83 percent of females currently fail to limit salt below recommended levels.

Follow the recommendations to ensure healthy amounts of minerals in the diet. The following list includes basic recommendations for mineral content in the diet:

- Minerals in amounts equal to the RDAs should be consumed in the diet each day.
- Pregnant females and postmenopausal females should consider taking a daily calcium supplement.
- A diet containing the food servings recommended for carbohydrates, proteins, and fats will more than meet the RDA standards.
- Extra servings of green and yellow vegetables, citrus and other fruits, and other nonanimal sources of foods high in fiber, vitamins, and minerals are recommended as a substitute for high-fat foods.

Dietary Recommendations for Water and Other Fluids

Water is a critical component of a healthy diet. Though water contains no calories, provides no energy, and provides no key nutrients, it is crucial to health and survival. Water is a major component of most of the foods you eat, and more than half of all body tissues are composed of it. Regular water intake maintains water balance and is critical to many body functions. Though a variety of fluid-replacement beverages are available for use during and following exercise, replacing water is the primary need.

Beverages other than water are part of many diets, but some beverages can have an adverse effect on good health. Coffee, tea, soft drinks, and alcoholic beverages are often substituted for water. Too much caffeine consumption has been shown to cause symptoms such as irregular heartbeat in some people. Tea has not been shown to have similar effects, though this may be because tea drinkers typically consume less volume than coffee drinkers, and tea has less caffeine per cup than coffee. Many soft drinks also have caffeine, though coffee typically contains two to three times the caffeine of a typical cola drink. One very recent study indicates that excessive consumption of diet drinks increases the risk of stroke among females over 50.

The consumption of alcohol is common throughout the world and is incorporated into meals in many cultures. Evidence supports the benefits of moderate alcohol consumption for reducing the risk for some types of cardiovascular disease; however, those who do not drink should not begin to drink alcohol because of potential health benefits. The recommendation from the 2020–2025 Dietary Guidelines Advisory Committee actually encouraged a tightening of alcohol consumption, but the *Dietary Guidelines* retained the traditional levels of two drinks for males and one for females on days when alcohol is consumed.

Minimizing alcohol consumption makes sense for many reasons but, from a nutrition perspective, excessive consumption of alcoholic beverages contributes extra calories and may replace other nutrient-dense foods in the diet. Alcohol consumption during pregnancy is associated with low birth weight, fetal alcoholism, and other damage to the fetus. Therefore, it should not be consumed during pregnancy.

Follow the recommendations to ensure healthy amounts of water and other fluids in the diet. Low water consumption has been linked to chronic conditions such as diabetes, obesity, hypertension, and metabolic syndrome among older adults. Lack of adequate water consumption can cause dehydration that can also have negative health consequences, especially in hot and humid environments and among physically active people. A common recommendation for water consumption is eight glasses (8 ounces each) per day. However, there is little research to support the 8 x 8 rule. Following the 8 x 8 rule may ensure adequate hydration, however, not all people need this amount of water. Individuals that are physically active will need more water to replace that lost in sweat. The color of the urine is a good indicator of hydration (transparent = overhydrated and dark or orange = underhydrated). The following list includes basic recommendations for water and other fluids in the diet:

- Choose water as the principal source of fluids in your diet.
- Limit daily servings of beverages containing caffeine to no more than three.
- Limit sugar-sweetened soft drinks that contain excess calories.
- If you are an adult and you choose to drink alcohol, do so in moderation.

Understanding Contemporary Nutrition Terms, Issues, and Trends

The term *functional foods* can be interpreted in different ways. The term *functional foods* is often used to refer to foods or dietary components that provide a health benefit beyond basic nutrition. Nutrient-rich foods such as fruits and vegetables are considered to be functional foods because they are loaded with a variety of powerful phytochemicals that have been shown to have potential health benefits. The relative importance to health of each compound is difficult to determine because the compounds may act synergistically with each other (and with antioxidant vitamins) to promote positive outcomes. For examples, the documented benefits of moderate alcohol consumption, as well as health benefits of chocolate and coffee, stem from the phytochemicals in these foods. The potential benefits of various phytochemicals are summarized in Table 3, but these are just examples.

Other examples of functional foods include the beneficial types of fiber and beta glucan in whole grains, the isoflavones in soy products, the omega-3 fatty acids in coldwater fish, and the probiotic yeasts and bacteria in yogurts and other cultured dairy products. Fortified foods and supplements containing vitamins, minerals, probiotics, and fiber are also classified as functional foods; however, the current dietary guidelines emphasize the consumption of healthier foods instead of targeting specific nutrient requirements. This is because there are many components of foods that combine to influence our health and well-being. By adopting healthy eating patterns, most people will obtain the benefits from sufficient intake of vitamins and minerals as well as the ancillary benefits from these other functional foods.

Table 3 ▶ Examples of Functional Foods and Potential Benefits

Carotenoids	Potential Benefits
Beta-carotene: found in carrots, pumpkin, sweet potato, cantaloupe	May bolster cellular antioxidant defenses
Lutein, zeaxanthin: found in kale, collards, spinach, corn, eggs, citrus	May contribute to healthy vision
Lycopene: found in tomatoes, watermelon, red/pink grapefruit	May contribute to prostate health
Flavonoids	**Potential Benefits**
Anthocyanins: found in berries, cherries, red grapes *Flavanones:* found in citrus foods *Flavonols:* found in onions, apples, tea, broccoli	May bolster antioxidant defenses; may maintain brain function and heart health
Isothiocyanates	**Potential Benefits**
Proanthocyanidins: found in cranberries, cocoa, apples, strawberries, grapes, peanuts	May contribute to maintenance of urinary tract health and heart health
Sulforaphane: found in cauliflower, broccoli, brussels sprouts, cabbage, kale, horseradish	May enhance detoxification of undesirable compounds; may bolster cellular antioxidant defenses
Phenolic Acids	**Potential Benefits**
Caffeic/ferulic acids: found in apples, pears, citrus fruits, some vegetables, coffee	May bolster cellular antioxidant defenses; may contribute to maintenance of healthy vision
Sulfides/Thiols	**Potential Benefits**
Sulfides: found in garlic, onions, leeks, scallions *Dithiolthiones:* found in cruciferous vegetables	May enhance detoxification of undesirable compounds; may contribute to maintenance of heart health and healthy immune function

Vegetarian diets are endorsed for health benefits, but people adhere to this practice for a variety of reasons. Awareness and acceptance of vegetarian diets has increased in recent years. The percentage of people reporting to be vegetarian is still relatively low (approximately 5–8 percent), but larger numbers label themselves as *flexitarian* and consume less meat. The health benefits of vegetarianism can be attributed to the greater consumption of fruits and vegetables and reductions in saturated fats, but individuals choosing this dietary pattern have to ensure that their food choices meet overall nutritional requirements. Vegetarian diets provide ample sources of protein as long as a variety of protein-rich food sources are included in the diet. According to the Academy of Nutrition and Dietetics, well-planned vegetarian diets "are appropriate for all stages of the life cycle, including during pregnancy and lactation," and can "satisfy the nutrient needs of infants, children, and adolescents." You can get plenty of protein and nutrients on a vegetarian diet. **Vegans** must supplement the diet with vitamin B-12 because the only source of this vitamin is food from animal sources. **Lacto-ovo vegetarians** do not have the same concerns because vitamin B-12 can be obtained in dairy products.

Vegetarian diets are widely endorsed by dietitians and were described in the U.S. dietary guidelines as one of the recommended "healthy eating patterns"; however, vegetarians may choose this pattern for a variety of reasons. Some may choose it for religious, ethical, or animal-rights reasons. Others may choose it for philosophical reasons (e.g., not wanting to eat flesh). Still others may pursue it because of the ancillary benefits on the environment. Societal awareness of vegetarianism is still evolving, but there are now more vegetarian food options in grocery stores and restaurants.

Organic foods are more expensive, but some people are willing to pay the extra cost to ensure how their food is produced. Organic food differs from conventionally produced food primarily in the way it is grown, handled, and processed. Organic food is produced without conventional pesticides and using natural fertilizers. Organic meat, poultry, eggs, and dairy products come from animals that are given no antibiotics or growth hormones. To be labeled as "organic," a food must be produced by a certified grower that follows USDA guidelines. Currently, a government-approved

Vegans Strict vegetarians, who exclude not only all forms of meat from the diet but also dairy products and eggs.
Lacto-Ovo Vegetarians Vegetarians who include dairy and eggs in the diet.

certifier must inspect the farm where the food is grown or produced to ensure that the farmer is following the rules necessary to meet USDA organic standards. Companies that handle, process, or sell organic food must also be certified, but inspections and certifications are not required for farmers who sell less than $5,000 worth of foods each year. Thus, foods at local farmers' markets may claim to be organic but they may or may not meet standards.

Organically produced food is not considered to be more nutritious than conventionally produced food. A recent review reported significant health benefits in individuals consuming more organic foods; however, it is not possible to definitively attribute the outcomes to the way the food was produced. This is because individuals that consume organic foods tend to have healthier dietary practices overall and lower levels of overweight and obesity. However, consumers also choose organic foods to reduce exposure to pesticides and to support more sustainable and environmentally friendly agricultural practices. The climate crisis has further increased interest in regenerative and organic farming practices (see A Closer Look).

Gluten intolerance is a common dietary concern. *Gluten intolerance* is actually an umbrella term that can refer to a number of digestive health problems, including celiac disease and wheat allergies. Gluten is a family of proteins found in certain grains, but most people associate it with wheat. Gluten is responsible for the satisfying texture of baked goods, but some individuals report fatigue, headaches, and abdominal problems after eating foods with gluten. However, many people who think they are gluten intolerant actually are not. The prevalence of true glucose intolerance is about 1 percent of the population, but approximately 25–30 percent of the population report trying to avoid gluten. Some individuals have other challenges digesting carbohydrates (e.g., those with irritable bowel syndrome), but it is likely that many people avoid carbohydrates because of misconceptions or because they perceive it to be a healthier choice.

Use of genetically engineered foods is common, but labeling laws remain controversial. A genetically modified organism (GMO) is a plant, animal, or microorganism that has been altered so that its genetic structure (DNA) contains genes not typically found in the organism. GMOs have allowed increased crop yields because the organisms (e.g., corn, wheat, soybeans) are genetically modified to resist diseases, insects, heat, cold, and drought. GMOs have also been modified to have higher levels of some nutrients (e.g., calcium, folate, protein), and they provide us with innovations such as seedless grapes and watermelon. The scientific consensus is that the use of GMOs is completely safe and that the use of GMO technology is essential to maximize food production for the population. However, the issue of labeling is more contentious. New labeling laws will require a label on foods with specific levels of GMO ingredients and reference that it is *bioengineered*. The official ruling states that "bioengineered food . . . shall not be treated as safer, or not as safe as, a non-bioengineered counterpart." Thus, the new labels are simply designed to be informative and not indicative of safety or nutrition.

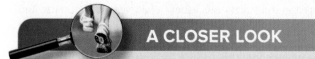

A CLOSER LOOK

Benefits of Regenerative Farming

A new movement in agriculture and farming offers promise for both improving soils and addressing climate change. Currently, agriculture accounts for more than 10 percent of U.S. greenhouse gas emissions. However, advocates of "regenerative farming" practices emphasize that it can actually help capture carbon in the soil, thereby helping reverse climate change. Regenerative farming is not a new idea but rather a traditional way of farming that focuses on enriching soil quality, improving watersheds, and rebuilding the natural ecosystem as part of the practice. A healthier landscape requires fewer pesticides and herbicides and prevents soil erosion. By building up soil microbes, carbon can also be trapped in the soil where it can be put back to good use. The evidence supporting the practice is clear but the challenges come in promoting and incentivizing widespread adoption.

Do the benefits of regenerative farming for climate change surprise you? Can consumers influence change by indirectly supporting regenerative farming practices?

HELP   Health is available to Everyone for a Lifetime, and it's Personal

What Do *Healthy* and *Natural* Really Mean?

Many food manufacturers label their products as *healthy* or *natural* to attract consumer interest. However, these terms may mean different things to different people. As nutritional guidelines change, the definitions of healthy foods have also shifted. The FDA has issued guidelines about the designation of *healthy* on food labels to help provide some form of standardized meaning, but it isn't regulated and enforced. There is also minimal guidance on the use of the term *natural*. Thus, consumers should be wary and check food labels and ingredients to make informed decisions.

Do the words healthy *or* natural *on a food product catch your attention when you shop? How do you make decisions about food products when given many options?*

Table 4 ▶ Comparing the Quality of Similar Food Products

Food Product	Less Desirable Option	More Desirable Option	Benefit of More Desirable Option in Nutrition Quality
Bread	White bread	Whole-wheat bread	More fiber
Rice	White rice	Brown rice	More fiber
Juice	Sweetened juice	100% juice	More fiber and less high fructose corn syrup
Fruit	Canned	Fresh	More vitamins, more fiber, less sugar
Vegetables	Canned	Fresh	More vitamins, less salt
Potatoes	French fries	Baked potato	Less saturated fat
Milk	2% milk	Skim milk	Less saturated fat
Meat	Ground beef (high fat)	Ground sirloin (low fat)	Less saturated fat
Oils	Vegetable oil	Canola oil	More monounsaturated fat
Snack food	Fried chips	Baked chips	Less fat/calorie content, less trans fat

Sound Eating Practices

Consistent eating patterns (with a daily breakfast) are important for good nutrition. Eating regular meals every day, including a good breakfast, is wise. Many studies have shown breakfast to be an important meal, but many people still skip it. Skipping breakfast impairs performance because blood sugar levels drop in the long period between dinner the night before and lunch the following day. Eating every 4 to 6 hours reduces risk of low blood sugar levels.

Minimize your consumption of overly processed foods. Several foods available in grocery stores have been highly processed to enhance shelf life and convenience. In many cases, the processing of foods removes valuable nutrients and includes other additives that may compromise overall nutrition. Processing of grains, for example, typically removes the bran and germ layers, which contain fiber and valuable minerals. In regard to additives, there has been considerable attention on the possible negative effects of high fructose corn syrup, as well as the pervasive use of hydrogenated vegetable oils containing trans fatty acids. Table 4 compares food quality in each of the main food categories. To improve your diet, you should aim to choose foods in the "more desirable" category instead of those in the "less desirable" category.

Moderation is a good general rule of nutrition. It is likely that some of your favorite foods may not be among the healthiest choices, but it is possible to still enjoy them in moderation. Eating smaller amounts of these foods or eating them less frequently is one way. 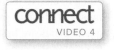 Balancing out high-calorie snacks or desserts with lower-calorie foods or meals is another good strategy.

Minimize your reliance on fast foods. Most consumers understand that many fast food options are relatively poor nutritional choices. Hamburgers are usually high in fat, as are french fries (because they are deep fat fried, often in saturated fat). Even chicken and fish 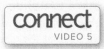 are often high in fat and calories because they may be cooked in fat and covered with high-fat/high-calorie sauces.

Shift toward a plant-based diet. Plant-based diets offer clear advantages for health. Current guidelines recommend that half of your plate should be filled with fruits and vegetables. A population shift toward a plant-based diet would also provide benefits to the environment. Conservative estimates indicate that livestock have a greater negative impact on greenhouse gas emissions than cars and trucks.

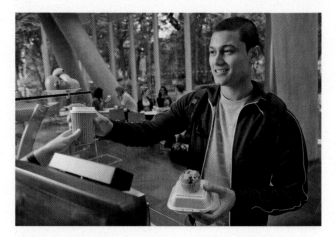

Healthy eating on campus requires good decision making.
Dirk Lindner/Image Source

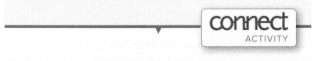

Technology Update

Start Simple with MyPlate

There are a variety of apps and web-based tools available to help consumers monitor their diet. However, many are overly complicated and tedious to use. The new USDA's Start Simple with MyPlate app offers a number of compelling, easy-to-use features to support healthy eating. Rather than focusing on tracking specific nutrients or portions, the app helps you set and monitor simple process-related goals (e.g., eating more fruit). The app includes tips to support your desired changes and built-in gaming features with basic challenges to reward your efforts and achievement of your goals over time. The app is also simple to use. (Visit www.myplate.gov or see the link in the Suggested Resources and Readings).

Have you used other apps to monitor your diet? Do you like the concept of the Start Simple app?

connect
ACTIVITY

Make better decisions when choosing snacks. Small snacks of appropriate foods can help maintain energy levels throughout the day. As with your total diet, the best snacks are nutritionally dense. Unfortunately, many widely available snack foods are high in calories, fats, simple sugar, and salt. Even foods sold as "healthy snacks," such as granola bars, are often high in fat and simple sugar. Some common snacks, such as chips, pretzels, and even popcorn, may be high in salt and may be cooked in fat. Look for options lower in salt or fat and consider other healthier snack options such as fresh fruits, vegetables, and nuts.

Nutrition and Physical Performance

Some basic dietary guidelines exist for active people. In general, the nutrition principles described in this Concept apply to all people, whether active or sedentary, but additional considerations apply to athletes and regular exercisers. Because active people often expend calories in amounts considerably above normal, they need extra calories in their diet. To avoid excess fat and protein, complex carbohydrates should constitute as much as 70 percent of total caloric intake. A higher amount of protein is generally recommended for active individuals (1.2 grams per kg of body weight) because some protein is used as an energy source during exercise. Extra protein is obtained in the additional calories consumed. Current protein guidelines range from 10 to 35 percent to provide flexibility but intakes above 15 percent are not typically necessary.

It is best to give your body time to digest foods before performing vigorous exercise. The body shunts blood to the digestive system to process the food we eat, so cramping may occur if you try to exercise too soon after eating. Athletes learn to select foods on the basis of experience, but easily digested carbohydrates are generally well tolerated. Fat intake should be minimal because fat digests more slowly; proteins and high-cellulose foods should be kept to a moderate amount prior to prolonged events to avoid urinary and bowel excretion. Drinking fluids with meals and prior to exercise is important to ensure adequate hydration. The consumption of simple carbohydrates (e.g., candy or sugary drinks) immediately prior to exercise is not recommended since it can lead to spikes in blood sugar that negatively influence performance.

Carbohydrate intake is important for endurance athletes. Athletes and vigorously active people must maintain a high level of readily available fuel to perform aerobic exercise. Consumption of complex carbohydrates is the best way to ensure this. Athletes competing in endurance events lasting more than 2 hours (e.g., marathon) consume high-carbohydrate foods 1 or 2 days before an event, a strategy known as **carbohydrate loading.** This helps build up maximum levels of stored carbohydrate (**glycogen**) in the muscles and liver so it can be used during exercise. The key in carbohydrate loading is not to eat a lot but, rather, to eat a higher percentage of carbohydrates than normal.

Ingesting carbohydrate beverages during sustained exercise can also aid performance by preventing or delaying muscle glycogen depletion. Fluid-replacement drinks containing 6–8 percent carbohydrates are very helpful in preventing dehydration and replacing energy stores. A number of companies also make concentrated carbohydrate gels that can be easily consumed during exercise (e.g., Powergel and Gu). Energy bars, such as Powerbars and Clif bars, are also commonly eaten during or after exercise to enhance energy stores. The consumption of supplemental carbohydrates has been shown to enhance performance in events longer than an hour but do not help for shorter bouts. To most effectively rebuild glycogen stores, it is best to consume carbohydrates 30–60 minutes after completing a workout or race. However, research has also documented the importance of replacing proteins since they play a role in regulating fuel consumption and energy production. The best recommendation is to consume nutrient-dense foods containing carbohydrates and protein to enhance recovery.

The frequency and composition of meals are important to gain muscle mass. To increase muscle mass, the body requires a greater caloric intake. The challenge is to provide enough extra calories for the muscle without excess amounts going to fat. An increase of 500–1,000 calories a day will help most people gain muscle mass over time. Smaller, more frequent meals are best for weight gain, since they tend to keep the metabolic rate high. The majority of extra calories should come from complex carbohydrates. Breads, pasta, rice, and fruits such as bananas are good sources. Granola, nuts, juices

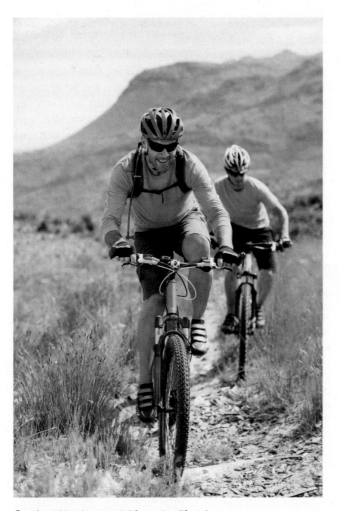

Good nutrition is essential for active lifestyles.
Paul Bradbury/Tony Talle/Alamy Stock Photo

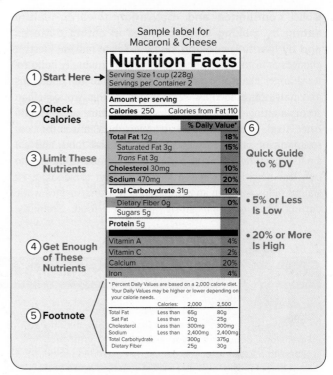

Figure 4 ▶ Tips for reading a food label (sample based on macaroni and cheese dinner).
Source: U.S. Food and Drug Administration.

(grape and cranberry), and milk also make good high-calorie, healthy snacks.

Protein supplements are marketed to strength athletes interested in gaining muscle but are not particularly effective. The body doesn't have a way to store extra protein, so extra protein is just converted to other fuels. As discussed in the Concept on Muscle Fitness and Resistance Exercise, there are no shortcuts to gaining muscle mass and body weight. Following the recommended training principles and a healthy diet remain the best approach.

Using Self-Management Skills

Build a base of nutrition knowledge and apply consumer skills to make more informed food choices. One of the best ways to enhance your nutrition knowledge and improve your eating patterns is to pay attention to food labels at grocery stores and nutrition content posted on restaurant menus. Reading food labels helps you be more aware of what you are eating and can help you make healthier choices when shopping for foods or dining out. The sample

label in Figure 4 highlights key nutritional information emphasized in the new dietary guidelines and described in this Concept. Try to get in the habit of evaluating and comparing foods based on "added sugar" or the percentage of saturated fat content. Research has supported the utility of the labels for enhancing consumer awareness, but you have to commit to reviewing the label to personally benefit.

Apply self-monitoring skills and relapse prevention skills to stay focused on healthy eating patterns. Making healthy food choices over time requires good self-management skills and a commitment to use them. In most cases, the unhealthy choice is the easier, tastier, and cheaper option, so restraint and self-control are very important. Learning to self-monitor (and regulate) aspects of your diet can help you make better decisions on a daily basis. For example, tracking fruit and vegetable consumption during the day can help you develop habits that include more of these foods. Relapse prevention skills can help remind you that a "diet" refers to a healthy pattern of eating. It is perfectly normal (and healthy) to incorporate sweets and desserts into your diet as long as you maintain a healthy overall pattern of eating over time.

Carbohydrate Loading The extra consumption of complex carbohydrates in the days prior to sustained performance.

Glycogen A source of energy stored in the muscles and liver necessary for sustained physical activity.

Build confidence and motivation toward healthy eating by making small changes in eating patterns and by learning cooking skills. A key to making lifestyle changes is to focus on small changes that gradually build toward larger changes over time. The many recommendations and nutrition guidelines summarized in this Concept can seem daunting, but the principles of good nutrition are pretty basic (e.g., eat more fruits and vegetables, minimize consumption of saturated fat, consume less fast food, and eat smaller portions). Making a positive choice can often lead to one less negative choice. Substituting fruit for cookies or snacks helps you gain an extra serving of fruits/veggies while cutting back on high-calorie, processed food. Similarly, cooking one more meal at home can translate to one fewer meal at a fast food restaurant.

As you make a few small changes you will notice that you may be more open to others. For example, if you start eating brown rice, you might find that it has more flavor and better texture than white rice. Similarly, shifting to products with lower fat (e.g., skim milk instead of 2 percent milk) or low-added sugar (e.g., 100 percent juice instead of juice drinks), may shift your palate and preferences to healthier options. By taking small steps to cook for yourself, you can also gain a deeper understanding of food and a greater appreciation for the ingredients that go into it. Like other skills, cooking skills take time to develop, but they can be learned and improved over time with practice.

Strategies for Action: Lab Information

An analysis of your current diet is a good first step in making future decisions about what you eat. Many experts recommend keeping a log of what you eat over an extended period, so you can determine the overall quality of your diet. In Lab 14A, you will have an opportunity to track your diet over several days. In addition to computing the amount of carbohydrates, fats, and proteins, you will also be able to monitor your consumption of fruits and vegetables. A number of online tools and personal software programs can make dietary calculations for you and provide a more comprehensive report of nutrient intake. Whether you use a web-based tool or a paper-and-pencil log doesn't really matter—the key is to monitor and evaluate the quality of your diet.

Making small changes in diet patterns can have a big impact. Nutrition experts emphasize the importance of making small changes in your diet over time rather than trying to make comprehensive changes at one time. Try cutting back on sweets or soft drinks. Adding a few more fruits and vegetables to your diet can also lead to lower consumption of less healthy foods and improve the overall diet quality. In Lab 14B, you will be given the opportunity to compare a "nutritious diet" to a "favorite diet." Analyzing two daily meal plans will help you get a more accurate picture as to whether foods that you think are nutritious actually meet current healthy lifestyle goals.

connect
ACTIVITY

Suggested Resources and Readings

The websites for the following sources can be accessed by searching online for the organization, program, or title listed. Specific scientific references are available at the end of this edition of *Concepts of Fitness and Wellness.*

- Academy of Nutrition and Dietetics. Eatright. Functional Foods.
- American Heart Association. Saturated Fat.
- Center for Science in the Public Interest. Eating Healthy.
- Centers for Disease Control and Prevention. Get the Facts: Added Sugars and Consumption.
- Hamdy, O. (2021, March 9). "How Are Fat Substitutes Such As Olestra (Olean) Used to Prevent Obesity?" *Medscape.*
- International Food Information Council Foundation.
- Link, R. (2020, January 17). "What Are Functional Foods? All You Need to Know." *Healthline.*
- McEvoy, M. (2019, March 13). "Organic 101. What the USDA Organic Label Means." U.S. Department of Agriculture.
- Meier, B., Dillard, A., & Lappas, C. (2019, August 2)."Why the Term 'Natural' Is So Seductive—and Possibly Misleading." *Stat+.*
- Nourish by WebMD.
- Olatunbosun, S. T. (2020, July 8). "What Is Glucose Intolerance?" *Medscape.*
- U.S. Department of Agriculture. History of the *Dietary Guidelines.*
- U.S. Department of Agriculture. *Start Simple with MyPlate* App.
- U.S. Department of Agriculture and U.S. Department of Health and Human Services. (2020). *Dietary Guidelines for Americans, 2020-2025,* 9th ed. (pdf)
- U.S. Department of Health and Human Services. FoodSafety.gov.
- The Vegan Society. Statistics.

Lab 14A Nutrition Analysis

Name	**Section**	**Date**

Purpose: To learn to keep a dietary log, to determine the nutritional quality of your diet, to determine your average daily caloric intake, and to determine necessary changes in eating habits.

Procedures

1. Record your dietary intake for 2 days using the Daily Diet Record sheets that follow. Record intake for 1 weekday and 1 weekend day. You may wish to make extra copies for future use.
2. Include the actual foods eaten and the amount (size of portion in teaspoons, tablespoons, cups, ounces, or other standard units of measurement). Be sure to include all drinks (coffee, tea, soft drinks, etc.). Include *all* foods eaten, including sauces, gravies, dressings, toppings, spreads, and so on. Estimate your caloric consumption for each of the 2 days using the information in Appendix B. Various online tools and apps are available for use by consumers and these could also be used. An online search using a statement such as "calorie content of ___" can also help in capturing data on food.
3. List the number of servings from each food group by each food choice.
4. Estimate the proportion of complex carbohydrate, simple carbohydrate, protein, and fat in each meal and in snacks, as well as for the total day.
5. Answer the questions in Chart 1 using information for a typical day based on the Daily Diet Record sheets. Score 1 point for each "yes" answer. Then use Chart 2 to rate your dietary habits (circle rating).
6. Complete the Conclusions and Implications section.

Results

Record the number of calories consumed for each of the 2 days.

Weekday [   ] calories   Weekend [   ] calories

Conclusions and Implications: In several sentences, discuss your diet as recorded in this lab. Explain any changes in your eating habits that may be necessary. Comment on whether the days you surveyed are typical of your normal diet.

Chart 1 Dietary Habits Questionnaire

Yes	No	Answer questions based on a typical day (use your Daily Diet Records to help).
○	○	1. Do you eat at least three healthy meals each day?
○	○	2. Do you eat a healthy breakfast?
○	○	3. Do you eat lunch regularly?
○	○	4. Does your diet contain 45–65 percent carbohydrates with a high concentration of fiber?*
○	○	5. Are less than one-fourth of the carbohydrates you eat simple carbohydrates?
○	○	6. Does your diet contain 10–35 percent protein?*
○	○	7. Does your diet contain 20–35 percent fat?*
○	○	8. Do you limit the amount of saturated fat in your diet (no more than 10 percent)?
○	○	9. Do you limit salt intake to acceptable amounts?
○	○	10. Do you get adequate amounts of vitamins in your diet without a supplement?
○	○	11. Do you typically eat 6–11 servings from the bread, cereal, rice, and pasta group of foods?
○	○	12. Do you typically eat 3–5 servings of vegetables?
○	○	13. Do you typically eat 2–4 servings of fruits?
○	○	14. Do you typically eat 2–3 servings from the milk, yogurt, and cheese group of foods?
○	○	15. Do you typically eat 2–3 servings from the meat, poultry, fish, beans, eggs, and nuts group of foods?
○	○	16. Do you drink adequate amounts of water?
○	○	17. Do you get adequate minerals in your diet without a supplement?
○	○	18. Do you limit your caffeine and alcohol consumption to acceptable levels?
○	○	19. Is your average caloric consumption reasonable for your body size and for the amount of calories you normally expend?
		Total number of "yes" answers

*Based on USDA standards.

Chart 2 Dietary Habits Rating Scale

Score	Rating
18–19	Very good
15–17	Good
13–14	Marginal
12 or less	Poor

Daily Diet Record

Day 1

Breakfast Food	Amount (cups, tsp., etc.)	Calories	Food Servings				Estimated Meal Calories %
			Bread/Cereal	Fruit/Veg.	Milk/Meat	Fat/Sweet	
							☐ % Protein
							☐ % Fat
							☐ % Complex carbohydrate
							☐ % Simple carbohydrate
							100% Total
Meal Total	✕						

Lunch Food	Amount (cups, tsp., etc.)	Calories	Food Servings				Estimated Meal Calories %
			Bread/Cereal	Fruit/Veg.	Milk/Meat	Fat/Sweet	
							☐ % Protein
							☐ % Fat
							☐ % Complex carbohydrate
							☐ % Simple carbohydrate
							100% Total
Meal Total	✕						

Dinner Food	Amount (cups, tsp., etc.)	Calories	Food Servings				Estimated Meal Calories %
			Bread/Cereal	Fruit/Veg.	Milk/Meat	Fat/Sweet	
							☐ % Protein
							☐ % Fat
							☐ % Complex carbohydrate
							☐ % Simple carbohydrate
							100% Total
Meal Total	✕						

Snack Food	Amount (cups, tsp., etc.)	Calories	Food Servings				Estimated Snack Calories %
			Bread/Cereal	Fruit/Veg.	Milk/Meat	Fat/Sweet	
							☐ % Protein
							☐ % Fat
							☐ % Complex carbohydrate
							☐ % Simple carbohydrate
Meal Total							**100% Total**

Estimated Daily Total Calories %

☐ % Protein
☐ % Fat
☐ % Complex carbohydrate
☐ % Simple carbohydrate
100% Total

Daily Totals	✕						
		Calories	Servings	Servings	Servings	Servings	

Daily Diet Record

Day 2

Breakfast Food	Amount (cups, tsp., etc.)	Calories	Food Servings				Estimated Meal Calories %
			Bread/Cereal	Fruit/Veg.	Milk/Meat	Fat/Sweet	
							☐ % Protein
							☐ % Fat
							☐ % Complex carbohydrate
							☐ % Simple carbohydrate
							100% Total
Meal Total	✕						

Lunch Food	Amount (cups, tsp., etc.)	Calories	Food Servings				Estimated Meal Calories %
			Bread/Cereal	Fruit/Veg.	Milk/Meat	Fat/Sweet	
							☐ % Protein
							☐ % Fat
							☐ % Complex carbohydrate
							☐ % Simple carbohydrate
							100% Total
Meal Total	✕						

Dinner Food	Amount (cups, tsp., etc.)	Calories	Food Servings				Estimated Meal Calories %
			Bread/Cereal	Fruit/Veg.	Milk/Meat	Fat/Sweet	
							☐ % Protein
							☐ % Fat
							☐ % Complex carbohydrate
							☐ % Simple carbohydrate
							100% Total
Meal Total	✕						

Snack Food	Amount (cups, tsp., etc.)	Calories	Food Servings				Estimated Snack Calories %
			Bread/Cereal	Fruit/Veg.	Milk/Meat	Fat/Sweet	
							☐ % Protein
							☐ % Fat
							☐ % Complex carbohydrate
							☐ % Simple carbohydrate
							100% Total
Meal Total							**Estimated Daily Total Calories %**
Daily Totals	✕						☐ % Protein
		Calories	Servings	Servings	Servings	Servings	☐ % Fat
							☐ % Complex carbohydrate
							☐ % Simple carbohydrate
							100% Total

Lab 14B Selecting Nutritious Foods

Name		Section	Date

Purpose: To learn to select a nutritious diet, to determine the nutritive value of favorite foods, and to compare nutritious and favorite foods in terms of nutrient content.

Procedures

1. Select a favorite breakfast, lunch, and dinner from the foods list in Appendix B. Include between-meal snacks with the nearest meal. If you cannot find foods you would normally choose, select those most similar to choices you might make. Calorie and nutrient information is also available in NutritionCalc Plus, a diet analysis tool available in Connect. Launch it by clicking the NutritionCalc Plus link on the Resources list on your Connect class home page.
2. Select a breakfast, lunch, and dinner from foods you feel would make the most nutritious meals. Include between-meal snacks with the nearest meal.
3. Record your "favorite foods" and "nutritious foods" in the "Favorite" Versus "Nutritious" Food Choices for Three Daily Meals chart that follows. Record the calories for proteins, carbohydrates, and fats for each of the foods you choose.
4. Total each column for the "favorite" and the "nutritious" meals.
5. Determine the percentages of your total calories that are protein, carbohydrates, and fat by dividing each column total by the total number of calories consumed.
6. Comment on what you learned in the Conclusions and Implications section.

Results: Record your results. Calculate percentage of calories from each source by dividing total calories into calories from each food source (protein, carbohydrates, or fat).

Food Selection Results

Source	Favorite Foods Calories	Favorite Foods % of Total Calories	Nutritious Foods Calories	Nutritious Foods % of Total Calories
Protein				
Carbohydrates				
Fat				
Total 100%		100%		100%

Conclusions and Implications: In several sentences, discuss the differences you found between your nutritious diet and your favorite diet. Discuss the quality of your nutritious diet as well as other things you learned from doing this lab.

"Favorite" Versus "Nutritious" Food Choices for Three Daily Meals

Breakfast Favorite	Food Choices				Breakfast Nutritious	Food Choices			
Food	Cal.	Prot. Cal.	Carb. Cal.	Fat Cal.	Food	Cal.	Prot. Cal.	Carb. Cal.	Fat Cal.
Totals					Totals				

Lunch Favorite	Food Choices				Lunch Nutritious	Food Choices			
Food	Cal.	Prot. Cal.	Carb. Cal.	Fat Cal.	Food	Cal.	Prot. Cal.	Carb. Cal.	Fat Cal.
Totals					Totals				

Dinner Favorite	Food Choices				Dinner Nutritious	Food Choices			
Food	Cal.	Prot. Cal.	Carb. Cal.	Fat Cal.	Food	Cal.	Prot. Cal.	Carb. Cal.	Fat Cal.
Totals					Totals				
Daily Totals (Calories)					Daily Totals (Calories)				
Daily % of Total Calories					Daily % of Total Calories				

Principles of Effective Weight Control

LEARNING OBJECTIVES

After completing the study of this Concept, you will be able to:

► Explain the principles for weight control and the concept of energy balance.

► Identify the features of an obesogenic environment that influence our behavior.

► Outline guidelines for weight loss treatments.

► Describe and apply, when appropriate, guidelines for losing body fat.

► Utilize healthy shopping and eating strategies and guidelines.

► Evaluate fast food options.

Various management strategies for eating and performing physical activity are useful in achieving and maintaining optimal body composition.

Jack Hollingsworth/Blend Images LLC

Why It Matters!

The fact that nearly 70 percent of adult Americans are classified as overweight or obese is evidence that weight control is a vexing problem for the majority of the population. People often resort to fad diets or follow flawed advice or regimens they see online or in consumer magazines. Too often the focus is placed on appearance and "weight loss" rather than on health and fat loss. In attempts to lose weight, the energy intake side of the energy balance equation (i.e., eating) is typically emphasized to a greater extent than the energy expenditure side of the equation (i.e., physical activity). Effective long-term weight control requires the adoption of healthy eating patterns *and* regular physical activity. This Concept will separate fact from fiction and provide strategies to help you establish lifestyles conducive to long-term weight control. Following appropriate lifestyle practices may not allow you to achieve the body you want, but it can promote health and wellness and help you attain a size appropriate for your genetics and body type.

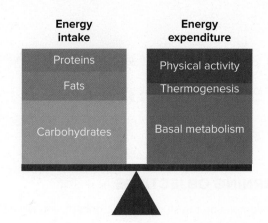

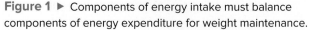

Figure 1 ▶ Components of energy intake must balance components of energy expenditure for weight maintenance.

Factors Influencing Weight and Fat Control

Long-term weight control requires a balance between energy intake and energy expenditure. The relationships governing energy balance are very simple: the number of calories expended must match the number consumed. There may be subtle differences on a daily basis, but if intake exceeds expenditure over a period of time, a person will store the extra calories as body fat. The average person gains 1 pound of weight (i.e., fat) for every year over the age of 25. This may sound like a lot—or a little—depending on your perspective. However, when extrapolated across a year, it represents a calorie difference of only 10 kcal per day (approximately the calories found in a cracker or potato chip). This subtle difference shows the precise regulation of intake and expenditure that is normally in effect when a person maintains his or her body weight. The built-in regulation system is based on our appetite, which guides us when we might be running low on energy.

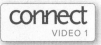

Energy intake comes from the three major nutrients in our diet (carbohydrates, fats, and proteins) as well as from alcohol. Energy expenditure can be divided into three major components as well. Basal metabolism accounts for the bulk of daily energy expenditure (60–75 percent) and this refers to the calories expended to maintain basic body functions

while the body is at rest. A second category, called thermogenesis, captures the energy expended processing the food we eat (approximately 10 percent of total daily energy expenditure). The third and most variable component of energy expenditure rate is physical activity (typically accounting for 10–30 percent of total energy expenditure in most people). To maintain a healthy weight, a person's overall energy expenditure must offset energy intake. Figure 1 shows the hypothetical balance between energy intake and expenditure.

A basic understanding of your overall calorie needs is important for weight control. Calorie requirements are unique to each person and are influenced by your gender, age, body size, and physical activity level. A simple but crude estimate of your **basal metabolic rate (BMR)** is about 10 calories per pound of body weight. For a 150-pound person, the contribution of basal metabolism (as shown in Figure 1) would be approximately 1,500 calories. If you have a moderately active lifestyle, you can multiply your BMR by 1.75 to provide a reasonable estimate of your total daily energy expenditure. Using the example, your total daily energy needs would be approximately 2,625 calories (i.e., $1,500 \times 1.75 = 2,625$). The World Health Organization refers to this multiplier value as a *physical activity level (PAL)*. Sedentary people typically have PAL values ranging from 1.4 to 1.7 while moderately active people might have PAL values ranging from 1.7 to 2.0. Your personal needs will depend on your actual activity level, which can vary from day to day. This method is intended to give you a basic estimate to guide weight control efforts. For example, you may think twice about that 1,000-calorie sandwich after realizing that it accounts for almost 40 percent of your daily calorie needs. To estimate your energy expenditure more precisely, refer to Lab 13C in the Concept on body composition.

Physical activity contributes to energy balance in a number of ways. By maintaining an active lifestyle, you can burn off extra calories, keep your body's metabolism high, and prevent the decline in basal metabolic rate that typically occurs with aging (due to reduced muscle mass). All types of physical activity can be beneficial to weight control. Moderate physical activity is especially effective because people of all ages and abilities can perform it. It can be maintained for long periods of time and results in significant calorie expenditure. Long-term studies show that 60 or more minutes of moderate activity such as walking is very effective for long-term weight loss and maintenance.

Vigorous physical activity can also be effective in maintaining or losing weight since it burns more calories throughout the day. This contributes to additional energy expenditure after the workout is done. There is now considerable evidence showing that muscle fitness exercise also contributes to maintaining a healthy body weight. Muscle fitness exercise expends calories and increases muscle mass, leading to an increase in basal metabolic rate. Clearly, all forms of physical activity can contribute to long-term weight control.

The accumulation of light physical activity can help burn extra calories. Most of the emphasis thus far has been on moderate and vigorous forms of physical activity. The category of "light" physical activity falls between rest and moderate physical activity on the energy expenditure continuum (1.5–3 METs). Research indicates that light activities may help reduce risks associated with excessive time spent being sedentary (e.g., sitting). The accumulation of light activity can also contribute to weight control by burning more calories. As noted in an earlier Concept, the term **NEAT (non-exercise activity thermogenesis)** is often used to refer to the accumulation of activity from low-intensity movements throughout the day. Light activity may account for as little as 15 percent of total daily energy expenditure in sedentary people and up to 50 percent in people with more active jobs and lifestyles. The weight maintenance benefits of light or NEAT activity are greatest when the activities replace sedentary activities such as sitting (e.g., TV watching and computer use). To further take advantage of NEAT, many people have started using active workstations that allow them to walk slowly on a treadmill or lightly pedal a bike while working at a computer.

Paying attention to appetite and hunger can help in weight control. The body has built-in regulatory systems that help in weight regulation. Hunger and appetite are the cues that should regulate calorie intake, but many people develop unhealthy habits and eat when they are not hungry. For example, food is often consumed as a source of comfort when feeling sad, anxious, or bored. This has been termed *emotional eating* since the consumption of food is directly tied to our emotions. Recent research has shown that a number of other factors influence our appetite and our food intake. For example, studies demonstrate that lack of sleep can alter hormones that regulate appetite. Learning about the factors that influence your personal eating patterns can help with long-term weight control (see In the News).

Basal Metabolic Rate (BMR) The minimal number of calories needed to perform your body's most basic (basal) functions (typically expressed and assessed as resting metabolic rate).

Non-Exercise Activity Thermogenesis (NEAT) Caloric expenditure attributed to the accumulation of light activity, such as standing.

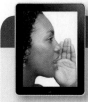

In the News

Strategies for Avoiding Emotional Eating

Emotional eating (characterized as eating in response to stress or an emotional state rather than to hunger) proved to be a major contributor to weight gain during the COVID-19 pandemic. While the isolation and time at home enabled some to adopt healthier eating habits, many found it harder to eat well and to maintain a healthy weight. Experts suggest that it is a normal response to confinement and not a sign of weakness. Learning how to make healthy food choices under challenging situations can help you build capacity for improved weight control in the future.

Did you experience challenges with emotional eating during the COVID-19 pandemic? What insights did you gain from your own experiences that might help with future weight control efforts?

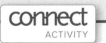

Confronting an Obesogenic Environment

An obesogenic environment makes it hard to maintain a healthy weight. While weight control is a personal issue, your ability to maintain a healthy weight is also strongly influenced by various environmental factors. The notion of social determinants of health and the Social-Ecological Model were introduced in the Concept on the determinants of lifelong health, wellness, and fitness. A simplified model is depicted in Figure 2 to show the specific environmental factors that influence weight control. The essence of the model is that we are continually confronted with environments that make it easy to consume large quantities of energy-dense food and limit our physical activity. On the energy-intake side, we have easy access to large quantities of low-cost, highly palatable, high-calorie foods almost everywhere we go. The convenience and large portion sizes lead to increases in daily energy intake. On the energy-expenditure side, we live in a world dominated by sedentary (computer-based) jobs and lifestyles dominated by automobiles and inactive recreation. These factors lead to reductions in daily energy expenditure. Small increases in energy intake combined with small decreases in energy expenditure lead to the storage of fat. While most people are aware of these general influences, it can still be hard to find ways to overcome them. Surprisingly, evidence suggests that food insecurity (i.e., lack of food availability because of inadequate resources) also contributes to obesity (see A Closer Look).

Societal changes are needed to create healthier environments. As shown in Figure 2, aspects of our environment are influenced by larger societal and economic forces. For example, it is unrealistic to expect changes in menu choices

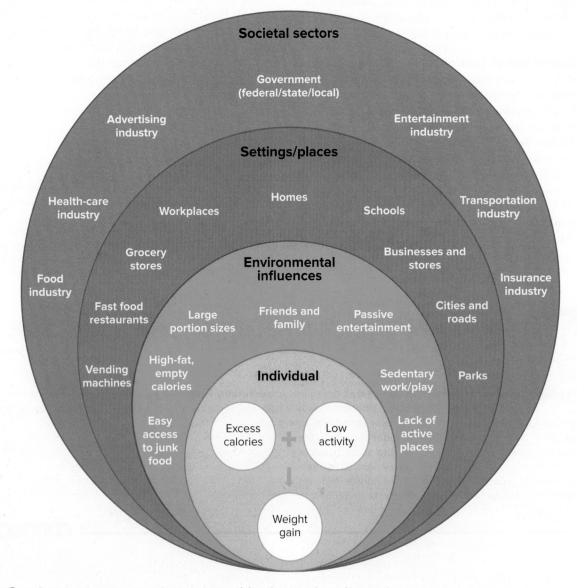

Figure 2 ▶ Social and environmental components of the obesogenic environment.

A CLOSER LOOK

Food Insecurity and Obesity

Food insecurity refers to a lack of adequate food due to inadequate resources. It may be hard to accept that food insecurity exists in a culture characterized by seemingly easy access to food. However, approximately 1 in 10 families in the United States reports sometimes not having enough food to eat. And what may seem even more surprising is that food insecurity has also been directly linked with obesity, primarily attributed to the fact that the cheapest and most accessible foods are often the least healthy. Although food insecurity is most directly caused by unemployment or financial constraints, it can also be due to a lack of access or mobility challenges.

Does it surprise you that food insecurity is linked to obesity? What does this suggest about how our environment influences our lifestyles?

connect
ACTIVITY

in a local fast food restaurant since it receives its food from the corporate supply chain, which in turn receives ingredients from other larger food conglomerates. To reverse the epidemic of obesity, experts contend that coordinated systemwide approaches are needed. Examples of recent or pending public policy changes aimed at addressing obesity are listed. (Also see the Trust for America's Health 2020 report in the Suggested Resources and Readings for more information.)

- *Posting nutritional content on menus in restaurants.* Legislation by the FDA requires chain restaurants to post calorie and other nutrition values for the foods they serve. The FDA has also extended the labeling rules to vending machines. Posting food values has been shown to be effective in reducing calorie consumption in people eating at fast food restaurants.

- *Improving access to healthy food in schools.* Policy guidelines from the USDA have improved quality and access to healthy school lunches, imposed restrictions on available foods in vending machines, and banned marketing of junk food in schools and on sports scoreboards. Results have shown promising increases in fruit and vegetable consumption with reduced food waste.

- *Incentivizing businesses to increase access to healthy food options and safe places to be physically active.* Components of the Affordable Care Act have been aimed at providing incentives to worksites that adopt worksite wellness programming. These efforts can benefit individual employees and also companies by enhancing employee productivity and controlling health-care costs.

- *Implementing taxes or subsidies to encourage healthier food choices.* There have been numerous calls and proposals for

a tax on foods low in nutritional density, such as sweetened soft drinks, candy, and fast food. Advocates of this type of tax propose that the proceeds go to campaigns to improve nutrition and increase activity levels, but others argue that policy changes such as "soda taxes" or "fat taxes" infringe on personal liberties. Subsidies to reduce costs of healthier foods is also an option that would more directly incentivize healthier choices.

- *Including bolder statements and communication on food labels.* Research has supported the effectiveness of revised food labels on promoting awareness of healthy eating. For example, the larger font showing calorie content of foods may help people reconsider choosing high-calorie foods. Some health experts have proposed further additions that would report the amount of physical activity needed to burn off the calories. For example, a food label for a candy bar that shows 200 calories in the serving would be accompanied by a note that it would take 37 minutes of brisk walking to expend the 200 calories. This is not likely to take effect anytime soon, but remembering this type of conversion may help in resisting extra snacks.

Guidelines for Losing Body Fat

Following appropriate weight loss guidelines is important for the best long-term results. Fat, weight, and body proportions are all factors that can be changed, but people often set goals that are impossible to achieve. Starting with small goals and aiming 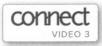 for reasonable rates of weight loss (1 to 2 pounds a week) are recommended. Setting unrealistic goals may result in eating disorders, failure to meet goals, or failure to maintain weight loss over time. Table 1 provides a summary of weight loss guidelines from the American College of Sports Medicine.

Process (behavioral) goals are more effective than product (outcome) goals. Many people make weight loss goals based on the amount of weight they want to lose or the size they want to attain. However, focusing only on **outcome goals** can lead to frustration if the targets aren't achieved as quickly as hoped. A focus on **behavioral goals** is more effective since it is within your control. By targeting specific diet changes or setting specific goals for physical activity, you will have better long-term success, even if the outcome goal of weight loss comes at a slower rate than desired.

Outcome Goal Statement of intent to achieve a specific test score or a specific standard associated with good health or wellness—for example, "I will lower my body fat level by 3 percent."

Behavioral Goal Statement of intent to perform a specific behavior (changing a lifestyle) for a specific period of time—for example, "I will reduce the calories in my diet by 200 a day for the next 4 weeks."

Table 1 ▶ Guidelines for Weight Loss—Common Questions

Questions	Recommendations
Who should consider weight loss?	Individuals with a BMI of >25 or in the marginal or overfat zone should consider reducing their body weight—especially if it is accompanied by abdominal obesity. Individuals with a BMI of >30 are encouraged to seek weight loss treatment.
What types of goals should be used?	Overweight and obese individuals should target reducing their body weight by a minimum of 5–10 percent and should aim to maintain this long-term weight loss.
What about maintenance?	Individuals should strive for long-term weight maintenance and the prevention of weight regain over the long term, especially when weight loss is not desired or when attainment of ideal body weight is not achievable.
What should be targeted in a program?	Weight loss programs should target both eating and exercise behaviors, as sustained changes in both behaviors have been associated with significant long-term weight loss.
How should diet be changed?	Overweight and obese individuals should reduce their current intake by 500–1,000 kcal/day to achieve weight loss (<30 percent of calories from fat). Individualized levels of caloric intake should be established to prevent weight regain after initial loss.
How should activity be changed?	Overweight and obese individuals should progressively increase to a minimum of 150 minutes of moderate-intensity physical activity per week for health benefits. However, for long-term weight loss, the program should progress to higher amounts of activity (e.g., 200–300 minutes per week or >2,000 kcal/week).
What about resistance exercise?	Resistance exercise should supplement the endurance exercise program for individuals undertaking modest reductions in energy intake to lose weight.
What about using drugs for weight loss?	Pharmacotherapy (medicine/drugs) for weight loss should be used only by individuals with a BMI >30 or those with excessive body fatness. Weight loss medications should be used only in combination with a strong behavioral intervention that focuses on modifying eating and exercise behaviors.

Source: American College of Sports Medicine.

A combination of physical activity and a healthy, low-calorie diet is the best approach for long-term weight control. The most effective diet for fat loss is a low-calorie diet that you can stick with over time. Reduced-calorie diets result in meaningful weight loss, regardless of the composition of the diet (e.g., carbohydrates, fats, proteins). Diets high in grains, fruits, and vegetables are generally recommended because they are typically low in calories and easy to maintain over time. Research also clearly indicates that regular exercise is crucial to long-term fat loss. Weight loss programs that do not include physical activity are likely to fail.

A major advantage of physical activity in a weight loss program is that it can help maintain basal metabolic rate and prevent the decline that occurs with calorie sparing. Studies have shown that programs that include physical activity promote greater loss of body fat than programs based solely on dietary changes. The total weight loss from the programs may be about the same, but a larger fraction of the weight comes from fat when physical activity is included. In contrast, programs based solely on diet result in greater loss of lean muscle tissue. A healthy diet and regular physical activity are both essential for long-term weight control. Small changes, such as eating a few hundred calories less per day or walking for 30 minutes every day, can make a big difference over time. The important point is to strive for permanent changes that can be maintained in a normal daily lifestyle (see Table 1).

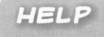 **Health is available to Everyone for a Lifetime, and it's Personal**

What Is the Secret for Long-Term Weight Control?

The National Weight Control Registry (NWCR) has tracked behaviors and outcomes for more than 10,000 people who have lost significant amounts of weight—and have kept it off. Insights from NWCR annual surveys are used to identify key strategies used by those people who have been successful in maintaining their weight loss. While there are a variety of reported strategies, most success stories include a low-calorie, low-fat diet and a high amount of physical activity. Approximately 78 percent eat breakfast every day, 75 percent weigh themselves at least once a week, 62 percent watch less than 10 hours of TV per week, and 90 percent exercise, on average, about 1 hour per day. Search "National Weight Control Registry" online to learn more.

What strategies do you find most helpful for maintaining a healthy weight?

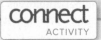

Table 2 ▶ Guidelines for Healthy Shopping and Eating in a Variety of Settings

Guidelines for Shopping	• Shop from a list to avoid purchasing foods that contain empty calories and other foods that will tempt you to overeat. • Shop with a friend to avoid buying unneeded foods. For this technique to work, the other person must be sensitive to your goals. In some cases, a friend can have a bad, rather than a good, influence. • Shop on a full stomach to avoid the temptations of snacking on and buying junk food. • Check labels to avoid foods that are excessively high in fat or saturated fat.
Guidelines for How You Eat	• When you eat, do nothing else but eat. If you watch television, read, or do some other activity while you eat, you may be unaware of what you have eaten. • Eat slowly. Taste your food. Pause between bites. Chew slowly. Do not take the next bite until you have swallowed what you have in your mouth. Periodically take a longer pause. Be the last one finished eating. • Do not eat food you do not want. Some people do not want to waste food, so they clean their plate even when they feel full. • Follow an eating schedule. Eating at regular meal times can help you avoid snacking. Spacing meals equally throughout the day can help reduce appetite. • Leave the table after eating to avoid taking extra, unwanted bites and servings. • Eat meals of equal size. Some people try to restrict calories at one or two meals to save up for a big meal. Eating several small meals helps you avoid hunger (fools the appetite), and this may help prevent overeating. • Avoid second servings. Limit your intake to one moderate serving. If second servings are taken, make them one-half the size of first servings. • Limit servings of salad dressings and condiments (e.g., catsup). These are often high in fat and sugar and can amount to greater caloric consumption than expected.
Guidelines for Controlling the Home Environment	• Store food out of sight. Avoid containers that allow you to see food. Limit the accessibility of foods that tempt you and foods with empty calories. Foods that are out of sight are out of mouth. • Do your eating in designated areas only, such as the kitchen and dining room, so you do not snack elsewhere. It is especially easy to eat too much while watching television. • If you snack, eat foods high in complex carbohydrates and low in fats, such as fresh fruits and carrot sticks. • Freeze leftovers so that it takes preparation to eat them, helping you avoid temptation.
Guidelines for Controlling the Work Environment	• Bring food from home rather than eating from vending machines or catering trucks. • Do not eat while working and take your lunch as a break. Do something active during breaks, such as taking a walk. • Avoid food provided by coworkers, such as snacks in work rooms, birthday cakes, or candy. • Have drinking water or low-calorie drinks available to substitute for snacks.
Guidelines for Eating on Special Occasions	• Practice ways to refuse food. Knowing exactly what to say will help you avoid being talked into eating something you do not want. • Eat before you go out, so you are not as hungry at parties and events. • Do not stand near food sources, and distract yourself if tempted to eat when you are not really hungry. • Limit servings of nonbasic parts of the meal, such as alcohol, soft drinks, appetizers, and desserts.
Guidelines for Eating at Restaurants	• Make healthy selections from the menu. Choose chicken without skin, fish, or lean cuts of meat. Grilled or broiled options are better than fried. Choose healthier options for dessert, as many decadent desserts can have more calories than the whole dinner. • Ask for the condiments (e.g., butter, mayonnaise, salad dressings) on the side, allowing you to determine how much to put on. • Do not feel compelled to eat everything on your plate. Many restaurants serve exceptionally large portions to try to please the customers. • Ask for a to-go box to divide big portions before eating. • Order à la carte rather than full meals to avoid multiple courses and servings. • Avoid supersizing your meals if eating at fast food restaurants, as this can add unwanted calories. Opt for the child-sized meal if possible.

Making minor changes in eating patterns can have major benefits. Evidence suggests that small restrictions in caloric intake sustained over time are more effective than drastic short-term changes. This is likely because they can more easily be incorporated into your lifestyle. Research has suggested that the size of plates and the dimensions of glasses can influence how much we eat and drink. In general, using smaller plates and drinking from taller glasses may trick our minds into

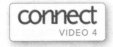

thinking that we ate or drank more than we did. By better understanding cues that lead us to eat, we can set habits and create environments that help us eat less. Table 2 provides specific guidelines for making good selections when purchasing and preparing food at home as well as when you are away from home. Other simple and effective changes in eating patterns are listed below:

• *Eat breakfast every day.* Studies show that skipping breakfast is associated with an increased risk of obesity.

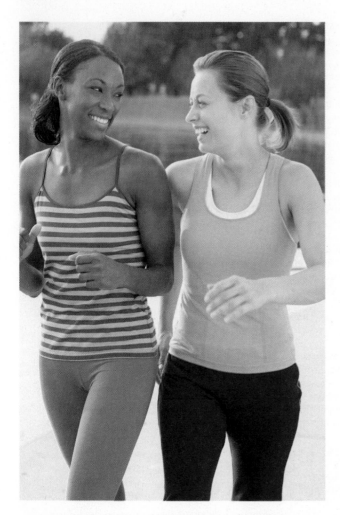

An active, healthy lifestyle is critical for long-term weight control.
Laura Doss/Fancy Collection/SuperStock

- *Consider eating smaller and more frequent meals in a day.* A common strategy in guided weight loss programs is to consume healthy, high-protein snacks to help curb hunger and excess consumption at meals.

- *Eat less fat.* Research shows that a reduction of fat in the diet results not only in fewer calories consumed (fats have more than twice the calories per gram as carbohydrates or proteins) but also in greater body fat loss as well.

- *Increase water consumption.* Drinking more water can help curb your appetite while also helping minimize consumption of sweetened, calorie-laden beverages.

- *Restrict consumption of* **empty calories**. Foods that provide little nutrition often account for an excessive proportion of daily caloric intake. Examples of these foods are candy, chips, and cookies.

- *Increase complex carbohydrates.* Foods high in fiber, such as fresh fruits and vegetables, contain few calories for their volume. They are nutritious and filling, and they are especially good foods for a fat loss program.

Facts about Fad Diets and Clinical Approaches to Weight Loss

Fad diets are not likely to be effective. Consumers are barraged with products and advertisements that claim easy weight loss solutions. Various fad diets capitalize on the consumer's concern about weight and a general lack of knowledge about diet and exercise. Proponents of fad diets often take some small fact about nutrition and claim they have uncovered a magic solution to weight loss that wasn't previously known. Consumers often believe the claims because they have a history of failing with past efforts to control their weight.

A strategy often used in fad diets is to restrict carbohydrates. Because water is required to store carbohydrates, reductions in carbohydrate intake leads to reductions in water storage—and weight. The person who restricts carbohydrates may see a reduction in weight (not fat!) and assume the diet worked when it

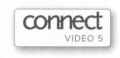

didn't. Regardless of the approach, fad diets provide little hope since they typically can't be maintained over time. When in doubt, avoid programs that promise fast and easy solutions, extreme diets that favor specific foods or eating patterns, and any product that makes unreasonable claims about easy ways to stimulate your metabolism or "melt away fat."

Avoid extreme diets that require severe caloric restriction. Some diet plans advocate severe caloric restriction and exercise programs that require exceptionally large caloric expenditure. These diet plans can be effective in fat loss over a short period but are seldom maintained for a lifetime. Studies show that extreme programs for weight control, designed to "take it off fast," result in long-term success rates of less than 5 percent. One reason extremely low-calorie diets are ineffective is that they may promote "calorie sparing." When caloric intake is 800–1,000 or less, the body protects itself by reducing basal and resting metabolism levels (sparing calories). This results in less fat loss, even though the caloric intake is very low. Cycles of losing and gaining weight, known as "yo-yo" dieting, tend to make it harder to achieve long-term weight control. Evidence suggests that this type of dieting leads to metabolic changes that make it harder to lose fat.

Artificial sweeteners and fat substitutes do not provide a long-term weight loss solution. Artificial sweeteners are frequently used in soft drinks and food to reduce the calorie content. Because they have few or no calories, these products would be expected to help people with weight control. However, evidence suggests that individuals using these products end up consuming just as many calories per day as people consuming products with real sugar or sweeteners. Similar conclusions have been reached with the use of fat substitutes in foods. These findings reinforce the recommendations in the dietary guidelines that emphasize replacing unhealthy foods with healthier choices (rather than seeking alternative versions with artificial sweeteners or fats).

A variety of appetite suppressants are available, but all of them have limitations. Because long-term weight control is difficult, many individuals seek simple solutions from various non-prescription weight loss products. Many negative reactions and multiple deaths were attributed to the use of ephedra, and this led the FDA to ban the sale and use of any products containing this compound. A concern among public health officials is that many supplement products are still not labeled accurately. Manufacturers of supplements also switch to other compounds that may present similar health risks. Consumers should be wary of dietary supplements, due to the unregulated nature of the industry.

A number of prescription drugs have been approved by the FDA for treatment of obesity, but long-term effects aren't known. The various drugs approved for supervised weight loss work in different ways, so it is important to know mechanisms and side effects. Orlistat (used in prescription Xenical and over-the-counter Alli) enhances weight loss by inhibiting the body's absorption of fat. Studies have confirmed that it can help patients lose more weight, but it also blocks the absorption of fat-soluble vitamins. Phenterimine (found in Qsymia) suppresses hunger but has several known side effects and presents specific risks for pregnant females. A related drug called lorcaserin (found in Belviq) was recently banned by the FDA since safety trials revealed an increased risk of cancer. Instead of suppressing hunger, other classes of drugs are designed to work by increasing perceptions of satiety or fullness. The use of a drug called Saxenda is approved for long-term use, but related drugs containing sibutramine (found in Meridia) were recently removed from the market due to greater risk for cardiovascular disease. The bottom line is that the long-term effects of most drugs are not known. They are designed for use only by obese patients (or overweight adults with other comorbidities) and are considered to be adjuncts to lifestyle modification. Consultation with a physician is recommended.

Programs emphasizing lifestyle change offer the best promise for long-term weight control. While magazines and web-based resources promise easy solutions to weight loss, the research evidence documents that there are no simple solutions. The benefits of sensible, lifestyle-based weight loss programs were documented in a recent comparison of randomized controlled trials of commercial programs. Weight Watchers (now known as WW) and Jenny Craig programs yielded the strongest long-term effects. The benefits were attributed to the focus on social support and learning self-management skills. While structured commercial programming may help some, research also supports the use of "motivational interviewing" and health coaching to build motivation and skills for lifestyle change. Many worksites offer health coaching, and many communities offer behavioral training as part of other programs (e.g., the Diabetes Prevention Program).

Using Self-Management Skills

Overcome barriers to weight loss by adopting new ways of thinking about food, eating, and weight control. Although many people struggle with weight control, some of the challenges are self-imposed. By changing your perspectives about food and eating, you can be more successful.

- *Establish realistic perceptions and goals.* Don't compare yourself to models or actors on television or images in magazines or social media. Focus on adopting healthy eating and physical activity habits by setting behavioral goals instead of targeting specific goals to achieve a certain weight or to have a specific measurement.

- *View the word* diet *from a lifestyle perspective.* The word *diet* has negative connotations that typically imply caloric restriction and suffering. Avoid thinking of a diet as something temporary that you go "on," since the only place to go is "off." Instead, view your "diet" as a healthy pattern of eating that you possess and live daily.

- *Learn the difference between craving and hunger.* Hunger is a physiological signal that helps promote an organism's drive to eat when energy supply gets low. A craving is simply a desire to eat something, often a food that is sweet or high in calories. When you feel the urge to eat, ask yourself, "Is this real hunger or a craving?"

- *Change your relationship with food.* Too often people consume food simply because it tastes good. While eating is an important part of our culture and a pleasurable experience, it may help to view food primarily for what it provides: sustenance and energy for healthy living.

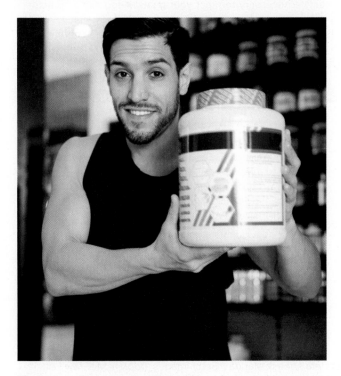

There are no shortcuts to improved nutrition or enhanced appearance.
Iakov Filimonov/Shutterstock

Empty Calories Calories in foods considered to have little or no nutritional value.

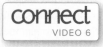

Technology Update

Can Smartphone Apps Help with Weight Control?

Maintaining a healthy weight requires discipline on both sides of the energy balance equation. A variety of smartphone apps are available to assist consumers in tracking both energy intake and energy expenditure (e.g., MyFitnessPal). However, it's still up to the individual to make healthy decisions. Research supports using self-planning and self-monitoring skills, and apps can assist in building these skills. However, there are many to choose from so it is important to consider the various options. Start with a quality review and then compare the features of competing apps to narrow the choices before committing to them. (See Suggested Resources and Readings.)

Do you use smartphone apps to help you track your personal diet or physical activity behaviors? How important are they for your personal weight control efforts?

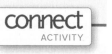
ACTIVITY

Build and engage your social support network to reinforce behavior change and long-term weight control. Family and friends can help you adopt and maintain healthy eating practices and participate in regular physical activity. However, it is important to ensure that they provide the type of support that you need. Sometimes, friends and family can intervene too much, resulting in the opposite effect if it is perceived as an attempt to control your behavior. Therefore, engage your social support network in ways that reinforce and support your behavior rather than control it.

connect
VIDEO 6

Adopt relapse prevention strategies to address minor setbacks. It is common for moods and motivations to cycle during efforts to lose weight. Some people become too compulsive in their behaviors and then overreact if they experience a minor setback or revert back to their old ways. For example, giving in and having a dessert or treat can lead some to go completely off their weight loss plan. Don't let one setback lead to relapse. Instead, view it as a minor setback and then get back to your efforts. Long-term weight control requires a lifetime commitment to healthy lifestyles. By following established principles of relapse prevention, you will be better prepared to get back on track.

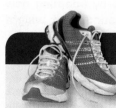

Strategies for Action: Lab Information

Knowing guidelines for controlling body fat is important; but it is more important to learn ways to follow them. The guidelines in this Concept work only if you use them. In Lab 15A, you will identify guidelines that may help you in the future.

Record keeping is important in meeting fat control goals and making moderation a part of your normal lifestyle. It is easy to fool yourself when determining the amount of food you have eaten or the amount of exercise you have done. Once fat control goals have been set, whether for weight loss, maintenance, or gain, keeping a diet log and an exercise log can help you monitor your behavior and maintain the lifestyle necessary to meet your goals. A log can also help you monitor changes in weight and body fat levels. Lab 15B will help you learn about the actual content of fast foods, so you can learn to make better choices when eating out.

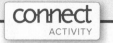
ACTIVITY

Suggested Resources and Readings

The websites for the following sources can be accessed by searching online for the organization, program, or title listed. Specific scientific references are available at the end of this edition of *Concepts of Fitness and Wellness.*

- Academy of Nutrition and Dietetics. www.eatright.org.
- Bird, E. (2020, September 24). "Food Insecurity in the U.S. Is Increasingly Linked to Obesity." *Medical News Today.*
- The Center for Mindful Eating. www.tcme.org.
- Elliott, B. (2020, June 17). "The 10 Best Weight Loss Apps That Help You Meet Your Goals." *Healthline.*

- Healthy Food America. www.healthyfoodamerica.org/.
- Trust for America's Health. *The State of Obesity 2020: Better Policies for a Healthier America.*
- Tucker, M. (2015, January 16). "New U.S. Obesity Guidelines: Treat the Weight First." *Medscape.*
- U.S. Department of Agriculture. Food and Nutrition Information Center.
- U.S. Food and Drug Administration. Menu and Vending Machine Labeling.
- U.S. Food and Drug Administration. Menu Labeling Requirements.
- Wadyka, S. (2019, December 31). "9 Ways to Follow a Healthier Diet in 2020." *Consumer Reports.*

Lab 15A Selecting Strategies for Managing Eating

Name	**Section**	**Date**

Purpose: To learn to select strategies for managing eating to control body fatness.

Procedures

1. Read the strategies listed in Chart 1.
2. Check the box beside 5 to 10 of the strategies that you think will be most useful for you.
3. Answer the questions in the Conclusions and Implications section.

Chart 1 Strategies for Managing Eating to Control Body Fatness

✔	Check 5 to 10 strategies that you might use in the future.
	Shopping Strategies
	Shop from a list.
	Shop with a friend.
	Shop on a full stomach.
	Check food labels.
	Consider foods that take some time to prepare.
	Methods of Eating
	When you eat, do nothing but eat. Don't watch television or read.
	Eat slowly.
	Do not eat food you do not want.
	Follow an eating schedule.
	Do your eating in designated areas, such as kitchen or dining room only.
	Leave the table after eating.
	Avoid second servings.
	Limit servings of condiments.
	Limit servings of nonbasics, such as dessert, breads, and soft drinks.
	Eat several meals of equal size rather than one big meal and two small ones.
	Eating in the Work Environment
	Bring your own food to work.
	Avoid snack machines.
	If you eat out, plan your meal ahead of time.
	Do not eat while working.
	Avoid sharing foods from coworkers, such as birthday cakes.
	Have activity breaks during the day.
	Have water available to substitute for soft drinks.
	Have low-calorie snacks to substitute for office snacks.

✔	Check 5 to 10 strategies that you might use in the future.
	Eating on Special Occasions
	Practice ways to refuse food.
	Avoid tempting situations.
	Eat before you go out.
	Don't stand near food sources.
	If you feel the urge to eat, find someone to talk to.
	Strategies for Eating Out
	Limit deep-fat fried foods.
	Ask for information about food content.
	Limit use of condiments.
	Choose low-fat foods (e.g., skim milk, low-fat yogurt).
	Choose chicken, fish, or lean meat.
	Order à la carte.
	Ask early for a to-go box and divide portions.
	If you eat desserts, avoid those with sauces or toppings.
	Eating at Home
	Keep busy at times when you are at risk of overeating.
	Store food out of sight.
	Avoid serving food to others between meals.
	If you snack, choose snacks with complex carbohydrates, such as carrot sticks or apple slices.
	Freeze leftovers to avoid the temptation of eating them between meals.

Conclusions and Implications

1. In several sentences, discuss your need to use strategies for effective eating. Do you need to use them? Why or why not?

2. In several sentences, discuss the effectiveness of the strategies contained in Chart 1. Do you think they can be effective for people who have a problem controlling their body fatness?

3. In several sentences, discuss the value of using behavioral goals versus outcome goals when planning for fat loss.

Lab 15B Evaluating Fast Food Options

Name	Section	Date

Purpose: To learn about the energy and fat content of fast food and how to make better choices when eating at fast food restaurants.

Procedures

1. Select a fast food restaurant and a typical meal that you might order. Then use an online food calculator to determine total calories, fat calories, saturated fat intake, and cholesterol for each food item.
2. Record the values in Chart 2.
3. Sum the totals for the meal in Chart 2.
4. Record recommended daily values by selecting an amount from Chart 1. The estimate should be based on your estimated needs for the day.
5. Compute the percentage of the daily recommended amounts that you consume in the meal by dividing recommended amounts (step 4) into meal totals (step 3). Record the percentage of recommended daily amounts in Chart 2.
6. Answer the questions in the Conclusions and Implications section.

Chart 1 Recommended Daily Amounts of Fat, Saturated Fat, Cholesterol, and Sodium

	2,000 kcal	3,000 kcal
Total fat	65 g	97.5 g
Saturated fat	20 g	30 g
Cholesterol	300 mg	450 mg
Sodium	2,400 mg	3,600 mg

Results

Chart 2 Listing of Foods Selected for the Meal

Food Item	Total Calories	Total Fat (g)	Saturated Fat (g)	Cholesterol (mg)
1.				
2.				
3.				
4.				
5.				
6.				
Total for meal (sum each column)				
Recommended daily amount (record your values from Chart 1)				
Calculate % of recommended daily amount (record your calculated %)				

Consult an online fast food calculator to estimate calorie content of menu choices (see www.fastfoodnutrition.org). Calorie and nutrient information is also available in NutritionCalc Plus, a diet analysis tool available in Connect. Launch it by clicking the NutritionCalc Plus link on the Resources list on your Connect class home page.

Conclusions and Implications

1. Describe how often you eat at fast food restaurants and indicate whether you would like to reduce how much fast food you consume.

2. Were you surprised at the amount of fat, saturated fat, and cholesterol in the meal you selected?

3. What could you do differently at fast food restaurants to reduce your intake of fat, saturated fat, and cholesterol?

Stress and Health

LEARNING OBJECTIVES

After completing the study of this Concept, you will be able to:

▶ Identify major sources and types of stress.

▶ Explain the ways in which the body responds to stress.

▶ Understand the function of the autonomic nervous system and mechanisms of stress.

▶ Identify common physical, emotional, and behavioral consequences of stress.

▶ Understand individual differences in both physiological and cognitive responses to stress.

▶ Describe personal characteristics that influence consequences of stress.

▶ Identify personal sources of stress and your approach to dealing with stressful life events.

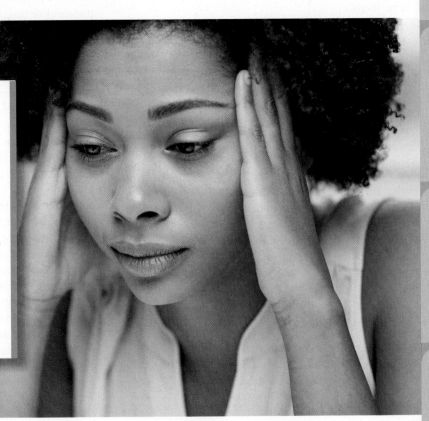

Stress can motivate us to succeed, but it can also overwhelm us and lead to physical and emotional health problems. Understanding personal sources of stress and your unique stress response can help facilitate optimal health.

dolgachov/123RF

Why It Matters!

Stress affects everyone to some degree. Approximately 75 percent of adults say they have experienced moderate to high levels of stress in the past month, and younger generations (Millennials and Gen Z) report higher levels of stress than older adults. This Concept will help you understand the causes and consequences of stress in your life. You will learn about common stressors and the physiological responses to stress. You will also gain a deeper appreciation about the impact of stress on both physical and mental health. Finally, you will learn about individual differences in responses to stress and the implications for health and wellness. Having knowledge of the effects of stress can help you adapt and, in some cases, use stressful situations to enhance healthy living.

Table 1 ▶ Ten Common Stressors in the Lives of College Students and Middle-Aged Adults

College Students	Middle-Aged Adults
1. Troubling thoughts about the future	1. Concerns about weight
2. Not getting enough sleep	2. Health of a family member
3. Wasting time	3. Rising prices of common goods
4. Inconsiderate smokers	4. Home maintenance (interior)
5. Physical appearance	5. Too many things to do
6. Too many things to do	6. Misplacing or losing things
7. Misplacing or losing things	7. Yard work or outside home maintenance
8. Not enough time to do the things you need to do	8. Property, investments, or taxes
9. Concerns about meeting high standards	9. Crime
10. Being lonely	10. Physical appearance

Source: Kanner et al.

Sources of Stress

It is important to understand the difference between stress and stressors. Stress is a nonspecific response of the body that helps the body maintain equilibrium in response to any demand. **Stressors** are things that cause stress. Stress can be motivating or debilitating. Stressors—those that evoke a stress reaction—come in many

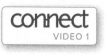

forms, and both positive and negative life events can increase our stress levels.

The first step in managing stress is recognizing the causes and being aware of the symptoms. Identify the factors in your life that make you feel "stressed out." Everything from minor irritations, such as traffic jams, to major life changes, such as births, deaths, or job loss, can be a stressor. A stress overload of too many demands on your time can make you feel that you are no longer in control. Recognizing the causes and effects of stress is important for learning how to manage it.

Stress has a variety of sources. There are many kinds of stressors. Environmental stressors include heat, noise, overcrowding, pollution, and secondhand smoke. Physiological stressors include things like drugs, caffeine, tobacco, injury, infection or disease, and physical effort.

Emotional stressors are the most frequent and important stressors. Some people refer to these as *psychosocial stressors*. A national study of daily experiences indicated that more than 60 percent of all stressful experiences fall into a few areas (see Table 1).

Stressors vary in severity. Major stressors create major emotional turmoil or require tremendous amounts of adjustment. This category includes personal crises (e.g., major health problems or death in the family, divorce/separation,

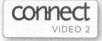

financial problems, legal problems) and job-/school-related pressures or major age-related transitions (e.g., college, marriage, career, retirement). Daily hassles are generally viewed as shorter term or less severe. This category includes events such as traffic problems, peer/work relations, time pressures, and family conflict. In school, pressures such as grades, term papers, and oral presentations would likely fall into this category. Major stressors can alter daily patterns of stress and impair our ability to handle the minor stressors of life, while daily hassles can accumulate and create more significant problems. It is important to be aware of both types of stressors.

Negative, ambiguous, and uncontrollable events are usually the most stressful. Although stress can come from both positive and negative events, negative ones generally cause more distress because negative stressors usually have harsher consequences and little benefit. For example, many dealt with fear, changes and limitations in resources, and a loss of control during the COVID-19 pandemic, which contributed to higher levels of stress. Positive stressors, on the other hand, usually have enough benefit to make them worthwhile. For example, the stress of starting a new job may be tremendous, but it is not as bad as the negative stress from losing a job.

Ambiguous stressors are harder to accept than more clearly defined problems. In most cases, if the cause of a stressor or problem can be identified, measures can be taken to improve the situation. For example, if you are stressed about a project at work or school, you can use specific strategies to complete the task on time. Stress brought on by a relationship with friends or coworkers, on the other hand, may be harder to understand. In some cases, it is not possible to determine the primary source or cause of the problem.

Stress in Contemporary Society

Americans report high levels of stress. The American Psychological Association (APA) commissions an annual survey (Stress in America) to monitor perceptions of stress in the United States. Although results from this national survey indicate that population levels of stress have decreased in the past 8 years, adults continue to report overall levels of stress that they believe are unhealthy, and 29 percent of adults reported increased stress in the past 5 years, compared to only 18 percent who reported a decrease. Money, work, and the economy continue to be the biggest sources of stress, and the most common symptoms include irritability/anger, nervousness or anxiety, and lack of interest/motivation. Although the majority of adults recognize that stress management is important, most do not believe they are managing their stress well.

The sources and consequences of stress are similar for males and females, but there are also some important differences. Females tend to report higher levels of stress, but they also tend to engage more actively in stress management. In the APA's annual reports, males tend to report less concern about managing stress and are more likely than females to say that they are doing enough to manage their stress. Females, in contrast, tend to report that they feel they are not doing enough despite engaging in more active efforts to cope.

College presents unique challenges and stressors. Although the college years are often thought of as a break from the stresses of the real world, college life has its own stressors. Students are often living independently of family for the first time and face new responsibilities with managing time, money, relationships, and their lifestyles. Unique social pressures evolve through new relationships with roommates, dating partners, friends, and classmates. Academic pressures include keeping up with homework, taking exams, speaking in public, and becoming comfortable with talking to professors. The freedom and autonomy of college life can be empowering and enjoyable, but it also presents additional sources of stress.

In addition to the traditional challenges of college, the new generation of students faces stressors that were not typical for college students in the past. More

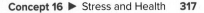

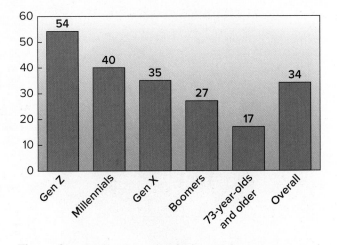

Figure 1 ▶ Adults who report feeling anxious or nervous at least once in the past month.

Source: American Psychological Association Stress in America 2018.

students now work, and many go back to school after spending time in the working world. More of today's college students are the first in their family to attend college. Adding to these challenges, with the onset of the COVID-19 pandemic in early 2020, college students had to quickly adapt to remote learning for many if not all their courses, and recent studies indicate increased stress related to this change. Perhaps as a result of some of these factors and the pressures that they create, rates of mental health problems among college students have increased dramatically in recent years, even prior to the onset of the pandemic. In one recent survey by Chegg, more than half of students reported at least moderate concern about their mental health, with roughly half reporting depressive symptoms, one-third reporting anxiety, and nearly one-fourth saying that they knew someone who had suicidal thoughts since the onset of the pandemic. Independent of college issues, evidence suggests that Millennials and Gen Zers have higher levels of reported stress than other age groups (see Figure 1.)

Some sources of stress are shared by entire communities, cultures, or societies. Although the stressors that individuals experience are often unique to their particular circumstances, there are times when entire

Stress The nonspecific response (generalized adaptation) of the body to any demand made on it in order to maintain physiological equilibrium. This positive or negative response results from emotions that are accompanied by biochemical and physiological changes directed at adaptation.

Stressors Things that place a greater than routine demand on the body or evoke a stress reaction.

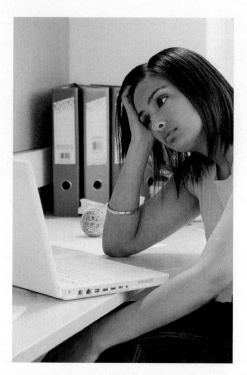

Daily hassles can contribute to stress.
Jasper White/Image Source

communities, cultures, or even countries have shared experiences of severe stress. While there are many examples, the COVID-19 pandemic is perhaps the most obvious recent example of a shared experience of stress. With hundreds of millions of cases and millions of deaths worldwide, no country has failed to feel the impact. Within the United States, although the timing of outbreaks differed by state, virtually every state experienced one or more periods of heightened risk.

Experiences of discrimination are a significant source of stress. In a meta-analysis of 134 previous studies, researchers found that higher levels of perceived discrimination were associated with both negative physical and psychological health outcomes. Perceived discrimination was also associated with more negative physiological and psychological stress responses, more negative health behaviors (e.g., smoking), and fewer positive health behaviors (e.g., exercise). With respect to physiological response, a study of white and African American females found that higher levels of perceived discrimination were associated with higher levels of visceral fat, a known risk factor for cardiovascular disease. Regarding health risk behaviors, a study of college students found that students who reported more discrimination experiences had more negative moods, were more likely to drink as a way to cope with negative emotions, and were more likely to be heavy drinkers. Recent high-profile instances of social injustice

have highlighted systemic racism and have increased stress among individuals at high risk for exposure to discrimination (see A Closer Look).

Social media and technology keep us connected, but they may also create stress. Advances in technology have changed the way we communicate and connect. This is especially true for young adults, as reports suggest that nearly 96 percent own and actively use smartphones. Although smartphones may facilitate organization and time management, excessive use may negatively impact well-being. One recent study found that the more time people spend on their smartphones, the higher their levels of stress. Excessive use in the evenings may be particularly harmful. A study of business managers found that late-night use of smartphones for business purposes was associated with poor sleep quality and quantity and reduced work performance the following day. A study of college students similarly found that those who texted more on their smartphones took longer to fall asleep, got fewer hours of sleep, and reported feeling more tired the following day.

Reactions to Stress

All people have a general reaction to stress. In the early 1900s, Walter Cannon identified the fight-or-flight response to threat. According to his model, the body reacts to a threat by preparing either to fight or flee the situation. The body prepares for either option through the activation of the **sympathetic nervous system (SNS)**. When the SNS is activated, epinephrine (adrenaline) and norepinephrine are released to focus attention on the task at hand. Heart rate

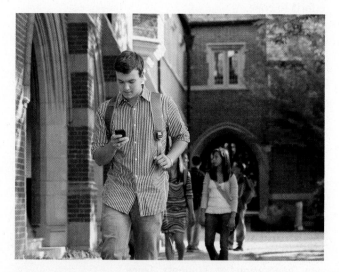

Smartphones can keep us connected, but they can also detract from "real" communication.
Ariel Skelley/Blend Images LLC

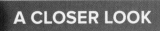

A CLOSER LOOK

Systemic Racism and Stress

A recent APA survey found that police violence and events related to the deaths of George Floyd, Breonna Taylor, and others have been sources of personal stress. Fifty-nine percent of U.S. adults reported that the issue of police violence was a significant source of stress, an increase from 36 percent in 2016. A similar proportion (64 percent) of Americans said that the U.S. government's response to these instances of racial injustice was a significant source of stress. Although these events have caused stress, they have also spurred

many into action and, in turn, have increased optimism about the potential for change. In the APA survey, 67 percent of those surveyed believed that recent efforts to address systemic racism and police brutality would lead to meaningful change in America.

Have police violence and racial injustice been a significant source of stress for you? What steps do you think we need take to address these issues?

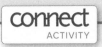

and blood pressure increase to deliver oxygen to the muscles and essential organs, the eyes take in more light to increase visual acuity, and more sugar is released into the bloodstream to increase energy level. At the same time, nonessential functions like digestion and urine production are slowed. Once the immediate threat has passed, the

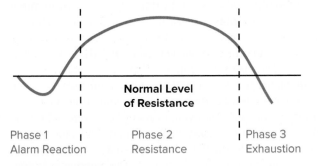

Phase 1: Alarm Reaction
Any physical or mental trauma triggers an immediate set of reactions that combat the stress. Because the immune system is initially depressed, normal levels of resistance are lowered, making us more susceptible to infection and disease. If the stress is not severe or long-lasting, we bounce back and recover rapidly.

Phase 2: Resistance
Eventually, sometimes rather quickly, we adapt to stress, and we tend to become more resistant to illness and disease. The immune system works overtime during this period, keeping up with the demands placed on it.

Phase 3: Exhaustion
Because the body is not able to maintain homeostasis and the long-term resistance needed to combat stress, we invariably experience a drop in resistance level. No one experiences the same resistance and tolerance to stress, but everyone's immunity at some point collapses following prolonged stress reactions.

Figure 2 ▶ Phases and depiction of the general adaptation syndrome.

parasympathetic nervous system (PNS) takes over in an attempt to restore the body to homeostasis and conserve resources. The PNS largely reverses the changes initiated by the SNS (e.g., slows heart rate and returns blood from the muscles and essential organs to the periphery).

Sometimes the fight-or-flight, or SNS, response is essential to survival, but when invoked inappropriately or excessively it may be more harmful than the effects of the original stressor. Hans Selye, another prominent scientist, was the first to recognize the potential negative consequences of this response. Selye suggested that this system could be invoked by mental as well as physical threats and that the short-term benefits might lead to long-term negative consequences. Based on these ideas, Selye described the general adaptation syndrome, which explains how the autonomic nervous system reacts to stressful situations and the conditions under which the system may break down (see Figure 2). The term *general* highlights the similarities in response to stressful situations across individuals. Selye's work led him to be referred to as the "father of stress."

The hypothalamic-pituitary-adrenal (HPA) axis plays a key role in the stress response. The chronic activation of the SNS has an influence on the development of physical disease, but negative impacts on health are influenced mainly by a system known as the hypothalamic-pituitary-adrenal (HPA) axis. The HPA axis is activated during stress, leading to the release of corticotropin-releasing hormone (CRH) and secondary activation of the pituitary gland. The pituitary releases a chemical called adrenocorticotropic hormone

Sympathetic Nervous System (SNS) The component of the autonomic nervous system that responds to stressful situations by initiating the fight-or-flight response.

Parasympathetic Nervous System (PNS) The component of the autonomic nervous system that helps bring the body to a resting state following stressful experiences.

In the News

The News Is Stressful!

The news has become an increasing source of stress for many, with stories about the COVID-19 pandemic, racial injustice, and political unrest playing prominently in the headlines. A study by the American Psychological Association suggests that the news is particularly stressful for Gen Zers, who report higher stress than older adults across a variety of current news topics including mass shootings, rising suicide rates, deportation, and sexual assaults. A more recent survey reported that Gen Z adults were the most likely generation to say that their mental health has worsened compared with before the pandemic. Approximately 46 percent of Gen Zers reported worsening health while 33 percent of Gen X adults felt the same.

Has the news been a major source of stress for you? Why do you think the news is more stressful for young adults than older adults?

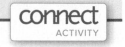

connect
ACTIVITY

(ACTH), which ultimately causes the release of an active stress hormone called cortisol. With chronic exposure to stress, the HPA system can become dysregulated, and both over- and underactivation of the system are associated with risk for negative health outcomes.

Stress Effects on Health and Wellness

Excessive stress has a negative impact on health. Moderate stress can motivate us to reach our goals and keep life interesting. However, when stressors are severe or chronic, our bodies may not be able to adapt successfully. Stress beyond the limits of **adaptation** can compromise immune functioning, leading to a host of diseases. In fact, stress has been linked to between 50 and 70 percent of all illnesses. Further, stress is associated with negative health behaviors, such as alcohol and other drug use, and to psychological problems, such as depression and anxiety.

Stress affects immune function and physical health. In addition to preparing the body for fight or flight, the stress-related activation of the SNS and the HPA axis slows down the functioning of the immune response. In the face of an immediate threat, mobilizing resources that will help in the moment is more important to the body than preventing or fighting infection. If the stress response is chronically activated, high levels of adrenaline and cortisol continue to tell the body to mobilize resources at the expense of immune functioning. This contributes to the tendency for people to become sick after experiencing high levels of stress.

Stress can lead to fatigue and can cause or exacerbate a variety of health problems. Exposure to chronic stress or repeated exposure to acute stress may lead to a state of fatigue. Fatigue may result from lack of sleep, emotional strain, pain, disease, or a combination of these factors. Both **physiological fatigue** and **psychological fatigue** can result in a state of exhaustion, with resultant physical and mental health

consequences. Chronic stress has been linked to health maladies that plague individuals on a daily basis, such as headaches, indigestion, insomnia, and the common cold. In fact, one study concluded that "out-of-control" stress is the leading preventable source of increased health-care costs in the workforce, roughly equivalent to the costs of the health problems related to smoking.

The effects of stress on health are not limited to minor physical complaints. Compelling evidence links psychological stress to a host of serious health problems, including cardiovascular disease, cancer, and HIV/AIDS. Stress may also increase the risk for upper respiratory tract infections, asthma, herpes, viral infections, autoimmune diseases, and slow wound healing. Reduced immune function due to negative emotions and stress appears to be a principal reason for these health problems. Stress may also increase the risk of early death. It is theorized that stress accelerates the aging process by shortening the telomeres in our chromosomes.

Stress can have mental and emotional effects. The challenges caused by psychosocial stress may lead to a variety of mental and emotional effects. In the short term, stress can impair concentration and attention span. Anxiety is an emotional response to stress characterized by apprehension. Because the response usually involves expending a lot of nervous energy, anxiety can lead to fatigue and muscular tension.

Anxiety may persist long after a stressful experience. For example, adverse childhood experiences (ACEs) such as physical and emotional abuse, neglect, poverty, and family stress can have long-term consequences. According to the CDC, ACEs contribute to risky health behaviors, chronic health conditions, low life potential, and early death. Risks tend to be proportional to the number and severity of ACEs; thus, public health emphasis is placed on preventing them before they happen.

Another long-term consequence of extreme stress is post-traumatic stress disorder (PTSD), a common problem among military veterans. Symptoms of PTSD include flashbacks of the traumatic event, avoidance of situations that remind the person of the event, emotional numbing, and an increased level of arousal. The associated mental health problems contribute to the high rates of depression and suicide among veterans. These consequences underscore the serious health consequences of excess stress.

Stress can alter both positive and negative health behaviors. In addition to direct effects on health, stress can contribute to negative health outcomes indirectly, through increased engagement in negative behaviors, such as smoking, alcohol use, and overeating. Stress may also decrease engagement in health-protective behaviors, such as exercise. During periods of increased stress, people may also get insufficient sleep and have sleep difficulties associated with the causes of stress. For example, an individual experiencing severe stress related to finances may pick up additional shifts at work, leaving less time for sleep. The person may also have difficulty sleeping due to worry associated with the financial situation. Unfortunately, reduced or disrupted sleep may exacerbate the problem. Studies have consistently found a link between sleep difficulties and stress-related physical and mental health problems, including cardiovascular disease and depression, and a recent study found a strong link between stress and sleep disturbances among college students.

Stress isn't all bad. We all need sufficient stress to motivate us to engage in activities that make our lives meaningful. Otherwise, we would be in a state of **hypostress**, which leads to apathy, boredom, and less than optimal health and wellness. An example of hypostress is a person working on an assembly line. Because the same task is repeated without variation, the level of stimulation is quite low and might lead to a state of boredom and job dissatisfaction. In fact, a certain level of stress, called **eustress**, is experienced positively. In contrast, **distress** is a level of stress that compromises performance and well-being. Each of us possesses a system that allows us to mobilize resources when necessary and seeks to find a homeostatic level of arousal (see Figure 3). Although we all have an optimal level of arousal, it varies considerably. What one person finds stressful another may find exhilarating. For example, riding a roller coaster is thrilling for some people, but stressful and unpleasant for others.

Individual Differences in the Stress Response

Individuals respond differently to stress. Individuals exposed to high levels of stress are most at risk for negative health consequences. However, not everyone exposed to severe or chronic stress will experience negative outcomes. The COVID-19 pandemic provides a vivid example of the very different reactions that people have to the same or similar stressors. Although everyone has been profoundly impacted, individual experiences and reactions have varied dramatically. Some individuals faced greater challenges than others as the pandemic impacted some occupations and families more than others. Thus, the same stressor can have different effects on people depending on their situation. However, some individuals also accepted the challenges of COVID-19 better than others by finding more positive ways to cope with the isolation and change in lifestyles. Although Americans reported high levels of stress related to COVID-19, they also showed great resilience, as more than 70 percent reported feeling hopeful about the future despite current challenges. Figure 4 depicts the role that stress appraisals play in mediating relations between stress and its emotional, physical, and behavioral consequences.

Reactions to stress depend on one's appraisal of both the event and the subsequent physiological response. Stressors by themselves generally do not cause problems unless they are perceived as stressful. As shown in Figure 4, two specific factors are thought to influence individual susceptibility to negative stress-related outcomes: stress appraisal and stress reactivity.

Stress appraisal refers to an individual's perceptions of a stressor and the person's resources for managing stressful situations. Appraisal usually involves consideration of the consequences of the situation (primary appraisal) and an evaluation of the resources available to cope with the situation (secondary appraisal). If one sees a stressor as a challenge that can be tackled, one is likely to respond in a more

Adaptation The body's efforts to restore normalcy.

Physiological Fatigue A deterioration in the capacity of the neuromuscular system as a result of physical overwork and strain; also referred to as *true fatigue*.

Psychological Fatigue A feeling of fatigue, usually caused by such things as lack of exercise, boredom, or mental stress, that results in a lack of energy and depression; also referred to as *subjective* or *false fatigue*.

Hypostress Insufficient levels of stress leading to boredom or apathy.

Eustress Positive stress, or stress that is mentally or physically stimulating.

Distress Negative stress, or stress that contributes to health problems.

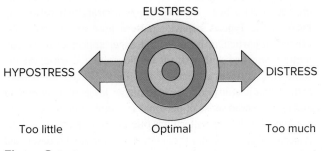

EUSTRESS

HYPOSTRESS ◀ ▶ DISTRESS

Too little · Optimal · Too much

Figure 3 ▶ Stress target zone.

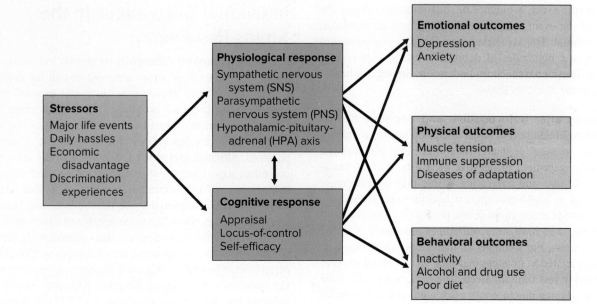

Figure 4 ▶ Reactions to stress.

positive manner than if the stressor is viewed as an obstacle that cannot be overcome. Individual differences in appraisal are due to inherited predispositions as well as our unique histories of experiencing and attempting to cope with stress.

Individual appraisal of the body's response to a stressful event is also important. Stress reactivity refers to the extent to which the sympathetic nervous system, or fight-or-flight system, is activated by a stressor. The degree of activation influences how one will react emotionally and behaviorally, but some react more than others. For example, public speaking is a situation that leads to significant autonomic arousal for most people. Those who handle these situations well probably recognize that these sensations are normal and may even interpret them as excitement about the situations. In contrast, those who experience severe and sometimes debilitating anxiety are probably interpreting the same sensations as indicators of fear, panic, and loss of control. The combination of individual differences in stress reactivity and cognitive responses (e.g. appraisals) may lead to characteristic ways of responding to stress that either confer risk or protect against risk for physical and mental health problems (See Figure 4). In fact, several different patterns of behavior (or personality styles) associated with stress responses have been clearly identified.

Type A and Type D personalities may increase risk for negative health outcomes.
The best-known "personality" style associated with risk for negative health outcomes is the **Type A behavior pattern**. Several decades ago, psychologists Friedman and Rosenman identified a subgroup of goal-oriented, or "driven," patients, whom they believed were at increased risk based on their pattern of behavior. These individuals demonstrated a sense of time urgency, were highly competitive, and

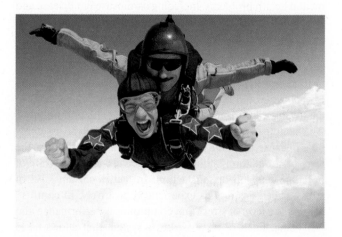

One person's stress is another's pleasure.
Sky Antonio/Shutterstock

tended to experience and express anger and hostility under conditions of stress. In contrast, individuals with the Type B behavior pattern were relatively easygoing and less reactive to stress. Although early research on Type A behavior demonstrated increased risk for heart disease, it now appears that certain aspects of the Type A behavior pattern pose greater risk than others. In particular, hostility and anger appear to be consistently associated with risk for cardiovascular disease. At the same time, certain aspects of the Type A behavior pattern (other than hostility) may lead to higher levels of achievement and an increased sense of personal accomplishment. Although the Type A behavior pattern has often been referred to as Type A personality, it was not the intention of those who developed the concept to identify a "personality type."

In contrast, the more recently identified **Type D,** or "distressed," **behavior pattern** is associated with two well-defined personality characteristics based on personality theory. Individuals with Type D personality are characterized by high levels of "negative affectivity," or negative emotion, and "social inhibition," or the tendency not to express negative emotions in social interactions. The combination of these characteristics appears to constitute risk for cardiovascular disease and other negative health outcomes. Converging evidence from recent research on both Type A and Type D behaviors has led some to conclude that negative affectivity, in general, is a more important risk for negative health outcomes than any emotion in particular. In other words, anger and hostility (Type A), as well as anxiety and depressed mood (Type D), pose a health risk. Several other well-established personality traits, including neuroticism and novelty seeking, have also been linked to greater stress and negative health outcomes. As an example, a recent study found that people with higher levels of neuroticism paid more attention to COVID-19-related information, worried more about potential negative outcomes, and experienced more negative emotion than those with lower levels of neuroticism.

Several personality traits are associated with resilience in the face of stress. Resilience refers not simply to an absence of risk factors, but also to the presence of protective factors that lead to adaptive functioning. The experience of positive emotion is one well-established protective factor. Individuals who experience more positive emotions are more likely to adopt healthy lifestyles, and their physical responses to stress are more adaptive than those who experience less positive emotion. For example, patterns of cortisol response, heart rate, and blood pressure under stress are all more favorable among individuals who experience higher levels of positive emotion. Positive emotion may also be an effective coping mechanism for managing acute stress. Positive moods have been shown to undo some of the cardiovascular effects associated with negative emotions. Individuals who have more positive moods are also more socially integrated and report higher levels of social support, both characteristics associated with health benefits. **Optimism** is a trait associated with more positive emotional experiences and a more positive outlook on the future. Extensive research demonstrates that optimistic individuals have better physical and mental health outcomes than pessimistic individuals.

An individual's **locus of control** can also have a significant impact on how the person responds to a stressful situation. Research has consistently found that having an internal locus of control is associated with better health outcomes. People with an internal locus of control are more likely to take steps to address the problems that created the stress, rather than avoiding them. Those with an external locus of control tend

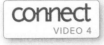

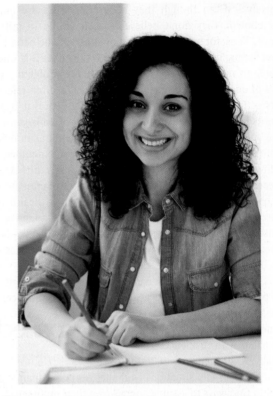

Resiliency and optimism can help with stress management.
Mediaphotos/iStockphoto/Getty Images

to use passive methods for managing stress. In addition, an external locus of control is related to higher perceived levels of stress, lower job satisfaction, and poorer school achievement.

Although an internal locus of control generally promotes health, this is not always the case. This truth is apparent in depressed individuals with a pessimistic explanatory style. They believe that their failures are due to internal factors, squarely placing the control of these events within

Type A Behavior Pattern Characterized by impatience, ambition, and aggression; Type A personalities may be more susceptible to the effects of stress but may also be more able to cope with stress.

Type D Behavior Pattern Characterized by high levels of negative emotion and the tendency to withhold expression of these emotions.

Resilience Positive outcomes in the face of stress or disadvantage.

Optimism The tendency to have a positive outlook on life or a belief that things will work out favorably.

Locus of Control The extent to which we believe the outcomes of events are under our control (internal locus) or outside our personal control (external locus).

themselves. Even though they believe stressors are under their control, they don't believe in their ability to initiate change. Thus, for an internal locus of control to be beneficial to well-being, it must be combined with the belief that one is capable of making changes to prevent future problems. The belief in one's ability to reach a desired goal is often referred to as **self-efficacy**. Studies have consistently shown health benefits of **conscientiousness,** the tendency to be organized, thoughtful, and goal directed. Highly conscientious individuals are at decreased risk for a range of negative outcomes, including asthma, stroke, depression, and panic attacks. It appears that conscientiousness contributes to better health outcomes, both through reduced engagement in health risk behaviors like alcohol use and through more adaptive responses to stressful experiences. For example, individuals higher in conscientiousness are more likely to exercise on days that they experience high levels of stress.

As noted earlier, individuals who possess characteristics that protect them from the negative health consequences of stress are said to be resilient. **Hardiness** is one constellation of characteristics associated with resilience. Hardy individuals are strongly committed to their goals, view difficult situations as challenges rather than stressors, and find ways to assume control over their problems.

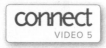
VIDEO 5

Technology Update

Challenges with Interpreting Online Information

According to Pew Research, 89 percent of Americans get at least some of their news from online sources. This may include websites for mainstream media outlets as well as social media sites where news stories are often posted or re-posted (such as Twitter). Because of this, social media outlets can also be a source of misinformation as well as "slanted" news information. This has resulted in many people distrusting the more mainstream media outlets. When asked about how much trust they had in the mainstream media to report the news "fully, accurately, and fairly," a Gallup poll found that 60 percent of Americans responded "not very much" or "none at all." "Fake news" has become a common phrase in online vocabulary, although interpreted differently based on the user. What may be "fake news" to one person may be perceived differently by another, which presents communication challenges.

Do you think that there is more "fake news" than there used to be? What do you think is the best way to tell the difference between fake news and real news?

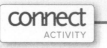
ACTIVITY

Using Self-Management Skills

Assess common sources of stress and evaluate how you typically respond. The first step to managing stress effectively is to understand the sources of stress in your life. For some, major life events may be the primary sources of stress, whereas for others, chronic everyday stressors may play a more important role. It is also important to understand the unique ways in which you react to stress. This may include both adaptive and maladaptive approaches. Once you know what "stresses you out" and how you typically react to stressful events, you can begin to find more effective ways to combat stress. The labs in this Concept can help with this step.

Learn how to balance your attitudes to moderate stress. While you can't always control your exposure to stressors, you can control your appraisal of stressful events. There are clearly some innate personality differences that may influence how you react to people and to stress. However, there are also a number of characteristics that can be

HELP | Health is available to Everyone for a Lifetime, and it's Personal

Telehealth Care for Stress

Mental health concerns among college students escalated as a result of anxiety, lockdowns, and disruptions in learning caused by the COVID-19 pandemic. A recent APA survey suggested associated gaps in care for their mental health issues. The majority of adults (61 percent) said they needed more emotional support than they received, and this number was even higher for Gen Zers (82 percent). Complications of in-person care led to greater reliance on telehealth options to help meet the demand. College counseling centers and other mental health providers have now built expertise to deliver effective support by phone or videoconference. During the peak of the pandemic, more than 75 percent of psychologists indicated that they were providing only remote services, but it is likely that many centers will retain this type of service over time.

Would telehealth support be an appealing approach for you to receive care for mental health concerns?

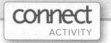
ACTIVITY

Self-Efficacy The belief in one's ability to take action that will lead to the attainment of a goal.

Conscientiousness Associated with high levels of organization, thoughtfulness, and goal-directed activity.

Hardiness A collection of personality traits thought to make a person more resistant to stress.

learned, emulated, or nurtured. For example, characteristics of resilience, optimism, conscientiousness, and hardiness all have been shown to help people become more resistant to stressful experiences. By paying attention to your attitudes and perceptions, you can develop a more stress-resistant personality.

Taking an optimistic perspective can build self-confidence and help you cope with stress. Optimists are hopeful about the future, while pessimists expect bad things to happen. Optimists see the glass as half full, while pessimists see the glass as half empty. Research also shows that optimists have a more positive physiological response to stress and respond more effectively to stress than do pessimists (see Figure 4).

If you are already an optimist, you'll reap the health benefits. If you tend to be more of a pessimist, you can take steps to adopt a more optimistic outlook. One way to see things from a more optimistic perspective is to build your self-confidence for handling difficult situations (a self-management skill). Here are some things you can do to increase your self-confidence and have a more optimistic outlook.

- *Set realistic goals for specific tasks.* Over time, setting goals that are too difficult leads to low confidence. Setting goals that are achievable leads to success and improved confidence.

- *Keep trying.* People with low confidence often give up when they don't have early success. They may think,

"I can't do it no matter how hard I try." Building self-confidence through continued effort promotes the feeling that "I can." Those who believe that "they can do it" are optimists.

- *Give yourself a break.* It is important to give yourself credit for giving effort. Effort pays off in the long run. Of course, not all attempts at performing a task will be successful. The key is to keep trying even when your initial efforts are unsuccessful.

- *Avoid evaluation when trying something new.* Anyone who has ever given a speech, performed before a large crowd, or taken an important test knows that stress levels increase when you are being evaluated. Trying something new while being evaluated is especially stressful and can undermine self-confidence. When trying something new, practice in private. This builds the confidence that you need prior to being evaluated or performing in public.

- *Don't sell yourself short.* "I'm not big enough to do that." "I have never done that." "I don't think I can do it." Societal stereotypes can make a task seem intimidating. Following the steps suggested above can help you succeed even in tasks that you think "are not for you."

- *Laugh it off.* Laughter has both short-term and long-term benefits for reducing stress and it is associated with both physical and mental health benefits. Some experts recommend watching a TV comedy or telling jokes with friends to create laughter and reduce stress. Give it a try!

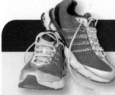

Strategies for Action: Lab Information

Self-assessments of stressors in your life can be useful in managing stress. To effectively manage stress, you first must identify the sources of stress in your life. In Lab 16A you will have the opportunity to evaluate your stress levels using the Life Experience Survey.

Learning to appraise stressful events in a more positive way can help you respond to stress more effectively. Personality characteristics have been associated with reactions to stress. Although overall personality structure has proven somewhat resistant to change, it is certainly possible to change your appraisal of stressful events and thereby diminish the resulting emotional, physical, and behavioral outcomes. In Lab 16B you can assess your hardiness and locus of control, characteristics associated with appraising and coping with stress.

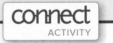

Suggested Resources and Readings

The websites for the following sources can be accessed by searching online for the organization, program, or title listed. Specific scientific references are available at the end of this edition of *Concepts of Fitness and Wellness.*

- American Psychological Association. (2020, April 14). Coping with COVID-19-Related Stress as a Student.
- American Psychological Association. Stress in America™ 2020: A National Mental Health Crisis.
- American Psychological Association. Stress Relief Is Within Reach.
- Anderson, G. (2020, September 11). "Mental Health Needs Rise with Pandemic." *Inside Higher Ed.*
- Center for Collegiate Mental Health. (2020, January). *2019 Annual Report* (Publication No. STA 20-244). Penn State University. (pdf)
- Greenberg, J. (2021). *Comprehensive Stress Management* (15th ed.). New York: McGraw-Hill Higher Education.
- O'Hara, D. (2020, October 30). "College Counselors Ensure Students Can Access Mental Health Services During COVID-19." American Psychological Association.
- Sharecare. Well-Being Index.

Design Element: (*magnifying glass*): Siede Preis/Getty Images; (*runners shoes*): Maridav/Getty Images; (*tablet*): McGraw Hill; (*woman*): GlobalStock/Getty Images; (*blue sports shoes*): chictype/Getty Images; (*smartphone*): Alexey Boldin/Shutterstock; (*Why It Matters*): MHHE

Lab 16A Evaluating Your Stress Level

Name		Section	Date

Purpose: To evaluate your stress during the past year and determine its implications.

Procedures

1. Complete the following Life Experience Survey based on your experiences during the past year. This survey lists a number of life events that may be distressful or eustressful. Read all of the items. If you did not experience an event, leave the box blank. In the box after each event that you did experience, write a number ranging from −3 to +3 using the scale described in the directions. Extra blanks are provided to write in positive or negative events not listed. Some items apply only to males or females. Items 48–56 are only for current college students.
2. Add all of the negative numbers and record your score (distress) in the Results section. Add the positive numbers and record your score (eustress) in the Results section. Use all of the events in the past year.
3. Find your scores on Chart 1 and record your ratings in the Results section.
4. Consider your scores and their implications for how you currently manage stress, as well as strategies you might use in the future. Provide your response in the Conclusions and Implications section.

Results

Sum of negative scores [　　] (distress)   Rating on negative scores [　　　　　]

Sum of positive scores [　　] (eustress)   Rating on positive scores [　　　　　]

Chart 1 Scale for Life Experiences and Stress

	Sum of Negative Scores (Distress)	Sum of Positive Scores (Eustress)
May need counseling	14+	
Above average	9–13	11+
Average	6–8	9–10
Below average	<6	<9

Scoring the Life Experience Survey

1. Add all of the negative scores to arrive at your own distress score (negative stress).
2. Add all of the positive scores to arrive at a eustress score (positive stress).

Conclusions and Implications: In several sentences, discuss your current stress rating and its implications.

Life Experience Survey

Directions: If you did not experience an event, leave the box next to the event empty. If you experienced an event, enter a number in the box based on how the event impacted your life. Use the following scale:

Extremely negative impact = –3
Moderately negative impact = –2
Somewhat negative impact = –1
Neither positive nor negative impact = 0
Somewhat positive impact = +1
Moderately positive impact = +2
Extremely positive impact = +3

1. Marriage
2. Detention in jail or comparable institution
3. Death of spouse
4. Major change in sleeping habits (much more or less sleep)
5. Death of close family member:
   a. Mother
   b. Father
   c. Brother
   d. Sister
   e. Child
   f. Grandmother
   g. Grandfather
   h. Other (specify) _____
6. Major change in eating habits (much more or much less food intake)
7. Foreclosure on mortgage or loan
8. Death of a close friend
9. Outstanding personal achievement
10. Minor law violation (traffic ticket, disturbing the peace, etc.)
11. Became pregnant or partner became pregnant
12. Changed work situation (different working conditions, working hours, etc.)
13. New job
14. Serious illness or injury of close family member:
    a. Father
    b. Mother
    c. Sister
    d. Brother
    e. Grandfather
    f. Grandmother
    g. Spouse
    h. Child
    i. Other (specify) _____
15. Sexual difficulties
16. Trouble with employer (in danger of losing job, being suspended, demoted, etc.)
17. Trouble with in-laws
18. Major change in financial status (a lot better off or a lot worse off)
19. Major change in closeness of family members (decreased or increased closeness)

20. Gaining a new family member (through birth, adoption, family member moving in, etc.)
21. Change of residence
22. Marital separation from mate (due to conflict)
23. Major change in church activities (increased or decreased attendance)
24. Marital reconciliation with mate
25. Major change in number of arguments with spouse (a lot more or a lot fewer arguments)
26. Change in partner's work (new job, loss of job, retirement, etc.)
27. Major change in usual type and/or amount of recreation
28. Borrowing more than $10,000 (buying a home, business, etc.)
29. Borrowing less than $10,000 (buying car or TV, getting school loan, etc.)
30. Being fired from job
31. Had an abortion or partner had an abortion
32. Major personal illness or injury
33. Major change in social activities, such as parties, movies, visiting (increased or decreased participation)
34. Major change in living conditions of family (building new home, remodeling, deterioration of home or neighborhood, etc.)
35. Divorce
36. Serious injury or illness of close friend
37. Retirement from work
38. Son or daughter leaving home (due to marriage, college, etc.)
39. Ending of formal schooling
40. Separation from spouse (due to work, travel, etc.)
41. Engagement
42. Breaking up with boyfriend/girlfriend
43. Leaving home for the first time
44. Reconciliation with boyfriend/girlfriend

Other recent experiences that have had an impact on your life: list and rate.

45. _____
46. _____
47. _____

For Students Only

48. Beginning new school experience at a higher academic level (college, graduate school, professional school, etc.)
49. Changing to a new school at same academic level (undergraduate, graduate, etc.)
50. Academic probation
51. Being dismissed from dormitory or other residence
52. Failing an important exam
53. Changing a major
54. Failing a course
55. Dropping a course
56. Joining a fraternity/sorority

Source: Sarason, I. G., Johnson, J. H., & Siegel, J. M. (1978). "Assessing the Impact of Life Changes: Development of the Life Experience Survey." *Journal of Consulting and Clinical Psychology, 46*(5).

Lab 16B Evaluating Your Hardiness and Locus of Control

Name		Section		Date

Purpose: To evaluate your level of hardiness and locus of control and to help you identify the ways in which you appraise and respond to stressful situations.

Procedures

1. Complete the Hardiness Questionnaire and the Locus of Control Questionnaire. Make an X over the circle that best describes what is true for you personally.
2. Compute the scale scores and record the values in the Results section.
3. Evaluate your scores using Chart 1, and record your ratings in the Results section.
4. Interpret the results by answering the questions in the Conclusions and Implications section.

Hardiness Questionnaire

	Not True	Rarely True	Sometimes True	Often True	Score
1. I look forward to school and work on most days.	1	2	3	4	
2. Having too many choices in life makes me nervous.	4	3	2	1	
3. I know where my life is going and look forward to the future.	1	2	3	4	
4. I prefer not to get too involved in relationships.	4	3	2	1	
Commitment Score, Sum 1–4					
5. My efforts at school and work will pay off in the long run.	1	2	3	4	
6. I just have to trust my life to fate to be successful.	4	3	2	1	
7. I believe that I can make a difference in the world.	1	2	3	4	
8. Being successful in life takes more luck and good breaks than effort.	4	3	2	1	
Control Score, Sum 5–8					
9. I would be willing to work for less money if I could do something really challenging and interesting.	1	2	3	4	
10. I often get frustrated when my daily plans and schedule get altered.	4	3	2	1	
11. Experiencing new situations in life is important to me.	1	2	3	4	
12. I don't mind being bored.	4	3	2	1	
Challenge Score, Sum 9–12					

Locus of Control Questionnaire

13. Hard work usually pays off.	1	2	3	4	
14. Buying a lottery ticket is not worth the money.	1	2	3	4	
15. Even when I fail I keep trying.	1	2	3	4	
16. I am usually successful in what I do.	1	2	3	4	
17. I am in control of my own life.	1	2	3	4	
18. I make plans to be sure I am successful.	1	2	3	4	
19. I know where I stand with my friends.	1	2	3	4	
Locus of Control, Sum 13–19					

Results

Hardiness

Commitment score	☐		Commitment rating	☐
+			+	
Control score	☐		Control rating	☐
+			+	
Challenge score	☐		Challenge rating	☐
=			=	
Total Hardiness score	☐		Hardiness rating	☐

Locus of Control

Locus of control score	☐		Locus of control rating	☐

Chart 1 Rating Chart

Rating	Individual Hardiness Scale Scores	Total Hardiness Score	Locus of Control Score
High	14–16	40–48	24–28
Moderate	10–13	30–39	12–23
Low	<10	<30	<12

Conclusions and Implications

1. In several sentences, discuss your commitment, control, and challenge ratings, as well as your overall hardiness rating. Are they what you expected? Do you think they are true indications of your hardiness? Explain.

2. In several sentences, discuss your locus of control rating. Is it what you expected (a high rating indicates an internal locus of control)? Do you think your rating is a realistic indicator of your locus of control? Explain.

Stress-Management Strategies

LEARNING OBJECTIVES

After completing the study of this Concept, you will be able to:

▶ Describe the stress-buffering effects of physical activity that contribute to positive psychological health.

▶ Identify behaviors that contribute to better sleep hygiene.

▶ Describe the benefits of recreation, leisure, and play to overall quality of life.

▶ Identify a variety of strategies for effective time management.

▶ Understand the unique benefits of cognitive-, emotion-, and problem-focused coping strategies.

▶ Describe the mental health benefits of mindfulness, spirituality, and emotional expression.

▶ Identify several relaxation techniques that can be used to effectively manage stress.

▶ Describe different types of social support and ways in which they facilitate effective stress management.

Although stress cannot be avoided, effective stress-management techniques can help reduce the impact of stress on your health and well-being.

Caiaimage/Robert Daly/Getty Images

Why It Matters!

Stress is a normal part of life so it is important to learn how to manage stress effectively. Healthy lifestyle behaviors and self-management skills are important for effective stress management. Exercising regularly is one way to manage stress as are getting sufficient sleep and allowing time for recreation. Time management is another self-management skill for balancing work and school demands and for ensuring that there is time for physical activity, sleep, and recreation. Developing active coping skills is especially important for managing stress and dealing with the demands of daily life. This Concept covers the importance of healthy lifestyle factors and the use of self-management skills for stress management.

Physical Activity and Stress Management

Regular activity can help you adapt to stressful situations. An individual's capacity to adapt to stress is not a static function but fluctuates as situations change. Physical activity is especially important for stress management because it conditions your body to function effectively under challenging physiological conditions. Unfortunately, participation in physical activity tends to be lower when people are under high stress, and that is when you may need physical activity the most. Therefore, it is important to build physical activity into your normal routine to effectively manage daily stress.

Physical activity can provide relief from stress and reduce muscle tension. Physical activity has been found to be effective at relieving stress and associated outcomes. For example, studies show that regular exercise decreases the likelihood of developing stress-related disorders and reduces the intensity of the stress response. It also shortens the period of recovery from an emotional trauma. Its effect tends to be short term, so exercise regularly for long-term benefits. Whatever your choice of exercise, it is likely to be more effective as an antidote to stress if it is something you find enjoyable.

Regular physical activity reduces reactivity to stress. Physical activity is associated with a physiological response that is similar, in many ways, to the body's response to psychosocial stressors. Individuals who are physically fit have a reduced physiological response to exercise. Therefore, it makes sense that someone who is physically fit will also have a reduced response to psychosocial stressors. Research supports this hypothesis, indicating that regular exercise reduces physiological reactivity to non-exercise stressors. For example, one recent study evaluated the impact of physical activity on responses to social stressors. The stress response was determined by monitoring levels of cortisol, a hormone released during stress. The social stressor led to a spike in cortisol

levels, but the magnitude of the cortisol response to stress was lower among those who were more physically active. Although regular exercise may protect against elevated cortisol levels, there is some evidence that intensive training and competition may lead to greater overall cortisol exposure. Thus, regular but not excessive exercise may be the most beneficial pattern for moderating your response to stress.

Physical activity has direct effects on mental health and also moderates the effect of stress on other health outcomes. Exercise can reduce anxiety, aid in recovery from depression, and assist in efforts to eliminate negative health behaviors, such as smoking. It also appears to buffer the effects of stress on cellular aging. Details about some of the major benefits for mental health are highlighted next:

- *Physical activity can reduce anxiety and depression.* The most recent edition of the *Physical Activity Guidelines for Americans* report indicates that "regular physical activity not only reduces the risk of clinical depression, but reduces depressive symptoms among people both with and without clinical depression." Other evidence indicates that aerobic exercise is comparable to medication in reducing depressive symptoms and decreasing risk for a recurrence of depression. A study of formerly depressed individuals found that exercise helped reduce the emotional consequences from negative mood states. This mechanism may explain the ability of exercise to reduce the recurrence of depression and reduce depressive symptoms among those without diagnosable depression. Physical activity can reduce the severity of those symptoms whether one has only a few or many. The *Physical Activity Guidelines* report also indicates that "regular physical activity reduces symptoms of anxiety, including both chronic levels of anxiety, as well as the acute feelings of anxiety felt by many individuals from time to time." Other research indicates that an exercise intervention can reduce anxiety among individuals with diagnosable anxiety disorders (e.g., panic disorder).

- *Physical activity buffers the effects of stress on obesity and health.* Recent analyses of data from the National Health and Growth Study found that adolescent females who reported more stress had larger increases in BMI during adolescence (aged 10–19). However stress-related increases were much smaller among those who engaged in regular physical activity.

- *Physical activity can help protect against the effects of stress on memory.* A recent study of older adults found that accumulated stress was associated with decreased volume in the hippocampus, a brain region implicated in memory. Stress effects on the brain were less significant for those who engaged in more frequent exercise. The *Physical Activity Guidelines* report indicates that physical activity also improves other components of cognition in addition to memory such as processing speed and overall focus.

- *Physical activity buffers the negative impact of stress on cellular aging.* Stress can reduce the length of telomeres (protective ends of DNA strands), leading to more rapid cell aging. Recent studies suggest that regular physical activity can prevent stress-induced damage to DNA. For example, one study found that sedentary individuals showed stress-induced decreases in telomere length, whereas those who engaged in at least 75 minutes of weekly exercise demonstrated no relationship between stress and telomere length.

Stress reduces engagement in exercise when we need it the most. Stress tends to increase engagement in negative health behaviors (e.g., smoking, alcohol use, other drug use) while also decreasing engagement in healthy lifestyles such as exercise. For example, data from more than 400,000 users of the smartphone app Argus across 187 countries showed a roughly 5 percent decrease in steps within 10 days of the COVID-19 pandemic declaration and a 27 percent decrease within 30 days. Reductions in physical activity corresponded with the timing of outbreaks in different countries and were more pronounced in countries with more restrictive quarantine rules. Further studies of lifestyles and stress related to COVID-19 will provide insights about these links. The takeaway message is to try to understand how stress interacts with your personal lifestyle and behaviors.

Stress, Sleep, and Recreation

Adequate sleep is critical to effectively managing stressful situations. Although there are individual differences in the number of hours of sleep needed, the average adult needs between 7 and 8 hours of sleep per night. Teenagers and young adults (those in their early 20s) may need slightly more sleep. Unfortunately, many do not get this amount of sleep. Full-time college students get an average of 8.6 hours of sleep on weekday nights. However, more than one-fifth of college students average 7 or fewer hours of sleep on weekdays. Thus, a substantial number of students fail to get adequate sleep. With insufficient sleep, many people resort to caffeine to stay awake, leading to an endless cycle of deficient sleep and caffeine use and compromised health and wellness. Table 1 presents guidelines for good sleep. The recent *Physical Activity Guidelines for Americans* report indicates that moderate to vigorous physical activity improves the quality of sleep both by reducing the length of time it takes to go to sleep and reducing awake time during the night. It can also increase the time in deep sleep and reduce daytime sleepiness.

All work and no play can lead to poor mental and physical health. Between 1860 and 1990, the number of hours typically spent working in industrialized countries decreased relatively dramatically. Although that trend has continued in most countries, work hours in the United States have increased considerably over the past two decades. A major reason for this increase is that more people now hold second jobs than in the past. Also, some jobs in modern society have increasing rather than decreasing time demands. The notion of 40 hour work weeks are the exception rather

Table 1 ▶ Guidelines for Good Sleep

- Be aware of the effects of medications. Some medicines, such as weight loss pills and decongestants, contain caffeine or other ingredients that interfere with sleep.
- Avoid tobacco use. Nicotine is a stimulant and can interfere with sleep.
- Avoid excess alcohol use. Alcohol may make it easier to get to sleep, but may be a reason you wake up at night and are unable to get back to sleep.
- You may exercise late in the day, but do not do vigorous activity right before bedtime.
- Sleep in a room that is cooler than normal.
- Avoid hard-to-digest foods late in the day, as well as fatty and spicy foods.
- Avoid large meals late in the day or right before bedtime. A light snack before bedtime should not be a problem for most people.
- Avoid too much liquid before bedtime.
- Avoid naps during the day.
- Go to bed and get up at the same time each day.
- Do not study, read, or engage in other activities in your bed. You want your brain to associate your bed with sleep, not with activity.
- If you are having difficulty falling asleep, do not stay in bed. Get up and find something to do until you begin to feel tired, and then go back to bed.

than the rule for many working professionals. It is common for most professionals to work much longer days and to continue to work while at home.

Experts have referred to young adults as "overworked Americans" because they work several jobs and maintain dual roles (full-time employment coupled with normal family chores), or they work extended hours in demanding professional jobs. A Gallup poll showed that the great majority of adults have "enough time" for work, chores, and sleep but not enough time for friends, self, spouse, and children. It is not yet clear how the move to working from home for many during the COVID-19 pandemic impacted work–life balance or attitudes related to work. Answers to this question will likely be important for many years to come. A recent Gallup poll showed that roughly two-thirds of Americans indicated a preference to work from home if given the opportunity.

Recreation and leisure are important contributors to wellness (quality of life). Leisure is generally considered to be the opposite of work and includes "doing things we just

Leisure Time that is free from the demands of work. Leisure is more than free time; it is also an attitude. Leisure activities need not be means to ends (purposeful) but are ends in themselves.

want to do," as well as "doing nothing." In contrast, **recreation** generally is something that is pursued for a specific purpose. The difference between leisure and recreation often depends on how it is perceived. Many people pursue recreational activities to contribute to fitness goals, but walking can also be a form of leisure for some. Reading and listening to music are common leisure activities, but both can be pursued for recreational purposes (if related to hobbies or for emotional, mental, and spiritual growth). Leisure and recreation both contribute to stress reduction and wellness, although leisure activities are not done specifically to achieve these benefits. The value of recreation and leisure in Western culture is evidenced by the emphasis public health officials place on the availability and accessibility of recreational facilities in communities.

Play is critical to development, and a sense of play in adult recreation contributes to wellness. Play is distinct from recreation in that it is typically intrinsically motivated and has an imaginative component. Play has been shown to be important to healthy brain development in humans, and there is considerable evidence for physical, social, and cognitive benefits of play. In children, "free play," or unstructured time for play, seems to be particularly important. This type of play has been linked to a number of positive outcomes, including increased attention in the classroom, better self-regulation, and improved social skills and problem solving. Although much less attention has been given to the value of play in adults, a recent literature review identified benefits of play in adults, including mood enhancement, skill development, and enhanced relationships. Clearly, benefits of play have the potential both to prevent stress and to facilitate effective coping with stress.

Principles of Stress Management

Stress-management skills can be learned. There is considerable evidence that stress-management training yields both physical and mental health benefits. Positive effects have been noted in a variety of populations. For example, a recent study found that stress-management training for patients with heart disease resulted in improved cardiovascular function, decreased depression, and lower levels of general distress. Similar results were found following a stress-management intervention provided to females following treatment for breast cancer. Interestingly, and perhaps of more relevance to college students, a recent meta-analysis of 43 studies documented consistent reductions in stress and anxiety from stress-management programs. Enrolling in available classes is a proactive step to help address personal stress.

Stress-management training focuses on teaching active coping strategies. There are a variety of effective stress-management approaches and which ones you choose

may depend on the outcome goal. The meta-analysis mentioned in the previous section showed that cognitive-behavioral therapy, coping skills, and social support interventions led to greater reductions in perceived stress, whereas relaxation training, mindfulness-based stress reduction, and psychoeducation led to a greater reduction in anxiety. Of course, using multiple approaches may result in the best outcomes. Another meta-analysis of studies of stress-management training in college students found that programs that incorporated both relaxation and more active strategies for managing stress had the most benefit.

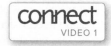

Active **coping** strategies are those that attempt to directly affect the source of the stress or to effectively manage the individual's reactions to stress, whereas passive coping strategies attempt to direct attention away from the stressor. Active coping strategies can be further classified into three basic categories: **appraisal-focused coping**, **emotion-focused coping**, and **problem-focused coping**. As indicated in Table 2, these coping strategies target the cognitive, emotional, physiological, and behavioral aspects of stress. Whereas each of these strategies is effective in various circumstances, the fourth one listed in the table (**avoidant coping** strategies) is likely to be ineffective for almost everyone. This includes strategies such as ignoring or escaping the problem or suppressing negative emotions.

A CLOSER LOOK

Weathering the Storm

Weathering is a term used to describe health disparities that may result from cumulative socioeconomic disadvantage. Dr. Arline Geronimus first used the term to describe discrepancies in reproductive outcomes of Black versus white females, but the term is now used more broadly to refer to health disparities in Black populations. A contributing factor to this weathering is systemic racism, a topic that has garnered increased attention in the United States following the deaths of George Floyd and other Black Americans. Forms of discrimination and marginalization slowly chip away at a person, causing those who are on the receiving end to have compromised health or premature death. The concept of weathering provides a way to understand a root cause of health disparities in our society.

What steps should individuals take to address systemic racism and unjust weathering?

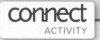

Table 2 ▶ Strategies for Stress Management

Category	Description
Appraisal-Focused Strategies	**Strategies That Alter Perceptions of the Problem or Your Ability to Cope Effectively with the Problem**
• Cognitive restructuring	• Changing negative or automatic thoughts leading to unnecessary distress
• Seeking knowledge or practicing skills	• Finding ways to increase your confidence in your ability to cope
Emotion-Focused Strategies	**Strategies That Minimize the Emotional and Physical Effects of the Situation**
• Relaxing	• Using relaxation techniques to reduce the symptoms of stress
• Exercising	• Using physical activity to reduce the symptoms of stress
• Expressing your feelings	• Talking with someone about what you are feeling or writing about your emotional experiences
• Spirituality	• Looking for spiritual guidance to provide comfort
Problem-Focused Strategies	**Strategies That Directly Seek to Solve or Minimize the Stressful Situation**
• Systematic problem solving	• Making a plan of action to solve the problem and following through to make the situation better
• Being assertive	• Standing up for your own rights and values while respecting the opinions of others
• Seeking active social support	• Getting help or advice from others who can provide specific assistance for your situation
Avoidant Coping Strategies	**Strategies That Attempt to Distract the Individual from the Problem**
• Ignoring	• Refusing to think about the situation or pretending no problem exists
• Escaping	• Looking for ways to feel better or to stop thinking about the problem, including eating or using nicotine, alcohol, or other drugs
• Suppressing	• Actively trying to suppress emotional experiences or emotional expression
• Ruminating	• Focusing on your negative emotions and what they mean without taking efforts to address the problem

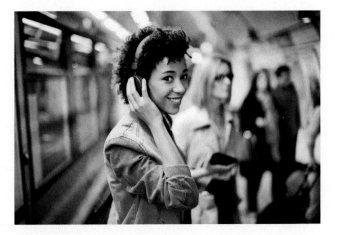

Using appropriate coping strategies can help manage stress.
Paul Bradbury/Getty Images

Active coping strategies affect stress in different ways. Appraisal-focused coping strategies are based on changing the way one perceives the stressor or changing one's perceptions of resources for effectively managing stress. In contrast, emotion-focused coping strategies attempt to regulate the emotions resulting from stressful events. Both appraisal- and emotion-focused coping can be considered "emotion regulation" strategies, but the difference between the two approaches is in the timing: Appraisal-focused coping attempts to change the initial emotional experience, whereas emotion-focused coping attempts to manage the emotional experiences that follow appraisal. Efforts to positively reappraise stressful experiences can reduce initial emotional reactions to a stressor, but additional strategies may be needed to manage these emotions. Problem-focused strategies act very differently. They do not influence emotional responses to stress but rather focus on helping address or remove the underlying source of the stress.

Recreation *Recreation* means creating something anew. We refer to it as something that you do for amusement or for fun to help you divert your attention and to refresh yourself (re-create yourself).

Play Activity done of one's own free will. The play experience is fun and intrinsically rewarding, and it is a self-absorbing means of self-expression. It is characterized by a sense of freedom or escape from life's normal rules.

Coping A person's constantly changing cognitive and psychological efforts to manage stressful situations.

Appraisal-Focused Coping Adapting to stress by changing your perceptions of stress and your resources for coping.

Emotion-Focused Coping Adapting to stress by regulating the emotions that cause or result from stress.

Problem-Focused Coping Adapting to stress by changing the source or cause of stress.

Avoidant Coping Seeking immediate, temporary relief from stress through distraction or self-indulgence (e.g., use of alcohol, tobacco, or other drugs).

HELP   Health is available to Everyone for a Lifetime, and it's Personal

Dealing with College Stress

College campuses offer a range of resources to help students with stress management. Resources include academic offices to help with time management and scholastic difficulties as well as counseling centers for anxiety, depression, relationships, and other problems. Issues with COVID-19 led to increases in mental health issues and heightened stress. Loneliness and social isolation were clear contributors to these issues, indicating the importance of social interactions for health and well-being. Clinicians and counselors have adapted to provide options to help students get the help they need. However, an important first step to treatment is to understand your personal mental health needs (and the needs of others close to you).

Did you notice impacts of social isolation on your mental health? Are you aware of where to find mental health services on your campus?

connect ACTIVITY

Effective coping strategies are described in detail in the following section, followed by guidelines on time management and effective social support. Although you should take

steps to minimize stress, it is critical to learn ways to effectively cope with it when it occurs.

Effective Coping Strategies

Coping with most stress requires a variety of thoughts and actions. Stress forces the body to work under less than optimal conditions, yet this is the time when we need to function at our best. Effective coping may require some efforts to regulate the emotional aspects of the stress and other efforts to solve the problem. For example, if you receive a bad grade on an exam, how you view the situation and interpret its meaning will have a major impact on how you feel. You will have to eventually accept your current grade and manage the emotions that accompany this reality. Then, you will need to take active steps to improve your performance on the next exam. It does no good to worry about past events so, instead, you look forward. Thus, coping with this situation can require the use of all three coping strategies.

Appraisal-focused coping strategies can be effective for certain situations. The way you think about stressful situations (see Table 3) can dramatically influence your emotional experiences. Research has demonstrated that cognitive reappraisal leads to down-regulation of the autonomic and endocrine systems, leading to physical and mental health benefits. Fortunately, even those of us who do not typically engage in reappraisal can learn to use this approach.

Table 3 ▶ Types of Distorted Thinking

Type	Description
1. All-or-none thinking	You look at things in absolute, black-and-white categories.
2. Overgeneralization	You view a negative event as a never-ending pattern of defeat.
3. Mental filter	You dwell on the negatives and ignore the positives.
4. Discounting the positives	You insist that your accomplishments and positive qualities don't count.
5. Jumping to conclusions	(a) Mind reading—you assume that others are reacting negatively to you when there is no definite evidence of this. (b) Fortune telling—you arbitrarily predict that things will turn out badly.
6. Magnification or minimization	You blow things out of proportion or shrink their importance inappropriately.
7. Emotional reasoning	You reason from how you feel: "I feel like an idiot, so I must be one." "I don't feel like doing this, so I'll put it off."
8. "Should" statements	You criticize yourself or other people with "shoulds" or "shouldn'ts." "Musts," "oughts," and "have tos" are similar offenders.
9. Labeling	You identify with your shortcomings. Instead of saying, "I made a mistake," you tell yourself, "I am a jerk," "a fool," or "a loser."
10. Personalization and blame	You blame yourself for something that you weren't entirely responsible for, or you blame other people and overlook ways that your own attitudes and behaviors might have contributed to the problem.

Source: Burns, D. D., (1999). *The Feeling Good Handbook.* New York, New York Penguin Group.

Research on cognitive therapy approaches for treating anxiety and mood disorders has shown that people can readily learn this skill, and learning to change the way you think can reduce emotional distress. Further, a recent meta-analysis showed that single-session reappraisal interventions lead to less subjective distress following exposure to an acute stressor. Thus, the way you think about stressful situations can be as important as how you respond to them.

At one time or another, virtually all people have distorted thinking, which can create unnecessary stress. Distorted thinking is also referred to as negative or automatic thinking. To alleviate stress, it can be useful to recognize some common types of distorted thinking (see Table 3). If you can learn to recognize distorted thinking, you can change the way you think and reduce your stress levels.

If you have ever used any of the 10 types of distorted thinking described in Table 3, you may find it 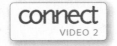 useful to consider different methods of "untwisting" your thinking to change negative thinking to positive thinking (see Table 4). To try this, think of a recent situation that caused stress. Describe the situation on paper, and see if you used distorted thinking in the situation (see Table 3). If so, write down which types of distorted thinking you used. Finally, determine if any of the guidelines in Table 4 would have been useful. If so, write down the strategy you could have used. When a similar situation arises, you will be prepared to deal with it. Repeat this technique, using several situations that have recently caused stress.

Emotion-focused coping strategies are helpful for issues or problems that are not within your control. 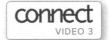 Relaxation techniques and/or coping strategies can help reduce the negative impact of both physical and emotional consequences of stress. These approaches can slow

Table 4 ▶ Ten Ways to Untwist Your Thinking

Way	Description
1. Identify the distortion.	Write down your negative thoughts, so you can see which of the 10 types of distorted thinking you are involved in. This will make it easier to think about the problem in a more positive and realistic way.
2. Examine the evidence.	Instead of assuming that your negative thought is true, or if you feel you never do anything right, you can list several things that you have done successfully.
3. Use the double standard method.	Instead of putting yourself down in a harsh, condemning way, talk to yourself in the same compassionate way you would talk to a friend with a similar problem.
4. Use the experimental technique.	Do an experiment to test the validity of your negative thought. For example, if, during an episode of panic you become terrified that you are about to die of a heart attack, you can jog or run up and down several flights of stairs. This will prove that your heart is healthy and strong.
5. Think in shades of gray.	Although this method might sound drab, the effects can be illuminating. Instead of thinking about your problems in all-or-none extremes, evaluate things on a range from 0 to 100. When things do not work out as well as you had hoped, think about the experience as a partial success, rather than a complete failure. See what you can learn from the situation.
6. Use the survey method.	Ask people questions to find out if your thoughts and attitudes are realistic. For example, if you believe that public speaking anxiety is abnormal and shameful, ask several friends if they have ever felt nervous before giving a talk.
7. Define terms.	When you label yourself "inferior," "a fool," or "a loser," ask, "What is the definition of 'a fool'?" You will feel better when you see that there is no such thing as a fool or a loser.
8. Use the semantic method.	Simply substitute language that is less colorful or emotionally loaded. This method is helpful for "should" statements. Instead of telling yourself, "I *shouldn't* have made that mistake," you can say, "It would be better if I hadn't made that mistake."
9. Use reattribution.	Instead of automatically assuming you are "bad" and blaming yourself entirely for a problem, think about the many factors that may have contributed to it. Focus on solving the problem instead of using up all your energy blaming yourself and feeling guilty.
10. Do a cost–benefit analysis.	List the advantages and disadvantages of a feeling (such as getting angry when your plane is late), a negative thought (such as "No matter how hard I try, I always screw up"), or a behavior pattern (such as overeating and lying around in bed when you are depressed). You can also use the cost–benefit analysis to modify a self-defeating belief, such as "I must always be perfect."

Source: Burns, D. D., (1999). *The Feeling Good Handbook.* New York, New York Penguin Group.

your heart and respiration rate, relax tense muscles, clear your mind, and help you relax mentally and emotionally. Perhaps most important, these techniques can improve your outlook and help you cope better with the stressful situation. In Lab 17B, you will try several relaxation techniques. However, performing the exercises only once will not prepare you to use relaxation techniques effectively. You must practice learning to relax.

Conscious relaxation techniques reduce stress and tension by directly altering the physical symptoms. When you are stressed, heart rate, blood pressure, and muscle tension all increase to help your body deal with the challenge. Conscious relaxation techniques reduce these normal effects and bring the body back to a more relaxed state. These approaches can also help you manage the negative emotions that result from stressors and your appraisal of those stressors. Most techniques use the "three *R*s" of relaxation to help the body and mind relax: (1) reduce mental activity, (2) recognize tension, and (3) reduce respiration. Some relaxation techniques include:

- *Deep breathing and mental imagery.* One of the quickest ways to experience relaxation is through deep breathing. A simple version involves inhaling deeply through your nose for about 4 seconds and then letting the air out slowly through your mouth (for about 8 seconds). Repeating these steps for several minutes can help you control your body's reaction to stress and slow your breathing. (See Lab 17B for more detailed instructions about diaphragmatic breathing.) The main advantage of this method is that it can be used in any setting and takes very little time to induce a relaxation response.

- *Jacobson's progressive relaxation method.* You must be able to recognize how a tense muscle feels before you can voluntarily release the tension. In this technique, you sequentially contract and then relax various muscles to improve perceptions of tense and relaxed muscles. Special emphasis is placed on the importance of relaxing eye and speech muscles, because these muscles are thought to trigger or influence tension in other muscles.

- *Biofeedback.* Biofeedback training uses machines that monitor certain physiological processes of the body and provide visual or auditory evidence of what is happening to normally unconscious bodily functions. The evidence, or feedback, is then used to help you decrease these functions. This technique is often combined with autogenic training (self-guided relaxation training that involves deep breathing and imagery) to help promote relaxation.

- *Stretching and rhythmical exercises.* After working long hours at a desk, release tension by getting up frequently to stretch, taking a brisk walk, or by performing "office exercises." One popular activity that uses stretching and rhythmic exercise (as well as

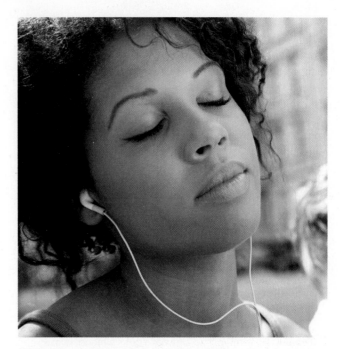

Taking time to relax can help you manage stress.
Oliver Rossi/Corbis/Getty Images

breathing techniques) is yoga. Many find it beneficial in reducing stress, and research has found both physical and mental health benefits associated with yoga.

Spirituality and mindfulness can help you cope with stress and daily problems. In addition to managing the body's physical response to stress, one must deal with the impact of stress on thoughts and emotions. Although relaxation strategies are helpful, additional approaches may be necessary to adequately manage these aspects of the stress response.

- *Spirituality.* Studies have shown that spirituality can decrease blood pressure, be a source of internal comfort, and have other calming effects associated with reduced distress. It can also provide confidence to function more effectively, thereby reducing the stresses associated with ineffectiveness at work or in other situations. One study of college students found that spirituality moderated the relationship between stress and health outcomes. For those low in spirituality, stress was associated with higher levels of negative emotion and physical symptoms of illness. Among those higher in spirituality, the link between stress and health outcomes was much weaker.

- *Mindfulness meditation.* While most relaxation techniques seek to distract attention away from distressing emotions, mindfulness meditation encourages the individual to experience their emotions in a nonjudgmental way. The individual brings full attention to the internal and external experiences that are occurring "in the moment."

Online Stress-Management Resources

There are many online resources available to help you manage your stress. A training program called SMART (Stress Management and Resiliency Training) provides interactive training exercises that teach users to monitor stress, regulate emotions, relax, think flexibly, be realistic, and take effective action to deal with stressors. Other commercially available apps include Headspace, Happify, and Personal Zen. Some of these apps allow you to track your body sensation to gain better control over your physiological responses to stress. For example, Elite HRV allows you to track your heart rate variability and see how it responds to stress reduction approaches like guided breathing exercises.

Would you consider using a stress-management app that utilizes biofeedback for stress management? Why or why not?

connect ACTIVITY

A meta-analysis of stress-management approaches in college students found that mindfulness-based approaches are effective in reducing anxiety and depressive symptoms, as well as cortisol levels. As an example, a study of Koru (a mindfulness approach) found that just four sessions resulted in increases in mindfulness, decreases in perceived stress, and a reduction in sleep problems. Mindfulness meditation may also be one way of fostering the health-protective effects of spirituality. One study found that changes in mindfulness were directly associated with reported gains in spirituality and quality of life. The nonjudgmental aspect of awareness in mindfulness is critical to the success of this approach. Mindfulness meditation can counter the tendency for people to focus excessively on negative outcomes (often referred to as *rumination*). Research has shown that rumination leads to negative psychological adjustment, including increased risk for depression.

Appropriately expressing emotion can help you reduce distress. The ability to control emotional outbursts is an adaptive skill that develops with age. As a society, we socialize our children to develop these skills, as they are critical to adaptive functioning in adulthood. At the same time, complete suppression of emotion has long been recognized as potentially harmful to our health. Among college students, emotional suppression has been related to increased anxiety sensitivity, depression, and poor social adjustment. The results demonstrate that to minimize the potential negative impact of our emotions, we need to find appropriate ways to express them.

We often turn to others to provide an outlet for us to "vent" or "get it off our chest." Although this is a perfectly good way to express emotion, we can also benefit from writing about our stressful experiences. Expressive writing has shown benefits for a wide range of outcomes, from faster wound healing to better adaptation following traumatic events. Writing also seems to help reduce the effects of stress related to discrimination. For example, a recent study of gay male college students found that writing about stresses related to sexual orientation led to better adjustment 3 months later. Although many of the early studies on the therapeutic benefits of writing focused on traumatic or stressful events, more recent "self-affirmation" approaches focus on writing about personal values. These self-affirmations are believed to counter threats to the self, which include threats related to discrimination and physical health problems. In adolescents and college students, self-affirmative writing has been shown to decrease the achievement gap between majority and minority students, and low versus high socioeconomic students. A recent study also showed that expressive writing led to improvements in symptoms of PTSD and depression among health-care workers dealing with stress related to the COVID-19 pandemic. In the physical health domain, self-affirmative writing has been shown to increase medication compliance and exercise among individuals with hypertension and heart disease. Thus, writing about both challenges and important core values may allow individuals to cope more effectively with stress.

Problem-focused coping is most effective in dealing with controllable stressors. While appraisal- and emotion-focused coping may be the most effective means for coping with situations beyond one's control, a problem under personal control may best be addressed by taking action to solve the problem. A technique called "systematic problem solving" has been shown to improve the likelihood of problem resolution.

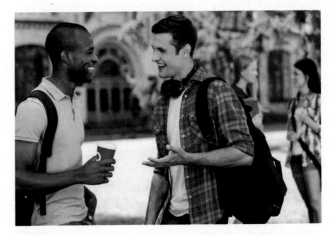

Finding ways to gain social support and express your feelings can reduce distress.
G-Stock Studio/Shutterstock

The first step is brainstorming, generating every possible solution to the problem. During this stage, do not limit the solutions you generate in any way. Even silly and impractical solutions should be included. After generating a comprehensive list, narrow your focus by eliminating any solutions that do not seem reasonable. Reduce the number of solutions to a reasonable number (four or five), and then carefully evaluate each option. Consider the potential costs and benefits of each approach to aid in making a decision. Once you decide on an approach, carefully plan the implementation of the strategy, anticipating anything that might go wrong and being prepared to alter your plan as necessary.

In some cases, directly addressing the source of stress involves responding assertively. For example, if the source of stress is an employer placing unreasonable demands on your time, the best solution to the problem may involve talking to your boss about the situation. This type of confrontation is difficult for many people concerned about being overly aggressive. However, you can stand up for yourself without infringing on the rights of others. Many people confuse assertiveness with aggression, leading to passive responses in difficult situations. An aggressive response intimidates others and fulfills one's own needs at the expense of others. In contrast, an assertive response protects your own rights and values while respecting the opinions of others. Once you are comfortable with the idea of responding assertively, practice or role-play assertive responses with a trusted friend before trying them in the real world. Your friend may provide valuable feedback about your approach, and the practice may increase your self-efficacy for responding and your expectancies for a positive outcome.

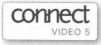

Effective Time-Management Skills

Effective time management is a self-management skill that helps you adapt to the stresses of modern living. Lack of time is cited by both the general public and experts as a source of stress and a reason for failing to implement healthy lifestyle changes.

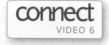

For college students, managing time is critical to academic success as well as overall well-being. Managing time effectively has become even more of a challenge for college students in recent years, as more and more students are working part- or full-time jobs to support their education (see Figure 1). The following strategies may help you learn to manage your time more effectively.

- *Prioritize.* Many people feel that there are not enough hours in the day to do everything that needs to be done. The truth is, they are probably right. If you think about all the things that have to get done, it can seem unmanageable. That is why it is important to prioritize. Many time-management experts advocate the ABC approach as a way to prioritize

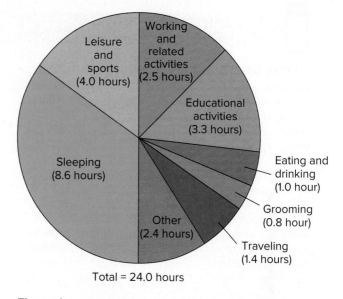

Total = 24.0 hours

Figure 1 ▶ Time use on an average weekday for full-time university and college students.

Note: Data include individuals, aged 15–49, who were enrolled full time at a university or college. Data include averages for non-holiday weekdays.

Source: Bureau of Labor Statistics, American Time Use Survey.

tasks effectively. Create three lists of things you need to do, with list A including the most urgent tasks and list C containing the least urgent. To help you remember the ABC approach, remember that A tasks *A*bsolutely must get done, B tasks had *B*etter get done, and C tasks *C*ould get done. See Table 5 for a brief description of the ABC approach.

Table 5 ▶ The ABC System for Time Management

Level of Importance	Description
A	*A tasks* are those that *must* be done, and soon. When accomplished, A tasks may yield extraordinary results. Left undone, they may generate serious, unpleasant, or disastrous consequences. Immediacy is what an A priority task is all about.
B	*B tasks* are those that *should* be done soon. While not as pressing as A tasks, they're still important. They can be postponed, but not for too long. Within a brief time, though, they can easily rise to A status.
C	*C tasks* are those that *could* be done. These tasks could be put off without creating dire consequences. Some can linger in this category almost indefinitely. Others—especially those tied to distant completion dates—will eventually rise to A or B levels as the deadline approaches.

Source: Mancini, M.

- *Plan.* One of the most important steps in effective time management is to plan your daily activities. This includes keeping a daily planner to remember your schedule, tracking important events and deadlines, and maintaining lists (using the ABC approach) to help you remember your goals and priorities. Computers and apps allow you to keep all of this information in one place.

- *Set SMART goals.* In addition to knowing how you spend your time, it is important to know what things need to get done. This includes everything from small tasks that need to get done today to important long-term goals. When setting goals, make sure they are SMART (specific, measurable, attainable, realistic, and timely). You want to set yourself up for success by setting goals that are realistic and attainable, and you need a system for tracking your progress. Thus, your goals need to be specific and measurable. Some tasks may be more easily accomplished if they are broken down into a series of smaller tasks, each with its own deadline. Setting specific deadlines for the completion of goals increases the likelihood that you will follow through.

- *Build recreational activities into your schedule.* Although it may seem that scheduling fun takes away from the enjoyment, you may not find this to be true. By scheduling your free time, you can fully enjoy it rather than worrying about other things you "should" be doing.

- *Make the most of the time you have.* To get the most out of your time, know when you do your best work and under what conditions. If you are sharpest in the morning, schedule the most important work to be done during this time. If you study most effectively when you are alone in a quiet place, schedule your studying at a time when you can create that environment. It is also important not to let time that could be productive go to waste. Try to take advantage of small periods of time (e.g., between classes).

- *Regularly self-assess and monitor your time-management skills in order to manage your time effectively.* Where does your time go? The answer to this question is the first step toward better time management. Most of us are not fully aware of how we spend our time. Periodic self-monitoring of your time usage can help you learn how to focus your time on the most important things and identify where you could spend less time. You probably need to do this for at least a week to get a good indication of where your time is going. Then reevaluate over time to track your progress, identify areas in need of further improvement, and adapt your plan to improve your chances of success.

- *Avoid procrastination.* Virtually all of us procrastinate at one time or another, but for many, procrastination can significantly decrease performance and increase stress. A number of causes of procrastination have been identified, including both internal and external influences. Understanding the causes of procrastination can help you find ways to prevent it in the future (see Figure 2). One of the simplest solutions to procrastination is simply to "get started." The first step toward completing a project is often the most difficult. Once people take the first step, they often find that the task becomes easier.

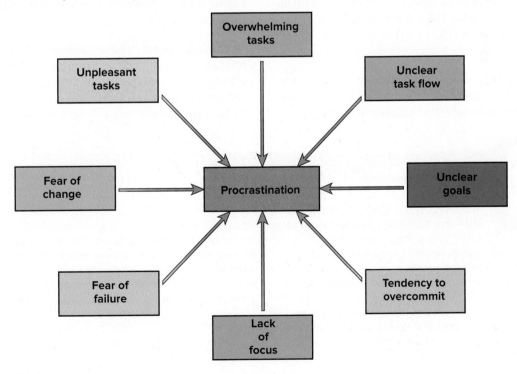

Figure 2 ▶ Causes of procrastination.

Source: Mancini, M. (2003). *Time Management.* The McGraw-Hill Companies, Inc.

Effective Social Support

Eliciting social support is an important self-management skill for stress management. **Social support** can play a role in coping with stress, and it has been linked to better physical and mental health outcomes among individuals with chronic stress-related illnesses. For example, in a large group of patients with coronary artery disease, participation in a social support group was associated with lower systolic blood pressure, better social functioning, and better mental health. Social support may also be critical to managing stress in academic settings. A recent study found that a lack of social support from family, teachers, and peers was associated with a lack of academic motivation and subsequent academic failure.

Social support may be particularly important for females. Females may be particularly likely to seek and provide social support when stressed. A paradigm called the "tend or befriend" model suggests that females have a unique stress response. Females respond to stress by tending to others (nurturing) and affiliating with a social group (befriending). This response is helpful in reducing the risk for the negative health consequences of stress.

Social support has various sources. Everyone needs someone to turn to for support when feeling overwhelmed. Support can come from friends, family members, clergy, a teacher, a coach, or a professional counselor. Different sources provide different forms of support. Even pets have been shown to be a good source of social support, with consequent health and quality-of-life benefits. The goal is to identify and nurture relationships that can provide this type of support. In turn, it is important to look for ways to support and assist others.

There are many types of social support. Social support has three main components: informational, material, and emotional. Informational (technical) support includes tips,

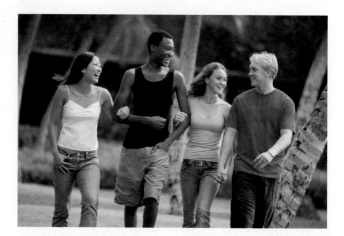
Social support is important for stress management.
Don Hammond/Design Pics

strategies, and advice that can help a person get through a specific stressful situation. For example, a parent, friend, or coworker may offer insight into how he or she once resolved similar problems. Material support is direct assistance to get a person through a stressful situation—for example, providing a loan to help pay off a short-term debt. Emotional support is encouragement or sympathy that a person provides to help another cope with a particular challenge.

Regardless of the type of support, it is important that it fosters autonomy. Social support that helps you become more self-reliant because of increased feelings of competence is best for developing autonomy. Social support that is controlling or leads to dependence may increase rather than decrease stress over time.

Obtaining good social support requires close relationships. Although we live in a social environment, it is often difficult to ask people for help. Sometimes the nature and severity of our problems may not be apparent to others. Other times, friends may not want to offer suggestions or

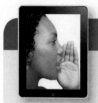

In the News

The Misinformation Superhighway

Americans are increasingly relying on social media as a primary news source. A recent Pew study found that 18 percent of respondents got most of their political and election news from social media. This is slightly higher than the percentage who get their news from cable television (16 percent) or local television (16 percent). This can cause problems because of the overwhelming volume of information on social media, and the tendency for social media users to affiliate with others who share their views (homopholy),

leading to "echo chambers" that protect people from opposing viewpoints. The result is often confirmation of what a person already believes, with limited efforts to fact-check the information they find. Several social media sites flag inaccurate or misleading information. Although many applaud these efforts, others suggest that such labeling suppresses free speech.

Do you think social media platforms should label posts that contain misinformation, or is this a violation of free speech?

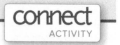

insight because they do not want to appear too pushy. To obtain good support, one must develop quality personal relationships. Although having a large social support network is helpful, quality is more important than quantity. Many individuals report feeling lonely despite having large social networks, and loneliness is associated with negative health behaviors, including smoking and lack of exercise.

Social support is especially critical during periods of high stress. Although social support helps us deal with daily stressors, it is especially important when we experience severe or chronic stress. The COVID-19 pandemic revealed the links between stress and social isolation as quarantines cut off many people from family members and other critical sources of social support. As a consequence, rates of mental health problems and substance use increased substantially during the latter half of 2020. Fortunately, people are resilient and found other ways to connect with those close to them (e.g., videoconferencing).

Using Self-Management Skills

Understanding distinctions among self-management skills can help you employ them. Coping skills and time-management skills are considered "enabling factors" that help you adopt healthy lifestyles. As applied to stress management, these skills can help you avoid stress and take effective action to manage or cope with stress. Seeking social support is categorized as a "reinforcing factor" that helps reinforce healthy behaviors. The key is to build your social support network and to learn how to effectively elicit and use support when needed. As you begin to use and practice these self-management skills, try to evaluate how effective they are in managing your stress. Not all approaches will work for all people, so there is no point in continuing to use strategies that do not work for you. If it works, keep practicing until you master the approach.

Sometimes professional help is necessary to deal with problems related to stress. This Concept introduces principles for effective stress management, but sometimes stress creates problems that require professional help. If you think you might be suffering from an anxiety or mood disorder (e.g., PTSD, depression), there are well-established treatments that can help you function more effectively. Sometimes, professionals can also be helpful in efforts to change negative health behaviors such as alcohol and drug use or problematic patterns of eating. Thankfully, stigma associated with these problems has decreased, leading many more people to seek professional services. In addition, the COVID-19 pandemic has accelerated the adoption of teletherapy via videoconferencing, further increasing the accessibility of mental health services.

Practicing self-management skills can help you manage stress more effectively. This Concept has described a variety of self-management skills that are important for preventing, managing, and coping with stress. One useful way to organize these different approaches is to think about their respective roles both prior to and after the experience of a stressful event. *Protective strategies* are those that help prepare your mind and body for a positive response even before a stressful event occurs. Once you have experienced a stressor, you can engage in efforts to directly address the source of the stress (*primary control strategies*) as well as efforts to effectively manage the consequences of the stressor (*secondary control strategies*). The distinctions are described next.

Protective strategies:

- *Time management.* Learning to prioritize tasks (see Table 5) and plan for effective use of time (see Lab 17A) are effective steps for reducing the amount of stress you experience. Stress is often the result of a failure to plan effectively. (See the "Effective Time-Management Skills" section for more strategies.)

- *Exercise and recreation.* Part of effectively managing stress is about being physically healthy and keeping a work–life balance. Regular physical exercise will allow your body to respond to stress more effectively, and recreation will help with work–life balance.

- *Good sleep hygiene.* Your body will respond most effectively to stress if you get enough good quality sleep. In the busy lives of young people, it can be difficult to find enough time to sleep, but it is essential to do so. Using the time-management approaches outlined in this Concept can help leave sufficient time for sleep. Also see Table 1 for tips on good sleep hygiene.

- *Relaxation techniques.* Regular practice of relaxation techniques helps keep the stress systems in the body in homeostasis so that a new stressor does not overwhelm your physical resources. A variety of approaches are available, and several are outlined in the emotion-focused strategies earlier in the Concept.

Primary control strategies:

- *Systematic problem solving.* Primary control strategies are best employed when there is an opportunity to directly address the source of the stress. For example, a conflict with a coworker may be addressable if you have an effective strategy.

Secondary control strategies:

- *Reappraisal.* In many cases the source of stress may not be something you can directly change (e.g., a poor grade or the end of a relationship), but you can always change the way you think about the event. For example, a poor test grade

Social Support The behavior of others that assists a person in addressing a specific need.

can be defeating, or it can be used as a source of motivation to excel on the next exam. Tables 4 and 5 can help you identify self-defeating thoughts and develop approaches to think in ways that lead to more effective responses to stress.

- *Social support.* When you experience events that are beyond your control, just talking to someone who understands your experience can make a big difference. Friends and family can also help you effectively use the other approaches outlined in this Concept. For example, exercising with a companion is often more enjoyable.

- *Protective coping strategies can also help with secondary control.* In addition to preparing your body and mind prior

to the experience of a stressor, several of the protective approaches outlined previously can help with managing the acute consequences of a stressor. For example, exercise and relaxation techniques can help your body recover from the acute physiological consequences of the stress response.

Although these categories may serve as a useful way to think about which approach to use in different circumstances, it is important to remember that not all strategies will work for all people. So, you have to find the approaches that work best for you. There is no point in continuing to use strategies that are not working. When you find approaches that do work, keep practicing until you master them.

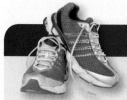

Strategies for Action: Lab Information

Performing a self-assessment of current time use can help you manage time effectively. Lab 17A provides you with an opportunity to take a careful look at your current use of time. The results of the self-assessment can help you develop a schedule that will allow you to focus on your priorities and use your time effectively.

Effectively using relaxation exercises requires practice. Relaxation exercises are a type of performance skill that can be

used to manage stress. Like any skill, they require practice to be effective. Lab 17B gives you the opportunity to practice several different relaxation exercises and to perfect the skills for future use in coping with stress.

Assessing your level of social support is the first step in improving it. Lab 17C gives you the opportunity to assess your current level of social support. After performing the self-assessment, use your scores to help you find social support if results indicate a need for improvement.

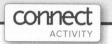

Suggested Resources and Readings

The websites for the following sources can be accessed by searching online for the organization, program, or title listed. Specific scientific references are available at the end of this edition of *Concepts of Fitness and Wellness.*

- The American Institute of Stress.
- Dierdorff, E. (2020, January 29). "Time Management Is About More Than Life Hacks." *Harvard Business Review.*
- Erdman, S. (2021). "Relaxation Techniques: Learn How to Manage Stress." *WebMD.*
- Genewick, J. (2020, December 31). "Setting SMART Goals for Success." Mayo Clinic Health System.
- LeBlanc, N., & Marques, L. (2019). "Anxiety in College: What We Know and How to Cope." *Harvard Health Publishing.*
- Mayo Clinic (2019). "Spirituality and Stress Relief: Make the Connection."
- Mayo Clinic (2020). "Exercise and Stress: Get Moving to Manage Stress."
- Mayo Clinic (2020). "Social Support: Tap This Tool to Beat Stress."
- Mitchell, A., et al. (2020, July 30). "Americans Who Mainly Get Their News on Social Media Are Less Engaged, Less Knowledgeable." Pew Research Center.
- National Institutes of Health. (2016). Relaxation Techniques for Health.
- Robinson, L., & Smith, M. (2020, September). "Social Media and Mental Health." *HelpGuide.org.*
- Sandoiu, A. (2021, February 26). "'Weathering': What Are the Health Effects of Stress and Discrimination?" *Medical News Today.*
- Scott, E. (2020, March 27). "The Benefits of Journaling for Stress Management." *Verywell Mind.*
- Scott, E. (2021, April 3). "Using Stress Relief Apps to Transform Your Life." *Verywell Mind.*
- Stress Management Society. From Distress to De-stress.
- Telehealth.HH.gov. Health Care from the Safety of Our Homes.
- U.S. Bureau of Labor Statistics. American Time Use Survey.
- Villines, Z. (2020, April 20). "Teletherapy: How It Works." *Medical News Today.*

Design Element: (*magnifying glass*): Siede Preis/Getty Images; (*runners shoes*): Maridav/Getty Images; (*tablet*): McGraw Hill; (*woman*): GlobalStock/Getty Images; (*blue sports shoes*): chictype/Getty Images; (*smartphone*): Alexey Boldin/Shutterstock; (*Why It Matters*): MHHE

Lab 17A Time Management

Name	**Section**	**Date**

Purpose: To learn to manage time to meet personal priorities.

Procedures

1. Follow the four steps outlined in the Results section and provide your responses at each step.
2. Complete the Conclusions and Implications section.

Results

Step 1: Establish Priorities

1. Check the circles that reflect your priorities in the following list. Add priorities as necessary.
2. Rate each of the priorities you checked. Use a 1 for highest priority, 2 for moderate priority, and 3 for low priority.

Check Priorities	Rating	Check Priorities	Rating	Check Priorities	Rating
◯ More time with family		◯ More time with boyfriend/girlfriend		◯ More time with spouse	
◯ More time for leisure		◯ More time to relax		◯ More time to study	
◯ More time for work success		◯ More time for physical activity		◯ More time to improve myself	
◯ More time for other recreation		◯ Other _____		◯ Other _____	

Step 2: Monitor Current Time Use

1. On the following daily calendar, keep track of daily time expenditure.
2. Write in exactly what you did for each time block.

7–9 A.M.	9–11 A.M.	11 A.M.–1 P.M.	1–3 P.M.
3–5 P.M.	**5–7 P.M.**	**7–9 P.M.**	**9–11 P.M.**

Step 3: Analyze Your Current Time Use by Using the ABC Method (See Table 5 in the Concept)

A Tasks That *Absolutely* Must Get Done	B Tasks That Had *Better* Get Done	C Tasks That *Could* Get Done

Step 4: Make a Schedule: Write in Your Planned Activities for the Day

Time	Activities	Time	Activities
6:00 A.M.		3:00 P.M.	
7:00 A.M.		4:00 P.M.	
8:00 A.M.		5:00 P.M.	
9:00 A.M.		6:00 P.M.	
10:00 A.M.		7:00 P.M.	
11:00 A.M.		8:00 P.M.	
Noon		9:00 P.M.	
1:00 P.M.		10:00 P.M.	
2:00 P.M.		11:00 P.M.	

Conclusions and Implications: In several sentences, discuss how you might modify your schedule to find more time for important priorities.

Lab 17B Relaxation Exercises

Name	**Section**	**Date**

Purpose: To gain experience with specific relaxation exercises and to evaluate their effectiveness.

Procedures

1. Choose two of the relaxation exercises included in Chart 1 of this lab and read through the written instructions until you have a basic understanding of the exercises. Think through the specific aspects of the exercise until you have the process figured out.
2. Find a quiet place to try one of the exercises and follow the procedures as best you can. It is not possible to provide detailed instructions, but the information should be sufficient to give you a basic understanding of the exercises.
3. On another day try a different exercise.
4. Answer the questions in the Results section. Then complete the Conclusions and Implications section.

Results

1. Which of the two exercises did you try? (List them below.)

2. Have you done either of the exercises before?　◯ Yes　◯ No

3. Was one relaxation exercise more effective or better suited to you than the other? If so, which one?

Conclusions and Implications: In several sentences, discuss whether or not you feel that relaxation exercises will be a part of your wellness program. In what ways might you benefit from relaxation training? If you do not think you have a problem with relaxation, explain why.

Chart 1 Descriptions of Relaxation Exercises

A. Progressive Relaxation

Progressive relaxation uses active (conscious) mechanisms to achieve a state of relaxation. The technique involves alternating phases of muscle contraction (tension) and muscle relaxation (tension release). Muscle groups are activated one body segment at a time, incorporating all regions of the body by the end of the routine. Begin by lying on your back in a quiet place with eyes closed. Alternately contract and relax each of the muscles—following the procedures described. Begin with the dominant side of the body first; repeat on the nondominant side.

1. Hand and forearm—Make a fist.
2. Biceps—Flex elbows.
3. Triceps—Straighten arm.
4. Forehead—Raise your eyebrows and wrinkle forehead.
5. Cheeks and nose—Wrinkle nose and squint.
6. Jaws—Clench teeth.
7. Lips and tongue—Press lips together and tongue to roof of mouth, teeth apart.
8. Neck and throat—Tuck chin and push head backward against floor (if lying) or chair (if sitting).
9. Shoulder and upper back—Hunch shoulders to ears.
10. Abdomen—Suck abdomen inward.
11. Lower back—Arch back.
12. Thighs and buttocks—Squeeze buttocks together, push heels into floor (if lying) or chair rung (if sitting).
13. Calves—Pull instep and toes toward shins.
14. Toes—Curl toes.

Muscle contraction phase: Inhale as you contract the designated muscle for 3–5 seconds. Use only a moderate level of tension.

Muscle relaxation phase: Exhale, relaxing the muscle and releasing tension for 6–10 seconds. Think of relaxation words such as *warm, calm, peaceful,* and *serene.*

Relax every muscle in your body at the end of the exercise.

B. Diaphragmatic Breathing

This exercise will help improve awareness of using deep abdominal breathing over shallower chest-type breathing. To begin, lie on your back with knees bent and feet on the floor. Place your right hand over your abdomen and left hand over your chest. Your hands will be used to monitor breathing technique. Slowly inhale through the nose by allowing the abdomen to rise under your right hand. Concentrate on expanding the abdomen for 4 seconds. Continue inhaling another 2 seconds allowing the chest to rise under your left hand. Exhale through your mouth in reverse order (for about 8 seconds, or twice as long as inhalation). Relax the chest first, feeling it sink beneath the left hand and then the abdomen, allowing it to sink beneath the right hand. Repeat 4–5 times. Discontinue if you become light-headed.

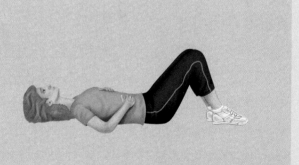

C. Tai Chi Basic Form

The basic principles of tai chi are to maintain balance, use the entire body to achieve movement, unite movement with awareness (mind) and breathing (chi), and to keep the body upright. Tai chi involves holding the body in specific positions, or "forms." To execute the basic form, stand straight, feet shoulder-width apart and parallel with one another. Your knees should be bent and turned outward slightly with knees over the foot. Your hands are on belly button with palms facing body (men place hands right on left and women left on right), fingers are straight, spread slightly and relaxed.

1. Bring arms in front of body at a 30-degree angle to the plane of the back, palms facing downward. Reach up to shoulder height with arms moving up and to the sides. (Breathe in, allowing belly to move out as you raise arms upward.)
2. When hands reach shoulder height, turn palms up and move hands to head, allowing wrists to drop down. Imagine energy (chi) flowing from palms to top of head. (Continue breathing in.)
3. Imagine energy flowing down through a central line of the body. Follow the energy with hands, point fingers toward one another, palms down, move arms downward in front of the midline of face and chest. (Breathe out as arms lower.)
4. Two inches below belly button stop, cross palms, and move hands together.
5. Lower hands toward sides. (Complete breathing out.)
6. Repeat.

Lab 17C Evaluating Levels of Social Support

Name	Section	Date

Purpose: To evaluate your level of social support and to identify ways that you can find additional support.

Procedures

1. Answer each question in Chart 1 by placing a check in the box for Not True, Somewhat True, or Very True. Place the number value of each answer in the score box to the right.
2. Sum the scores (in the smaller boxes) for each question to get subscale scores for the three social support areas.
3. Record your three subscores in the Results section on the next page. Total your subscores to get a total social support score.
4. Determine your ratings for each of the three social support subscores and for your total social support score using Chart 2.
5. Reflect on your social support and provide your response in the Conclusions and Implications section.

Chart 1 Social Support Questionnaire

These questions assess various aspects of social support. Base your answer on your actual degree of support, not on the type of support that you would like to have. Place a check in the space that best represents what is true for you.

Social Support Questions	Not True 1	Somewhat True 2	Very True 3	Score
1. I have close personal ties with my relatives.				
2. I have close relationships with a number of friends.				
3. I have a deep and meaningful relationship with a spouse or close friend.				
		Access to social support score:		
4. I have parents and relatives who take the time to listen to and understand me.				
5. I have friends or coworkers whom I can confide in and trust when problems come up.				
6. I have a nonjudgmental partner or close friend who supports me when I need help.				
		Degree of social support score:		
7. I feel comfortable asking others for advice or assistance.				
8. I have confidence in my social skills and enjoy opportunities for new social contacts.				
9. I am willing to open up and discuss my personal life with others.				
		Getting social support score:		

Results

Scores and Ratings

(Use Chart 2 to obtain ratings.)

Access to social support score [   ]   Rating [   ]

Degree of social support score [   ]   Rating [   ]

Getting social support score [   ]   Rating [   ]

Total social support score
(sum of three scores) [   ]   Rating [   ]

Chart 2 Rating Scale for Social Support

Rating	Item Scores	Total Score
High	8–9	24–27
Moderate	6–7	18–23
Low	Below 6	Below 18

Conclusions and Implications

1. In several sentences, discuss your overall social support. Do you think your scores and ratings are a true representation of your social support?

[   ]

2. In several sentences, describe any changes you think you should make to improve your social support system. If you do not think change is necessary, explain why.

[   ]

The Use and Abuse of Tobacco and Other Nicotine Products

LEARNING OBJECTIVES

After completing the study of this Concept, you will be able to:

▶ Identify the most widely used forms of tobacco and other nicotine products, and the contents of tobacco and other nicotine products that contribute to negative health outcomes.

▶ Describe the negative health and economic costs of cigarette and cigar smoking and smokeless tobacco use.

▶ Describe secondhand smoke and identify the negative health consequences of secondhand smoke exposure.

▶ Understand trends in the prevalence of tobacco use and concerns about increased rates of vaping, particularly among young people.

▶ Identify important factors contributing to recent reductions in tobacco use and efforts by the tobacco industry to maintain higher rates of smoking and use of other nicotine products.

▶ Identify effective prevention and intervention approaches designed to reduce usage rates of tobacco and other nicotine products.

Tobacco use is the number one cause of preventable disease and is associated with the leading causes of death in our culture.

Gary Bus/Taxi/Getty Images

Why It Matters!

Tobacco is the number one cause of preventable death in the United States, and it is linked to most of the leading causes of death. Although rates of smoking in the United States have decreased in recent decades due to better awareness and a changed social norm, smoking is still a major public health problem. More than 34 million adults in the United States currently smoke (roughly 14 percent of the population). More than two-thirds of current smokers want to quit, but they find it extremely difficult to succeed. In addition, the use of various forms of e-cigarettes (or "vapes") is widespread and the health consequences and risk for nicotine dependence related to these products is still being determined. This Concept will help you understand risk factors for the use and abuse of tobacco and other nicotine products so you can avoid the negative consequences that result from their use.

Tobacco: Components and Implications of Use

Tobacco and its smoke contain over 400 noxious chemicals, including 200 known poisons and 50 carcinogens. Tobacco smoke contains both gases and particulates. The gaseous phase includes a variety of harmful gases, but the most dangerous is carbon monoxide. This gas binds onto hemoglobin in the bloodstream and thereby limits how much oxygen can be carried in the bloodstream. As a result, less oxygen is supplied to the vital organs of the body. While not likely from smoking, overexposure to carbon monoxide can be fatal. The particulate phase of burning tobacco includes a variety of carbon-based compounds referred to as tar. Many of these compounds found in tobacco are known to be **carcinogens**. Nicotine is also inhaled during the particulate phase of smoking. Nicotine is a highly addictive and poisonous chemical. It has a particularly broad range of influence and is a potent psychoactive **drug** that affects the brain and alters mood and behavior.

Nicotine is the addictive component of tobacco. When smoke is inhaled, the nicotine reaches the brain in 7 seconds, where it acts on highly sensitive receptors and provides a sensation that brings about a wide variety of responses throughout the body. At first, heart and breathing rates increase. Blood vessels constrict, peripheral circulation slows down, and blood pressure increases. New users may experience dizziness, nausea, and headache. Regular smokers often experience tension reduction and increased attention and energy, effects that reinforce continued use. However, after a few minutes, these positive feelings wear off and a

rebound, or **withdrawal**, effect occurs. The smoker may feel depressed and irritable and have the urge to smoke again. **Physical dependence** occurs with continued use. Nicotine is one of the most addictive drugs known, even more addictive than heroin or alcohol.

Smoked Tobacco: Health and Economic Costs

Tobacco use is the most preventable cause of death in our society. The 1964 landmark Surgeon General's report first called attention to the negative health consequences of smoking. It is now well established that tobacco use is the leading cause of death in the United States (accounting for nearly one in five of all deaths). It contributes to 7 of the 10 leading causes of death and also contributes to negative outcomes and death from COVID-19. The life expectancy of smokers is 10 or more years less than nonsmokers. It is estimated that between 80 and 90 percent of all deaths related to lung cancer and obstructive lung disease are caused by smoking, and risk for coronary disease and stroke is two to four times higher among smokers. Further, the World Health Organization indicates that as many as 14 percent of Alzheimer disease cases worldwide may be attributed to smoking. The report suggests that exposure to secondhand smoke may be sufficient to increase risk for dementia. Thus, the number of diseases resulting from tobacco use is much more extensive than previously thought (see Figure 1).

One way to highlight the health risks associated with smoking is to examine the health benefits associated with smoking cessation. Estimates suggest that reducing serum cholesterol to recommended levels can increase life expectancy by about 1 week to 6 months. In contrast, smoking cessation may increase life expectancy by 2½ to 4½ years. The earlier people quit, the more years of life they save, with roughly 3 years saved for those who quit at 60 years of age, 6 years for those who quit at 50, and 9 years for those who quit at 40. The most effective way to reduce health risks associated with smoking is clearly to quit; however, reducing how much one smokes also makes a difference. In one study, rates of lung cancer dropped by 27 percent among those who reduced their smoking from 20 or more to less than 10 cigarettes a day.

The health risks from tobacco are directly related to overall exposure. In the past, tobacco companies denied there was conclusive proof of the harmful effects of tobacco products. However, in the face of overwhelming medical evidence, tobacco officials have conceded that tobacco is harmful to health. It is clear that the more you use the product (the more doses), the greater the health risk. Several factors determine the dosage: (1) the number of cigarettes smoked, (2) the length of time one has been

Brain: Increases risk of stroke

Eyes: Increases risk of cataracts and macular degeneration

Lungs: Increases risk of lung cancer, bronchitis, emphysema, tuberculosis, pneumonia, and asthma

Kidneys, Colon, Liver, Bladder, Pancreas: Increases risk of cancer and increases diabetes risk

Stomach/Abdomen: Increases risk of stomach cancer, peptic ulcers, and abdominal aortic aneurysm

Mouth/Throat: Increases risk of cancers of the mouth, throat, larynx, and esophagus and causes gum disease

Heart: Increases risk of coronary artery disease and atherosclerosis

Reproductive System: Increases risk of breast and cervical cancer, erectile dysfunction, birth complications, unhealthy babies, and sudden infant death syndrome in babies of smokers

Blood: Impairs immune system, increases risk of leukemia, and decreases HDL

Figure 1 ▶ Unhealthy effects of smoking.

smoking, (3) the strength (amount of tar, nicotine, etc.) of the cigarette, (4) the depth of the inhalation, and (5) the amount of exposure to other lung-damaging substances (e.g., asbestos). The greater the exposure to smoke, the greater the risk.

Although risks clearly increase with the amount of exposure, recent studies suggest that even low levels of smoking have negative consequences. Unfortunately, despite decreases in overall rates of smoking in recent years, rates of nondaily smoking have increased. These "chippers" or "social smokers" have lower risk relative to regular smokers, but there are negative health consequences of even low levels of smoking. For example, one study found that smoking one to four cigarettes per day nearly triples the risk of death from heart disease. Short-term physical consequences of smoking include increased rates of respiratory infections and asthma, impairment of athletic performance, and reduced benefits and enjoyment associated with recreational exercise.

Cigar and pipe smokers have lower death rates than cigarette smokers but are still at great risk. Cigar and pipe smokers usually inhale less and, therefore, have less risk for heart and lung disease. However, cigarette smokers who switch to cigars and pipes tend to continue inhaling the same way. As the number of cigars smoked and the depth of smoke inhalation increase, the risk for death from cigar smoking approaches that of cigarette smoking. Cigar and pipe smoke contains most of the same harmful ingredients as cigarette smoke, sometimes in higher amounts. It may also have high nicotine content, leading to no appreciable difference between cigarette and pipe/cigar smoking with respect to the development of nicotine dependence. Cigar and pipe smokers also have higher risks for cancer of the mouth, throat, and larynx relative to cigarette smokers. Pipe smokers are especially at risk for lip cancer.

Secondhand smoke poses a significant health risk. When smokers light up, they expose those around them to **secondhand smoke**. Secondhand smoke is a combination of **mainstream smoke** (inhaled and then exhaled by the smoker) and **sidestream smoke** (from the burning end of the cigarette). Because sidestream 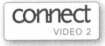 smoke is not filtered through the smoker's lungs, it has higher levels of carcinogens and is therefore more dangerous. There is evidence that secondhand smoke exposure has been reduced in recent years and that smoke-free policies have been effective. Still, millions of people are exposed, often against their wishes, and experience health and economic consequences. Consequences of exposure to secondhand tobacco smoke include:

- Increased risk of cancer, respiratory, and cardiovascular diseases and stroke among adults.

- Increased risk of chronic diseases among adolescents, increased risk of metabolic syndrome, and an increased likelihood of becoming a smoker.

- Increased health risks in infants and children (e.g., ear infections, SIDS, asthma, bronchitis, pneumonia).

- An annual economic cost of $5.6 billion (e.g., loss of productivity).

Carcinogens Substances that promote or facilitate the growth of cancerous cells.

Drug Any biologically active substance that is foreign to the body and is deliberately introduced to affect its functioning.

Withdrawal A temporary condition precipitated by the lack of a drug in the body of an addicted person.

Physical Dependence A drug-induced condition in which a person requires frequent administration of a drug in order to avoid withdrawal.

Secondhand Smoke A combination of mainstream and sidestream smoke.

Mainstream Smoke Smoke that is exhaled after being filtered by the smoker's lungs.

Sidestream Smoke Smoke that comes directly off the burning end of cigarette, cigar, or pipe.

Technology Update

Are There "Safer" Cigarettes?

In 2020, the FDA authorized the marketing and sale of a "modified risk tobacco product" (MRTP) called IQOS (pronounced eye-koss) Tobacco Heating System. The name IQOS is a marketing acronym thought to stand for "I Quit Original Smoking." Produced by Phillip Morris International (a large cigarette manufacturer), the new "heat not burn" product is designed to reduce the production of harmful chemicals present in burned tobacco. Like e-cigarettes, the MRTP product delivers nicotine. The FDA is careful to indicate that these products are not safe nor are they FDA approved. They are authorized for sale as a risk modification device with less risk than burned tobacco. There is some evidence to support claims that IQOS is less harmful than traditional cigarettes, but critics argue that more and longer-term studies are needed to examine the product's safety. There is also concern that IQOS marketing using social media (similar to those for e-cigarettes) targets teens to attract them to trying the new tobacco/nicotine delivery system.

Do you believe Phillip Morris's claims of "safer" cigarettes or is this just another way to promote nicotine addiction?

connect ACTIVITY

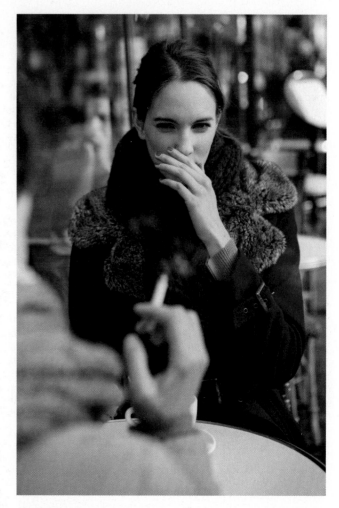

Awareness about the risks of secondhand smoke has contributed to changed social norms.
Image Point Fr/Shutterstock

Thirdhand smoke can also be harmful to health. Thirdhand smoke refers to smoke present in the environment, even when smokers are not present (producing secondhand smoke). Smoke clings to furniture, carpets, clothing, and hair. One study found that babies of parents who only smoked outdoors had levels of cotinine (a nicotine byproduct) seven times higher than babies of nonsmokers. These findings have led to public health efforts to involve pediatricians in smoking cessation efforts, as parents generally see their child's pediatrician more often than their own doctor. Parents may also be more responsive to the message if they learn that smoking can hurt their children.

Smoking while pregnant is harmful to the unborn child. Although not technically considered secondhand exposure, smoking during pregnancy harms a developing fetus. Children of smoking mothers typically have lower birth weight and are more likely to be premature, placing them at risk for a host of health complications. There is also a well-established relationship between maternal smoking and risk for sudden infant death syndrome (SIDS). Finally, children of mothers who smoke are at increased risk for later physical problems (respiratory infections and asthma) and behavioral problems (attention deficit hyperactivity disorder). The best way to reduce risk for pregnant mothers and their children is to quit smoking altogether. However, there is some evidence that reductions in smoking also have benefits.

Smoking has tremendous economic costs. In addition to the cost of human life, medical costs and lost productivity related to smoking-related illnesses in the United States exceed $300 billion annually. Over and above the costs at the societal level, there are significant financial costs for the individual, particularly with increased taxes on tobacco products. In an effort to help smokers appreciate the financial burden of smoking, the website wwwsmokefree.gov has a tool that allows users to see how much they spend on cigarettes. For someone who smokes a pack a day for 10 years, the total would be more than $25,000, based on typical cigarette prices.

Other Nicotine Products: Health and Economic Costs

Electronic cigarettes deliver a heated aerosol that is inhaled. Electronic cigarettes have many different names including e-cigarettes, e-cigs, vapes, vape pens, ENDS (electronic nicotine delivery system), mods, and hookahs. Using e-cigarettes is often referred to as vaping or Juuling (after a brand-name e-cigarette). E-cigarettes have a liquid holder, a battery, and a heating element. The battery charges the heating element that heats the liquid that is then delivered by the device as an aerosol. The aerosol is inhaled from the delivery device (e.g., pen, pipe, stick). The legal commercial form delivers nicotine, but they can also be used to deliver marijuana and other drugs. The exhaled aerosol can be inhaled by bystanders much like secondhand smoke from cigarettes.

Electronic cigarette use has increased dramatically in recent years, especially among youth. Although a form of e-cigarette was patented in 1965, it was not until the early 2000s that they began to be popular. Currently 4.5 percent of adults and nearly 20 percent of teens are e-cigarette users. About 24 percent of e-cigarette users have never smoked cigarettes, 40 percent formerly smoked cigarettes, and 36 percent use both cigarettes and e-cigarettes. The percentage of e-cigarette users who never smoked traditional cigarettes is highest among teens.

There are significant health risks associated with e-cigarette use. According to the CDC, e-cigarettes include potentially harmful substances in addition to nicotine. Among these are a form of flavoring that contains a chemical (diacetyl) linked to lung disease, other cancer-causing chemicals, heavy metals, volatile organic compounds, and ultrafine particles that can be inhaled into the lungs. Because e-cigarettes are relatively new, there is little research concerning long-term health effects. The CDC notes that because e-cigarettes contain nicotine, they are addictive. Nicotine can be harmful to pregnant adults and toxic to fetuses. It can also impair brain development among teens and young adults. An additional danger of e-cigarettes is accidental burns associated with the heating unit and burns to the lungs. This condition, referred to as EVALI (e-cigarette or vaping product use associated lung injury), has contributed to 60 deaths. It is concerning that a survey of teen vapers found that 63 percent did not know that e-cigarettes contained nicotine.

Smokeless chewing tobacco comes in a variety of forms. Types of chewing tobacco include loose leaf, twist, and plug forms. Rather than being smoked, the dip, chew, or chaw stays in the mouth for several hours, where it mixes with saliva and is absorbed into the bloodstream. Smokeless tobacco contains about seven times more nicotine than cigarettes, and more of it is absorbed because of the length of time the tobacco is in the mouth. It also contains a higher level of carcinogens than cigarettes.

Snuff, a form of smokeless tobacco, comes in either dry or moist form. Dry snuff is powdered tobacco and is typically mixed with flavoring. It is designed to be sniffed, pinched, or dipped. Moist snuff is used the same way, but it is moist, finely cut tobacco in a loose form and is sold in tea-bag-like packets.

The health risks and economic costs of smokeless tobacco use are similar to those of other forms of tobacco. Some smokers switch to smokeless tobacco, thinking it is a safe substitute for cigarette, cigar, and pipe smoking. While smokeless tobacco does not lead to the same respiratory problems as smoking, the other health risks may be even greater because smokeless tobacco has more nicotine and higher levels of carcinogens. Because it comes in direct contact with body tissues, the health consequences are far more immediate than those from smoking cigarettes. One-third of teenage users have receding gums, and about half have precancerous lesions, 20 percent of which can become oral cancer within 5 years. Some of the health risks of smokeless tobacco are listed in Table 1. The economic costs of smokeless tobacco use are not well defined. However, given the health risks associated with its use, direct costs (e.g., medical treatments, health care) and indirect costs (e.g., lost productivity) are substantial.

Table 1 ▶ Health Risks of Smokeless Tobacco

Smokeless tobacco increases the risk for the following:

- Oral cavity cancer (cheek, gum, lip, palate); it increases the risk by 4 to 50 times, depending on length of time used

- Cancer of the throat, larynx, and esophagus

- Precancerous skin changes

- High blood pressure

- Rotting teeth, exposed roots, premature tooth loss, and worn-down teeth

- Ulcerated, inflamed, infected gums

- Slow healing of mouth wounds

- Decreased resistance to infections

- Arteriosclerosis, myocardial infarction, and coronary occlusion

- Widespread hormonal effects, including increased lipids, higher blood sugar, and more blood clots

- Increased heart rate

Marketing and Use of Tobacco and Other Nicotine Products

At one time, smoking was an accepted part of our culture, but the social norm has changed. Although smoking has always been a part of our culture, the industrialization and marketing in the middle of the 20th century led to tremendous social acceptance of smoking. As odd as it may sound, cigarettes were once provided free to airline passengers when they boarded planes. Aggressive and well-funded anti-smoking campaigns and increases in cigarette prices have contributed to reductions in smoking in the United States in recent years.

As noted earlier, rates of smoking have declined in recent years from a high of 50 percent in 1950 to the current level of 14 percent. Rates among young people (high school students) have dropped even more dramatically, from 36 percent to 5.8 percent (see Figure 2). These declining trends in youth smoking are encouraging, but the increase in other tobacco-related products such as e-cigarettes is on the rise. Also troubling is the fact that e-cigarette use is generally viewed much more positively by the general public than cigarette smoking or smokeless tobacco use. Interestingly, while rates of smoking have been decreasing in the United States, they have been increasing in many other countries, particularly developing countries. Prevalence rates in China and many European countries greatly exceed those in the United States.

Most users begin during adolescence and find it hard to quit. The initiation of smoking and vaping is viewed as a pediatric problem by most public health experts. Ninety percent of adults who smoke cigarettes daily tried smoking prior to age 18. In the United States, nearly 200 youth start smoking every day. One in 13 American teens aged 17 or younger will die an early death related to smoking. E-cigarette use is most frequently initiated in the adolescent years, but there is evidence of an ever-lowering age of first use. Smokeless tobacco use also begins early in life. Almost 50 percent of users report that they started before age 13.

The media play a role in promoting and preventing use of tobacco and other nicotine products. Much of the blame for tobacco use among youth has been attributed to media campaigns of tobacco companies that have targeted this age group. Marketing campaigns have focused on flavored tobacco products in both cigarettes and e-cigarettes. Of teens who use tobacco products, 85 percent use products that are flavored. Fortunately, regulations now make it more difficult for companies to directly market their products to anyone under the age of 18, at least for cigarettes. Settlements from lawsuits against tobacco companies have also helped fund smoking prevention programs and public education campaigns (Figure 3). However, consumers need to be aware of continued efforts by tobacco companies to introduce young people to smoking and other nicotine products.

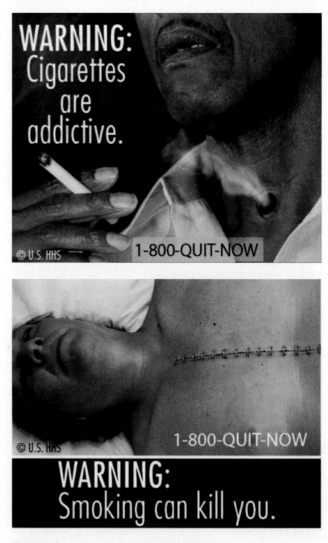

Figure 3 ▶ Warning label images.
Both: Food Collection/Alamy Stock Photo

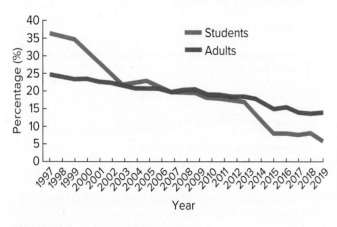

Figure 2 ▶ Trends in cigarette smoking.
Source: Centers for Disease Control and Prevention.

Public policy can affect use of tobacco and other nicotine products. A number of states have passed special tax laws to fund anti-tobacco efforts. In addition to efforts at the state level, federal taxes have increased by roughly $1 per pack. These tax increases have contributed to the dramatic decreases in smoking in recent years. There is, however, wide variability in state tax (per pack) ranging from less than $0.50 in some states to nearly $5 in others. In 2016, e-cigarettes were ruled a tobacco product regulated in ways similar to other tobacco products. Eighteen states currently levy a tax on e-cigarettes. Higher state tax rates have been shown to help reduce cigarette smoking rates. Data are not yet available on the effects of taxes on e-cigarette use, although there is some concern that such taxes might lead to increases in traditional cigarette use.

Public health campaigns and policies influencing access have also been very effective in reducing smoking. States that have aggressive anti-tobacco campaigns report rates of tobacco use well below those without them. According to the Substance Abuse and Mental Health Services Administration (SAMHSA), efforts to cut down on tobacco sales to minors have also been extremely effective. The overall reductions in access have been correlated to usage, so the policies seem to have had a positive effect. Bans on indoor smoking have also been important for reducing access and exposure. A total of 27 states, as well as Washington, DC, Puerto Rico, and the U.S. Virgin Islands, now ban smoking in all nonhospitality restaurants, bars, and workplaces. Thousands of cities and counties have local mandates that ban indoor smoking. A recent review confirms that public smoking bans decrease rates of heart disease and heart attacks. Some cities have approved bans on e-cigarettes in restaurants and workplaces; however, most have yet to affect policy decisions relating to e-cigarettes.

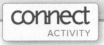

HELP Health is available to Everyone for a Lifetime, and it's Personal

Outdoor Smoking Bans

Indoor smoking bans are in place in most states, and outdoor smoking bans are becoming increasingly common, particularly on college campuses. There are now more than 2,500 smoke-free campuses in the United States, up from almost 500 in 2010. These policies reflect the changing social norms about smoking in the United States. More recently, some college campuses have also begun to ban e-cigarette use.

Is your campus smoke-free? Does this include e-cigarettes? Do you support outdoor smoking bans that include e-cigarettes, or is this taking things too far?

connect ACTIVITY

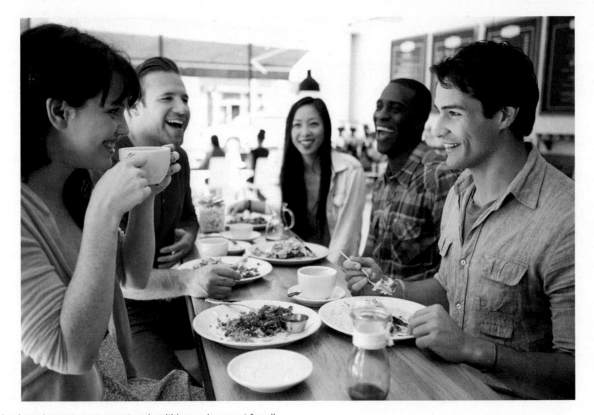

Smoking bans in restaurants create a healthier environment for all.
monkeybusinessimages/Getty Images

Tobacco companies are finding new ways to recruit users. Following a legal settlement in 1998, the tobacco industry responded by dramatically increasing its spending on advertising and promotion. Each year tobacco companies spend nearly $25 million per day to market tobacco products. 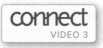 The vast majority of this spending is for price discounts meant to directly undermine the tax increases that have led to reduced smoking rates. The tobacco industry has also introduced new products and packaging to target young people. First it introduced flavored cigarettes, followed by dissolvable tobacco in pill form (e.g., Camel Orbs). Most recently, the industry has invested heavily in e-cigarettes and other smokeless tobacco products. Although companies manufacturing these products argue that they are a healthy alternative to smoking, the U.S. Food and Drug Administration (FDA) is not convinced, and many people are concerned that e-cigarette use will be a gateway to traditional cigarette use.

Another approach to targeting young people is through Internet-based sales. Although store sales to minors have decreased dramatically in recent years, it is relatively easy for minors to obtain cigarettes online. 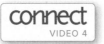 A Surgeon General's report noted that 8 out of 10 minors who placed online cigarette orders were able to fill their orders, and only 1 in 10 was asked to provide proof of age. Another study showed that more than 75 percent of teens were able to obtain e-cigarettes purchased through online vendors.

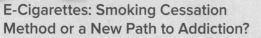

A CLOSER LOOK

E-Cigarettes: Smoking Cessation Method or a New Path to Addiction?

There is considerable controversy about the impact and effects of electronic cigarettes (e-cigarettes). There is research evidence that e-cigarettes help some people to stop smoking cigarettes. However, rates of e-smoking have increased dramatically in recent years, particularly among young people who have never smoked conventional cigarettes. Government statistics indicate that 1 in 4 people of all ages who vape did not smoke before becoming an e-cigarette user. Moreover, those who use e-cigarettes are nearly twice as likely to have intentions to try conventional cigarettes compared to those who have not used e-cigarettes. Some experts also suggest that vaping can be a gateway to illicit drug use.

Are e-cigarettes a healthier alternative or a way for tobacco companies to recruit new smokers? Do you think that e-cigarettes provide a new path to illicit drug use?

connect ACTIVITY

Various factors influence a person's decision to begin using tobacco and other nicotine products. The reasons for starting to use tobacco and other nicotine products are varied but are strikingly similar to reasons given for using alcohol and other drugs. Common reasons that influence young people include peer influence, social acceptance, or desires to be "mature" or to seem "independent." Some young females begin smoking because they believe it will help them control their weight and negative mood states, and current smokers often fear they will gain weight if they quit. Young people identify their enjoyment of the different flavors (e.g., apple pie, watermelon) as a reason for vaping. Also, those who smoke report higher levels of stress, and stress has been shown to be a maintaining factor among current smokers and a barrier to quitting among those who want to stop smoking. Some vapers note that they find it stress reducing. The stress-management approaches covered in other Concepts may help with managing stress more effectively during quit attempts.

People who smoke cigarettes also tend to use alcohol, cannabis, and hard drugs. Alcohol has often been considered a gateway to other drug use, and marijuana/cannabis is often thought of as a gateway to other drugs, such as cocaine and heroin. Although tobacco use has been studied less extensively as a gateway drug, there is strong evidence that smoking is associated with increased risk for the use of both alcohol and illicit drugs. The combination of smoking and drinking is particularly common in college students. Results of a nationally representative study of college students indicated that 97 percent of college smokers drink, while other national data report that 80 percent of all college students drink. Those who drink also report higher levels of smoking. Rates of smoking among college drinkers range from 44 to 59 percent (compared with a national average rate of under 30 percent). The combination of alcohol use and smoking poses an even greater risk to physical health.

The addictive nature of nicotine makes it difficult to quit using tobacco and other nicotine products. Salient examples of the power of nicotine addiction are high rates of continued use among those with serious smoking-related health consequences and low 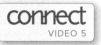 rates of success for quit attempts. In a study in 15 European countries, over half of adults who suffered from serious medical problems known to be associated with smoking (e.g., heart attack, bypass surgery) continued to smoke 1 year later. Data from the CDC found that nearly 7 in 10 smokers want to quit and slightly more than half have tried to quit. Unfortunately, most of these attempts are unsuccessful. Most people make more than three serious attempts before they succeed. Withdrawal symptoms and craving for nicotine are often-cited reasons for failed quit attempts. Many former smokers report nicotine craving months and even years after quitting. The good news is that when you quit you may feel better right away and your body will heal. You will feel more energetic, the

In the News

Tobacco-Use Controversies

Life insurance companies charge reduced rates to nonsmokers and those who do not use tobacco products. And some employers prohibit smoking not only in the workplace but also in all aspects of life. Some tobacco users have suggested that these rules violate personal rights. Also controversial was the decision to allow tobacco users earlier access to the COVID-19 vaccine. Evidence from a prominent study in the *Journal of the American Medical* *Association* documented that smokers were more likely to be hospitalized and die from COVID-19. However, many questioned the fairness of giving smokers earlier access to preventive vaccines.

Do you think tobacco users are discriminated against by insurance companies or unfairly advantaged by public health policies (e.g., vaccine access)?

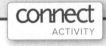

coughing will stop, you will begin to taste food again, and your sense of smell will return. Your lungs will eventually heal and look like the lungs of a nonsmoker. Your risk for lung cancer will return to that of the nonsmoker in about 15–20 years. If you aren't successful at first, keep trying, as there are now more former smokers in the United States than current smokers.

Because e-cigarettes typically deliver nicotine, they can be as addictive as smoking cigarettes. Reports from Johns Hopkins indicate that vaping is less harmful than smoking, but still not safe, partially because of the addictive nature of the nicotine in e-cigarettes. The addiction causes you to want to vape more and withdrawal symptoms result if you ignore the urge to vape.

Using Self-Management Skills

Building self-confidence and motivation is important in quitting. Although quitting tobacco use or use of other nicotine products may be one of the most difficult things a person ever has to do, there are established behavioral strategies that can help you or someone you know succeed. Multiple quit attempts may be necessary, but evidence suggests that people learn valuable behavioral skills through the process and this may help

them eventually succeed. Table 2 provides some concrete self-management skills that can be used to successfully quit.

Building knowledge and changing beliefs can help you take action. There are a variety of resources available to help those who want to stop smoking. A number of national organizations provide telephone hotlines to help with quit attempts. These include the American Cancer Society (1-800-227-2345) and the National Cancer Institute (1-800-QUIT-NOW). In addition, an online smoking program sponsored by several federal agencies is now available at www.smokefree.gov, and the U.S. Public Health Service (USPHS) has published a consumer's guide to quitting smoking (https://dcp.psc.gov/OSG/tobacco/).

Exercise and medication can help overcome barriers to quitting. People trying to adopt healthy lifestyles face many challenges and this is especially true for those trying to quit smoking. Adopting a counter habit of exercise can help shift focus and priorities and facilitate behavior change. Evidence also suggests that physical activity reduces the likelihood of relapse among those who quit. Nicotine

---

Table 2 ▶ Strategies for Quitting Smoking and Vaping

- You must want to quit. The reasons can be for health, family, money, and so on.

- Remind yourself of the reasons. Each day, repeat to yourself the reasons for not using tobacco.

- Decide how to stop. Methods to stop include counseling, attending formal programs, quitting with a friend, going "cold turkey" (abruptly), and quitting gradually. More succeed with "cold turkey" than with the gradual approach.

- Remove reminders and temptations (ashtrays, tobacco, etc.).

- Use substitutes and distractions. Substitute low-calorie snacks or chewing gum, change your routine, or try new activities.

- Do not worry about gaining weight. If you gain a few pounds, it is not as detrimental to your health as continuing to smoke.

- Get support. Try a formal "quit smoking" program for professional help and seek support from friends and relatives.

- Consider a product that requires a prescription, such as a nicotine transdermal patch, Zyban tablets, or nicotine chewing gum.

- Develop effective stress-management techniques. The single most frequently cited reason for difficulty in quitting smoking is stress.

replacement products (patches, gum, nasal sprays, pouches) and medications such as Zyban and Chantix have also helped many smokers quit. For those who don't like using medications, there are also a variety of behavioral strategies that can help them quit, even without medications.

Developing coping skills can help you stick to your plan to quit. A number of apps and text-messaging tools are available to specifically help with smoking cessation. For example, smokefree.gov now includes a text-messaging service (www.smokefree.gov/smokefreetxt). Smokers complete a brief online questionnaire that includes their quit date, and the program sends 1–5 texts per day over a 6- to 8-week period. The text messages provide encouragement, advice, and tips to help the smoker succeed. Users can also text keywords to get additional support. For example, on the day before the identified quit date, the smoker might receive the message "*Tomorrow is quit day! Toss your pack in the trash & get plenty of sleep. For extra support, text these keywords at any time: Crave, Mood, or Slip.*" The cues and prompts can help in facing temptations and give smokers the boost they need to quit. The program is provided at no cost to the user other than any data or texting fees from the user's cell phone provider.

Because both cigarette and e-cigarette users have a similar addiction, programs to help smokers quit can be effective for people addicted to e-cigarettes. However, new programs specifically for e-cigarette users are starting to emerge. For example, the Truth Initiative recently developed a text-messaging program to help teens and young adults quit using e-cigarettes. All you have to do is text DITCHJUUL to 88709.

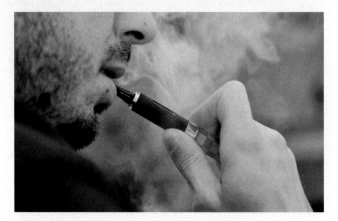

Self-management skills can help a person successfully quit bad habits.
Martina Paraninfi/Moment/Getty Images

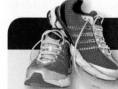

Strategies for Action: Lab Information

If you are a smoker or use other nicotine products like e-cigarettes or smokeless tobacco, an honest assessment of your background and exposure is an important first step to quitting. Lab 18A will help you evaluate your potential risks and need for behavior change. If you score in the "high risk" or "very high risk" category, the website www.smokefree.gov provides a list of questions that can help motivate you to quit (https://smokefree.gov/quitting-smoking/prepare-quit).

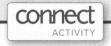

Suggested Resources and Readings

The websites for the following sources can be accessed by searching online for the organization, program, or title listed. Specific scientific references are available at the end of this edition of *Concepts of Fitness and Wellness*.

- American Nonsmokers' Rights Foundation.
- American Nonsmokers' Rights Foundation. (2020). *Smokefree and Tobacco-Free U.S. and Tribal Colleges and Universities*. (pdf)
- American Nonsmokers' Rights Foundation. (2021). Lists and Maps: U.S. Tobacco Control Laws Database©.
- Campaign for Tobacco-Free Kids.
- Campaign for Tobacco-Free Kids. (2021, February 1). *Public Education Campaigns Reduce Tobacco Use*. (pdf)
- Centers for Disease Control and Prevention. Smoking and Tobacco Use.
- Conley, G. (2018, August 28). "Don't Let Fearmongering Guide Vaping Debate." *USA Today*.
- Johns Hopkins Medicine. "5 Vaping Facts You Need to Know."
- Kodjak, A. (2017, November 27). "In Ads, Tobacco Companies Admit They Made Cigarettes More Addictive." *NPR*.
- National Academies of Sciences, Engineering, and Medicine. (2018). *Public Health Consequences of E-cigarettes*. (pdf)
- QuitAssist®.
- Rodriguez, A. (2021, February 3). "People Who Smoke Are Prioritized to Get the COVID-19 Vaccine before the General Population." *USA Today*.
- Truth Initiative (2019, January 19). Quitting E-cigarettes.
- U.S. Food and Drug Administration. (2020, July 7). FDA Authorizes Marketing of IQOS Tobacco Heating System with "Reduced Exposure" Information.
- U.S. Food and Drug Administration. (2020, September 17). Vaporizers, E-cigarettes, and Other Electronic Nicotine Delivery Systems (ENDS).
- WebMD. Smoking Cessation Health Center.
- World Health Organization. (2020). Fact Sheet: Tobacco.

Design Element: (*magnifying glass*): Siede Preis/Getty Images; (*runners shoes*): Maridav/Getty Images; (*tablet*): McGraw Hill; (*woman*): GlobalStock/Getty Images; (*blue sports shoes*): chictype/Getty Images; (*smartphone*): Alexey Boldin/Shutterstock; (*Why It Matters*): MHHE

Lab 18A Use and Abuse of Tobacco and Other Nicotine Products

Name	**Section**	**Date**

Purpose: To understand the risks of diseases associated with the use of tobacco and other nicotine products (as well as exposure to tobacco by-products).

Procedures

1. Read the Tobacco Use Risk Questionnaire (Chart 1).
2. Answer the questionnaire based on your tobacco use or exposure.
3. Record your score and rating (from Chart 2) in the Results section.
4. Complete the Conclusions and Implications section.

Results

What is your tobacco risk score? [ ] (total from Chart 1)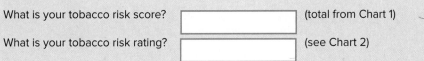

What is your tobacco risk rating? [ ] (see Chart 2)

Chart 1 Tobacco Use Risk Questionnaire

Circle one response in each row of the questionnaire. Determine a point value for each response using the point values in the first row of the chart. Sum the numbers of points for the various responses to determine a Tobacco Use Risk score.

	Points				
Categories	**0**	**1**	**2**	**3**	**4**
Cigarette use	Never smoked		1–10 cigarettes a day	11–40 cigarettes a day	>40 cigarettes a day
E-cigarette use	Never vaped	50 hits a day (0.5 milliliter bottle)	100 hits a day (1 milliliter bottle)	150 hits a day (1.5 milliliter bottles)	200 hits a day (2 milliliter bottles)
Pipe and cigar use	Never smoked	Pipe—occasional use	Cigar—infrequent daily use	Cigar or pipe—frequent daily use	Cigar—heavy use
Smoking style	Don't smoke		No inhalation	Slight to moderate inhalation	Deep inhalation
Smokeless tobacco use	Don't use	Occasional use: not daily	Daily use: one use per day	Daily use: multiple uses per day	Heavy use: repetitious, multiple uses daily
Secondhand or sidestream smoke	No smokers at home or in workplace	Smokers at workplace but not at home	Smokers at home but not at workplace	Smokers at home and at workplace	
Years of tobacco use	Never used	1 or less	2–5	6–10	>10

Note: Different forms of tobacco use pose different risks for different diseases. This questionnaire is designed to give you a general idea of risk associated with use and exposure to tobacco by-products. E-cigarette use based on 16 milligram per milliliter bottles; bottles vary in level in nicotine per bottle.

Chart 2 Tobacco Use Risk Questionnaire
Rating Chart

Rating	Score
Very high risk	16+
High risk	7–15
Moderate risk	1–6
Low risk	0

Conclusions and Implications

1. In several sentences, discuss your personal risk. If your risk is low, discuss some implications of the behavior of other people that affect your risk, including what can be done to change these risks. If your risk is above average, what changes can be made to reduce your risk?

2. In several sentences, discuss how you feel about public laws designed to curtail tobacco use. Discuss your point of view, either pro or con.

The Use and Abuse of Alcohol

LEARNING OBJECTIVES

After completing the study of this Concept, you will be able to:

- ▶ Understand the effects of alcohol on the body.

- ▶ Describe different patterns of alcohol use and problems, including alcohol use disorders.

- ▶ Identify the negative physical, psychological, and behavioral consequences of excess alcohol consumption.

- ▶ List factors that have contributed to declining rates of driving under the influence of alcohol.

- ▶ Explain biological and environmental factors associated with increased risk for alcohol problems.

- ▶ Determine aspects of the college environment that contribute to heavy drinking among students.

- ▶ Describe effective approaches for preventing and treating alcohol-related problems.

- ▶ Identify steps you can take to protect yourself and others.

John Foxx/Stockbyte/Getty Images

Alcohol is among the most widely used and destructive drugs. Abstaining from alcohol is the surest way to prevent negative consequences, but learning to drink in moderation can significantly reduce risk.

Alcohol and Alcoholic Beverages

Alcoholic beverages contain ethanol (ethyl alcohol), an intoxicating and addictive drug that is often misused. The active **drug** in alcoholic beverages (ethanol) is a toxic chemical, but unlike methanol (wood alcohol) and isopropyl (rubbing alcohol), it can be consumed in small doses. As a drug, it is classified as a depressant. However, this classification does not capture the full range of alcohol's effects. The effects experienced by the drinker depend, in part, on whether the drinker's blood alcohol concentration (BAC) is rising or falling. Alcohol is classified as a depressant due to the sedative effects experienced as levels of blood alcohol fall. However, primarily stimulant effects are experienced by the user as blood alcohol concentrations rise.

Humans have consumed alcoholic beverages for thousands of years. Unfortunately, many people in our culture view drunkenness as a rite of passage and an expectation. Indeed, there are more synonyms for the word *drunk* or **intoxication** than for any other word in the English language. This illustrates the importance we give to overconsumption. Fortunately, as people mature and responsibilities such as work and family become more important, most reduce their consumption.

Alcoholic beverages have varying concentrations of alcohol, but many have similar amounts per serving. Beverages are usually served in proportions such that a drink of any one of the three categories (beer, wine, or liquor) contains the same amount of alcohol. Beer is usually served in a 12-ounce can, bottle, or mug. A typical glass of wine holds 5 ounces, and a shot of liquor is 1.5 ounces. Even though the percentage of alcohol in the beverages differs, the drinks

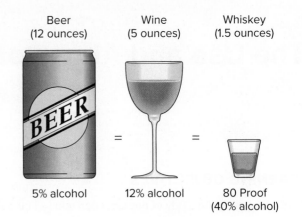

Beer (12 ounces) — 5% alcohol
Wine (5 ounces) — 12% alcohol
Whiskey (1.5 ounces) — 80 Proof (40% alcohol)

Figure 1 ▶ Alcohol content of drinks.

Source: National Institute on Alcohol Abuse and Alcoholism.

would be equivalent in alcohol because each would contain about 14 g of alcohol (see Figure 1). Keep in mind that these comparisons assume that the liquor contains 40 percent ethanol (80 proof), and beer and wine contain 5 and 12 percent ethanol, respectively. With the increased popularity of microbrewed beers, alcohol content is more variable, with many microbrews containing 6–10 percent (rather than 5 percent) ethanol. It's also important to realize that differences in the ways that different types of alcohol are consumed may lead to differences in blood alcohol concentrations. For example, because liquor is often consumed more quickly than beer or wine, blood alcohol concentrations rise more quickly.

Alcohol's effects on the body depend on many factors. Alcohol is absorbed directly into the bloodstream, primarily in the small intestines. It then concentrates in various organs in proportion to the amount of water each contains. The brain has a high water content, so much of the alcohol goes there. Once it is absorbed, alcohol is metabolized primarily by the liver. An enzyme in the liver, called alcohol dehydrogenase (ADH), converts alcohol to acetaldehyde, which is then converted by acetate and other enzymes into carbon dioxide and water. Individuals differ with respect to their ability to metabolize alcohol, but a healthy adult takes 1–1.5 hours to metabolize one standard drink.

Although the basic processes of alcohol absorption and metabolism are the same for everyone, the effects of alcohol depend on a number of additional factors including stomach contents, body size/weight, rate of consumption, beliefs about alcohol effects, and drinking context (e.g., bar vs. home). There are also important sex differences in alcohol response. Because females have lower amounts of body water, a given amount of alcohol represents a greater percentage of the volume of the blood in their bloodstream. Females also have lower amounts of the enzymes needed to process alcohol.

Because the rate of alcohol consumption is often greater than the rate at which it is processed, the alcohol concentration in the bloodstream begins to increase. Blood alcohol concentration (BAC) is measured as a percentage and is used by law enforcement officials to determine if a driver is legally intoxicated.

Table 1 ▶ Terms and Criteria for Patterns of Alcohol Use

Term	Criteria
Moderate drinking (NIAAA)	Males: ≤2 drinks/day Females: ≤1 drink/day Over 65: ≤1 drink/day
At-risk drinking (NIAAA)	Males: >14 drinks/week or >4 drinks/occasion Females: >7 drinks/week or >3 drinks/occasion
Heavy-episodic drinking/binge drinking (NIAAA)	Males: 5 or more alcoholic drinks consumed in a 2-hour period Females: 4 or more alcoholic drinks consumed in a 2-hour period
Alcohol use disorder (APA)	Maladaptive pattern of alcohol use leading to clinically significant impairment or distress, manifested within a 12-month period by two or more of the following: (mild: 2–3 symptoms, moderate: 4–5 symptoms, severe: 6 or more symptoms) • Use of larger amounts or over a longer time period than intended • Persistent desire or unsuccessful attempts to cut down or control use • Great deal of time spent obtaining, using, or recovering from use • Craving, or a strong desire or urge to use • Recurrent use leading to failure to fulfill role obligations at work, school, or home • Continued use despite alcohol-related social or interpersonal problems • Important social, occupational, or recreational activities given up or reduced due to use • Recurrent use in hazardous situations • Use despite knowledge of alcohol-related physical or psychological problems • Tolerance (either increasing amounts used or diminished effects with the same amount) • Withdrawal (withdrawal symptoms or use to relieve or avoid symptoms)

Note: NIAAA, National Institute on Alcohol Abuse and Alcoholism; APA, American Psychiatric Association.
Source: O'Conner and Schottenfeld.

Alcohol Consumption and Alcohol Abuse

Risks and benefits of alcohol use depend on the amount and pattern of consumption. Making statements about the consequences of alcohol consumption is difficult because the consequences vary depending on the amount consumed and the pattern of consumption. Moderate alcohol consumption has been shown to provide some benefits for reducing risk of heart disease, though some recent studies call this conclusion into question. Moreover, considerable risks occur when consumed in excess. Risks for alcohol consumption are not the same for everyone, so it is important to understand the relative risks and benefits of various levels of alcohol consumption.

Patterns of alcohol consumption are characterized in a variety of ways. Roughly two-thirds (66.3 percent) of the U.S. population over the age of 18 report alcohol use in the past year. This 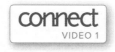 makes alcohol the most widely used drug of abuse in this country. Most who choose to drink (about 95 percent) develop a pattern of light or moderate drinking. The National Institute on Alcohol Abuse and Alcoholism (NIAAA) characterizes "moderate consumption" as one drink per day or less for females and two drinks per day or less for males (see Table 1). Those who exceed these standards are often described as at-risk drinkers. Heavy-episodic drinking (commonly referred to as binge drinking) is common among at-risk drinkers. It is defined as five or more standard alcoholic drinks (for males), and four or more for females (see Table 1) within a 2-hour period. Using this standard, approximately 24 percent of the U.S. population aged 12 or older (more than 66 million people) report binge drinking in the past month. Rates are even higher among young adults with a rate of 28 percent for non-students and a rate of 33 percent for college students. More than half of the roughly 88,000 alcohol-related deaths in the United States each year and 77 percent of the annual economic costs of alcohol use are a result of binge drinking.

Binge drinkers are also at increased risk for developing **alcohol use disorders (AUDs)** (see Table 1 for characteristics). Two key signs of alcohol use disorders are **alcohol tolerance** and **alcohol withdrawal**. Unfortunately, many people seem to

Drug Any biologically active substance that is foreign to the body and is deliberately introduced to affect its functioning.

Intoxication Also referred to as drunkenness; a blood alcohol level of 0.08 percent.

Alcohol Use Disorder (AUD) A psychiatric condition characterized by alcohol-related problems that cause significant impairment or distress.

Alcohol Tolerance The phenomenon of requiring more and more alcohol over time to achieve the desired effect.

Alcohol Withdrawal Symptoms that occur when alcohol is withdrawn after a period of prolonged heavy use. Symptoms include sweating, anxiety, tremors, and seizures.

In the News

Has COVID-19 Increased or Decreased Drinking?

There is no question that the COVID-19 pandemic has been a major source of stress. In the height of the pandemic, college students found themselves socially isolated while having to adapt to online classes. Interestingly, studies of the impact of COVID-19 on college drinking have been mixed, with some showing increases and others decreases. Although the stress associated with the pandemic and more flexible schedules could have contributed to increased drinking, reduced access to social events where drinking often occurs (e.g., parties, bars) may have led to decreases for some.

Do you think restrictions caused by the COVID-19 pandemic will lead to more lasting changes in societal and campus attitudes toward parties and large social gatherings?

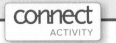

think that tolerance is a good sign, as evidenced by statements such as "I can hold my liquor" and "I'm not a lightweight." The reality is that tolerance has mostly negative implications. There is also recent evidence that those who have a natural, or "innate," tolerance to alcohol effects are at increased risk for developing AUDs. With the heavier use that comes with the development of tolerance, withdrawal symptoms may develop when alcohol is not consumed regularly. Withdrawal symptoms include anxiety, increased heart rate, sweating, hand tremor, nausea, and vomiting. In more severe cases, withdrawal can lead to hallucinations and seizures.

Health and Behavioral Consequences of Alcohol Use

Heavy alcohol use is associated with an increased risk for a variety of negative health and social outcomes. The most well-established health risk associated with alcohol consumption is liver disease. Alcohol consumption is the leading cause of disease and death from liver dysfunction, with roughly half of all liver disease deaths related to excess alcohol consumption. Although the liver is capable of metabolizing moderate amounts of alcohol on a regular basis, persistent, heavy drinking may lead to swollen liver cells, a condition called **fatty liver**. If drinking is stopped or significantly reduced at this point, the damage to the liver is likely reversible. With continued heavy drinking, the individual is likely to develop **alcoholic cirrhosis**, or permanent scarring of the liver.

Heavy drinking is also a risk factor for other life-threatening diseases. Figure 2 depicts all causes of mortality risk as well as mortality risk for several specific diseases by level of alcohol consumption, with values less than 1 reflecting decreased risk and values greater than 1 reflecting increased risk. Although moderate alcohol consumption may protect against coronary heart disease (CHD), as outlined later in this Concept,

heavier use of alcohol may increase the risk for CHD and other cardiovascular disease. Specifically, heavy drinking is associated with increased risk for hypertension, cardiomyopathy, cardiac arrhythmia, and congestive heart failure. Alcohol consumption increases the risk for cancer, including cancer of the oral cavity and pharynx, esophagus, liver, larynx, colon, and female breast. There is also evidence that heavy drinking may impair immune functioning, leading to increased risk for infectious diseases, including pneumonia and tuberculosis. Finally, heavy alcohol use has both acute and long-term effects on cognitive functions including memory, and increases risk for psychiatric disorders that often occur with alcohol problems (e.g., mood and anxiety disorders).

Although many health risks of alcohol use are directly related to the effects of alcohol on the body, others are related to the intoxicated behavior of the drinker. For example, heavy episodic drinking increases risk for motor vehicle crashes, falls, burns, drownings, interpersonal violence, and sexually transmitted infections. Ambitious public health goals have been set for curtailing binge drinking in the United States. Although rates have been on a gradual

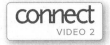

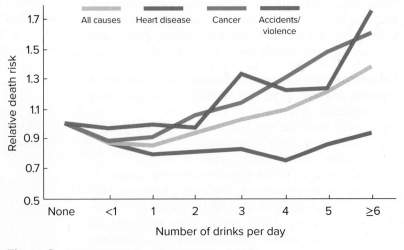

Figure 2 ▶ Alcohol consumption and death risk.

Source: American Cancer Society.

decline for the last two decades, rates remain well above public health goals for binge drinking.

Females appear to be especially susceptible to the negative health consequences of heavy drinking. At similar levels of alcohol consumption, females are more likely than males to experience liver, cardiovascular, and brain damage from drinking. Alcohol also increases risk of breast cancer and negatively impacts the reproductive system. Pregnant females should avoid alcohol because it can lead to fetal alcohol effects, including fetal alcohol syndrome (FAS), which is associated with low birth weight, physical defects, mental retardation, and stunted growth. In summary, the health risks of alcohol consumption are extensive and must be considered in relation to the potential benefits.

Whereas excessive drinking presents many risks, moderate consumption can provide some health benefits. There is some evidence that moderate alcohol consumption (one drink per day for females, up to two drinks per day for males) is associated with decreased risk for some risks of CHD, Type 2 diabetes, and certain types of stroke. A recent study that followed more than 300,000 people found that those who were light or moderate drinkers (but not heavy drinkers) were 20 percent less likely to die over an 8-year period, with most of the reduced risk attributable to lower cardiovascular disease mortality. However, another recent study found that, although alcohol use was associated with lower risk for myocardial infarction (e.g., heart attack), it was associated with increased risk for hypertension and stroke. The mechanism linking moderate alcohol use to reduced CHD risk is still not well understood. It is possible that light to moderate drinkers are simply at lower risk because they have other protective characteristics like higher education, better diet, and more regular exercise. Still, mechanisms for a causal role of alcohol use in protection against CHD are plausible. Recent evidence suggests that moderate alcohol use may also protect against cognitive declines with aging. Although the health benefits of moderate alcohol consumption have largely been attributed to wine consumption, beer appears to have similar benefits. In addition, there is some evidence that beer consumption may benefit bone strength because it has high levels of dietary silicon, which contributes to bone density. Beers with high levels of barley and hops have higher levels of silicon, but the health benefits do not justify drinking greater amounts of beer. It is important to recognize that even moderate alcohol consumption may not be safe for some people and that some are better off not drinking at all (see Table 2). Also note that the pattern of drinking is as important as the absolute level. A female who has seven drinks one time each week consumes an average of one drink per day but does not receive the same health benefits as a female who consumes one drink each day. Moderate

Table 2 ▶ People Who Should Consider Abstaining from Alcohol Use

- People under age 21 (legal age)
- Athletes striving for peak performance
- Females trying to get pregnant or who are pregnant or nursing
- People with an AUD or recovering from an AUD
- People with a family history of alcohol problems
- People with a medical or surgical problem and/or on medications
- People with psychiatric problems or persons experiencing severe psychosis
- People driving vehicles, operating dangerous machinery, or involved in public safety
- People conducting serious business transactions or study

consumption of alcohol can be safely incorporated into a healthy lifestyle, but heavy drinking cannot.

The greatest danger of alcohol occurs when the drinker gets behind the wheel of a motor vehicle. Alcohol-related traffic crashes are the leading cause of death and spinal cord injury for young Americans. Approximately one-quarter of fatal injury traffic accidents involve alcohol use by one or more drivers. The driver's likelihood of causing

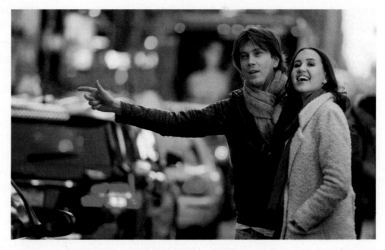

Choosing not to get behind the wheel is the only responsible choice for those who drink.
Florin Prunoiu/Image Source/Getty Images

Fatty Liver Swelling of the cells of the liver.

Alcoholic Cirrhosis Permanent scarring of the liver, resulting in reduced blood flow and buildup of toxins in the body.

Table 3 ▶ The Effects of Blood Alcohol Concentration (BAC) on Driving Performance and Function

BAC 0.02%
- Vision is impaired: less ability to see objects in motion; less ability to monitor multiple objects.
- Attention span is lower.
- Reaction time slows.

BAC 0.05–0.06%
- Inhibitions are reduced (unnecessary chances may be taken).
- Visual abilities decrease; side vision is impaired by 30 percent.
- Judgment is the first function to be impaired.
- Braking distance is extended.
- Coordination is impaired.
- Driving performance is impaired at moderate speed.

BAC 0.08%
- Vision is seriously impaired, especially at night.
- Driver is overconfident in driving ability.
- Driver is less able to concentrate.
- Judgment is dulled; driver is more careless.
- Muscle control and coordination are hindered.
- Driving performance is impaired at low speeds.
- Driver increases the use of the accelerator and brake.

BAC 0.15%
- Driver experiences gross motor impairment and lack of physical control.
- Blurred vision and loss of balance occur.

BAC 0.20%
- Driver is disoriented and has difficulty walking.
- Nausea and vomiting occur.
- Anesthesia occurs.
- Driver may have impaired gag reflex.
- Driver may suffer blackouts.

BAC 0.30%
- Stupor and decreased respiration occur.
- Driver may lose consciousness.

BAC 0.40%
- Coma may occur.
- Death is possible, due to respiratory arrest.

Source: Mothers Against Drunk Driving.

Table 4 ▶ Approximate BAC Values (%) Based on the Number of Drinks Consumed over a 2-Hour Period

Number of Drinks	Females		Males	
	120-Pound	180-Pound	140-Pound	200-Pound
1	0.02	0.004	0.007	0.001
2	0.06	0.03	0.04	0.02
3	0.10	0.06	0.07	0.04
4	0.15	0.09	0.10	0.06
5	0.19	0.12	0.13	0.08
6	0.23	0.15	0.16	0.10
7	0.27	0.17	0.19	0.13
8	0.31	0.20	0.22	0.15

Source: National Highway Traffic and Safety Administration (NHTSA), 1994.

even higher (roughly 20 percent) among young adults aged 21–25. Table 3 summarizes the effects of different BACs on physical and driving performance. Awareness of the impact of alcohol on impairment is important for avoiding problems. Table 4 provides estimated BACs for males and females at various weights. Lab 19A provides the formula for calculating BAC for your precise weight.

Stronger policies have contributed to decreases in alcohol-related traffic fatalities. Although alcohol-related traffic fatalities remain a major public health concern, policy changes, such as increasing the legal drinking age to 21 and decreasing the legal limit for intoxication to 0.08 percent, have led to dramatic decreases in impaired driving over the past 30 years. In 2019, alcohol-related fatalities reached their lowest point since 1982, although over 10,000 people still lost their lives (see Figure 3). In addition, after steep decreases over a 25-year period, rates have leveled off considerably in the last 10 years, suggesting the need for renewed efforts. Fortunately, new approaches are being developed, including ignition interlock devices that prevent a driver who is over the legal limit from starting their car. Most states require the interlock devices in the cars of at least some offenders, and studies show that they decrease re-arrest by almost 70 percent. Many states are considering interlock devices for all offenders, and car manufacturers are also working on developing alcohol sensors that can be installed in new cars. This would allow all drivers (not just offenders driving under the influence [DUI]) to know if they are driving impaired. Perhaps in response to stricter laws, many people are testing their own blood alcohol levels before getting behind the wheel. Sales of blood alcohol self-tests have increased dramatically in recent years.

a highway accident increases at a BAC of 0.04 percent (1–2 drinks for most people). The likelihood of a fatal or serious injury increases exponentially at a BAC of 0.08 or higher (the legal limit for intoxication in all 50 states).

In addition to injury risks associated with traffic accidents, those who drink and drive face significant legal, financial, and social costs. Although the short-term costs are significant, the long-term costs of a drunk driving arrest typically far outweigh the immediate financial burden. Having an offense on your record can lead to problems with schools, family, and future employers. Despite the potential short- and long-term costs, a recent survey conducted by the National Highway Traffic Safety Administration (NHTSA) found that about 11 percent of drivers in the United States drove under the influence in the previous year. Rates were

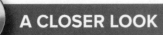

A CLOSER LOOK

Controversies over Alcohol Plus Cannabis

State-by-state decisions to legalize cannabis have been driven by many factors. Some have argued that cannabis use is safer than alcohol use and that cannabis use may lead to reductions in the use of alcohol. For example, one study reported that medical cannabis use was associated with decreased alcohol use and another found that abstinence from cannabis was associated with increased alcohol use. However, the combined use of these drugs has led to new public health concerns.

Studies have recently documented greater risks associated with the combined usage of cannabis and alcohol. The debates about legalization will likely continue, so it is important to stay informed.

Which drug is the greater problem? Does the evidence about a combined risk change your perceptions about the relative safety of cannabis or attitudes about legalization?

connect
ACTIVITY

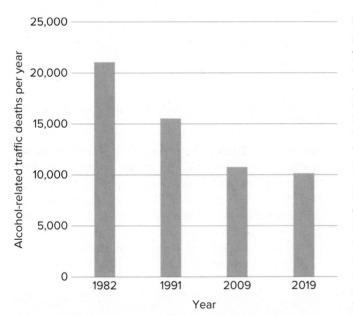

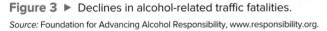

Figure 3 ▶ Declines in alcohol-related traffic fatalities.
Source: Foundation for Advancing Alcohol Responsibility, www.responsibility.org.

Risk Factors for Alcohol-Related Problems

Early age of drinking onset increases risk for later problems. Those who begin drinking at an earlier age are at risk for the development of alcohol use disorders. Although the nature of the relation between age of onset and later problems is not clear, many believe that early use interferes with a critical period of brain development. The part of the brain involved in emotion regulation and impulse control (the frontal lobe) is not fully developed until the mid-20s, so although physical maturation may be complete by age 18, cognitive abilities are still developing. Use of alcohol and other drugs during this important period of brain development may have long-term negative consequences for young people.

Having a family member with an alcohol problem places you at increased risk for developing a problem yourself. Experts have known for some time that the development of alcohol use disorder has a genetic component. Alcohol problems run in families, and it is estimated that genetics account for roughly half of the risk for AUD. In the future, we may find out exactly how genetic differences contribute to risk, but for now we know that genetics are important. Thus, if you have a family history of alcoholism, you should be especially careful about your drinking behavior.

Environment also plays a role in the initiation and escalation of alcohol use. During childhood, parents play a significant role in the socialization process, which includes socialization regarding alcohol use. Parents who talk to their kids about alcohol use, provide social support, and monitor their children's behavior are less likely to have children who drink excessively during adolescence. During adolescence, peers take on a powerful role in the development of alcohol problems. One of the best predictors of adolescent alcohol use patterns is the pattern of alcohol use among their close friends.

Broader environmental influences also play a key role in the development of alcohol use. The promotion of alcohol as a social lubricant leads to the development of positive beliefs about the effects of alcohol, referred to as "alcohol expectancies." These beliefs have been shown to develop even before personal experience with alcohol. Media portrayals of the benefits of drinking are believed to play an important role in the development of positive expectancies. Adolescents are bombarded with these messages from an early age. In one study of 1,000 13- to 20-year-olds, those who did not see any alcohol ads consumed about 14 drinks per month, whereas those who saw ads consumed an average of 33 drinks per month. The COVID-19 pandemic also highlights the potential role of the broader social environment. The combination of stress and isolation from quarantining contributed to significant increases in alcohol use, despite less access to establishments (restaurants and bars) where alcohol use often takes place. Consistent with this point, a recent study of over

800 adults found that those who experienced more COVID-19-related stress drank on more days and consumed more total drinks.

Alcohol Use in Young Adults

Excess alcohol consumption is a major problem on most college campuses. Students may view drinking alcohol as a "rite of passage" during college, but it is a very serious public health problem. Alcohol consumption by college students has been associated with hundreds of thousands of cases of injuries, violence, unsafe sexual behavior, sexual assaults, and numerous deaths (over 1,500 annually). About 25 percent of college students report academic problems caused by drinking, including lower grades, poor performance on exams and papers, and missed classes. Grade point average has also been found to be inversely related to the amount of alcohol consumed (see Figure 4).

The problems associated with alcohol are directly related to the amount consumed. As shown in Table 5, the proportion of various alcohol-related problems is considerably higher for people categorized as *frequent binge drinkers* than for *non-binge drinkers*.

Rates of binge drinking in college have remained high and rates of frequent binge drinking have increased, but there are also signs of progress. There have been consistent increases in the number of students who do not drink at all. Over the past 30 years, the percentage of students reporting no alcohol use in the past 30 days has increased approximately 20 percent since the early 1980s. This increase may be due, at least in part, to the greater number of first-generation college students and nontraditional college

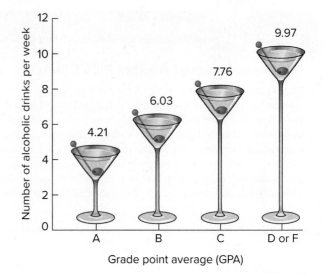

Figure 4 ▶ Average number of alcoholic drinks per week by GPA.

Source: Adapted from Core Institute.

students returning to college after spending time in the workforce.

The college environment plays a key role in heavy alcohol use among college students. Although many more college students today are not of traditional college age (18–25) and/or work full or part time, college remains a period of transition from adolescence to adulthood for many. Because this period is characterized by fewer adult responsibilities, some have referred to it as "extended adolescence" or "emerging adulthood." Regardless of the terminology, the

Table 5 ▶ Alcohol-Related Problems among College Students

Problems	All Students (%)	Non–Binge Drinkers (%)	Occasional Binge Drinkers (%)	Frequent Binge Drinkers (%)
Did something you regret	36.1	18.0	39.6	62.0
Missed a class	29.9	8.8	30.9	62.5
Drove after drinking	28.8	18.6	39.7	56.7
Forgot where you were or what you did	27.1	10.0	27.2	54.0
Argued with friends	22.5	9.7	23.0	42.6
Got behind in schoolwork	24.1	9.8	26.0	46.3
Engaged in unplanned sexual activities	21.6	7.9	22.3	41.5
Got hurt or injured	12.4	3.9	10.9	26.6
Damaged property	10.8	2.3	8.9	22.7
Had unprotected sex	10.3	3.7	9.8	20.4

Source: Wechsler et al.

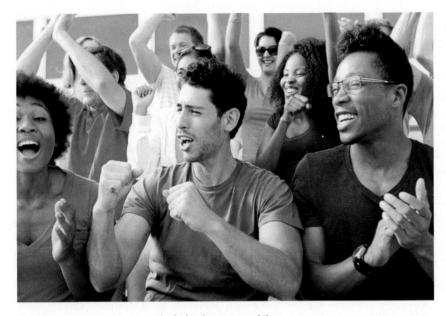

It's not necessary to consume alcohol to have a good time.
stockbroker/123RF

early 20s are clearly a period of heightened risk for engagement in risky behaviors, including alcohol and other drug use. It has been suggested that flexible schedules for college students contribute to this problem. In contrast to emerging adults in the work sector, college students can often avoid morning classes and Friday classes to extend the weekend.

Drinking games and pregaming place college students at high risk for negative consequences. Drinking games are common on college campuses, but studies show that students who engage in drinking games reach dangerously high blood alcohol concentrations and experience more negative consequences. Younger students are more likely to play drinking games and experience negative repercussions. This is probably due to the fact that younger drinkers have less tolerance and are therefore more impaired at comparable blood alcohol levels.

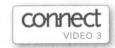

Pregaming (drinking prior to a social event or going to a drinking establishment) is also common among college students and places them at increased risk for negative consequences. One recent study of primarily young adults (mean age of 22) at bars found that roughly 80 percent reported pregaming with an average of three to four drinks consumed prior to going to the bar. Those who pregamed reached higher BACs and were more likely to be classified as problem drinkers. Thus, avoiding drinking games and pregaming can substantially decrease risk for negative consequences of alcohol use.

Mixing alcohol and energy drinks puts young people at risk. Many college students and other young adults mix alcohol with energy drinks (such as Red Bull or Monster), with one recent study finding that nearly one-third of young adults reported engaging in this behavior at least once in the past year. Because energy drinks may mask the depressant effects of alcohol, people may end up drinking more and reaching higher BACs. There is evidence that young adults who mix alcohol and energy drinks are more likely to engage in high-intensity drinking as well as risk behaviors, including unprotected sex and drunk driving.

Female college students are at particularly high risk for negative consequences of drinking. Females are at increased risk for a variety of acute negative behavioral outcomes of drinking, though unprotected or unwanted sexual behavior is perhaps the greatest concern. More than half of sexual assaults occur when either the perpetrator or victim (or often both) have been drinking. Risks are particularly high for young females in situations where high blood alcohol levels are likely. For example, females experience more negative consequences of drinking games because they drink at similar levels to males, leading to higher blood alcohol concentrations.

Misperceptions about peer attitudes and drinking behavior contribute to heavy drinking in college. Although increased attention to college drinking has led to increased education and prevention, rates of heavy use have not changed dramatically.

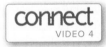

One contributing factor may be that attention to heavy drinking has led to the perception by college students that their peers are drinking more than they actually are. Research has shown that college students routinely overestimate use by their peers and that these misperceptions are associated with increases in drinking. In theory, students drink more to keep up with what they perceive to be the norm on campus. In addition to overestimating how much alcohol their peers consume, college students appear to overestimate how much alcohol their peers want them to consume. This may be particularly true for females. A recent study found that 71 percent of females believed males wanted them to consume alcohol excessively, and 17 percent thought that males would find them more sexually attractive if they had five or more drinks. In truth, the percentage of males who endorsed these beliefs was about half of what females perceived it to be.

Much like colleges, the military confronts high rates of alcohol use and abuse. Young males (as a group) are at high risk for heavy drinking and related problems, and the military is a major employer of this demographic (roughly

Alcohol Treatment Navigator

Deciding to get treatment for an alcohol problem is an important first step. However, finding effective treatment can also be challenging. The National Institute on Alcohol Abuse and Alcoholism (NIAAA) has a website called the Alcohol Treatment Navigator (https://alcoholtreatment .niaaa.nih.gov/) that guides users through a step-by-step process to find highly qualified treatment professionals. It also provides information about the types of treatments (including medications) that have been shown to be most effective. In response to the COVID-19 pandemic, the website added telehealth options as well.

Do you think medications should be included in treatment of alcohol problems? Would you support their use on your campus?

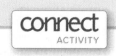

86 percent of active-duty military are male, and roughly 67 percent are between the ages of 18 and 30). Given these demographics, it is not surprising that active-duty military personnel report levels of binge drinking that are even higher than rates among college students. This risk is exacerbated by the stress associated with deployment and redeployment. Soldiers may turn to alcohol as a means to cope with the stresses of war or with symptoms of post-traumatic stress disorder related to their experiences in the field. For example, one study reported that nearly 15 percent of army soldiers returning from deployments in Iraq or Afghanistan met criteria for an AUD. Another report documented that demand for alcohol treatment programs increased more than 50 percent during the first 6 years after the beginning of the war in Iraq.

Effective Approaches for Alcohol Prevention and Treatment

New approaches to preventing heavy drinking among college students are showing promise. Efforts to prevent heavy drinking among college students have traditionally focused on education. Unfortunately, a task force developed by the NIAAA found that these approaches are largely ineffective. Confrontational approaches do not work well either, particularly with young people. Effective strategies include motivational and skills-based approaches. These approaches encourage young people to examine how their drinking behavior affects their lives and to consider ways that changing their behavior might benefit them. Skills training focuses on teaching young people strategies to moderate their consumption or to maintain abstinence in the face of social pressure to drink. Another promising approach that is

increasingly used on college campuses addresses students' misperceptions of drinking behavior on campus. Campuses often provide students with information about actual rates of alcohol consumption on campus to counter erroneous beliefs about heavy drinking. Students may perceive that "everyone" drinks, but data from nationally representative samples of college students indicate that about 38 percent do not report any alcohol use in the past 30 days. Overall, results from the longitudinal Monitoring the Future study show promising declines in various indicators of alcohol use by college students.

The options for treating alcohol use disorders have expanded in recent years. If you think you have (or someone you know has) a problem with alcohol, a number of options are available. Self-help groups, such as Alcoholics Anonymous (AA) and Rational Recovery, are widespread in the United States. Treatment centers are also readily available. Most treatment centers focus on abstinence using a 12-step approach consistent with AA. Although this approach works well for many, some are turned off by the strong religious component. A recent multisite clinical trial showed that cognitive-behavioral therapy and motivational enhancement yield similar results to 12-step approaches. These approaches can often be implemented in less time and place more emphasis on personal control over behavior, features that may appeal to young adults in particular. The medication naltrexone has also been shown to help those trying to abstain from or reduce their alcohol consumption, providing yet another alternative or adjunct to behavioral treatment.

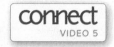
VIDEO 5

Technology Update

Apps to Treat Addiction?

Yes, there is an app for that too. Although some argue that smartphone use has become a new form of addiction, there are a number of apps designed to cure rather than create addictions. For example, reSET-O from Pear Therapeutics, the first mobile app for addiction approved by the Food and Drug Administration, provides a 12-week program with weekly check-ins and self-paced lessons and quizzes. A recent clinical trial found that use of the app nearly doubled rates of abstinence for those in treatment. Although reSET-O requires a prescription from your physician, a variety of other apps like Sober Grid, Nomo, and WEconnect are available for free. Although these apps might not be able to help those with severe addictions, they could potentially provide a useful tool for someone trying to get a handle on an addictive behavior before it gets out of control.

Would you recommend this type of app to a friend struggling with alcohol problems?

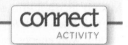

Using Self-Management Skills

Self-monitoring and self-assessment skills are important in reducing your risk for excess drinking. Moderate alcohol consumption is safe for many people and may even have some health benefits. However, many people who drink do so beyond safe levels. As excess alcohol consumption is associated with a variety of acute negative consequences (e.g., alcohol poisoning, injuries, unsafe sex, driving accidents), a key self-management strategy is to closely monitor consumption and use behavioral strategies to keep your BAC at a safe level. Protective strategies include eating before you drink, alternating between alcoholic and nonalcoholic drinks, going to a party later and/or leaving earlier, setting a reasonable drink limit that you will not exceed, and avoiding high-risk situations, like pregaming and drinking games. Studies have shown that students who use these strategies are at much lower risk for experiencing alcohol-related problems.

Honest self-assessment is important in detecting if you or your friends may have alcohol-related problems. The NIAAA created a website called "Rethinking Drinking" (www.rethinkingdrinking.niaaa.nih.gov/) to help you evaluate your behaviors and associated risks. The site also provides resources for those who wish to change their drinking behavior. The site is specifically targeted toward young adults with the goal of reducing harm associated with heavy drinking. While some people will need formal intervention to change, it is possible for many with alcohol problems to cut down on their drinking or quit on their own. The following list provides some tips to successfully quit or reduce your alcohol use:

- Make a list of reasons to stop drinking or cut down.
- Set a goal for yourself and make plans to meet it.
- Monitor your drinking—when, where, how much.
- Identify situations that trigger strong urges to drink.
- Spend less time in drinking settings (e.g., bars).

- Establish nondrinking days; offer to be a designated driver.
- Don't try to keep up with others.

Social support is important for avoiding problems associated with alcohol. You can reduce your risk by building a strong and supportive network of friends and by choosing activities that aren't tied to alcohol. If you do have friends that drink, make sure that they understand your preferences and limits. Clearly identify a designated driver if you are out. If you are hosting a party, you have a responsibility to prevent your friends from drinking too much. You also have a responsibility for making sure that they get home safely. Guidelines for being a responsible party host include:

- Have water, nonalcoholic beverages, and food available.
- Do not assume that everyone wants to drink.
- Do not continue to serve drinks to those who are clearly intoxicated.
- Close the bar an hour or two before the party ends.
- Secure safe transportation for those who are intoxicated.

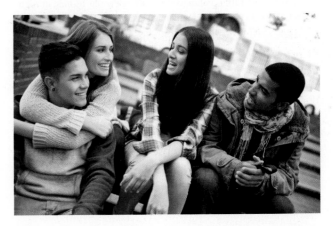

Friends can help each other make responsible choices related to alcohol use.
Peopleimages/iStock/Getty Images

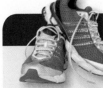

Strategies for Action: Lab Information

Although one of the greatest risks associated with alcohol use is driving under the influence, drinking to the legal limit for intoxication (0.08 percent) is associated with many other negative consequences. This includes physical fights, unwanted sexual behavior, and impaired academic performance. So, knowing how much you can drink without becoming intoxicated is critical. Lab 19A provides a formula to estimate your BAC at different levels of consumption over different periods of time so you can avoid drinking to intoxication.

The first step in protecting yourself from long-term problems with alcohol is to know your level of risk. In college, where students may be exposed to many heavy drinkers, students may underestimate their own levels of risk. Lab 19B provides an opportunity to evaluate your own behavior or the behavior of a friend to determine if a problem may exist. It is always better to identify a problem early and take steps to reduce risk for long-term negative consequences.

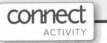

Suggested Resources and Readings

The websites for the following sources can be accessed by searching online for the organization, program, or title listed. Specific scientific references are available at the end of this edition of *Concepts of Fitness and Wellness*.

- American Addiction Centers. The Prevalence of Pregaming.
- Centers for Disease Control and Prevention. Alcohol and Caffeine.
- Centers for Disease Control and Prevention. Alcohol and Public Health.
- Centers for Disease Control and Prevention. Heavy Drinking among U.S. Adults, 2018.
- Earlenbaugh, E. (2021, January 11). "Cannabis Abstinence Is Tied to More Alcohol Use for Teens and Young Adults, Study Finds." *Forbes.*
- Food and Drug Administration. (2018, December 10). "FDA Clears Medical Mobile App to Help Those with Opioid Use Disorder Stay in Recovery Programs."
- Leonard, J. (2020, March 4). "What Happens When You Mix Weed and Alcohol?" *Medical News Today.*
- Magallon, G. (2021, February 10). "More People Turning to Alcohol, Drugs to Cope with Pandemic Anxiety: UC Merced Study." *ABC 30 Action News.*
- Mayo Clinic. (2019, October 26). "Alcohol Use: Weighing Risks and Benefits."
- National Highway Traffic Safety Administration. Drunk Driving.
- National Institute on Alcohol Abuse and Alcoholism:
  - Alcohol Facts and Statistics.
  - Binge Drinking.
  - College Drinking.
  - NIAAA Alcohol Treatment Navigator.
- Research Society on Alcoholism. (2021, March 19). "College Students' Alcohol Use Fell, Not Rose, during the Early COVID-19 Pandemic." *Newswise.*
- Responsibility.org. Drunk Driving Fatality Statistics.
- Schulenberg, J. E., et. al. (2020). *Monitoring the Future National Survey Results on Drug Use, 1975–2019: Volume II, College Students and Adults ages 19–60.* Ann Arbor: Institute for Social Research, The University of Michigan. (pdf)
- Sellman, D. (2020). "Alcohol Is More Harmful Than Cannabis." *New Zealand Medical Journal, 133*(1520).
- Siebert, A. (2020, November 30). "Cannabis as Harm Reduction? Study Shows Patients Who Use It Drink Less Alcohol." *Forbes.*
- Buddy, T. (2020, October 5). "How Teens Are Influenced by Alcohol Advertising." *Verywell Family.*
- Villa, L. (2021, February 15). "Top 6 Smartphone Addiction Recovery Apps." American Addiction Centers.

Design Element: (*magnifying glass*): Siede Preis/Getty Images; (*runners shoes*): Maridav/Getty Images; (*tablet*): McGraw Hill; (*woman*): GlobalStock/Getty Images; (*blue sports shoes*): chictype/Getty Images; (*smartphone*): Alexey Boldin/Shutterstock; (*Why It Matters*): MHHE

Lab 19A Blood Alcohol Level

Name   **Section**   **Date**

Purpose: To learn to calculate your (or a friend's) blood alcohol concentration (BAC).

Procedures

1. Assume a drink is a 12-ounce can or bottle of 5 percent beer, a 5-ounce glass (a small glass) of 12 percent alcohol (wine), or a mixed drink with a 1½-ounce shot glass of 80 proof liquor.
    Case A: Assume you consumed two drinks within 40 minutes.
    Case B: Assume you consumed two drinks over a period of 1 hour and 20 minutes.
    Case C: Assume you had two six-packs of beer (12 cans) over 5 hours.
    Case D: Same as C, but, if you weigh less than 150 pounds, assume you weigh 50 pounds more than you now weigh, and, if you weigh more than 150 pounds, assume you weigh 50 pounds less.

2. Divide 3.8 by your weight in pounds to obtain your "BAC maximum per drink," or refer to Table 4 in this Concept. You should obtain a number between 0.015 and 0.04 (based on one drink in 40 minutes). Use the formula below to determine BAC over time.

$$\text{Approximate BAC over time} = \frac{(3.8 \times \text{\# of drinks})}{(\text{body weight})} - \frac{[0.01 \times (\text{\# min} - 40)]}{40}$$

3. After 40 minutes have passed, your body will begin eliminating alcohol from the bloodstream at the rate of about 0.01 percent for each additional 40 minutes. Multiply the number of drinks you've had by your "BAC maximum per drink" and subtract 0.01 percent from the number for each 40 minutes that have passed since you began drinking—but don't count the first 40 minutes. Compute your BAC for cases A, B, C, and D.

    Example: Case A. Mary weighs 100 pounds. $\dfrac{3.8 \times 2}{100} = \dfrac{7.6}{100} = 0.076\%$ BAC

    Case B. Mary takes 80 minutes. $0.076\% - \dfrac{[0.01 \times (80 - 40)]}{40} = 0.066\%$ BAC

4. Record your results below by writing the formula and computing the BAC for each case.
5. Select whether each case would be able to legally drive with that level of BAC. Then complete the Conclusions and Implications Section to summarize your observations.

Results

Case A $\dfrac{(3.8 \times \underline{\quad} \text{ \# of drinks})}{\underline{\quad} \text{ lbs}} = \underline{\quad} - \% \text{ BAC}$

Case B $\dfrac{(3.8 \times \underline{\quad} \text{ \# of drinks})}{\underline{\quad} \text{ lbs}} - \dfrac{[0.01 \times (\underline{\quad} \text{ \# min} - 40)]}{40} = \text{BAC} (\quad) - (\quad) = \underline{\quad}\% \text{ BAC}$

Case C $\dfrac{(3.8 \times \underline{\quad} \text{ \# of drinks})}{\underline{\quad} \text{ lbs}} - \dfrac{[0.01 \times (\underline{\quad} \text{ \# min} - 40)]}{40} = \text{BAC} (\quad) - (\quad) = \underline{\quad}\% \text{ BAC}$

Case D $\dfrac{(3.8 \times \underline{\quad} \text{ \# of drinks})}{\underline{\quad} \text{ lbs}} - \dfrac{[0.01 \times (\underline{\quad} \text{ \# min} - 40)]}{40} = \text{BAC} (\quad) - (\quad) = \underline{\quad}\% \text{ BAC}$

Would you (or your friend) be able to drive legally according to your state's laws? Place an X over your answer.

Case A   (Yes) (No)

Case B   (Yes) (No)

Case C   (Yes) (No)

Case D   (Yes) (No)

Conclusions and Implications: In several sentences, discuss what you have learned from doing this activity.

Lab 19B Perceptions about Alcohol Use

Name	Section	Date

Purpose: To better understand perceptions about drinking behaviors.

Procedures

1. Think of a person you care about. Do not identify this person on this lab report.
2. Answer each of the questions below as honestly as possible, evaluating the behavior of the person you have identified. Calculate a total score and determine a rating (see Chart 1).
3. At another time, when you do not have to submit your results, you should answer the questions about yourself.
4. Answer the questions in the Conclusions and Implications section.

Results

	Never	Sometimes	Frequently	Too Often	Add Score
1. How often does the person drink?	0	1	2	3	
2. How often does the person have six or more drinks on one occasion?	0	1	2	3	
3. How often do friends of the person drink?	0	1	2	3	
4. How often has the person been unable to stop after starting to drink?	0	1	2	3	
5. How often does the person need a drink to get started in the morning?	0	1	2	3	
6. How often has the person been unable to remember previous events after drinking?	0	1	2	3	
7. How often does the person miss class or work associated with drinking?	0	1	2	3	
8. How often does the person have social or personal problems associated with drinking?	0	1	2	3	
9. How often does the person deny drinking too much (only for those whom you consider to drink too much)?	0	1	2	3	

Total Score

Chart 1 Drinking Behavior Rating Scale

Rating	Score
Alcohol abuse*	18+
Drinking problem	12–17
Potential problem	8–11
Low risk of problem	<8

*Professional help recommended.

Rating

377

Conclusions and Implications

1. In several sentences, discuss the drinking behavior of the person you identified. Do you think your ratings give an accurate picture of the person? Do you think the person you rated has a problem with alcohol?

2. In several sentences, discuss the drinking behavior of the person's friends. Do the friends promote drinking, or not?

3. In several sentences, discuss things you could do to help a friend or loved one solve a drinking problem.

The Use and Abuse of Other Drugs

LEARNING OBJECTIVES

After completing the study of this Concept, you will be able to:

► List the six major classes of illicit drugs and their effects.

► Describe the negative health, financial, and legal consequences of illicit drug use.

► Identify biological, psychological, and social factors that contribute to illicit drug use and abuse.

► Explain differences in prevalence of the various classes of drugs, including both illegal drugs and prescription drugs.

► Describe long-term and recent trends in use of different drugs.

► Identify signs of drug problems and available resources for addressing these problems.

Use of psychoactive drugs (both illicit and prescription) has serious health consequences and enormous personal, social, and economic costs. Preventing onset of psychoactive drug use and providing adequate treatment to individuals with substance use disorders is a public health priority.

Terry Vine/Blend Images LLC

Why It Matters!

Illicit drug use and misuse of prescription drugs are associated with a host of personal and societal costs, including overdoses, legal problems, and substance use disorders. Approximately 45 percent of college students report using illegal drugs in the past year. In fact, rates of use among young adults are higher than any other age group, with rates among college students even higher than similar-aged young adults not in college. Use of illicit drugs is usually preceded by use of alcohol and/or tobacco. However, other risk factors include exposure to substance-using peers and the belief that drug use will have more positive than negative consequences. This Concept summarizes six distinct categories of illicit drugs: depressants, opioids, stimulants, hallucinogens, cannabis, and designer drugs. Prevalence and consequences of each drug class are outlined along with risk factors for substance misuse so you can avoid or address these problems.

Classification of Illicit and Prescription Drugs

Psychoactive drugs can be classified in six major groups. Although there are hundreds of illicit drugs, they can generally be classified as depressants, opioids, stimulants, hallucinogens, cannabis, and designer drugs. Drugs in the same group have similar effects. Although opioids (also referred to as opiate narcotics) are actually depressants, with high levels of use and severe negative consequences (e.g., overdoses) they are generally given their own category. Across drug classes, effects are classified as either physiological or psychological (primarily affecting the body versus affecting behavior). The effects of these **psychoactive drugs** can vary with each individual and with different doses.

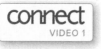

Depressant drugs include alcohol, tranquilizers, and barbiturates. Depressants come in the form of pills, liquids, and injectables (see Table 1). In small doses, they slow heart rate and respiration. In larger doses, they act as a poison and damage every organ system in the body. In large enough doses, they can dramatically depress heart rate and respiration enough to cause death, if quick intervention is not available. In terms of their effect on behavior, the user might at first feel stimulated, despite their depressant effects. Depression, loss of coordination, drop in energy level, mood swings, and confusion occur after prolonged use. Alcohol is the most widely used depressant.

Opioids include heroin, morphine, fentanyl, and oxycodone. Opioids are all opium poppy derivatives or synthetics that emulate them. They are often used clinically to treat pain; however, heroin has no legal medical use in the United States and has a high rate of addiction. It is three times stronger than many other medicinal opioids and induces different physiological effects. Opioids used for nonmedicinal purposes (i.e., narcotics) are smoked, injected, sniffed, or swallowed (see Table 2).

Every opioid, legal or illegal, is a potential poison. A single dose can be fatal. Deaths related to opioid abuse are typically caused by overdose, impurities of the drug, or mixing of the drug with other depressants, such as alcohol. The mixing of drugs in the same or similar categories can produce a heightened physiological effect known as synergism, or the **synergistic effect**. The combined use makes drug taking far more dangerous.

Stimulants include cocaine and methamphetamine as well as prescription drugs like Ritalin and Adderall. Cocaine comes in powder form (coke) and a rocklike form (crack). The timing and magnitude of effects of cocaine vary depending on whether it is inhaled, injected, or smoked. Combining cocaine and alcohol use leads to production of cocaethylene, which increases risk for overdose. Amphetamines and methamphetamines are also classified as stimulants due to their effects on the central nervous system.

Table 1 ▶ Depressants ("Downers," Sedatives)

Examples	Physiological Effects	Psychological Effects
Tranquilizers (e.g., Valium, Xanax, meprobamate, sleeping pills, methaqualone; also called tranks, downers, or candy)	In large doses, act as a poison and damage every organ system	Feelings of relaxation and euphoria; after prolonged use: depression, loss of coordination, drop in energy level, mood swings, confusion, euphoria
Barbiturates (e.g., Mebaral, Nembutal)	Quick sedation: vomiting; loss of motor and neurological control; combined with alcohol, can lead to coma and death	Amnesia

Table 2 ► Opioids

Examples	Physiological Effects	Psychological Effects
Codeine, morphine, synthetic opiates (e.g., Vicodin, OxyContin), methadone	Opioids (other than heroin): blockage of pain, chronic constipation, depressed respiration, redness and irritation of nostrils, nausea, lowered sexual drive, impaired immune system	Opioids (including heroin): euphoria and feeling of pleasure; nontherapeutic doses may result in mental distress, such as fear and nervousness; in heavy users, drowsiness and apathy may occur
Heroin (also called brown sugar, junk, or smack)	Heroin: blood clots, bacterial endocarditis, serum hepatitis, brain abscess, HIV infection (from shared needles); in pregnant users, high risk of miscarriage, stillbirths, birth defects, toxemia, addicted babies	

Table 3 ► Stimulants

Examples	Physiological Effects	Psychological Effects
Cocaine (also called coke, blow, snow, or crack)	Cocaine: sore throat, hoarseness, shortness of breath (leads to bronchitis and emphysema), dilated pupils, "lights" seen around objects	Powder cocaine causes an initial response of energy, feeling of confidence; as it wears off: depression, moodiness, irritability, severe mental disorders Crack causes intense euphoria, then crushing depression, intense feeling of self-hate; as it wears off: depression and sadness, intense anxiety about where to get more drugs, aggressiveness, paranoia
Amphetamines and powder methamphetamines (also called speed, uppers, or black beauties); diet and pep pills, Ritalin	Excite central nervous system; increase blood pressure, respiration, and heart rate (sometimes resulting in convulsions and stroke); reduce appetite; highly addictive; overdose is fatal; with increased use: dizziness, headaches, sleeplessness; with long-term use: progressive brain damage, malnutrition	Initially, feeling of being invincible, alertness, excitement; with increased use: feeling of anxiety; with long-term use: hallucinations, psychosis
Crystal methamphetamine (also called meth, crystal, crank, or ice)	Extreme energy, sleeplessness, seizures, flushed skin, constricted pupils	Euphoria, delusions of grandeur, feelings of invincibility, physical aggression, paranoia, mood swings, psychosis

Crystal methamphetamine (also known as ice, meth, or crystal) is a purified methamphetamine that also comes in rock form or powder. As a powder, it is usually smoked in a glass pipe or cigarette. It is a powerful stimulant, with an effect that lasts 8–30 hours. Much like crack cocaine, ice is a concentrated form of an already potent stimulant drug that is either smoked or injected. Ice also causes an intense "rush" or "flash," which is experienced as highly pleasurable. Because the initial rush lasts for only a few minutes, users need to administer the drug frequently to maintain the effects. Stimulants are often included in diet pills to reduce appetite; others (e.g., Ritalin) are used clinically to treat attention deficit hyperactivity disorder (ADHD; see Table 3).

Drugs that cause the user to have hallucinations are called hallucinogens, or psychedelics. PCP and LSD are common examples of hallucinogens, but other drugs in this category include mushrooms, and peyote cactus buttons, which have been used for ceremonial purposes by some indigenous groups for centuries.

Inhalants are sometimes classified separately from other hallucinogens because their effects are so serious. They reach the brain in seconds, and the effect lasts only a few minutes. There are three types: (1) solvents, such as glue, gasoline, paints, paint thinner, lighter fluid, shoe polish, and liquid wax; (2) aerosols, such as hair spray, air fresheners, insect spray, and spray paint; and (3) nitrites, such as nitrous oxide (laughing gas) and butyl nitrite (a liquid incense). Table 4 describes the effects of hallucinogens and pyschedelics (drugs that cause **hallucinations**).

Psychoactive Drug Any drug that produces a temporary change in the physiological functions of the nervous system, affecting mood, thoughts, feelings, or behavior.

Synergistic Effect The joint actions of two or more drugs that increase the effects of each.

Hallucinations Imaginary things seen, felt, or heard or things seen in a distorted way.

Table 4 ▶ Hallucinogens (Psychedelics)

Examples	Physiological Effects	Psychological Effects
Lysergic acid diethylamide (LSD; also called acid, boomers, or cubes)	Changes chromosomes and may result in birth defects of babies of users; bad trips, confusion, flashback	Vivid hallucinations, feelings of overlapping/merging of the senses, expanded consciousness and mystical experiences, stimulated awareness and desire, confusion, flashback
Phencyclidine (PCP)	Accumulates in fat cells and may remain in body longer than most drugs; impaired immune system, poor coordination, weight loss, speech problems, heart and lung failure, irreversible brain damage, convulsions, coma, death	Insensitivity to pain can lead to death; euphoria, depersonalization, hallucinations, delirium, amnesia, tunnel vision, loss of control, violent behavior
Inhalants (solvents, aerosols, and nitrites; also known as poppers, rush)	Slow reaction time, headache, nausea, vomiting, seizure, brain damage, suffocation, heart attack, death, double vision, sensitivity to light, dizziness, loss of coordination, weakness, numbness; irregular heartbeat, liver and kidney failure, bone marrow damage	Giddiness, overexcitement, less inhibition, feelings of being all-powerful; powerfulness soon fades and leaves irritability

Table 5 ▶ Cannabis (Subclass of Hallucinogens)

Examples	Physiological Effects	Psychological Effects
Cannabis (containing tetrahydrocannabinol, or THC; also called weed, pot, grass, blunt, herb, dabs, or wax)	Long-term use: bronchitis, emphysema and lung cancer, bloodshot eyes, heart disease, infertility, sexual dysfunction, permanent memory loss (brain damage)	May not hallucinate; pleasant, relaxed feeling; giddiness; self-preoccupation; less precise thinking; impaired task performance; inertia; with prolonged use: may be withdrawn and apathetic, have anxiety reactions, paranoia; eventually, decreased motivation and enthusiasm, reduced ability to absorb and integrate effectively, profoundly impaired scholastic performance

Cannabis is classified as a hallucinogenic, but its effects are less dramatic than those of other drugs in this class. The active ingredient in cannabis (delta-9-tetrahydrocannabinol-THC) is technically a hallucinogen (see Table 5). Flower cannabis (marijuana) use became widespread in the 1960s and then decreased steadily in the 1970s and 1980s before increasing dramatically in the 1990s and remaining relatively stable over the past 20 years. Cannabis is the most widely used illicit substance in the United States and takes multiple forms, including flower, concentrates (liquid or wax), and edibles (food products). Concentrates and edibles tend to have much higher concentrations of THC than flower. Cannabis use leads to a range of experiences, which differ from person to person.

Designer drugs, which are made in laboratories, have many of the same properties as the drugs they simulate, such as pain relievers, anesthetics, and amphetamines. Designer drugs (also called *club drugs*) are modifications of illegal or restricted drugs made by chemists working illicitly to create street drugs that are not specifically listed as controlled. They change the molecular structure of an existing drug to create a new substance. Since new drugs are being created all the time, their potential effects and associated risks are often unknown (see Table 6).

Prevalence and Consequences of Illicit Drug Abuse

Use of most illicit substances has decreased in the past decade, but rates of use remain high among adolescents and young adults. In the United States, rates of illicit drug use peaked in the 1970s followed by sharp decreases during the 1980s. Overall drug use by adolescents spiked upward in the early 1990s, primarily as a result of two- to threefold increases in cannabis use

Table 6 ▶ Designer Drugs

Examples	Physiological Effects	Psychological Effects
Date-rape drugs: • Rohypnol • Gamma hydroxybutyrate (GHB; also called Georgia homeboy or liquid ecstasy) • Ketamine (also called Special K)	Depression of the central nervous system, incapacitation, coma, seizures, tremors, nausea, sweating, high blood pressure, and potentially fatal respiratory problems	Negative mood states including depression and anxiety; amnesia and delirium; insomnia and impaired motor function
MDMA (3,4-methylenedioxymethamphetamine (also called ecstasy, or X)	Irregular heartbeat, intensified heart problems, liver and brain damage, depletion of serotonin in the brain, muscle tension, and dry mouth	Initial feelings of calm and euphoria may be followed by exhaustion or psychological burnout; increased risk for psychosis and depression; cognitive impairment
Synthetic cannabinoids (e.g., K2, Spice) and cathinones (also called bath salts)	Rapid heart rate, vomiting, agitation, confusion, high blood pressure, reduced blood supply to the heart, heart attack, kidney failure, dehydration	Elevated mood, relaxation, altered perception, anxiety, paranoia, hallucinations, panic attacks, delirium

(See figure 1). Rates of illicit drug use then began a steady but gradual decline during the first decade of the new century. Unfortunately, annual rates of illicit drug use in college students and other young adults have increased roughly 10 percent in the past 10 years, representing a proportional increase of more than 20 percent. In contrast to other illicit drugs, misuse of prescription drugs peaked in 2001 and rates remained high among twelfth graders through 2013. Fortunately, rates of prescription drug misuse have declined by more than 50 percent since that time. Still, the annual prevalence of 7.6 percent among twelfth graders makes prescription drugs the second most widely used drug class (not including alcohol and tobacco) in young people, trailing only cannabis use.

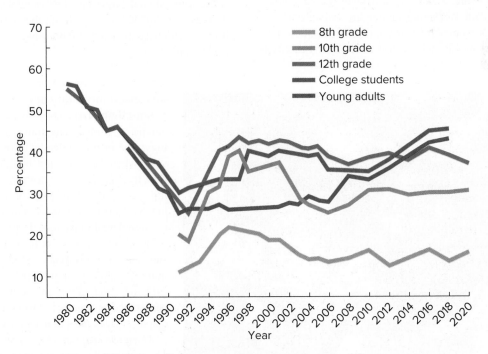

Figure 1 ▶ Trends in annual prevalence of an illicit drug use index across five populations.

Note: Use of "any illicit drugs" includes any use of cannabis, LSD, other hallucinogens, crack, other cocaine, or heroin, or any use that is not under a doctor's orders of other opiates, stimulants, barbiturates, methaqualone (excluded since 1990), or tranquilizers.

Source: National Institute on Drug Abuse.

Rates of illicit drug use among college students are among the highest of any age group. High rates of drug use in college are associated with a host of negative consequences, including impaired cognitive abilities and academic performance, increased risk of accidents and injuries, greater incidence of high-risk sexual behavior, and increased risk for substance use disorders (SUDs). Students who use drugs have less academic motivation and report lower involvement in religion, community service, and extracurricular activities on campus.

Much like alcohol, both direct and indirect peer influences are important predictors of use among college students. Students with friends who use cannabis are more likely to use it themselves. Misperceptions of normative behavior may also influence personal behavior. 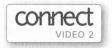 One study found that 98 percent of students incorrectly believed that the typical student on campus used cannabis at least once per year, despite the fact that most of the students reported no personal use of cannabis. Although both direct and indirect peer influences may contribute to drug use, these same influences can also deter use. One study found that peers exposed to a peer group with strong anti-drug attitudes were likely to conform to this norm.

The development of new drugs contributes to the maintenance of drug use in the United States. New drugs are always being manufactured, and new ways of administering old drugs often lead to a resurgence in use. Designer drugs provide examples of new drugs, and crack cocaine and crystal methamphetamine are examples of old drugs that became popular in new forms. When these new drugs become available, information about their benefits is generally spread immediately by word of mouth. In contrast, the risks associated with use are often unknown until the drug has been used for a number of years. This gives new drugs time to become popular before information that might deter their use is available. Ecstasy and crystal methamphetamine are good examples of this phenomenon. Fortunately, once the risks were well established, public campaigns by the National Institute on Drug Abuse (NIDA) and other agencies provided information about those risks and helped curb levels of use relatively quickly. Thirty-day prevalence of ecstasy use in high school seniors decreased from 3.6 to 1 percent in a 5-year period, and rates of crystal methamphetamine use decreased from 1.2 percent to 0.5 percent over a similar period of time. Unfortunately, efforts to protect the public are challenged by the constant production of new designer drugs. Recent examples include synthetic cannabinoids and cathinones (bath salts). These drugs emerged around 2010 and quickly led to a large number of calls to poison control centers. (See Table 6 for a description of negative drug reactions.) The Drug Enforcement Administration (DEA) acted swiftly to place bans on these products, and annual rates of synthetic cannabinoid use among teens subsequently decreased from 8.0 percent in 2012 to 3.1 percent in 2016. The current prevalence is 2.2 percent. Similarly, the use of salvia decreased from 3.6 to 1.4 percent between 2011 and 2014, and bath salts decreased from 0.9 to 0.5 percent between 2013 and 2017. In addition to the emergence of new drugs, there is a tendency to forget about the negative consequences of existing drugs after rates decrease—a phenomenon called **generational forgetting**. For example, after dramatic decreases in MDMA use following the peak in 2000, rates began to climb again, nearly doubling between 2005 and 2010 before stabilizing.

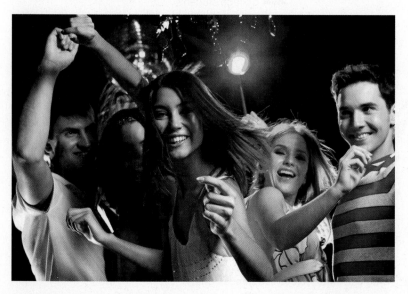

Social environments and peer pressure can influence decision making and drug behavior.
Pressmaster/Shutterstock

Drug use takes a human toll in terms of increased morbidity and mortality and lost productivity. Drug abuse leads to over 4 million emergency room visits annually and is the leading cause of injury deaths in the United States, surpassing traffic-related fatalities for the first time in 2011. This does not take into account the indirect effects of drug use on mortality, including deaths from accidents, homicides, and AIDS (acquired via intravenous drug use). Use of illicit drugs also increases risk for the development of **substance use disorders (SUDs)** that often require formal treatment. Because of problems with low productivity in the workplace, a large percentage of American businesses now conduct employee drug tests to detect usage.

Drug use also has significant economic costs. The economic costs of illicit drug abuse and misuse of prescription opioids is estimated at more than $270 billion a year. Approximately 8.3 million adults (about 3 percent of the

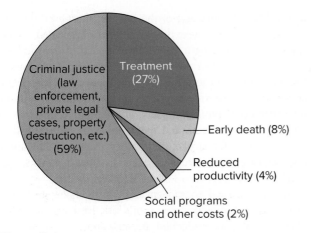

Figure 2 ▶ The estimated cost of drug abuse (percentage of total costs).

Source: U.S. Department of Justice National Drug Intelligence Center.

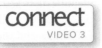

population) in the United States meet criteria for an illicit SUD (which includes illicit drugs and prescription opioids), but most of the national economic burden is not related to treatment (2 percent). More than half of the costs are associated with drug-related crime. Figure 2 illustrates the proportion of societal costs resulting from factors such as law enforcement expenditures, social programs, and reduced productivity.

Drug use can lead to significant legal problems, resulting in jail time and substantial fines. State laws regarding the possession and sale of illicit drugs vary considerably, and penalties within states vary based on the amount of the drug, the type of drug, and the type of offense (possession, sales, or production). Although 19 states have decriminalized cannabis for recreational use and others have legalized medical use, penalties for cannabis possession are still substantial in other states, and all states tend to have more severe penalties for drugs like cocaine, heroin, and methamphetamine. Penalties for the possession of small amounts are the least severe, with penalties for the sale or production of large amounts the most severe. In most states without recreational use laws, the maximum jail time for possession ranges from 6 months to 1 year for cannabis and from 1 to 7 years for cocaine, methamphetamine, and ecstasy. In addition, fines between $500 and $1,000 for cannabis and between $5,000 and $25,000 for other illicit drugs are typical.

Drug-Specific Prevalence and Consequences

Cannabis is the most widely used (illicit) drug in the United States and is associated with a host of physical health and social consequences. Estimates from national surveys suggest approximately 17.5 percent of people over the age of 12 used cannabis in the past year. Although many believe it is a relatively safe drug, and some favor decriminalization or legalization, a number of risks are associated with cannabis use. The Substance Abuse and Mental Health Services Administration (SAMHSA) outlines the many risks of cannabis use. With respect to health, chronic smoking of cannabis products leads to many of the negative consequences associated with cigarette smoking, including cardiovascular disease and lung cancer. One study showed that cannabis use also increases risk for stroke. Another study found that cannabis use leads to nearly a fivefold increase in acute risk for a heart attack, especially among those with existing cardiovascular risk. Cannabis use is also associated with impaired cognitive abilities. For example, adolescents who use cannabis heavily have been shown to have deficits in attention, learning, and processing speed. There is also direct evidence from neuroimaging studies for differences in brain function. In particular, areas of the brain associated with processing of emotional information appear to be affected. These findings are cause for concern, given evidence for increased risk for depression, anxiety, and psychosis among individuals who use cannabis.

A CLOSER LOOK

Cannabis/Marijuana Decriminalization

More than 30 states now have medical cannabis/marijuana laws, and 19 states have decriminalized or legalized cannabis/marijuana for recreational use (as of 2021). However, cannabis remains illegal and is classified as a Schedule 1 drug at the federal level. Research on the impacts of legalization shows both pros and cons. On the one hand, there are significant concerns about the safety of food products containing cannabis, and several states have reported increases in child poisonings following legalization. On the other hand, some studies suggest that opioid-related deaths are lower in states that have legalized medical cannabis use. It will be critical to continue closely monitoring changes in the public health impact of cannabis as laws change.

Do you support laws that allow for medical cannabis use? What about laws that allow for recreational use? What do you think are the biggest benefits and risks of legalization?

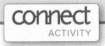

Generational Forgetting The tendency for individuals to forget about the risks of a particular drug over time, leading to a resurgence in its use.

Substance Use Disorder (SUD) The use of a drug to the extent that it impairs social, psychological, or physiological functioning.

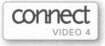

Although the debate is ongoing regarding the addictive (physical dependence) potential of cannabis, it is clear that one can become psychologically addicted to the drug. Psychological dependence is characterized by craving for the drug and continued use despite negative consequences. There is also emerging evidence that those who try to quit using cannabis experience withdrawal symptoms. For example, a recent study found that smokers of cannabis experienced withdrawal symptoms that were quite similar to those of tobacco smokers, including irritability, anxiety, and sleep difficulties. Based on the most recent national survey, roughly 2 percent of people aged 12 and older in the United States met the criteria for a cannabis use disorder in the past year.

Stimulants are among the most commonly used illicit drugs. Cocaine and methamphetamine are prominent examples of widely used stimulant drugs (see Figure 3). They share common characteristics and have similar effects and risks. First, both come in powder form as well as more concentrated crystal (ice) or rock (crack) forms. Crack cocaine was one of the most abused drugs in the United States during the peak rates of use in the early to mid-1980s, and crystal methamphetamine was at the center of the less dramatic increase in illicit drug use in the early 1990s. Crack and ice are

highly addictive. Because of the intense, short-lived high associated with using these drugs, patterns of repeated use develop quickly, leading to rapid development of dependence. Both drugs are also known to damage dopamine neurons in the brain and lead to a host of short- and long-term health consequences. Short-term effects that occur after the initial high include irritability, anxiety, and paranoia. In terms of long-term risk, cocaine and methamphetamine use lead to increased risk for stroke, respiratory problems (including respiratory failure), irregular heartbeat, heart attacks, and psychiatric symptoms.

Unique physical consequences of methamphetamine use include poor complexion and tooth loss. Ice has added risks associated with its production. Because some of the products used to produce meth (e.g., pseudoephedrine) have legitimate pharmaceutical uses, policies have been put in place to monitor their sale. If you go to your pharmacy to purchase an over-the-counter (OTC) decongestant, you may be asked to provide identification and a signature. In addition, you may have to purchase your medication at the pharmacy even though it is an OTC drug, and you may be limited to one or two packages.

The continued use of designer drugs is a concern, given strong evidence of their harmful effects. Designer drugs include ecstasy/Molly (MDMA), Rohypnol, GHB, ketamine, DOM, DOB, and NEXUS. Ecstasy (or Molly), a hallucinogen, is inhaled, injected, or swallowed. The drug was initially popular at all-night dance parties called raves, but its use quickly expanded beyond the club scene. Ecstasy alters brain levels of serotonin; negatively impacts memory; and affects the brain regions that regulate sleep, mood, and learning. This type of ecstasy is often referred to as "Molly." The negative effects of ecstasy/Molly may last as long as 7 years. Dealers often pass off other drugs as ecstasy, and they are often even more dangerous.

Rohypnol and GHB are predominately central nervous system depressants, like the other sedative drugs described previously. These drugs are odorless, colorless, and tasteless, so they can be added to food or beverages without the consumer detecting their presence. Because of these properties, Rohypnol and GHB are known as drug-assisted assault or date-rape drugs. In addition to incapacitating the user, these drugs lead to anterograde amnesia, or the inability to remember events that occur after consumption.

Inhalant use poses a serious risk to physical health, including risk for sudden death. Those who use inhalants are at risk for what is known as "sudden sniffing death." Sniffing inhalants can lead to irregular and rapid heart rhythms that can cause heart failure and rapid death. This can occur from a single episode of sniffing in an otherwise healthy adolescent.

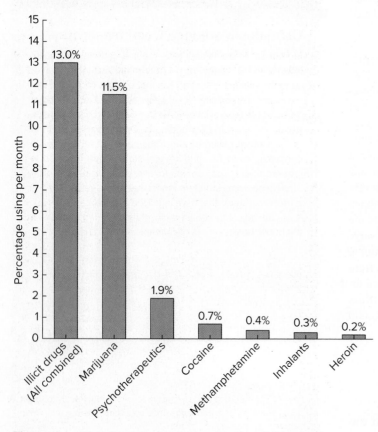

Figure 3 ▶ Illicit drug use among persons 12 and older, by drug (% per month).

Source: Substance Abuse and Mental Health Services Administration.

Misuse and abuse of OTC and prescription drugs has become an increasing problem. Prescription drugs are often used inappropriately. In fact, psychotherapeutic drugs are now the second most commonly abused class of drugs, trailing only cannabis (see Figure 3). Examples of psycho-therapeutic drug misuse include using prescriptions written for other people and using medicines for purposes other than as prescribed. Users may also obtain prescription drugs without prescriptions via the Internet, though most people who misuse prescription drugs indicate that they obtain them for free from friends or family members. Many fail to recognize the potential risks of prescription drug use, assuming that anything prescribed by a physician must be safe. The more commonly abused prescription drugs among college students include Adderall, Ritalin, Valium, and Xanax, as well as prescription pain medications such as Percocet, Vicodin, and OxyContin. Methadone use without a prescription also appears to be increasing. Methadone has been approved in the United States for the treatment of opiate dependence (primarily heroin) since 1972, but it is increasingly making its way into the hands of those without prescriptions.

Rates of misuse of ADHD drugs like Ritalin and Adderall are high among young people, particularly college students who often use the drugs in an effort to enhance academic performance. The most recent national data indicate that roughly 8.4 percent of college students report using Adderall, and 2.5 percent report using Ritalin without a prescription in the past year.

Overdoses from misuse of prescription drugs account for the vast majority of drug overdoses in the United States. Drug overdose deaths have nearly quadrupled in the past 20 years, largely due to increases in opioid use. Over 70 percent of drug-related overdoses are related to use of opioids (including synthetic opioids), with roughly 137 opioid overdose deaths in the United

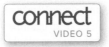
VIDEO 5

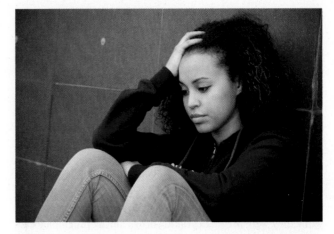

Misuse of prescription pain medications and ADHD drugs can lead to dependence and adverse outcomes.
paolo81/Getty Images

States each day. In fact, the recent increases in drug overdoses associated with prescription narcotics are even more dramatic than the increases seen when heroin and crack cocaine were first introduced. Although prescription drugs like Vicodin and OxyContin were important drivers of the early surge in opioid overdoses, more recent increases have been driven primarily by use of fentanyl and synthetic derivatives. Rates of overdose related to fentanyl are more than double that of all other opioids combined. This is not surprising as fentanyl, which is primarily prescribed for end-stage cancer, is 50–100 times more potent than morphine. The surge in opioid-related overdoses has led major public health organizations, including the CDC, to declare an opioid epidemic in the United States. Although rates are not as dramatic as for prescription opioids, ER visits related to nonprescription use of tranquilizers like Valium and Xanax have also increased dramatically beginning in 2005. Fortunately, after increasing for more than a decade, rates have started to decline in the last few years.

In the News

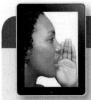

The Opioid Crisis: Who Is at Fault?

Deaths from drug overdoses have doubled over the past decade. The CDC has labeled the opioid crisis an epidemic, and the Council of Academic Advisors estimates the cost of the opioid epidemic at roughly half a trillion dollars. Many believe that major drug companies that produced and marketed highly addictive opiate drugs should bear responsibility for the opioid crisis. The courts seem to agree. In a prominent legal case, Purdue Pharma, the maker of OxyContin, agreed to an $8.3 billion settlement related to its production and marketing of the drug. Other court cases have implicated physicians for unethical distribution of opioids and one case included charges of murder related to prescribing practices.

Who do you think is most responsible for the opioid epidemic? Do you think legal actions against physicians and pharmaceutical companies will help reverse the problem?

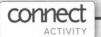
ACTIVITY

Accidental misuse of prescription drugs is another common problem. Examples of unwitting misuse of drugs include taking a medicine twice, taking the wrong medicine from unlabeled bottles, using outdated medicines, and taking multiple medications that negatively interact with one another. Thus, it is important to understand the nature of all the medications you are taking (including supplements, prescription drugs, and OTC drugs) and how they interact. Women who are pregnant, are nursing, or want to get pregnant should avoid drug use, including many prescription drugs. The most recent results of the National Pregnancy and Health Survey, conducted by NIDA, estimated that 5 percent of women who give birth each year in the United States use illegal drugs while they were pregnant. Taking drugs during pregnancy can result in various conditions, including premature separation of the placenta from the womb, fetal stroke, miscarriage, birth defects, low-birth-weight babies, babies born addicted to substances, and postnatal risks, including sudden infant death syndrome (SIDS) and learning disabilities.

Causes of Illicit Drug Abuse

Drug use generally begins with cigarette smoking and alcohol use. Of course, most people who smoke or drink will not go on to use illegal drugs, but it is rare for people who do not smoke or drink to use illegal drugs. The average age of first use of cigarettes, alcohol, and cannabis is roughly 16 among those who report using prior to age 21, suggesting that cannabis may also provide a pathway to use of other illicit drugs. In general, the younger a person is when they start using drugs, including nicotine and alcohol, the more likely they are to use illegal drugs and become physically dependent on them.

Most experts agree that drug use and abuse are complex phenomena that must be understood within a biopsychosocial model. The bio-psychosocial model suggests that biological, psychological, and social factors must be considered in under- 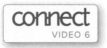 standing substance use and abuse. From this perspective, the potential for addiction depends on a host of factors, including genetic vulnerability, the type of drug used, the route of administration, attitudes toward drug use, expectations regarding drug effects, peer use, and ease of access.

Genetics play a role in susceptibility to drug addiction. Research has suggested that genetic factors explain as much as 50 percent of alcohol and nicotine addiction, and the same is likely true for other drugs of abuse. The effect of genetics (and susceptibility to addiction) depends on how the drug is used and how it affects the brain. Some drugs act on receptors in the brain that are specific to that drug (e.g., cannabinoid receptors for cannabis; opioid receptors for heroin and prescription opioids), whereas others act on more general neurotransmitters associated with reward (e.g., effects of

HELP   **Health is available to Everyone for a Lifetime, and it's Personal**

Preventing Drug-Impaired Driving

With an increasing number of states legalizing cannabis and rising rates of prescription drug misuse, efforts to reduce negative consequences of impaired driving have expanded beyond a focus on alcohol use. Although many perceive there is a lower risk for driving under the influence of other drugs, there is strong evidence that cannabis and prescription opioids lead to significant impairment in driving ability and increased crash risk. In addition, prevention may be more critical for other drugs because it is harder to enforce drug-impaired driving laws (e.g., no comparable standard to a BAC of 0.08). To address this need, researchers at the University of California–San Diego have developed a new program to reduce the risk for drug-impaired driving and are working to train law enforcement and health professionals to deliver the program.

Do you think it's important to establish standards for drug-impaired driving? Will education about impairment caused by cannabis and prescription drug use help reduce rates of drug-impaired driving?

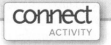

cocaine and methamphetamine on the dopamine system) and the regulation of mood and behavior (e.g., MDMA effects on the serotonin system). Because both the dopamine and opioid systems are directly related to the experience of reward, drugs like heroin and cocaine that affect these systems are particularly addictive. The route of administration also influences risk for addiction. For example, the likelihood of becoming addicted to methamphetamine is much higher if it is smoked rather than inhaled as powder.

Psychological factors such as personality traits, attitudes, perceptions of risk, and expectations of benefits can influence drug use. Individuals with higher levels of sensation seeking (e.g., need for a high level of stimulation) and impulsivity have been shown to be at increased risk for use of a range of illicit drugs. Those who believe drug use is acceptable and affiliate with others with similar views are also more likely to use drugs and to develop problems. These attitudes are influenced by both parental and peer attitudes as well as the attitudes of the broader culture. Perceptions of risk are also a strong predictor of drug use. In fact, national studies have consistently found that shifts in perceptions of risk related to specific drugs precede changes in rates of use of those drugs. Much like alcohol, those who believe drugs will have strong positive effects are more likely to use and abuse them. This is particularly true for those who believe that drug use is an effective way to cope with stress.

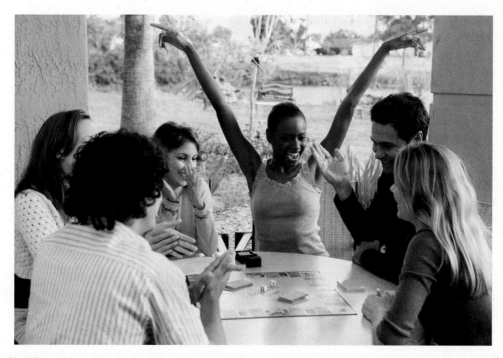

Connecting with the right social group can help you adopt positive lifestyles and behaviors.
Radius Images/Alamy Stock Photo

Social factors and social norms have important effects on drug use. People who live in areas where drugs are readily available are at increased risk for both use and abuse. Another major influence on drug use in young people is the extent to which their social group engages in drug use. Those who perceive that most of their peers use drugs are likely to use drugs themselves. Often these perceptions are not accurate and efforts to correct these misperceptions can aid in reducing drug use.

Technology Update

Vaping Technology and Cannabis

E-cigarettes and other vaporizing devices (vapes) were initially used primarily for vaping nicotine products. However, users quickly learned ways to vaporize cannabis concentrates (e.g., cannabis oil), and the vaping industry quickly developed new products (e.g., mods) to facilitate such use. Some may argue that vaping cannabis is safer than smoking it; however, a recent study noted that vaping cannabis caused more lung damage than smoking cannabis or smoking or vaping nicotine. In addition, vaped cannabis (e.g., cannabis oil) typically has a much higher THC content than flower cannabis (e.g., marijuana), which can lead to adverse effects. There is also concern that technology that facilitates cannabis vaping will lead to increased use because it makes it easier for people to use cannabis products in public places. In fact, the prevalence of vaping cannabis by teens has doubled over the last few years.

Do you think the widespread availability of vaping devices contributes to increases in cannabis use?

connect
ACTIVITY

Using Self-Management Skills

The best way to avoid problems associated with drug use is not to try illegal drugs and to be careful in the use of legal drugs. This Concept clearly indicates that taking a drug for reasons other than managing your own good health increases the risk of taking more drugs in the future. Although most people avoid illegal drugs, almost everyone will take medication sometime in their life. Monitor the use of medications to be sure that you are using them as directed and not with other medications that may result in dangerous synergistic effects.

You can also reduce your risk by knowing the true rates of drug use and learning skills to resist peer pressure. In general, college students overestimate the extent to which other students are using illicit drugs, which can lead to drug use in an effort to fit in with one's peers. Knowing true rates of illicit drug use can help protect you from trying to conform to a norm that is not accurate. Current rates of use of the different illicit drugs in U.S. college students are available at www.monitoringthefuture.org. Of course, some peers are actually using drugs and may invite you to join them. So, making responsible decisions about drugs in the face of peer pressure is also an important life skill. To combat peer pressure, the ability to clearly and effectively say no is necessary. One effective strategy is to choose friends whose values support, rather than undermine, your own.

People who have a problem with drugs need support and specific skills to quit using them. People who are struggling with a drug problem need to talk to someone they can trust, perhaps a friend or relative. If you know somebody with a drug problem, you may be able to help them seek assistance from a referral source, such as an employee assistance program, a family or university physician or hospital, or your city or county health department. These sources help get the person into a treatment program or support group. Some of the better-known nationwide programs include Alcoholics (or Narcotics or Cocaine) Anonymous and Al-Anon

Family Groups. Another option is to call the Substance Abuse and Mental Health Services Administration (SAMHSA) hotline and someone will direct you to help in your area. SAMHSA also has an online treatment locator to help you find local resources:

- SAMHSA National Hotline: 1-800-662-HELP (4357)
- SAMHSA Behavioral Health Treatment Services Locator: https://findtreatment.samhsa.gov/

If you think a fellow student might have a problem with illicit or prescription drugs, help is probably available within the counseling center at your school. Most colleges and universities have information on the school's website about available substance abuse services.

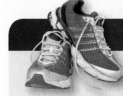

Strategies for Action: Lab Information

In order to help yourself or someone else with a drug problem, you first have to know how to identify when a problem exists. In Lab 20A, you will have the opportunity to evaluate the behavior of a friend or loved one to determine if he or she might need help. Think of somebody you know who uses illicit drugs or misuses

prescription medications and complete the lab to see if that person might need your help. At a later time, it might be a good idea to answer the questions in Lab 20A for yourself to determine if you need to reach out for help in managing your own substance use.

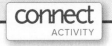
connect
ACTIVITY

Suggested Resources and Readings

The websites for the following sources can be accessed by searching online for the organization, program, or title listed. Specific scientific references are available at the end of this edition of *Concepts of Fitness and Wellness*.

- American Addiction Centers. (2020). Drug Offenses & Sentencing by State.
- American Addiction Centers. (2020). "Legalizing Marijuana Decreases Fatal Opiate Overdoses, Study Shows."
- Centers for Disease Control and Prevention. Fentanyl.
- Cirino, E. (2020, January 2). "Vaping, Smoking, or Eating Marijuana." *Healthline.*
- Johnston, L. D., et al. (2021). *Monitoring the Future National Survey Results on Drug Use 1975–2020: Overview, Key Findings on Adolescent Drug Use.* Ann Arbor: Institute for Social Research, University of Michigan. (pdf)
- Kneisel, K. (2020, December 18). "Driving under the Influence of Cannabis: What the Data Show." *MedPage Today.*
- National Center for Complementary and Integrative Health. Cannabis (Marijuana) and Cannabinoids: What You Need to Know.
- National Conference of State Legislatures. (2021). State Medical Marijuana Laws.

- National Institute on Drug Abuse:
  - Drugged Driving DrugFacts.
  - Overdose Death Rates.
  - Salvia.
  - Synthetic Cannabinoids (K2/Spice) DrugFacts.
  - Synthetic Cathinones ("Bath Salts") DrugFacts.
- National Institutes of Health. (2019, December 18). "Vaping of Marijuana on the Rise among Teens."
- Radcliffe, S. (2021, January 31). "Study Finds Lower Opioid Deaths in Counties Where Cannabis Is Legal." *Healthline.*
- Recovery Centers of America. Economic Cost of Substance Abuse in the United States, 2016.
- Sellman, D. (2020, August 21). "Alcohol Is More Harmful Than Cannabis." *The New Zealand Medical Journal.*
- Substance Abuse and Mental Health Services Administration. Behavioral Health Treatment Services Locator.
- Substance Abuse and Mental Health Services Administration. (2020). *Key Substance Use and Mental Health Indicators in the United States: Results from the 2019 National Survey on Drug Use and Health.* Rockville, MD: Center for Behavioral Health Statistics and Quality, Substance Abuse and Mental Health Services Administration. (pdf)
- Substance Abuse and Mental Health Services Administration. (2020). Know the Risks of Marijuana.

Lab 20A Risk for Problem Drug Use

Name	Section	Date

Purpose: To evaluate a friend or family member's behavior and potential for developing a problem with drugs; if this report is submitted to an instructor, be sure not to identify by name the person you are evaluating.

Procedures: Answer these questions to determine if the person you are evaluating has a problem with the misuse of medications. Place an X over the answer that applies.

A. Prescription Drug Problems.

(Yes) (No)　1. Does he/she take more medicine than prescribed per dosage?

(Yes) (No)　2. Does he/she feel more nervous than ever when the medicine wears off?

(Yes) (No)　3. Does he/she hoard medicine?

(Yes) (No)　4. Does he/she hide the amount of medicine taken from friends, family, or his/her doctors?

(Yes) (No)　5. Does he/she fail to provide his/her doctor with a complete list of medications he/she is taking from all sources (dentist, family physician, specialists)?

The more questions to which you answered "yes," the more likely he/she is to have a drug problem.

B. Risk Factors for Developing a Substance Use Disorder. (Remember that alcohol is a drug, too.)

(Yes) (No)　1. Have any members of his/her family ever had problems with drugs?

(Yes) (No)　2. Was he/she abused as a child, or did he/she go through other trauma during childhood?

(Yes) (No)　3. Is he/she now undergoing unusual stress or mental pain?

(Yes) (No)　4. Does he/she have easy access to drugs?

(Yes) (No)　5. Has he/she used or does he/she use drugs recreationally?

(Yes) (No)　6. If he/she has used or now uses drugs recreationally, did or does he/she choose the fastest method of getting a hit?

The more "yes" answers, the greater his/her risk of addiction.

C. Signs and Symptoms of a Drug Problem. (Remember that alcohol is a drug, too.)

(Yes) (No)　1. Does he/she use drugs as an escape or to cope with a stressful situation?

(Yes) (No)　2. Does he/she become depressed easily?

(Yes) (No)　3. Does he/she use drugs the first thing in the morning?

(Yes) (No)　4. Has he/she ever tried to quit and resumed using again?

(Yes) (No)　5. Does he/she do things under the influence of a drug that he/she would not normally do?

(Yes) (No)　6. Has he/she had any drug-related "close calls" with the police or any arrests?

(Yes) (No)　7. Does he/she think a party or social gathering isn't fun unless drugs are served/available?

(Yes) (No)　8. Does he/she feel proud of an increased tolerance to drugs?

(Yes) (No)   9. Does he/she use drugs when alone?

(Yes) (No) 10. Has or does he/she use a wide variety of drugs?

(Yes) (No) 11. Is he/she constantly thinking about being high?

(Yes) (No) 12. Does he/she avoid people or places that oppose usage?

(Yes) (No) 13. Have his/her friends, family, teachers, or employer expressed concern about his/her use?

(Yes) (No) 14. Is his/her usage causing him/her to neglect responsibilities?

(Yes) (No) 15. Has he/she ever had blackouts or lack of memory of drug use or other events?

(Yes) (No) 16. Has he/she stolen to get money for drugs?

(Yes) (No) 17. Has he/she seriously considered that he/she might have a drug problem?

The more "yes" answers, the more likely he/she is to have a serious problem with drugs.

Results

A. Does he/she misuse prescription drugs?   (Yes) (No)
    (Questions A: 1–5)

B. Is he/she at considerable risk a substance use disorder? (Yes) (No)
    (Questions B: 1–6)

C. Does he/she have a serious problem with drugs?   (Yes) (No)
    (Questions C: 1–17)

Conclusions and Implications: In several sentences, discuss a plan of action that could be taken by a person who has a problem with the misuse of over-the-counter drugs, prescription drugs, or illegal drugs. Discuss specific things you could do to help a person with a problem. At some point, you may want to answer the questions about yourself.

Preventing Sexually Transmitted Infections

LEARNING OBJECTIVES

After completing the study of this Concept, you will be able to:

▶ Identify the most common sexually transmitted infections (STIs).

▶ Define HIV and AIDS and indicate rates and trends in their prevalence.

▶ Describe common modes of HIV transmission and the HIV replication process.

▶ Understand the importance of testing and early intervention in preventing HIV/AIDS.

▶ Describe symptoms and consequences of common STIs, including HPV, chlamydia, gonorrhea, and syphilis.

▶ Identify less common STIs and their associated health risks.

▶ Describe important factors contributing to increased risk for STIs.

▶ Understand effective approaches to the prevention and treatment of STIs.

Safe sex and sound information about sexually transmitted infections are important to health and wellness.

Antonio Guillem/Shutterstock

Why It Matters!

Interpersonal relationships and sexual interactions strongly influence our moods and behaviors. They are basic to family life and fundamental to the reproduction of the human species. Approached responsibly, the human sexual experience contributes to wellness and quality of life in many ways. When approached irresponsibly, it can result in disease and personal and interpersonal suffering. Learning and adopting safe sex practices are critical for avoiding unwanted pregnancies and for reducing risks for various infections and diseases. This Concept provides information about the symptoms, causes, and treatments of various infections and diseases transmitted through sexual contact.

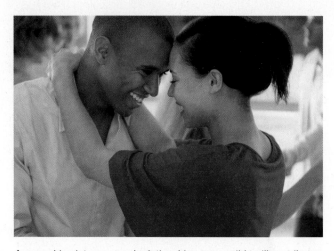

Approaching interpersonal relationships responsibly will contribute to wellness and quality of life.
Laura Doss/Getty Images

General Facts

The healthy sexual experience can contribute to wellness in many ways. All five wellness dimensions are involved in decisions concerning participation in, the meaningfulness of, and the long-term consequences of the sexual experience. The healthy sexual

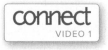

experience requires sensitive and thoughtful consideration of the consequences. When approached responsibly, sexual behavior can enhance quality of life in important ways. A study of over 1,500 college students identified 237 different reasons for engaging in sexual behavior. Although females tended to report more intimacy reasons and males tended to report more reasons related to physical pleasure, 20 of the top 25 reasons overlapped for males and females. The most common reasons across the full sample were love, pleasure, affection, romance, emotional closeness, arousal, excitement, adventure, experience, connection, celebration, curiosity, opportunity, and the desire to please. Although antisocial reasons for sexual behavior were less common, they have the potential for severe negative consequences. For example, one of the very infrequently endorsed reasons for sex was to intentionally infect a partner with an STI, and another was to break up a rival's relationship. Thus, as stated previously, sexual behavior can have both rewarding and costly effects.

Good physical health contributes to an active and satisfying sex life. Two population-based studies in the United States found that individuals who were in good or excellent health were more likely to be sexually active. Among those who were sexually active, good health was associated with greater interest in sex, more frequent sex, and a better-quality sex life. On average, being in good health increased the sexual life expectancy for males by 5–7 years and for females by 3–6 years.

***Sexually transmitted infections* is a broad term that refers to a number of different conditions.** The term *sexually transmitted disease (STD)* has been used to refer to these conditions, but the broader term *sexually transmitted infection (STI)* is now more accepted.

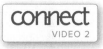

STI better reflects the fact that a period of infection typically occurs prior to the emergence of any associated disease symptoms. HIV/AIDS is an example of this, as one can be infected for many years before signs of disease begin to occur. In other cases, STIs never result in identifiable disease symptoms. **Human papillomavirus (HPV)** is an example of this type of STI. Although HPV can lead to cervical cancer in females, most females infected with HPV never experience disease symptoms. Although consequences vary, the major risks justify a strong emphasis on prevention of STIs.

Unsafe sexual activity can result in disease, poor health, and much pain and suffering. Until the 1940s, STIs were a leading cause of death. The discovery of penicillin and other antibiotics, and improved public health practices, lowered the death rate from STIs,

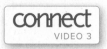

but they have remained a significant health problem. In 1991, STIs became 1 of the 10 leading causes of death in the United States, principally because of the high death rate from **acquired immune deficiency syndrome (AIDS)** caused by the **human immunodeficiency virus (HIV)**. The development of more effective treatments has reduced deaths from HIV/AIDS and moved STIs off the top 10 list.

HIV/AIDS

Of all the STIs, HIV/AIDS poses the greatest health threat to the world. Slightly more than 30,000 people in the United States are infected with HIV annually, with almost

1 million people currently infected. Worldwide, the problem is even more profound, with roughly 1.7 million people infected each year and a total of more than 38 million people currently living with HIV. The problem of HIV/AIDS is particularly bad in eastern and southern Africa, which accounts for over half of individuals living with HIV. Only 60 percent are aware of the fact that they are infected, which contributes to the spread of HIV. International health agencies have been working to address the gap in awareness and the limited access to treatments in these parts of the world. Fortunately, these efforts are starting to pay off, with a 60 percent decrease in HIV infections since the peak in 1998. More people are getting HIV medication, and the rate of new infections is decreasing. However, for the first time in two decades, a new strain of HIV was recently identified. Although the new strain is rare, it has caused concern especially for blood screening. Researchers indicate that while we are making advances in prevention and treatment, we have not yet defeated HIV.

There are three mechanisms for most HIV transmission.

The three primary mechanisms responsible for the transmission of HIV are sexual activity, contact with infected blood (needle sharing), and transmission from an infected mother to her child. Among males in the United States, the greatest number of new cases result from males having sex with males, though a significant number of cases result from heterosexual sex. Among females, risk of transmission is most frequent in heterosexual sex. Worldwide, the most common cause of AIDS is heterosexual sex.

Roughly 6 percent of new cases in the United States are the result of using contaminated needles to inject drugs. Transmission from infected mothers to their children used to account for roughly as many HIV infections as IV drug use. However, rates have decreased dramatically since the turn of the century. The latter mode of transmission could be largely prevented through the use of a specific drug (nevirapine) and with a cesarean delivery.

While HIV can be transmitted in multiple ways, it is important to understand that HIV is not transmitted through the air or in saliva, sweat, or urine. It does not spread by hugging, sharing foods or beverages, or casual kissing. Contact with phones, silverware, or toilet seats does not cause the spread of HIV. Although people who had blood transfusions before 1985 had an increased risk of HIV transmission, the safety of the blood supply has increased dramatically since that time, resulting in extremely low rates of risk from transfusion. The routes of transmission of HIV in the United States are summarized in Figure 1.

Incidence of HIV/AIDS is increasing disproportionately in women and minorities.

What was once thought to be a disease of males, especially gay males, is now increasingly a female condition. Females now represent roughly one-fourth of those living with HIV in the United States and nearly half of the global cases of HIV. Racial and ethnic minority groups in the United States are also disproportionately affected, with roughly 45 percent of new cases occurring among African

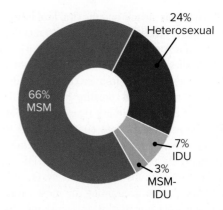

Figure 1 ▶ Routes of transmission for HIV in the United States.

Note: MSM = males who have sex with males; IDU = injection drug users; MSM-IDU = both MSM and IDU.

Source: Centers for Disease Control and Prevention (2018).

Americans and another 42 percent occurring among Latinx individuals. This discrepancy is largest among females, with a rate among African American females roughly 20 times that of white females.

HIV attacks the immune system and can lead to AIDS.

A test of **serostatus** can indicate if a person is seropositive. When a person tests seropositive for HIV, it means that a blood test has indicated the presence of HIV in the body. HIV invades the body's immune system cells, even killing them, which damages the immune system and the body's ability to fight infections. HIV causes immune suppression by directly invading and killing **CD4 helper cells** (also called **T helper cells**). When too many of these cells are destroyed, the body cannot fight **opportunistic infections** effectively.

Sexually Transmitted Infection (STI) An infection for which a primary method of transmission is sexual activity.

Human Papillomavirus (HPV) A group of more than 150 related viruses that represents the most prevalent STI and a cause of both genital warts and cervical cancer.

Acquired Immune Deficiency Syndrome (AIDS) An HIV-infected individual is said to have AIDS when they have developed certain opportunistic infections (for example, pneumonia, tuberculosis, yeast infections, or other infections) or when their CD4 cell count drops below 200.

Human Immunodeficiency Virus (HIV) A virus that causes a breakdown of the immune system in humans, resulting in the body's inability to fight infections. It is a precursor to AIDS.

Serostatus A blood test indicating the presence of antibodies the immune system creates to fight disease. A seropositive status indicates that a person has antibodies to fight HIV and is HIV positive.

CD4 Helper Cells (T Helper Cells) Cells that protect against infections and activate the body's immune response. HIV kills these cells, so a high count usually means better health.

Opportunistic Infections Infections that typically do not affect healthy people, but may lead to diseases in people whose immune systems have been compromised.

When T cell counts are low and the **viral load** is high, the immune system cannot function properly, thereby making the seropositive person more susceptible to various types of diseases and disorders. **Antibodies** in the blood that normally fight infections are ineffective in stopping HIV from invading the body.

HIV comes in many forms, creating unique challenges for treatment. There are two primary types of HIV (HIV1 and HIV2). HIV2 appears to be less contagious and to have a longer latency between infection and disease, but the vast majority (roughly 95 percent) of cases of AIDS are due to HIV1. There are four groups of HIV1 (M, N, O, and P), with the M, or "Major," type accounting for most cases. Within the M group, there are at least nine different subtypes, though subtype B (predominant in the United States and Europe) and subtypes A and C (predominant in southern and eastern Africa) account for the majority of the global epidemic.

An individual has AIDS when they are infected with HIV and develop opportunistic diseases because of impairment of the immune system. Examples of opportunistic diseases associated with AIDS are pneumonia, tuberculosis, **Kaposi's sarcoma**, yeast infections, and cervical cancer. Other symptoms include fatigue, swollen glands, rashes, weight loss, and loss of appetite. Once a person receives a diagnosis of AIDS, the diagnosis is maintained even if the individual becomes asymptomatic.

The risk of acquiring HIV/AIDS is reduced if exposure to the methods of transmission is avoided. Experts from the National Institutes of Health (NIH) have concluded that HIV transmission could be reduced if legislative barriers to needle exchange programs were lifted, if greater emphasis were given to youth education programs about HIV/AIDS, if greater funding were available for the treatment of people who abuse drugs, and if educational efforts among high-risk populations were increased. Worldwide, the money expended on treatment far exceeds the amounts spent on prevention. Taking personal responsibility for reducing risky behaviors is important for prevention on a personal level. Increasing awareness of these risks is important for national and international prevention.

Early detection is critical for controlling the spread of AIDS. Unfortunately, the majority of adults in the United States have never been tested for HIV. Although rates have increased gradually over the past decade, only about half of adults report having been tested for HIV. Further, the Centers for Disease Control and Prevention (CDC) estimates that about 13 percent of individuals with HIV are unaware that they are infected and that roughly one-third are diagnosed so late that they develop AIDS within a year of their HIV diagnosis. To facilitate early identification of HIV, the CDC now recommends testing for everyone between the ages of 13 and 64 at least once as part of routine health care. The American College of Physicians also recommends that physicians encourage all of their patients to get tested for HIV, regardless of their level of risk.

HELP   Health is available to Everyone for a Lifetime, and it's Personal

CDC Campaigns to Prevent STIs

The CDC has launched several publicity campaigns designed to help prevent the spread of STIs in the United States. (*Note: The* CDC still uses the term *sexually transmitted diseases, or STDs*.) The most recent is the "Let's Stop HIV Together" campaign that is part of the "Ending the HIV Epidemic (EHE) plan for America." The campaign focuses on overcoming the stigma of HIV, increased testing and prevention efforts, and increased research to find a cure. The CDC's three Ts campaign (Talk, Test, and Treat) is more broadly focused on preventing all STIs. Talk refers to having open discussions about STIs with partners and health-care providers. Test refers to getting tested because it is the only way to know for sure if you have an STI. Treat refers to seeking medical care to ensure that you have the right medicine for treating your infection. The CDC publicity campaigns also emphasize the dangers of allowing STIs to go untreated. (See Suggested Resources and Readings for links to "Let's Stop HIV Together" and "Talk, Test, and Treat.")

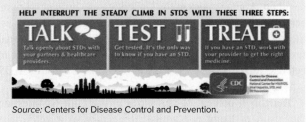

Source: Centers for Disease Control and Prevention.

How effective do you think publicity campaigns are in preventing STIs including HIV?

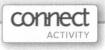

Testing for HIV and other STIs can be either confidential or anonymous. When a test is confidential, there is a written record of the test results, but there is also assurance that this information will be kept private by the health-care provider. An anonymous test is one for which there is no written record, and the results cannot be connected to a name or other identifiable information. Clinics throughout the country provide both confidential and anonymous (in most states) testing at no cost. Self-testing kits can be purchased at drugstores and mailed to labs for analysis so you do not have to see a health-care provider. The tests are noninvasive, requiring the use of a swab to collect cells from inside the mouth.

There is no cure for AIDS, but treatments have improved. For those infected with HIV/AIDS, there is no known cure. However, treatments have been developed to suppress or slow the progress of the disease process. HIV is a type of virus (retrovirus) and is treated with drugs called antiretrovirals. These treatments target various stages in the

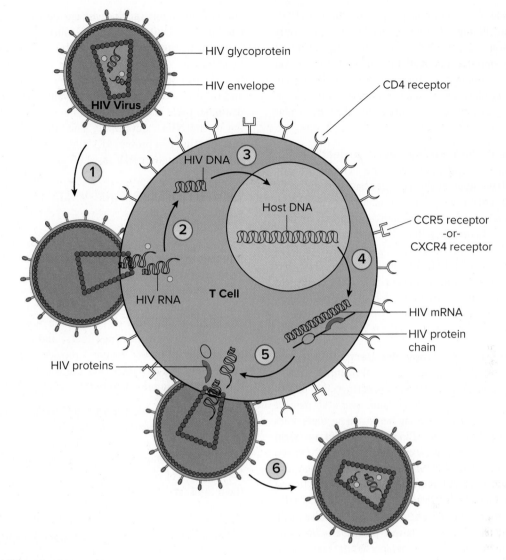

Figure 2 ▶ HIV replication cycle.

Source: Adapted from U.S. Department of Health and Human Services.

replication process of the HIV virus (see Figure 2). In the first step, the virus must enter T cells in the body (1). Once HIV enters these cells, HIV RNA is translated into DNA through a process called reverse transcription (2). Once the HIV RNA has been converted, an enzyme called integrase facilitates the integration of HIV DNA into the host DNA of the cell (3). The HIV DNA is then able to generate new protein sequences (4) necessary to create new copies of the virus (5). In the final step (6), the HIV protein called protease separates the protein sequence into its components so that these proteins can combine to form new viruses.

There are at least six classes of antiretroviral (ART) drugs that are used in combination to target different stages in the progression of HIV infection. The four most common are described here. Fusion inhibitors are a class of drugs that operate in the first stage of the process by interfering with the virus's ability to enter the host cell. Reverse transcriptase inhibitors operate at the second stage by disrupting reverse transcription so that HIV RNA cannot be converted into DNA or integrated into the DNA of the host cell. Integrase inhibitors operate at the final stage by interfering with the protease enzyme, which prevents the HIV DNA from being separated into the components needed to create a mature (infectious) virus.

A combination of several drugs referred to as "drug cocktails" have been the most common form of HIV treatment, but the FDA has also approved "once a day" pills that

Viral Load The level of virus (HIV) in the blood.

Antibodies Proteins in the bloodstream that react to overcome bacterial and other agents that attack the body.

Kaposi's Sarcoma A type of cancer evidenced by purple sores (tumors) on the skin.

combine multiple drugs into a single pill. In 2021 the FDA approved an injectable drug regimen that requires only monthly injections. Experts believe that the single pill and injectable drug options may lead to better adherence and lower rates of hospitalization. Individuals with HIV are encouraged to work closely with their physicians to decide on the best drug or combination of drugs for their particular circumstances.

Early treatment dramatically reduces death rates. Numerous studies have demonstrated the benefits of early treatment for HIV. Public health agencies have responded by promoting and encouraging greater access to treatment. Whereas the CDC used to recommend treatment only for individuals with a CD4 count less than 350, it now recommends treatment for all individuals with HIV, regardless of CD4 count. Similarly, the World Health Organization (WHO) has moved from recommending treatment at a CD4 count less than 500 to recommending treatment for all children, adolescents, and adults, including all pregnant and breastfeeding females living with HIV, regardless of CD4 cell count.

Early treatment with ART may also decrease rates of HIV transmission. Although antiretroviral treatment (ART) does not eliminate the risk for HIV among partners of individuals who are HIV positive, one study found over a 96 percent reduction in risk for infection among the sexual partners of individuals started on ART, relative to those who did not begin ART. A drug referred to as "pre-exposure prophylaxis" (PrEP) has also proven effective in preventing infection among those at risk. Current recommendations by WHO support offering PrEP to selected people at substantial risk of acquiring HIV. Combining the approaches of routine testing, preventive medication, and early treatment may have a particularly dramatic impact. Mathematical models have supported the potential of universal voluntary testing combined with immediate ART for those infected with HIV. Using South Africa as a basis for calculations, the mathematical model suggested that the incidence and mortality associated with HIV could be reduced to 1 in 1,000 cases within 10 years of full implementation. Although these are only theoretical models, trials of the test and treat approach in sub-Saharan Africa have shown promising results with 20 to 30 percent decreases in HIV incidence.

The search for a vaccine for HIV is well under way, though no vaccine is currently available. HIV medicines and treatments such as ART have allowed individuals living with HIV to stay healthy for many years. However, the ultimate goal is to develop vaccines that can prevent a person from getting HIV in the first place. Vaccines typically work by teaching the body's immune system how to recognize and defend against harmful viruses or bacteria. Successful vaccines have been developed for many diseases, including polio, chicken pox, measles, mumps, rubella, influenza (flu), and COVID-19, but effective vaccines for HIV have proven elusive. More than 100 vaccines have been tested in humans or

animals, and many vaccines are currently undergoing clinical trials in the United States and abroad. For example, the National Institutes of Health (NIH) is currently supporting two late-stage, multinational vaccine clinical trials called Imbokodo and Mosaico. Vaccines have proven to be the safest and most cost-effective way to prevent illness, disability, and death, so there is considerable interest in this work. According to the NIH, "developing safe, effective, and affordable vaccines that can prevent HIV infection in uninfected people is the NIH's highest HIV research priority."

Common Sexually Transmitted Infections

Roughly 26 million people in the United States are infected with one or more STIs each year. The CDC indicates that there has been a "steep and sustained" rise in STIs in recent years. Although HIV is the deadliest of the sexually transmitted infections, it is not among the most common in the United States. Table 1 lists some of the most common STIs in terms of both incidence (new cases) and prevalence (cumulative number of cases). Figure 3 provides a graphic depiction of the trends in STI rates over the past 30 years. Details for specific STIs are presented in the sections that follow.

The human papillomavirus (HPV) is a very common STI in young people. An estimated 13 million people become infected with HPV each year, making this the most commonly transmitted STI. The virus is responsible for the development of genital warts, but most people do not develop them and are therefore unaware that they are infected.

Table 1 ▶ Rankings of Incidence and Prevalence of Common STIs

STI	Rank of Incidence (Number of New Cases of the Condition)	Rank of Prevalence (Number of People with Condition)
Chlamydia	3	4
Gonorrhea	4	6
Herpes (HSV)	5	2
Human Immunodeficiency Virus (HIV)*	7	5
Human Papillomavirus (HPV)	1	1
Syphilis	6	7
Trichomoniasis	2	3

Source: Centers for Disease Control and Prevention.

Ages 13 and older.

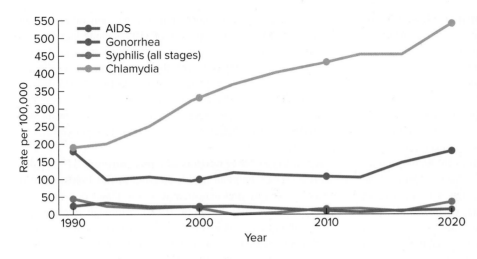

Figure 3 ▶ Trends in STI rates in the United States.
Source: Centers for Disease Control and Prevention.

Although the disease is asymptomatic in the short term, it leads to significantly increased risk for cervical cancer in females. In fact, HPV is the leading cause of cervical cancer. Two strains are particularly dangerous, accounting for approximately 70 percent of cases of cervical cancer. There is also recent evidence that oral HPV can be contracted through oral sex, which increases risk for oropharyngeal (throat) cancer. Prevalence of oral HPV is considerably higher for males than females.

Federal guidelines initially recommended that all young females (aged 11–12) be vaccinated, but the CDC now recommends that all young males be vaccinated as well. For those who were not fully vaccinated in childhood, the CDC recommends that anyone under the age of 26 be vaccinated. Although most adults 27 and over do not need to get vaccinated, because most will have already been exposed and because the vaccine is less effective in older adults, some adults aged 27–45 years may benefit from getting the vaccine based on discussion with their clinician. Several states have mandated vaccinations and a number of other states provide vaccinations at no cost or provide education programs designed to increase vaccination rates.

Advocates argue that vaccinations save lives, whereas opponents have argued that providing the vaccine will encourage casual sexual behavior. A long-term study published in *JAMA Internal Medicine* concluded that "HPV was not associated with increases in STIs in a large cohort of females, suggesting that vaccination is unlikely to promote unsafe sexual activity." Also, many females (35 percent) are now fully vaccinated, and rates of HPV in young females decreased dramatically in the early 2000s. In recent years there have been gradual decreases in multiple forms of HPV. Rates of vaccination among male adolescents are much lower overall, although they are increasing. It is important to note that the vaccine will not help those already infected with HPV. However, routine Pap tests can identify the early cell changes associated with HPV and help prevent the development of cervical cancer.

Genital herpes is among the most commonly spread STIs because of a lack of awareness of infection. Genital herpes, one of the most commonly reported STIs, is caused by the herpes simplex virus (HSV). Although fewer new cases of genital herpes are reported annually than cases of chlamydia, the number of individuals currently infected is much higher. This is because chlamydia is treatable. In contrast, once someone contracts genital herpes, he or she will always carry the virus. Genital herpes causes lesions or blisters on the penis, vagina, or cervix usually occurring 2–12 days after infection and often lasting a week to a month. Swollen glands and headache may also occur.

No cure exists for genital sores caused by HSV, though some prescription drugs can help treat the disease symptoms. Episodic antiviral therapy is taken at the first sign of an outbreak, and suppressive antiviral therapy is taken daily to prevent outbreaks from occurring. HSV can remain dormant in the body for long periods, and as a result, symptoms can recur at any time, especially after undergoing stress or illness.

Genital herpes is especially contagious when blisters are present. Condom use or abstinence from sexual activity when symptoms are present can reduce the risk of transmission of the disease. Although genital herpes is less infectious when there are no symptoms present, the infection can still be spread to other partners. Condoms provide some protection, but they are not totally effective in preventing infection because they do not cover all genital areas. Herpes is more dangerous for women than men because of the association between genital herpes and cervical cancer and the risk of transmitting the disease to the unborn.

Trichomoniasis is the third most common STI in the United States. More than 2.5 million people in the United States are infected with trichomoniasis each year. It is caused by a parasite and if untreated can result in increased risk of transmission of other STIs and health problems, including birthing problems, transmission to the baby, and low baby birth weight. Many males and females who are infected have no symptoms. When symptoms are present, they include genital redness, burning and itching, painful urination, and discharge from the vagina or penis. A lab test is required for an accurate diagnosis. It can be treated with medication taken in pill form (e.g., metronidazole, tinidazole).

Genital Herpes A viral infection that can attack any area of the body but often causes blisters on the genitals.

Chlamydia is a common STI, but it is often difficult to detect. About 1.7 million new cases of **chlamydia** are reported in the United States each year. Chlamydia is known as the "silent" STI because about three-fourths of infected females and about half of infected males have no symptoms. Cases are most frequent in the 15–24 age group. Thus, routine screening is essential for detecting most cases of chlamydia. If symptoms do occur, it is typically in the first 3 weeks following infection. For males who experience symptoms, the most common are discharge from the penis and a burning sensation when urinating. Common symptoms in females include abnormal vaginal discharge, a burning sensation when urinating, lower abdominal or back pain, pain during intercourse, and bleeding between menstrual periods. If chlamydia is left untreated, the health consequences can be extensive, particularly for females. The disease has been linked to increased risk of **pelvic inflammatory disease (PID)**, as well as a number of other secondary health problems, including urethritis, cervicitis, ectopic pregnancy, infertility, and chronic pelvic pain.

As a result of the high levels of risk for young females (more than three-fourths of cases in females are among those under age 25), guidelines from the U.S. Preventive Services Task Force suggest that sexually active females under the age of 25 and females 25 and older who are at increased risk undergo routine screening for chlamydia. Although rates of screening have increased, less than half of females in this age group are screened annually. Fortunately, chlamydia is very treatable, and its long-term health consequences can be prevented if the infection is identified quickly. Treatment with antibiotics can clear up the infection within a week to 10 days.

Early detection is critical for effective treatment of gonorrhea. **Gonorrhea** is a bacterial infection that can be treated with modern antibiotics if detected early. Sexual activity is the principal method of disease transmission. Penile and vaginal gonorrhea are the most common types. Symptoms usually occur within 3–7 days after bacteria enter the system. Among males, the most common symptoms are painful urination and penile drip or discharge. Symptoms are less apparent among females, though painful urination and vaginal discharge are not uncommon. Other types of gonorrhea often have fewer symptoms. Chills, fever, painful bowel movements, and sore throat are the most common. Early detection by a culture or smear test at the site or sites of sexual contact is how the disease is diagnosed. Early cure is especially important for females because gonorrhea can lead to PID, which can result in infertility. Like other STIs, the rate of gonorrhea in the United States has increased in recent years and has doubled among males.

Hepatitis B can lead to chronic liver disease. Like other STIs, **hepatitis B (HBV)** is typically spread through unprotected sex with an infected partner, intravenous drug use, or transmission from an infected mother to her baby. Although rare, HBV can be spread through blood transfusion or any other contact with infected blood. Symptoms of HBV include jaundice, fatigue, abdominal pain, loss of appetite, and nausea. Among those chronically infected with the virus, chronic liver disease typically develops, leading to premature death in 15–25 percent of cases. Fortunately, a vaccine for HBV has been available since 1982, and rates have decreased since then from over 260,000 cases to slightly more than 3,000 cases per year.

Syphilis is another serious but less common STI. **Syphilis** was a serious national health problem in the 1940s, when it was much more prevalent than it is now. Cases of syphilis declined significantly during the 1990s. Although rates remain lower than they were in 1990, rates of primary and secondary syphilis (considered a good index of incidence) in the United States have increased in recent years with an increase of 76 percent since 2012. These increases appear to be driven primarily by males who have sex with males, a group that now accounts for more than half of new cases in the United States each year. However, it is important to note that rates have also increased among females. The CDC also reports that syphilis continues to have a disproportionate effect on African Americans and people living in the southern United States.

Like gonorrhea, syphilis is a bacterial infection that can be effectively treated with antibiotics. The symptoms of syphilis include **chancre** sores that generally appear at the primary site of sexual contact, then change from a red swelling to a hardened ulcer on the skin. Even if not treated, the sores disappear after 1–5 weeks. It is important to get treatment even after this primary phase of the disease because the disease is still present and contagious. After several weeks or longer, secondary symptoms occur, such as a rash, loss of hair, joint pain, sore throat, and swollen glands. Even after these symptoms go away, untreated syphilis lingers in a latent phase. Serious health problems may result, including blindness, deafness, tumors, and stillbirth.

Early detection is important and can be diagnosed from chancre discharge or a blood test several weeks after the appearance of chancres. There is an association between syphilis and the spread of HIV. Evidence suggests that the presence of chancres increases the risk of transmitting HIV during sexual activity.

Although health risks are not as severe, lesser-known STIs are highly prevalent and cause significant distress. Genital warts, pubic crab lice, and chancroid are examples of lesser-known but prevalent STIs (see Table 2). Genital warts are caused by the strains of the human papillomavirus, discussed earlier. Fortunately, the strains of HPV associated with genital warts tend to be relatively low risk. The most significant consequence to the individual is often psychological, due to concern about the appearance of the warts and the potential consequences associated with them. Because HPV is so common, the chance of developing genital warts is relatively high, even with a small number of sexual partners. Fortunately,

Table 2 ▶ Facts about Lesser-Known STIs

Genital Warts (Condylomas)

- Constitute approximately 5 percent of all reported STIs
- Are most prevalent in ages 15–24
- Are caused by HPV
- Are hard and yellow or gray on dry skin
- Are soft and pink, red, or dark on moist skin
- Are treated by the prescription drug Podophyllin

Pubic Crab Lice

- Are pinhead-sized insects (parasites) that feed on the blood of the host
- Are transmitted by sexual contact and/or contact with contaminated clothes, bedding, and other washable items
- Have symptoms that include itching, but some people have no symptoms
- Can be controlled by using medicated lotion and shampoos and by washing contaminated bedding
- Do *not* transmit other STIs

Chancroid

- Is caused by bacteria
- Is more commonly seen in males than in females, particularly uncircumcised males
- Has symptoms including one or more sores or raised bumps on the genitals
- Can result in progressive ulcers occurring on the genitals; sometimes the ulcers persist for weeks or months
- Can be successfully treated with certain antibiotics

there are several effective treatments for genital warts, including remedies that can be self-administered by patients in their own homes. Pubic lice can be highly distressing to the individual, but effective over-the-counter treatments are available to eliminate pubic lice in a matter of days. Although individuals with genital warts and pubic lice may have few long-term effects from these infections, studies have found that both groups tend to have more sexual partners and are at higher risk for other STIs, including gonorrhea and chlamydia. Therefore, these individuals should be routinely tested for other STIs. Most patients with chancroid in the United States, where it is uncommon, contract it during travels to countries where it is more common. Chancroid is a known risk factor for HIV and should therefore be treated promptly.

Factors That Contribute to Sexual Risks

Sexually explicit media influence teen sexual behavior. There has been considerable concern about the impact of explicit sexual content in the media (music, magazines, television, movies, and Internet) on teen sexual behavior. A recent study found that adolescents exposed to sexually explicit content on the Internet had more permissive attitudes toward sex and were more likely to have multiple sexual partners and to have engaged in anal sex. Another study evaluating exposure to sexually explicit content found that early exposure predicted permissive sexual norms and an increase in oral sex and sexual intercourse two years later. This research shows the powerful impact of media on teen sexual behavior.

Misperceived norms may contribute to sexual risk. Many teens engage in sex because they believe that "everybody is doing it." The media portrayals discussed in the previous section may contribute to these inaccurate beliefs, though they may also be driven by inaccurate communication. In a study of males between ages 15 and 22, 45 percent reported that they were virgins, although 23 percent indicated that they told others they were not. Overall, 60 percent reported that they lied about something related to sex to appear experienced and more popular. Interestingly, they said that girls who were more sexually experienced were perceived as less popular. Young people need to be aware of the true norms for sexual behavior and not get caught up in perceptions based on inaccurate information.

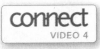

College students are at risk for HIV and other STIs due to the practice of serial monogamy. Many college students are sexually active, yet most do not use condoms on a consistent basis. This is partly due to perceptions that they are in committed relationships and therefore at low risk for infection. Such perceptions are problematic for several reasons. First, some college students

Chlamydia A bacterial infection, similar to gonorrhea, that attacks the urinary tract and reproductive organs.

Pelvic Inflammatory Disease (PID) An infection of the urethra (urine passage), which can lead to infertility among females.

Gonorrhea A bacterial infection of the mucous membranes, including the eyes, throat, genitals, and other organs.

Hepatitis B (HBV) An infection of the liver caused by the hepatitis B virus, which is often sexually transmitted and can lead to long-term liver disease.

Syphilis An infection caused by a corkscrew-shaped bacteria that travels in the bloodstream and embeds itself in the mucous membranes of the body, including those of the sexual organs.

Chancre Sore or lesion commonly associated with syphilis.

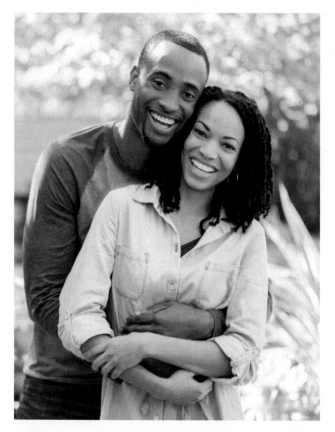

Healthy relationships depend on trust and good communication.
Sam Edwards/Glow Images

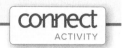

Technology Update

"Hook-Up" Apps May Contribute to Risky Sex and STIs

Dating websites and apps, such as Match.com and Hinge, are designed to help users find potential partners, but other smartphone apps are often used to find sexual partners rather than dating partners. Well-known apps include Tinder, Bumble, and Grindr (specifically for gay and bisexual males). Research has shown that males who used Grindr and similar smartphone apps were 25 percent more likely to contract gonorrhea and 37 percent more likely to contract chlamydia relative to males who did not use these apps. The risks are not restricted to gay and bisexual males. Another study of heterosexual college students found that nearly 40 percent reported using dating apps like Tinder, and those who did were more likely to report having sex after using drugs and alcohol as well as unprotected vaginal or anal sex. Some, but not all, companies have worked with advocacy groups and departments of health to encourage STI testing, to provide testing site locators, and to send alerts about STI outbreaks.

Do you think apps that help people find casual sexual partners should be regulated to prevent harm, or might they provide opportunities to intervene with those at greatest risk?

connect ACTIVITY

define a regular partner as someone they have been with for as little as 1 month, and most define a regular partner as someone they have been with for less than 6 months. Second, most college students do not get tested on a regular basis, if at all. Third, when students perceive that they are in a committed relationship, the likelihood of condom use decreases dramatically. This is particularly true when an alternative form of birth control, primarily birth control pills, is being used. One study found that 93.7 percent of sexually active college females were using contraception to prevent pregnancy, but only 23 percent used contraception to prevent STIs. The common result is unprotected sexual intercourse

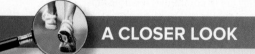

A CLOSER LOOK

Sexual Misconduct on Campus

The issue of sexual violence on college campuses has received considerable media attention in recent years and rightfully so. According to Rape, Abuse & Incest National Network (RAINN), 1 in 4 undergraduate females and 1 in 15 undergraduate males experience rape, sexual assault through physical force, violence, or incapacitation. Rates are even higher when verbal coercion and lack of consent are included. Recent high-profile cases of sexual misconduct in sports (e.g., Larry Nassar, USA Gymnastics team physician), business (e.g., financier Jeffrey Epstein), and entertainment (e.g., Bill Cosby, Harvey Weinstein) have brought unwanted sexual behavior into the spotlight. The

Me Too movement on various social media platforms brought attention to the large percentage of people—both females and males—who have experienced unwanted sexual advances. Many believe that these disclosures have the potential to lead to long-term changes in cultural norms that could reduce the incidence of sexual assault. RAINN has a 24/7 national (free and confidential) hotline available to assist those who have experienced sexual assault (1-800-656-HOPE).

How can campaigns such as the Me Too movement help reduce sexual assault issues on campus?

connect ACTIVITY

between two people who have known one another for a short time and who are unaware of each other's STI status. Many students go through multiple committed relationships during the college years. This type of serial monogamy places college students at increased risk for HIV and other STIs.

Sexting can have many negative consequences. Though "sexting" (defined as sending or receiving sexually suggestive, nearly nude, or nude photos by text message or email) does not involve physical contact, it has led to problems for many—from teens to prominent politicians. Between 50 and 70 percent of college students have reported sending explicit pictures or videos to their partners, with a sizable percentage sharing them with strangers. Although the phenomenon may reflect a new social media form of intimacy, many people find the concept of sexting objectionable, and laws in some states make it illegal to send or forward sexually explicit images.

Prevention and Early Intervention of STIs

Early prevention can increase understanding of risk and strategies for practicing safe sex. Some argue that abstinence-only education is best, while others believe that young people also need to be educated about ways to protect themselves in the event that they are or will become sexually active. Between 2001 and 2009, the federal government allocated over a billion dollars to abstinence-only sex education programs. Proponents of this strategy point to decreases in sexual intercourse among teens during this period (from 54 percent in 1991 to 47 percent in 2005). However, most of the decrease occurred before 2001, with virtually no change in the rate between 2001 and 2013. Since 2013, rates have dropped by more than 5 percent. Rates of teen pregnancy also decreased between 2001 and 2009, but again this reduction appears to reflect a general linear decrease that has been ongoing since 1991.

The declines in rates of sexual intercourse and teen pregnancy are encouraging, but studies have not demonstrated conclusively that abstinence-based programming caused the trend. In contrast, evidence does support the effectiveness of comprehensive prevention programs that both promote abstinence and teach safe sex practices. These approaches are shown to be effective in reducing sexual activity, pregnancy, and STIs.

Regular screening and notification of partners who may be infected can reduce the spread of STIs. Because many STIs are treatable with antibiotics, catching them early can reduce the negative health consequences associated with infection. For those 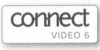 who are sexually active with partners of unknown STI status, yearly testing is a good idea. Even more frequent testing may be appropriate for those at very high risk (e.g., intravenous drug users and those previously diagnosed with an STI). When an individual is identified with a sexually transmitted infection, it is important that he or she notify his or her sexual partners so that they can also receive treatment. This helps reduce the spread of the infection. For more support and information, contact the following national HIV and STI hotlines:

- CDC HIV hotline (English): 1-800-448-0440
- CDC STD (STI) hotline: 1-800-232-4636

Using Self-Management Skills

A variety of self-management skills are relevant for preventing STIs. Self-management skills are important for all facets of health, wellness, and fitness, but there are unique considerations with sexual activity since your actions are directly influenced by and linked to others. Abstaining from sexual activity is the safest option, but if you do engage in sex,

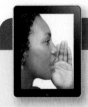

In the News

Condom Use Resistance and STIs

Over 25 million new STIs occur each year in the United States, and nearly half of males report not using a condom the last time they had sex. A recent study determined that condom use resistance was most often related to sexual pleasure; however, among males, techniques to avoid condom use can be noncoercive or coercive. Examples of noncoercive techniques include stating "I don't have an STI" and "sex would feel better without a condom." Coercive techniques may include threats, such as "insisting on using a condom is making me angry" and deception such as "stealthing"

(nonconsensually removing a condom). Coercive behavior is more common among males who have been drinking and those with aggressive personality traits. Research indicates that females also use techniques to avoid condom use, but less often (e.g., untruthfully claiming to be on birth control). Understanding factors influencing resistance is important to reversing the problem.

Do rates of STIs influence perceptions of risk? What do you think can be done to reduce condom use resistance?

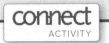

do so responsibly and with appropriate consideration of both your needs and your partner's. Many people do not fully consider the serious, life-changing consequences of unsafe sex, so it is important to enter into sexual relationships with appropriate care. Remember that condoms are for STI prevention as well as pregnancy prevention, even if your partner is using another form of birth control. Use condoms if your partner has not been tested or you do not know his or her sexual history. Following sound consumer guidelines is recommended to further decrease your risks:

- Talk with your partner about his or her and your own sexual history before initiating sexual behavior.
- Limit sexual activity to a noninfected partner. A lifetime partner who has never had sex with other people and has never used injected drugs (unless medically administered) is the only completely safe partner.
- Avoid sexual activity or other activity that puts you in contact with another person's semen, vaginal fluids, or blood.
- Properly use a new condom (latex) every time you have sex, especially with a partner who is not known to be safe.

- Use a water-based lubricant with condoms because petroleum-based lubricants increase risk for condom failure.
- Abstain from risky sexual activity, such as anal sex and sex with high-risk people (prostitutes, people with HIV or other STIs).
- Use a condom or dental dam when engaging in oral sex.
- Do not inject drugs.
- Never share a needle or drug paraphernalia.

Self-monitoring and regular testing can help detect STIs and reduce complications from these infections. A self-assessment, such as the one provided in Lab 21A, can be helpful in identifying potential STI risk. However, it is not a substitute for medical testing. If symptoms are present, such as those described in this Concept, medical testing is warranted—sooner rather than later. As noted in this Concept, some home tests are available but, in many cases, tests must be performed and interpreted by a health-care professional, and prompt treatment can reduce many of the long-term negative consequences of STIs.

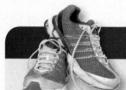

Strategies for Action: Lab Information

The first step in protecting yourself is understanding your level of risk. More than half of all STIs occur in people under age 25. Both teens and college students are at high risk, although they often fail to recognize their level of risk. In Lab 21A, you will evaluate the risk of a friend or loved one. You may also want to evaluate your own risk using the questionnaire in the lab. Adequate knowledge of risk is likely to increase your practice of behaviors that reduce risk for STIs.

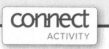

Suggested Resources and Readings

The websites for the following sources can be accessed by searching online for the organization, program, or title listed. Specific scientific references are available at the end of this edition of *Concepts of Fitness and Wellness*.

- Avert. Global Information and Education on HIV and AIDS.
- Centers for Disease Control and Prevention:

  - Ending the HIV Epidemic.
  - HIV.
  - HIV and COVID-19.
  - *Incidence, Prevalence, and Cost of Sexually Transmitted Infections in the United States.* (2021). (pdf)

  - Let's Stop HIV Together.
  - Sexually Transmitted Diseases (STDs).
  - Talk. Test. Treat.
  - Vaccines and Preventable Diseases: Human Papillomavirus (HPV).
- CNN Films. *The Hunting Ground.* (2015).
- Me Too. You are not alone.
- U.S. Department of Health and Human Services. HIV.gov:

  - HIV Vaccines. What Are Vaccines and What Do They Do?
  - What Is *Ending the HIV Epidemic in the U.S.?*
- Vagianos, A. (2017, April 5). "30 Alarming Statistics That Show the Reality of Sexual Violence in America." *Huff Post.*
- WebMD. (2020, July 28). Antiretrovirals: HIV and AIDS Drugs.

Lab 21A Sexually Transmitted Infection Risk Questionnaire

Name	**Section**	**Date**

Purpose: To help you understand the risks of contracting a sexually transmitted infection.

Procedures

1. Read the Sexually Transmitted Infection Risk Questionnaire (Chart 1).
2. Answer the questionnaire based on information about someone you know who might be at high risk of contracting an STI.
3. Record the scores in the Results section for the person for whom the questionnaire was answered but do *not* include the person's name on the lab sheet. Use the scores to make a rating (Chart 2) and draw conclusions.
4. You may also wish to answer the questionnaire based on your own information but do *not* record your personal results on the lab sheet. Use these scores strictly for your own personal information.

Chart 1 Sexually Transmitted Infection Risk Questionnaire

Place an X over one response in each row of the questionnaire. Determine a point value for each response using the values in the circles. Sum the numbers of points for the various responses to determine an STI risk score.

	Points				
Categories	**0**	**1**	**3**	**5**	**8**
Feelings about prevention	Able to talk with future partner about STIs ⓪	Finds it hard to discuss STIs with a possible partner ①			
Behaviors	Never engages in sexual activity ⓪		Sexual activity with one partner, well known to them ③	Sexual activity with one partner, not well known to them ⑤	Sexual activity with multiple partners and/or high-risk individuals ⑧
Behavior of friends	Most friends do not engage in unsafe sexual activity ⓪	Many friends engage in unsafe sexual activity ①			
Contraception	Not sexually active ⓪	Would use condom to prevent STI ①		Would sometimes use condom to prevent STI ⑤	Would never use condom to prevent STI ⑧
Other	Does not use drugs ⓪				Uses injected drugs in unsafe manner ⑧

Chart 2 STI Risk Questionnaire Rating Chart

Rating	Score
High risk	9+
Above average risk	7–8
Moderate risk	4–6
Low risk	0–3

Results

What is the person's STI risk score? [   ] (Total from Chart 1)

What is the person's STI rating? [   ] (See Chart 2)

Conclusions and Implications: Of course, risk varies with different types of STIs. However, this questionnaire will give you an idea of an individual's "general" risk for most STIs. Answer the following questions about the risk of the person you scored and rated.

1. In several sentences, explain which STI you think this person should be especially concerned about. Why?

2. What specific recommendations would you have for the person for whom you filled out this questionnaire?

Cancer, Diabetes, and Other Health Threats

LEARNING OBJECTIVES

After completing the study of this Concept, you will be able to:

▶ Describe the general nature of cancer and its various forms and indicate the frequency of each form of cancer in the population.

▶ Outline screening guidelines, lifestyle changes for prevention, and early warning signals for cancer.

▶ Describe the general nature of diabetes and its various forms and indicate the frequency of diabetes in the population.

▶ Outline screening guidelines, lifestyle changes for prevention, and early warning signals for diabetes.

▶ Describe the general nature of Alzheimer disease/dementia and mental health conditions that impact the population.

▶ Identify risks of injuries, infectious diseases, and other health threats.

▶ Learn self-management skills and self-exams that can help you assess your personal risk for cancer and other health threats.

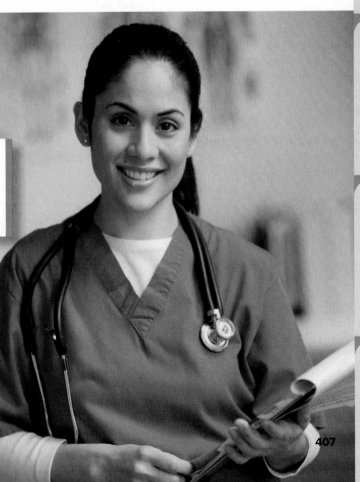

Many health problems that cause pain, suffering, and premature death are associated with unhealthy lifestyles.

Jose Luis Pelaez Inc/Blend Images LLC

Cancer

Cancer is a group of more than 100 different diseases. According to the American Cancer Society, cancer is a group of many different conditions characterized by abnormal, uncontrolled cell growth that will ultimately invade the blood and lymph tissues and spread throughout the body if not treated. Throughout the body, new cells are constantly being created to replace older ones. For reasons unknown, abnormal cells capable of uncontrolled growth sometimes develop. **Benign tumors** are generally not considered to be cancerous because a protective membrane restricts their growth to a specific area of the body. Treatment is important because any tumor can interfere with normal body functioning. Once removed, a benign tumor typically will not return.

Malignant tumors are capable of uncontrolled growth that can cause death to tissue. Approximately 85 percent of malignant tumors are carcinomas, or tumors of the epithelial cells of the inner and outer linings of the body (e.g., lungs, skin). Other malignant tumors include adenocarcinomas (glands such as breast tissue) and sarcomas (bones, muscles, connective tissue, and blood). Malignant cells invade healthy tissues, deplete them of nutrition, and interfere with a multitude of tissue functions. In the early stages of cancer, malignant tumors are located in a small area and can be more easily treated or removed. In advanced cancer, the cells invade the blood or lymph systems and travel throughout the body (**metastasize**). When this occurs, cancer becomes much more difficult to treat.

Figure 1 provides a more detailed illustration of the stages in the spread of cancer. It illustrates how an abnormal cell can divide to form a primary tumor (a), get nourishment from new blood vessels (b), invade the blood system (c), and escape to form a new (secondary) tumor (d). The four stages of cancer range from I to IV, with I being the early stage and IV being most advanced. The early stage is characterized by containment only in the layers of cells where they developed. When cancer spreads beyond the original layers (see Figure 1), it is considered to be invasive and is rated at a higher stage. Early detection is very important in the treatment and cure of cancer. One method of detecting a tumor is to take a **biopsy** of suspicious lumps in the breasts, testicles, or other parts of the body.

Cancer is not only a leading killer but also a cause of much suffering. In a typical year, one of every four deaths in the United States is caused by some form of cancer. About 4 out of every 10 people (40 percent of males and 39 percent of females) will have cancer at some time during their lifetimes, accounting for the billions of dollars spent on health care and the billions more in lost earnings. Of the over 100 forms of cancer, 4 of them (sometimes referred to as the Big 4) account for approximately half of all illness and death (see Figure 2). Because of the high incidence of these types of cancers (lung, colon-rectal, breast, and prostate), they are discussed in more detail here. In addition, three forms of cancer for which college students have relatively high risk—skin, ovary, and uterus—are discussed.

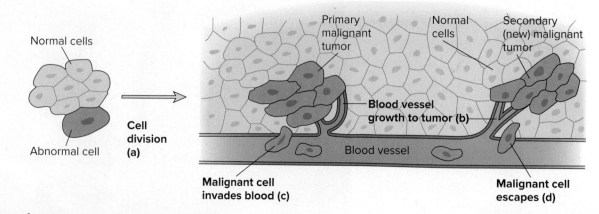

Figure 1 ▶ The spread of cancer (metastasis).

Cancer type

Death rank/%	New cases rank/%	Cancer type
1. 23%	2. 13%	lungs/bronchus
2. 10%	1. 21%	prostate
3. 9%	3. 9%	colon-rectal
4. 8%	10. 3%	pancreas
5. 6%	*	liver
6. 4%	9. 4%	leukemia
7. 4%	*	esophagus
8. 4%	4. 7%	urinary/bladder
9. 4%	7. 5%	non-Hodgkin's lymphoma
10. 3%	*	brain/nervous system
*	5. 7%	skin
*	6. 5%	kidney
*	8. 4%	oral/pharynx

Males   **Females**

Death rank/%	New cases rank/%	Cancer type
1. 22%	2. 12%	lungs/bronchus
2. 15%	1. 30%	breast
3. 9%	3. 8%	colon-rectal
4. 8%	9. 3%	pancreas
5. 5%	*	ovary
6. 4%	4. 4%	uterine
7. 4%	10. 3%	leukemia
8. 3%	*	liver
9. 3%	7. 5%	non-Hodgkin's lymphoma
10. 3%	*	brain/nervous system
*	5. 4%	thyroid
*	6. 4%	skin
*	8. 3%	kidney

*Not in top 10.

Figure 2 ▶ Cancer incidence (new cases) and death by site and sex (percentage).

Note: COVID-19 was among the top 10 causes of death in 2020 and 2021. Rankings are for non-COVID-19 years.

Source: American Cancer Society.

While some forms of cancer are equally threatening to both sexes (e.g., lung and colon-rectal), others are more specific to one sex or the other (see Figure 2). It is also important to note that incidence rates are different from death rates. Skin cancer is an example of a form of cancer that is high in incidence (fifth for males and sixth for females) but relatively low in death rate (not in the top 10 for males or females). This is because it can be treated with early detection, and steps can be taken to prevent it. In Lab 22A you will have the opportunity to assess your risk for the major forms of cancer.

Breast Cancer

Breast cancer is the most prevalent form of cancer among females, but lung cancer causes more deaths. Symptoms of breast cancer include lumps and/or thickening or swelling of the breasts. Breast pain may also exist but is more often a symptom of benign tumors. Risk becomes greater as you grow older. Other risk factors include sex at birth (females have higher risk), family history of disease, early menstruation, hormone supplementation, breast implantation, use of oral contraceptives, late childbirth or no children, excessive use of alcohol, poor eating habits, and sedentary living. The discovery of a "breast cancer gene" provides a possible explanation of the hereditary risks. Because a number of factors influence breast cancer risk, follow appropriate screening procedures to detect the possible presence of the disease.

In recent years there have been fewer deaths from breast cancer partly because of improved early diagnosis resulting from screening and more effective treatments. Though breast cancer is not as common among males, both males and females should do regular screening. Like colon-rectal and lung cancers, breast cancer is most prevalent among African Americans (more than twice as frequent) and least prevalent among Asians and Hispanics.

Early detection steps include regular self-exams of the breasts (see Lab 22B), breast exams by a physician, and regular mammograms. In many cases, lumps are present before they can be detected with self-exams. This is one reason for regular **mammograms** (breast X-rays).

The American Cancer Society (ACS) recommends that mammogram screening for females with "average risk" should begin at age 45 (see Table 1). Average risk is defined as a

Benign Tumors Slow-growing tumors that do not spread to other parts of the body.

Malignant Tumors Malignant means "growing worse." Malignant tumors are tumors that are considered to be cancerous and will spread throughout the body if not treated.

Metastasize The spread of cancer cells to other parts of the body.

Biopsy The removal of a tissue sample that can be checked for cancer cells.

Mammograms X-rays of the breast.

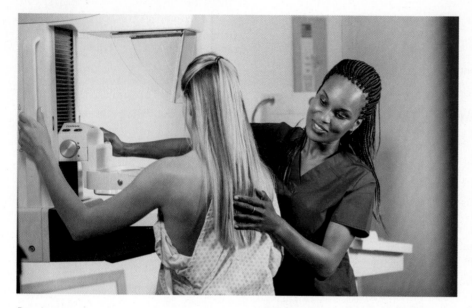

Regular screenings are important for detecting cancer in early stages when it can be treated more effectively.
John Foxx/Getty Images

person with no previous history or strong family history of breast cancer, no genetic mutations (e.g., *BRCA* gene), and no chest radiation therapy before age 30. Screening for females aged 40–44 may still be warranted and recommended by physicians. The choice to begin screening at age 40 is an individual one and should take into account both benefits and risks of screening. The primary benefit is early detection of cancer that is very important for aggressive breast tumors. The risks cited by the various organizations include false positives (test results indicate possible cancer when it is not present), unnecessary biopsies, and overtreatment. There is evidence that digital mammography may be more effective than traditional film mammography. Digital "3D" mammography is still being refined but may cut down on false positive tests.

Standard "local" treatments for breast cancer include lumpectomy (removal of the tumor and surrounding lymph nodes), mastectomy (removal of breast and surrounding lymph nodes), and local radiation. More "systemic" treatments include chemotherapy, hormone therapy, and targeted therapies that directly target the cells that cause cancer to grow out of control.

Colon-Rectal Cancer

Colon-rectal cancer is the third-leading killer of both males and females (see Table 1). In recent years, colon-rectal cancer rates have declined by about one-third. During this same period, there has been a similar increase in colon-rectal cancer screening, suggesting that testing helps reduce risk. Risk is highest among African Americans; whites have slightly less risk. Risk among Asians and Hispanics is less than half that of Blacks. Lifestyle risk factors include diet, use of alcohol, family history, physical activity patterns, and smoking (see Lab 22A). A high-fiber diet and physical activity can decrease the risk.

Colon-rectal cancer is most common among those over 50 years of age. When caught early, 90 percent of colon-rectal cancers can be cured. Unfortunately, only 59 percent of adults over the age of 50 report having regular screening. Symptoms include cramping in the lower stomach, change in the shape of the stool, urge to have a bowel movement when there is no need to have one, and blood in the stool. A variety of tests are available for early detection of colon-rectal cancer. All of the tests are designed to detect either the presence of polyps that can turn into cancer, or polyps (or cancers) that are bleeding. The ACS recommends that colon-rectal screening begin at age 45 for people with "average risk." Average risk is defined as people with no personal or family history of colon-rectal cancer, no other cancer-related bowel disease, and no history of abdominal radiation therapy. After age 75, screening should be done based on personal preference and a physician's recommendation. No screening is recommended after age 85.

As shown in Table 1, the ACS recommends one of two plans for colon-rectal cancer screening: visual exams and stool-based tests. Visual exams include one of three medically focused screening options: a colonoscopy, a virtual colonoscopy, or a flexible sigmoidoscopy. The *colonoscopy* is often considered to be the "gold standard" because it checks for polyps and lesions in the entire colon. If polyps are found during a colonoscopy, they can be removed immediately without an additional procedure. The *virtual colonoscopy* provides a less invasive alternative to the conventional colonoscopy. It uses a CT scan that creates two- and three-dimensional images of the colon. These images allow the colon to be viewed from several different angles, something that is difficult to do with a conventional colonoscopy. Research shows that the procedure identifies 90 percent of large polyps. However, two major disadvantages are that the procedure requires exposure to radiation, and if a positive test occurs (polyps found), a regular colonoscopy must be done to remove them. The *sigmoidoscopy* tests only the lower one-third of the colon, and if polyps are found, a follow-up colonoscopy is recommended. While not as comprehensive as a colonoscopy, a recent study found that having one sigmoidoscopy between the ages of 55 and 64 can cut the risk of colon cancer by 43 percent.

Stool-based tests involve more independent screening with follow-up treatment if warranted. A variety of tests are available, but each requires you to wipe stool samples on a test card to be sent to a lab for testing or for home analysis (with home test kits). A simple *fecal immunochemical test (FIT)* detects blood in the stool and does not require any special preparations. A related test called the *fecal occult blood test (FOBT)* requires

Table 1 ▶ Cancer Screening Guidelines

Cancer Type	Test or Procedure	Age	Frequency
Males and Females			
General Cancer-Related Checkup	Exam for thyroid, oral cavity, skin, lymph nodes, testes, and ovaries as part of periodic health exam	20+	With health exam
Colon-Rectal Cancer	Choose from visual exams and stool-based tests		
	Visual exams: Colonoscopy -or- CT colonography (virtual colonoscopy) -or- Flexible sigmoidoscopy	45+	Every 10 years Every 5 years (colonoscopy if +) Every 5 years (colonoscopy if +)
	Stool-based tests: Multi-stool fecal immunochemical test (FIT), -or- Multi-stool fecal occult blood test (FOBT), -or- Stool DNA test	45+	Annual (colonoscopy if +) Annual (colonoscopy if +) Every 3 years (colonoscopy if +)
Skin Cancer[a]	Self-exam	Any age	Monthly
	Exam by health-care provider	Any age	With symptoms
Lung Cancer	Low-dose computed tomography (LDCT) scan	55–74 or high risk	Personal choice after consultation with health-care provider
Females			
Breast Cancer	Breast self-exam	Any age	Know feel and look of breasts; consult health-care provider if changes occur
	Clinical breast exam	Any age	Performed by health-care provider if changes occur
	Mammogram	40–44 45–54 55+	Annual, self-choice Annual Every 2 years, or choose annual
	Breast MRI (for those with high risk)	40+	Consult health-care provider
Cervical Cancer[b]	Pap test Pap and HPV tests Women (normal prior results) Women (history of precancer)	21–29 30–65 65+ 65+	Every 3 years Every 5 years (Pap every 3 years) No tests Continued Pap testing for 20 years
Uterine Cancer	Information about symptoms and risks	Menopause	Consult health-care provider
Males			
Prostate Cancer	Consider pros and cons of testing (2 main options) Digital rectal exam (DRE) -or- Prostate-specific antigen (PSA) test	40+ with very high risk (several relatives with disease); 45+ African Americans and high risk (one relative with disease; 50+ those with average risk	Consult health-care provider; PSA frequency depends on past PSA results. Those with high previous PSA may need more frequent testing. Very high PSA values may warrant a biopsy.
Testicular Cancer[a]	Self-exam	20+	Monthly

[a]The American Cancer Society (ACS) has no current recommendation, but many doctors recommend monthly self-exams.

[b]Exams should begin at age 21; females under age 21 should not be tested.

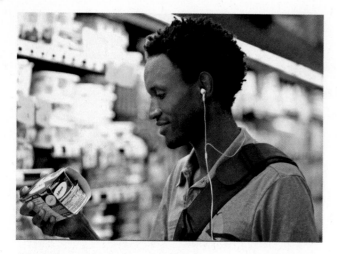

Adopting a healthy diet can help decrease risk for many cancers.
Rob Melnychuk/Fuse/Getty Images

some dietary modifications and restriction of medication since a specific chemical is used in the detection. Consumer test kits such as Cologard® detect mutated DNA in the stool, but this test requires a prescription. These screening tests each require follow-up colonoscopies if positive tests occur.

Lung Cancer

Lung cancer is the leading cause of cancer death in males and females. Lung cancer rates have dropped in the past decade, a change attributable in part to declines in smoking. Smoking rates among youth and young adults have increased, however, suggesting that lung cancer deaths may increase in the years ahead. Incidence and death rates are much higher among African Americans than whites, with considerably lower rates among Asians and Hispanics. Females have lower lung cancer death rates than males, but the gap between the two groups has narrowed in recent years.

By far, the greatest risk factor for lung cancer is smoking. Environmental tobacco smoke (ETS) has been shown to be a potent risk factor. According to the ACS, nonsmoking spouses of smokers have a 30 percent greater risk of developing lung cancer than do spouses of nonsmokers. A number of other carcinogens, including radon, asbestos, and pollution, have been linked to lung cancer, so nonsmokers can also get lung cancer.

Symptoms of lung cancer include persistent cough, chest pain, recurring pneumonia or bronchitis, and sputum (spit) streaked with blood. Lung cancer can spread to other organs and tissues before symptoms are evident, so it is important to pay attention to possible symptoms.

A recent study (National Lung Screening Trial) found that screening with low-dose computed tomography (LDCT) scans can lower the risk of dying from lung cancer. The LDCT uses lower doses of radiation than standard CT or CAT scans and does not use intravenous dye. The ACS guidelines reference LDCT but recommend consultation with your health-care provider prior to screening (see Table 1). Like mammograms, LDCT has some risks, including radiation exposure, false positives, and unnecessary additional treatments. Other detection steps include monitoring for symptoms, regular chest X-rays, and analysis of sputum samples. Standard treatments include surgery, radiation, and chemotherapies.

Prostate Cancer

Prostate cancer is the most common form of cancer in males accounting for 10 percent of all cancer deaths. One in every eight males will get prostate cancer during their lifetime. The death rate from prostate cancer is highest among older people and African Americans. Risks of prostate cancer increase dramatically after age 50. Symptoms of prostate cancer are urination problems (weak or interrupted stream, inability to start or stop, pain, high frequency of urination at night, and/or presence of blood in the urine).

The two principal screening techniques include a digital rectal exam (DRE) by a physician (to detect an enlarged prostate gland) and a prostate-specific antigen (PSA) blood test. A PSA threshold of 4 nanograms per milliliter was previously

In the News

Cancer Screening Guidelines

Early detection is critical for effective cancer treatment, but screening guidelines have proven difficult for consumers to follow. The U.S. Preventive Services Task Force (USPSTF) provides recommendations and resources to help doctors and patients decide together whether screening tests or preventive medicines are appropriate for a person's needs. The recommendations are based on critical reviews of scientific evidence and separate sections are available for both clinicians and consumers. Considerations such as the typical age of onset, the cost of unnecessary screening, and the risks and anxiety associated with false positive tests factor into decisions about screening. The guidelines change as new evidence is available.

Does knowing current guidelines on cancer screening make you more likely to discuss prevention topics with your physician?

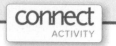

used as an indicator of potential risk, but other screening criteria are now being used. Research suggests that year-to-year changes in PSA are a better predictor, even if the score is lower than 4. A new autoantibody signatures test has promise for the future. If future research verifies early findings, this test may be used instead of, or in addition to, the PSA test. Preliminary studies with the new test show that it identifies 82 percent of cancers correctly.

Although research has shown that PSA screening does reduce prostate cancer deaths, there is debate about the age for beginning PSA screening. The ACS recommends males begin the discussion about a yearly PSA test with a health-care provider beginning at age 50 for those with average risk. However, those with very high and high risk should begin screening earlier (see Table 1).

Given that screening has reduced cancer risk, every male should consult with a health-care professional about when to begin screening and which methods are best for unique personal needs (e.g., age, current symptoms, family history). The discussion should consider the concerns related to testing, including false positives. Although false positives can lead to overtreatment and unnecessary worry, when to begin screening and frequency of screening is clearly a personal decision. As noted earlier, changes in PSA values are more important than absolute values in detecting prostate cancer; thus, an advantage of testing is that it provides a potential baseline measure for purposes of future comparison.

Current treatments for prostate cancer have been shown to be highly effective, and death rates due to prostate cancer have decreased. However, despite the progress, the ACS points out that there is no uniform agreement on treatment. Among the most common treatments is "watchful waiting" with no immediate treating since prostate cancer progresses slowly in some patients. Other treatments include surgery to remove the prostate; hormone therapy; radiation therapy, including implanting of radioactive seeds to kill the tumor; and chemotherapy. One recently approved medication called Provenge uses a patient's own immune system to fight advanced prostate cancer that is no longer responding to hormone therapy.

Uterine and Ovarian Cancers

Combined, uterine and ovarian cancers account for nearly 10 percent of all cancer deaths among females. Uterine cancer is of two different types: cervical cancer occurs when cancers develop in the cervix, or opening to the uterus, and endometrial cancer occurs when a tumor develops in the inner wall of the uterus. Ovarian cancer occurs when a cancer develops in an ovary. Symptoms of ovarian cancer include abdominal swelling and digestive disturbances. Vaginal bleeding can be a symptom of either uterine or ovarian cancer. Other vaginal discharge may be a symptom of uterine cancer. Understanding the risk factors for these female reproductive system cancers is important for prevention.

Established risk factors for cervical cancer include having sex at an early age, having sex with many partners, and a history of smoking. However, the most important risk factor for cervical cancer is infection by human papillomavirus (HPV), a sexually transmitted infection. The FDA has approved two "cervical cancer" vaccines (Cervarix and Gardasil) that have been shown to prevent the formation of precancerous genital lesions as well as genital warts attributed to HPV infection. While it is not effective against all forms of HPV, it is effective in preventing the form implicated in most cervical cancers and other HPV-related cancers. According to the CDC, each year there are thousands of cases of HPV-related cancer that could be prevented with the HPV vaccine. While HPV-related cancers are twice as common in females, the CDC recommends the HPV vaccine for preteen girls and boys.

The other form of uterine cancer, endometrial cancer, is less common and has a different mechanism of causation. The primary risk factors (early menarche, late menopause, infertility) are all associated with increased exposure to estrogen during the lifespan. However, other risks include obesity and a high-fat diet.

Risk factors for ovarian cancer include age, family history, and lack of pregnancy during the lifetime. One study showed that risk is considerably higher among those who have taken estrogen-progestin therapy, especially those who have taken it for 10 years or more. Those who have had breast cancer or who are at high risk for breast cancer have a relatively high risk for ovarian cancer.

A periodic and thorough pelvic exam is the best method of screening for cervical and ovarian cancers. A **Pap test** is an important part of the exam for detecting cervical cancer. This test (named for Dr. George Papanicolaou, who pioneered it) involves taking scrapings (samples) from the cervix and analyzing them under a microscope. Liquid-based Pap testing (sometimes referred to as ThinPrep) was thought to be more effective than previous Pap testing procedures, but recent research has shown the methods to be equally effective. The liquid-based test is more expensive but is preferred by labs because of the speed and ease of assessment. For this reason, some labs have stopped using the more conventional method. The liquid-based method allows for HPV testing from the same sample, and the ACS indicates that it can be done less frequently. Some home Pap smear kits are available, but these have not been shown to provide accurate information. As noted in Table 1, females should begin Pap testing at age 21 and should be tested every 3 years. Older females can be tested less frequently.

Treatments include surgery to remove one or both of the ovaries and fallopian tubes and/or removal of the uterus (hysterectomy). Radiation and chemotherapy are other options. DNA tests to find cancer-specific genes have been found to predict this form of cancer in a small percentage of the population, but this test has yet to receive governmental approval.

Pap Test A test of the cells of the cervix to detect cancer or other conditions.

Skin Cancer

While rates of cancer in general have decreased, skin cancer rates have increased in recent years. Each year more than 3 million people are treated for non-melanoma skin cancer. Skin cancer ranks high in new cases (fifth for males and sixth for females), but does not rank high as a cause of death. This is because it can be cured if caught early. Symptoms include darkly pigmented growths, changes in size or color of moles, changes in other nodules on the skin, skin bleeding or scaliness, and skin pain (see Figure 3).

The principal risk factor is exposure to ultraviolet light, such as sun exposure and indoor tanning. Other risk factors include family history, pale skin, exposure to pollutants, and radiation. Some people feel that tanning lights are safe, but research has shown the opposite. Research indicates that tanning dramatically increases risk of skin cancer. A federal tax has been imposed on tanning salons because of the growing evidence of a link between indoor tanning and skin cancer. The effect of sun exposure is illustrated by the fact that significantly more skin cancer is found on the left arm, the arm that is exposed to the sun when driving, than the right arm. **Melanoma** is 10 times more frequent in whites than African Americans, and a recent study showed an especially high rate of skin cancer among young white females who tan regularly. Unlike many other forms of cancer, skin cancer is not necessarily a disease of older adults. Young people who do not take preventive measures are at risk.

Early detection is essential to treatment, so regular screening is important. Screening techniques include self-exams of the skin followed by a physician's exam of suspicious lesions. A number of different cancer organizations recommend the ABCDE rule for self-exams (see Figure 3). *A* is for asymmetry: Does one half of a growth look different from the other half? *B* is for border irregularity: Are the edges notched, rugged, or blurred? *C* is for color: Is the color uniform, not varying in shades of tan, brown, and black? *D* is for any lesion with a diameter greater than 6 millimeters (about 1/4 inch). Beware of sudden or progressive growth of any lesion. *E* stands for evolution of a lesion (changes in shape or elevation of a lesion, scaliness, pain, itching, or bleeding). Some experts have recommended adding *F* to the list for friend (attentive friends may see changes before you do).

Nonmalignant basal and squamous cell cancers can be treated in a doctor's office using freezing, heat, or laser procedures. These milder forms of cancer have become more common among younger people in recent years. They occur on the head and neck in 90 percent of cases; however, with the increase in total body exposure and tanning practices, they are now much more common on other parts of the body. Once you have had one of these cancers, your risk of having another is high. Treatment for early melanoma involves the removal of affected cells and surrounding lymph tissues. Advanced cases require radiation and/or chemotherapies, or immunotherapy.

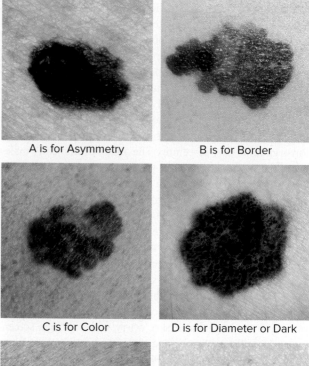
A is for Asymmetry

B is for Border

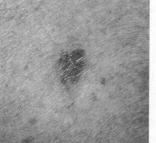
C is for Color

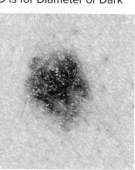
D is for Diameter or Dark

E is for Evolving (Before)

E is for Evolving (After)

Please note: Since not all melanomas have the same appearance, these photos serve as a general reference for what melanoma can look like. If you see anything NEW, CHANGING, or UNUSUAL on your skin, go get checked by a dermatologist.

Figure 3 ▶ **Warning signs for melanoma: Know your ABCDEs.** A. Asymmetry: One half does not match other half; B. Border irregularity: Ragged or notched edges; C. Color: Color uneven shades of tan, brown, or black and sometimes red, white, or blue; D. Diameter or Dark Diameter larger than ¼ inch (diameter of a pencil eraser) Note: Some cancers can be smaller. E. Evolving.

(a) National Cancer Institute (NCI); www.cancer.gov/CDC (b) National Cancer Institute (NCI)/CDC (c) Nasekomoe/Shutterstock (d) Australis Photography/Shutterstock (e) Kelly Nelson, National Cancer Institute (NCI); www.cancer.gov/CDC (f) National Cancer Institute (NCI)

Important preventive measures include limiting exposure to the sun or tanning devices, reducing exposure during midday hours, covering the skin when exposed to the sun (hat, long pants, long-sleeve shirts,

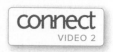
connect VIDEO 2

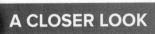 **A CLOSER LOOK**

FDA Proposes Safety Measures for Indoor Tanning Devices

There are many documented risks associated with the use of indoor tanning beds (e.g., eye injury, skin damage, skin cancer). For example, according to the CDC, use before age 35 increases future risk of melanoma by 75 percent. Although the World Health Organization has labeled indoor tanning devices as "cancer-causing," the public has not been deterred. More than one-third of all Americans say they have used a tanning bed at some point, and 13 percent have used one in the last year. More than 59 percent of college students have used a tanning bed, with 43 percent reporting use in the previous year. To help deter use, the FDA has proposed new safety measures.

Previous guidelines required labels on tanning devices indicating that they should not be used by people under age 18. However, new safety guidelines by the FDA will require indoor tanning facilities to inform adult users about the health risks of indoor tanning and to get signed "risk acknowledgment" from users. This rule will also directly prohibit use of indoor tanning facilities by people under 18.

Are these warnings sufficient to influence your feelings about indoor tanning? Do you agree with laws that limit tanning for children and teens?

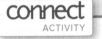

high collars on shirts, sunglasses), and using sunscreen on exposed skin. It is best to choose "broad spectrum" sunscreens that protect against both ultraviolet A radiation (UVA) and ultraviolet B radiation (UVB). Those with a family history of skin cancer and a history of sunburn or extensive sun exposure should be especially careful to minimize exposure.

Testicular Cancer

While not a leading cause of death, testicular cancer is a threat to males of all ages, including young males. As noted in Table 1, a monthly testicular self-exam is recommended (see Lab 22B for more information).

Cancer Prevention

Many factors are associated with increased risk for cancer, including unhealthy lifestyles. The malfunction of genes that control cell growth and development is responsible for all cancers. Five to ten percent of cancers result from an inherited faulty gene. Although genetics can't be altered, a variety of lifestyle and environmental factors also influence cancer. Environments or exposures that may be harmful include exposure to carcinogens at work (e.g., secondhand smoke, coal dust), exposure to geophysical factors (e.g., radon and radiation), exposure to polluted environments (e.g., poor air and water), exposure to certain industrial products (e.g., polychlorinated biphenyls [PCBs] produced in making plastics), and exposure to medical procedures (e.g., X-rays, CT scans). Some risks are hard to avoid, but minimizing exposure to the carcinogens related to environmental factors is an effective strategy for cancer prevention.

Making changes in lifestyles can also be important to cancer prevention. The World Cancer Research Fund (WCRF) and the American Institute for Cancer Research (AICR) released a definitive source of information concerning the importance of nutrition and physical activity in cancer

prevention. The primary recommendations of this report are included in Table 2.

Many forms of cancer can now be treated effectively. Cancer death rates (all forms of cancer) have decreased significantly each year since the beginning of this century. Many people have lived long, healthy lives after breast, skin, and many other forms of cancer. These people die from other

Table 2 ▶ Recommendations for Nutrition and Physical Activity to Prevent Cancer

- Be as lean as possible within the normal range of body weight. A Body Mass Index in the healthy range is recommended.

- Be physically active as part of everyday life. At least 30 minutes of moderate activity per day is recommended, with an increase to 60 minutes of moderate activity or 30 minutes of vigorous activity per day as fitness improves.

- Limit consumption of energy-dense foods (including fast foods), and avoid sugary drinks.

- Eat mostly foods from plant origin. Eat 5–9 servings of nonstarchy vegetables and fruits every day.

- Limit intake of red meat and avoid processed meat (no more than 30 g per week).

- Limit alcoholic drinks to no more than two drinks a day for males and one for females.

- Limit consumption of salt (less than 1.5 g per day).

- Aim to meet nutritional needs through diet alone. Dietary supplements are not recommended for cancer prevention.

Source: Adapted from WCRF/AICR.

Melanoma Cancer of the cells that produce skin pigment.

Table 3 ▶ Other Lifestyle Changes for Cancer Prevention

- Eliminate tobacco use (smoke and smokeless).
- Reduce sun and ultraviolet light exposure: use sunscreen, wear protective clothing, and avoid excess sun and tanning lights.
- Do regular self-screening and medical testing.
- Avoid excessive X-rays.
- Avoid breathing polluted air (e.g., exercise away from freeways and polluted air, check for pollution advisories).
- Minimize occupational and environmental pollutants when possible.

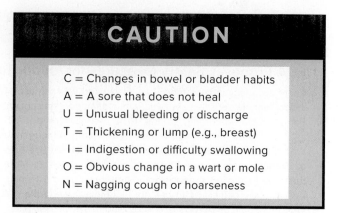

CAUTION

C = Changes in bowel or bladder habits
A = A sore that does not heal
U = Unusual bleeding or discharge
T = Thickening or lump (e.g., breast)
I = Indigestion or difficulty swallowing
O = Obvious change in a wart or mole
N = Nagging cough or hoarseness

Figure 4 ▶ Acronym for monitoring and early detection and treatment of cancer (CAUTION).

causes, and some observers would consider them to be "cured." Still, what constitutes a cure is elusive. Those who achieve 5-year survival after cancer now have a 70 percent survival rate, compared to 49 percent 45 years ago. Though people who survive for 5 years after detection may not be considered cured, the high survival rate illustrates that cancer can be treated, even for those with inherited faulty genes. Much of the increase in the 5-year survival rate is attributed to healthy lifestyle practices such as decreases in tobacco use and improved screening and treatment. Other recommendations for other lifestyle behaviors for cancer prevention are provided in Table 3.

Medical consultation is essential when considering hormone replacement therapy. For years, hormone replacement therapy (HRT) was prescribed to females to help prevent loss of bone density, reduce risk for heart disease, and reduce the symptoms of menopause (e.g., hot flashes, sleep disturbances, fatigue, poor concentration, and disruption of work and recreational activities). Research conducted in the early 2000s suggested that HRT increased the risk for some forms of cancer, was not effective in reducing heart disease, and increased the risk for blood clots. As a result, females were cautioned against HRT. The number of HRT prescriptions dropped from nearly 18 million in 2001 to less than 6 million by the late 2000s. However, more comprehensive studies are now providing clarity on the issue.

Several large-scale studies have been conducted on HRT and cancer risks. Results vary based on the type of HRT used. The ACS indicates that combined estrogen-progestin therapy (EPT) does not increase risk of uterine (endometrial), lung, or skin cancer. However, EPT has still been linked to a higher risk of breast cancer and ovarian cancer. Results are mixed for colon-rectal cancer. Those on EPT had lower risk of getting colon-rectal cancer but, when they got it, the cancer was at a more advanced stage.

The conflicting information on risks can be confusing to many females who wonder if HRT is safe for treating the very real symptoms of menopause. Experts agree that each case should be considered individually, with patient and doctor weighing all risks and benefits before choosing a course of action. In addition, other research suggests that low-dose HRT and HRT delivered by gels, patches, and creams may be effective in treating symptoms of menopause and are less likely to cause clotting than oral forms.

Recognizing early warning signals can help reduce the risk of cancer. There are many warning signs and symptoms of cancer. These include unusual fatigue, prolonged fever, abnormal weight loss, and changes in skin. Others are easily remembered using the acronym CAUTION (see Figure 4).

Diabetes

Diabetes presents major health risks, but it can be treated effectively. Diabetes mellitus, typically referred to as diabetes, is a disease that occurs when the blood sugar is abnormally high. The body relies on glucose as the primary source of energy, and complex regulatory processes help regulate levels of blood sugar. Low levels of blood sugar are clearly a problem, but other problems occur if blood sugar is too high. There are as many as 30 different reasons for high blood sugar; therefore, diabetes is really many different diseases, not just one. There is no cure for diabetes, but with proper medical treatment and healthy lifestyle modifications, the condition can be managed effectively.

There are two main forms of diabetes, and it is important to understand the differences. **Type 1 diabetes** (or *insulin-dependent diabetes mellitus [IDDM]*) is caused by the inability of the body to produce an adequate amount of **insulin**, a hormone produced by the pancreas that regulates glucose levels in the blood. Individuals with Type 1 diabetes must take daily doses of insulin (oral or injection) to help their body regulate blood glucose levels. This form is more genetically based and is not directly related to obesity or unhealthy lifestyles. A relatively small percentage of diabetics (5 percent) have Type 1 diabetes, and it is typically diagnosed before the age of 30. **Type 2 diabetes** is

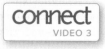
connect VIDEO 3

a far more common form that is caused by a lack of sensitivity to insulin. It is often called *non-insulin-dependent diabetes mellitus (NIDDM)* since the body loses sensitivity to insulin and cannot effectively take up and use the sugar in the blood. Unlike Type 1 diabetes, this form is caused primarily by unhealthy lifestyles (obesity and lack of physical activity). It was previously referred to as *adult-onset diabetes* because it tended to occur later in life, but children and adolescents can also develop the condition. A third and relatively rare form of diabetes is referred to as *gestational diabetes mellitus*. This form results when high blood sugar levels occur in pregnant females previously not known to have diabetes. This condition is present in about 3 percent of all pregnancies, can have implications for the fetus, and may or may not result in a diabetic state after pregnancy. Other forms of diabetes are rare.

An understanding of normal blood sugar levels and regulation is important for reducing risk of diabetes. Normal levels range from 50 to 100 mg per 100 mL of blood (measured in a fasted state). A condition known as **pre-diabetes** exists when blood glucose levels range from 101 to 125, and diabetes exists when blood glucose levels regularly exceed 125. Pre-diabetes was formerly known as *impaired glucose tolerance,* but the name was changed to help focus attention on the seriousness of this condition. Recent research has shown that pre-diabetes can result in long-term damage to the body similar to that of diabetes if not controlled. People who take steps to control pre-diabetes can delay or even prevent the development of Type 2 diabetes. More than 10 percent of all Americans have diabetes (about 34 million overall), and almost three times that many have pre-diabetes (about 80 million). Millions more are either pre-diabetic or diabetic and do not know it. Early screening is important for detecting and reversing pre-diabetes and diabetes.

Diabetes and related conditions are a leading cause of death in our society. Diabetes is the seventh-leading cause of death, and it is a leading killer in other Western nations, including Canada. People with diabetes have a shortened lifespan, as well as many short-term and long-term complications associated with the disease. A study of people in the Netherlands, England, and the United States indicated that longevity after 50 years of age is decreased by 7.5 years for males and 8.2 years for females for diabetics as opposed to nondiabetics.

African Americans, Hispanics, and Native Americans are especially at risk for diabetes. Unlike heart disease and cancer, which have shown recent decreases in incidence, the incidence of diabetes has increased in the last decade, with little progress being made in accomplishing national health goals for this disease.

People with diabetes have an increased risk for additional health problems. For example, diabetes is considered to be a risk factor for heart disease, high blood pressure, and COVID-19. Diabetics have a higher rate of kidney failure (including the need for kidney transplants

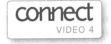

and kidney dialysis), a high incidence of blindness, and a high incidence of lower limb amputation. Females with diabetes also have a high rate of pregnancy complications. A national health goal is to increase the rate of diagnosis and to increase the number of diabetics who get regular blood lipid assessments, blood pressure checks, and eye examinations.

Screening for pre-diabetes and diabetes is essential for diagnosis and treatment. The symptoms of diabetes include frequent urination, excessive thirst, extreme hunger, unusual weight loss, increased fatigue, irritability, and blurry vision. Those who have recently gained large amounts of weight are also at risk. Early diagnosis as a result of attention to the symptoms can expedite treatment. Guidelines recommend screening for pre-diabetes and diabetes using one or more of several blood tests: a fasting plasma glucose (FPG) test, which measures levels of glucose in the blood after an overnight fast (values of 99 mg/dL or less are normal), or a 2-hour **oral glucose tolerance test (OGTT)**, which includes the FPG test but also tests glucose levels 2 hours after a person drinks a standard glucose solution (values of 140 mg/dl or less are normal). A blood test called A1C can also be performed (values of 5.7 percent or less are normal). The A1C test has the advantage of assessing your average blood glucose level of the past 2 or 3 months as opposed to your blood sugar level on a given day. Also, you do not have to fast prior to the test.

Guidelines recommend screening if symptoms exist. Regular screening is recommended beginning at age 45 for those potentially at risk. Because African Americans, Hispanics, American indigenous peoples, and Pacific Islanders have especially high risk, some experts recommend testing at age 30 or earlier for these groups. Others with diabetes risk factors and those with a Body Mass Index over 25 should also consider testing at an earlier age. Consider using the ADA diabetes risk calculator to see what your risk is. (Search "ADA Diabetes Risk Test" online.)

Lifestyle changes are needed for effective prevention and treatment of diabetes. Although diabetes presents significant health risks, it can be managed effectively. Consultation with a physician is essential to determine appropriate

> **Type 1 Diabetes** A chronic metabolic disease characterized by high blood sugar (glucose) levels associated with the inability of the pancreas to produce insulin; also called *insulin-dependent diabetes mellitus (IDDM)*.
>
> **Insulin** A hormone that regulates blood sugar levels.
>
> **Type 2 Diabetes** A chronic metabolic disease characterized by high blood sugar, usually not requiring insulin therapy; also called *non-insulin-dependent diabetes mellitus (NIDDM)*.
>
> **Pre-Diabetes** A condition in which fasting blood glucose levels are higher than normal but not high enough to be clinically diagnosed as diabetes.
>
> **Oral Glucose Tolerance Test (OGTT)** A test used to diagnose diabetes. It consists of a blood sugar measurement following the ingestion of a standard amount of sugar (glucose) after a period of fasting.

Table 5 ▶ Steps to Reduce Injuries
Reduce Motor Vehicle Accidents
• Do not drive while under the influence of alcohol.
• Use shoulder seat belts and drive cars that have air bags.
• Reduce driving speed.
• Use motorcycle helmets.
• Increase safety programs for pedestrians and cyclists.
• Establish more effective licensing for very young and older drivers.
Improve Home and Neighborhood Environments
• Require safety controls on handguns.
• Require sprinkler systems in homes with high risk of fire.
• Increase presence of functional smoke detectors in homes.
• Increase injury and poison education in schools.
• Wear effective safety gear in sports.
• Improve pool and boat safety education.
• Learn cardiopulmonary resuscitation.
• Properly mark poisons and prescription drugs.
• Require childproof packaging for poisons and prescription drugs.

Infectious Diseases and Other Health Threats

COVID-19 caused worldwide illness, death, and economic hardships. While scientists have warned about the potential of global pandemics, the world was clearly not prepared for the challenges presented by COVID-19. Named COVID-19 (*CO* stands for "corona," *VI* for "virus," *D* for "disease," and *19* for the year of its origin—2019), the virus was a novel (new) form of a virus known to cause SARS (severe acute respiratory syndrome). It was first identified in China in late 2019 and quickly spread throughout the entire world. Nearly 2 million deaths were reported worldwide in 2020, with nearly a quarter from the United States. The WHO indicates that 3 million is closer to the true number of cases worldwide in 2020. The pandemic (global epidemic) continued to escalate in 2021 as the virus mutated to produce more contagious and deadly strains—including the Delta variant that became dominant in the U.S. By the end of 2021, more than 40 million cases had been reported in the U.S. and deaths exceeded 700,000. In addition, hospitalizations from COVID-19 strained the medical and health care systems, sometimes requiring hospitals to suspend elective surgeries and ration health care. In some cases, hospitals were unable to take additional patients, requiring transferring patients to other hospitals, sometimes out of state.

Common symptoms of COVID-19 include fever/chills, cough, shortness of breath, fatigue, muscle or body aches, headache, loss of taste or smell, nasal congestion, nausea/vomiting, and diarrhea. However, some people are asymptomatic carriers, meaning that they do not exhibit symptoms but could unknowingly transmit the virus to others and make them sick. While most people recovered without treatment, many people infected by the virus experienced moderate to severe complications including pneumonia, acute respiratory stress syndrome (low oxygen levels), heart problems, blood clots, kidney injury, and organ failure. Death from COVID-19 has most frequently been the result of septic shock and multiple organ failure associated with pulmonary (lung) infection. People with risk factors for other chronic diseases such as high blood pressure, heart conditions, and obesity experience more severe symptoms and have greater risk of dying from COVID-19. As emphasized throughout this edition, maintaining healthy lifestyles helps prevent these risk factors and enhances immune function. While everyone is at risk of contracting COVID-19, those with healthy lifestyles tend to have fewer complications and better outcomes.

Personal responsibility is critical for minimizing the spread of infectious diseases. Guidelines for preventing the spread of HIV and other sexually transmitted infections have been established for decades, but the COVID-19 pandemic introduced new issues for minimizing the spread of respiratory conditions. It took time for researchers to identify the most effective methods of limiting transmission and

HELP
Health is available to Everyone for a Lifetime, and it's Personal

Personal Health Versus Public Health

Before the COVID-19 pandemic, many considered their health solely in "personal" terms (e.g., choosing what to eat or whether to exercise or not). The pandemic led to greater awareness of "public" health as collective efforts were needed to contain the virus. For example, the critical need to preserve public health led to local, state, and national lockdowns and policies for masks and social distancing all over the world. While individuals may have autonomy to make decisions impacting personal health, the mandates were needed to help promote health and safety for all. The public health issues evident throughout the pandemic reveal how the environment influences our health and how we also shape our environment.

Do you influence your environment in positive or negative ways? Does your environment shape you in positive or negative ways?

connect
ACTIVITY

treating COVID-19. Concerns about transmission through contact with contaminated solid surfaces led to dramatic changes in sanitation practices. However, the use of masks and social distancing were later emphasized to minimize exposure to airborne virus particles. Other sound prevention strategies included regular and thorough hand washing, the use of hand sanitizer, and avoiding touching the face and mouth with unclean hands. Retaining these habits can promote personal health as well as minimize spread of COVID-19, the flu, or other infectious diseases.

Vaccines provide a public health solution for the control of infectious diseases. The development and release of vaccines for COVID-19 were major news headlines for most of 2020 and 2021. The first two vaccines approved in the U.S. as safe and effective in clinical trials were the Pfizer-BioNTech and Moderna vaccines (both two shot vaccines), with a vaccine from Johnson & Johnson (one shot vaccine) being released shortly thereafter. By mid-2021, vaccines were available to all people aged 12 and older. Late in 2021, vaccines became available for children 5 years of age and older. In addition, a booster shot (a third shot) was recommended for those over 65 and those with existing health problems.

When the vaccine was first approved, many people got vaccinated as quickly as they could qualify. However, some resisted vaccination recommendations, delaying "herd immunity" needed to extinguish or greatly reduce the spread of COVID-19. The WHO indicates that a certain percentage of the population must be vaccinated or have immunity from a previous infection varies to achieve herd immunity. The percentage varies by disease. For measles a vaccination rate of 95% is required and for polio the rate is 80%. The percent required for COVID-19 is unknown. Late in 2021 COVID-19 spiked, as did hospitalizations and deaths, indicating that herd immunity had not yet been achieved in the U.S. Experts also suggest that mutations may necessitate ongoing vaccinations over time (similar to how flu shots are changed annually).

Infectious diseases present a continued threat to public health. In addition to the health consequences, COVID-19 resulted in economic hardships including unemployment associated with closing businesses (e.g., restaurants, entertainment venues), disruptions in education programs, and shutdowns in mass transit. Government subsidy programs were enacted to help prevent food insecurity, loss of housing, and other hardships, but the funds were not available or effective for all people. Minorities and people of color were disproportionately affected. The impact of the social determinants of health has been dramatically evident throughout the COVID-19 pandemic.

The effects of COVID-19 will be with us for many years to come, but the public health lessons will help prepare us locally and globally for future health problems and pandemics. For example, insights about the spread of infections and the utility of contact tracing will help better control the spread of diseases in the future. Similarly, insights on vaccine development will enhance future responsiveness to new public health threats (see the Technology Update).

Using Self-Management Skills

Self-assessments and medical exams done regularly can help you determine if you need help with various health problems. Just as the fitness assessments you completed earlier helped you build a profile that will help you improve your fitness, regular self-assessments can help you identify and prevent common health problems. Regular medical exams that include the tests outlined in Table 1 as well as those described in other sections of this Concept will help you identify problems that can be treated and cured with early diagnosis.

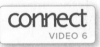

Staying current with new health information can help you identify and get treatment for health problems. Building knowledge about various health problems changes rapidly as new methods of treatment and prevention become

Technology Update

Drivers of COVID-19 Vaccine Development

The rapid development, evaluation, and release of vaccines to combat COVID-19 were amazing scientific and technological feats that required coordination and collaboration between researchers, pharmaceutical companies, and public health agencies. However, the work was also dependent on innovative technology that had been refined and tested in research studies over many years. The efficient application of this technology and the streamlined process of clinical testing document the importance of science to medicine and public health.

Did the rapid development of vaccines influence your perceptions of the importance of medical and public health research?

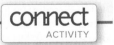

available. The information provided in this edition will get you started but, because new information is rapidly accumulating, it is important to learn ways to stay current on health topics. Information presented in the Concept on consumerism will help you develop skills for making good health, wellness, and fitness decisions.

Adhering to sound medical advice is important for disease prevention and treatment. Many conditions described in this Concept, especially cancer and diabetes, can be managed or cured with early diagnosis and proper treatment. Numerous people ignore early warning signs or symptoms, hoping that problems go away on their own. Some people fear disease and avoid medical advice because of this fear. An important key to good health is to note any irregularities in your health and to seek expert advice when needed. Establishing a regular habit of getting scheduled checkups and/or health screens is part of a healthy lifestyle because it helps ensure that your health is where it should be. Periodic checks can also help detect early signs of heart disease, cancer, diabetes, and other health threats, and this allows for more effective treatment. These checks become increasingly important as you age because people become vulnerable to a wider array of chronic conditions.

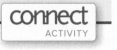

Strategies for Action: Lab Information

A risk questionnaire can help you identify your personal risk for diseases such as cancer. In Lab 22A you will have the opportunity to assess your cancer risk. Knowing your current risk level can be of value as you consult with your health-care professional as suggested in Table 1.

Self-assessments can be effective screening tools, but you need to follow up with a health-care provider if positive results are present. In Lab 22B you will learn to do self-exams to help you screen for breast and testicular cancer. A skin self-exam using the ABCDE rule is also advised. Home self-evaluation kits are now available for colorectal cancer screening. If irregularities are found, follow-up consultation with a health-care provider is essential.

connect ACTIVITY

Suggested Resources and Readings

The websites for the following sources can be accessed by searching online for the organization, program, or title listed. Specific scientific references are available at the end of this edition of *Concepts of Fitness and Wellness.*

- Alzheimer's Association. Types of Dementia.
- American Academy of Dermatologists. Skin Cancer Awareness: SPOT Skin Cancer.
- American Cancer Society. Guidelines for the Early Detection of Cancer.
- American Diabetes Association. Our 60-Second Type 2 Diabetes Risk Test.
- American Diabetes Association. *Understanding Diabetes.* (pdf)
- Centers for Disease Control and Prevention:
  - Alzheimer's Disease and Related Dementias.
  - Cancer: Screening Tests.
  - COVID-19: Contact Tracing.
  - COVID-19: How to Protect Yourself & Others.
  - Learn about Mental Illness.
- National Alliance on Mental Health. Depression.
- National Alliance on Mental Illness. Mental Illness Fact Sheets.
- National Institutes of Health. Menopausal Hormone Therapy Information.
- U.S. Food and Drug Administration:
  - FDA Proposes New Safety Measures for Indoor Tanning Devices: The Facts.
  - Sunscreen: How to Help Protect Your Skin from the Sun.
  - Tips to Stay Safe in the Sun: From Sunscreen to Sunglasses.
- U.S. Preventive Services Task Force. Browse Information for Consumers.
- U.S. Preventive Services Task Force. (2020, October 27). *U.S. Preventive Services Task Force Issues Draft Recommendation on Screening for Colorectal Cancer.* (pdf)

Lab 22A Determining Your Cancer Risk

Name	**Section**	**Date**

Purpose: To become aware of your risk for various types of cancer.

Procedures

1. Answer the questions in the six-part questionnaire for the various forms of cancer.
2. Record the number of "yes" answers for each form of cancer in the Results section.
3. Use Chart 1 to determine ratings and record the ratings in the Results section.
4. Answer the questions in the Conclusions and Implications section.

Results: Place an X over your answer to each question.

Skin Cancer Risk Factors

Do you frequently work or play in the sun for long periods?	Yes	No
Do you work or have you worked near industrial exposure (coal mine, radioactivity)?	Yes	No
Do you have a family history of skin cancer?	Yes	No
Do you have fair skin?	Yes	No

Lung Cancer Risk Factors

Do you smoke?	Yes	No
Do you work or have you worked near industrial exposure (coal mine, radioactivity)?	Yes	No
Do you have a family history of lung cancer?	Yes	No
Do you work in a place that allows smoking, such as a bar, or live in a home with smokers?	Yes	No

Colon-Rectal Cancer Risk Factors

Do you eat poorly, abuse alcohol, or smoke?	Yes	No
Are you African American or over 50 years of age?	Yes	No
Do you have a family history of colon or rectal cancer?	Yes	No
Have you noticed blood in your stool?	Yes	No

Breast Cancer Risk Factors

Do you have a family history of breast cancer?	Yes	No
Are you sedentary, do you eat poorly, or do you abuse alcohol?	Yes	No
Are you a female over 35 who has not had children?	Yes	No
Have you ever detected lumps or cysts in your breasts?	Yes	No

Uterine/Cervical Cancer Risk Factors* (Females)

Do you regularly have bleeding between periods?	Yes	No
Is your body-fat level high?	Yes	No
Did you have early intercourse and multiple sexual partners?	Yes	No
Have you had viral infections of the vagina, such as HPV?	Yes	No

Prostate Cancer Risk Factors (Males)

Do you eat a high-fat or low-fiber diet?	Yes	No
Are you a male over 50 years of age or African American?	Yes	No
Have you had a regular PSA test?	Yes	No
Has a digital rectal exam shown an enlargement of the prostate?	Yes	No

*Because of the personal nature of several questions, do not record results if turned in to an instructor.

Cancer Type	Score	Rating
Skin		
Breast (females)		
Lung		
Uterine/cervical (females)*		
Colon-rectal		
Prostate (males)		

*Do not record results if handed in to an instructor.

Chart 1 Cancer Risk Ratings

Rating	Score
High risk	4
Relatively high risk	3
Lower risk	2
Low risk	0–1

Conclusions and Implications: In several sentences, discuss the type or types of cancer for which you are at greatest risk and why. Also, discuss the lifestyles you could modify to reduce your risk.

Lab 22B Breast and Testicular Self-Exams

Name	**Section**	**Date**

Purpose: To learn to do breast or testicular self-exams.

Procedures

1. If you are female, read the procedures for breast self-exams. *Note:* Males should also be aware of abnormal lumps in their breasts.
2. If you are male, read the procedures for testicular self-exams.
3. After reading the directions, perform the self-exam. If you find lumps or nodules, contact a physician.
4. This procedure should be done monthly. The breast exam is best done a day or two after the end of menstrual flow. For this lab, it can be done at any time.
5. It is not necessary to record your results here. Do answer the questions in the Conclusions and Implications section.

Lying Breast Self-Exam (Males and Females)

1. Lie down with one arm behind your head. You can more easily detect lumps when lying as compared to standing or sitting because when lying the breast tissue is spread more evenly (see illustration).

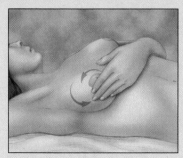

Brian Evans/Science Source

2. With the tips of the middle three fingers (see illustration) of the hand opposite the one behind your head, feel for lumps in the breast on the side of the raised arm. Use a circular pattern with the fingers. The large arrows illustrate the circular pattern but should be done with overlapping, *dime-sized,* circular motions of the finger pads to feel the breast tissue (see illustration).
3. Identify the spot for the overlapping, dime-sized, circular motions and feel for lumps using three levels of pressure. First apply light pressure to feel for lumps closest to the skin. Then apply medium pressure to feel for lumps deeper below the skin. Finally, to find lumps near the ribs and chest cavity, apply firm pressure. Then move to another spot and repeat the same procedure, applying all three levels of pressure. A firm ridge in the lower curve of each breast is normal. If you have questions about this procedure and how hard to press, talk with your doctor or medical professional.
4. To ensure full coverage of each breast, examine the entire area from your side up and to the middle of the sternum (breastbone) and from the clavicle (collarbone) down to the ribs below the breast.

5. Repeat the exam on the other breast, using the finger pads of the opposite hand.

Standing Breast Self-Exam (Females)

1. Stand in front of a mirror. Press down firmly on your hips with your hands. Look for any changes of size, shape, contour, or dimpling or redness or scaliness of the nipple or breast skin. (Pressing down on the hips contracts the chest wall muscles and enhances any breast changes.)
2. Examine each underarm with your arm slightly raised, so that you can easily feel in this area. Raising your arm straight up (too high) tightens the tissue in this area and makes it harder to examine.

Testicular Self-Exam (Males)

1. Using both hands, grasp one testicle between the thumb and first finger.
2. Roll the testicle gently with the thumb and first finger. Look and feel for lumps or rounded bumps as well as for changes in size, shape, and consistency of testicles.
3. Examine the other testicle using the same procedure.
4. If you find any of the symptoms (see number 2), consult a physician. The symptoms may not be associated with disease, but this can be determined only by a physician.

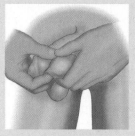

Monica Schroeder/Science Source

Conclusions and Implications: In several sentences, discuss the effectiveness of the procedure you performed. Do you think the directions provided were adequate for you to perform the self-exam effectively? Do you think you will perform this self-exam on a regular basis? Do you believe the screening procedures described in the lab are effective? Why or why not? What could be done to motivate you and others to do regular self-exams?

Additional Self-Exam Information

Several national health agencies maintain websites that include detailed breast and testicular self-exam information. These sites contain both written and pictorial descriptions of both self-exam procedures. For more information, visit the sites listed below.

American Cancer Society
www.cancer.org

Mayo Clinic
www.mayohealth.org

National Cancer Institute
www.nci.nih.gov

Early detection is critical for effective cancer treatment. The ACS notes that a "breast self-exam is an option for females starting in their 20s. Females should be told about the benefits and limitations of BSE. Females should report any changes in how their breasts look or feel to a health expert right away." Males should also be aware of changes in breast tissue. The ACS indicates that many physicians recommend a BSE each month. For those who do a BSE, it is wise to review the technique with a physician or medical professional. According to the ACS, finding a lump in the testicles at an early stage is important. It recommends a regular testicular exam by a physician and indicates that many doctors recommend testicular self-exams.

Body Mechanics and Care of the Back

LEARNING OBJECTIVES

After completing the study of this Concept, you will be able to:

▶ Identify and describe the anatomy and function of the spine.

▶ Identify and describe the anatomy and function of core muscles.

▶ Clarify the causes and consequences of back and neck pain.

▶ Describe how to prevent and rehabilitate back and neck problems.

▶ Explain why posture is important to back and neck health and ways to improve posture.

▶ Explain why good body mechanics are important to back and neck health and ways to improve body mechanics.

▶ Indicate the exercise guidelines for back and neck health and ways to implement the guidelines.

▶ Name questionable exercises and safer alternatives.

▶ Determine self-assessments to identify potential back, neck, and posture problems and risks, and plan a self-monitored personal program that includes exercises for reducing these problems.

The health, integrity, and function of the back and neck are influenced by modifiable as well as nonmodifiable factors. Maintaining a healthy back and neck can be attained by using good posture, good body mechanics, and safe exercise technique.

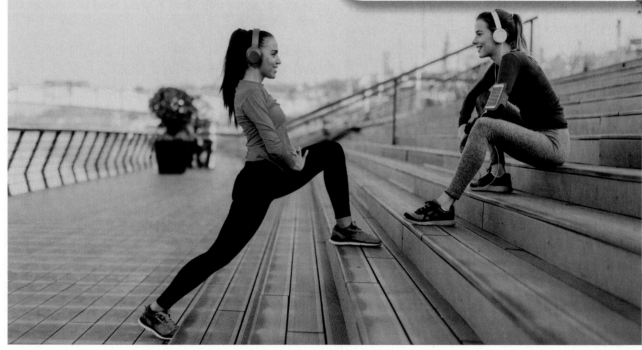

Anatomy and Function of the Spine

The spinal column is arranged for movement. The bones that make up the spine are called vertebrae. There are 33 vertebrae in the spine, and most are separated from one another by an **intervertebral disc** (see Figure 1). The vertebrae are divided into three main regions commonly referred to as cervical (neck), thoracic (upper back), and lumbar (low back). The fused vertebrae that form the tailbone are called the sacrum and coccyx. The connections among the vertebrae of the cervical, thoracic, and lumbar spine allow the trunk to move in complex ways. The spine is capable of flexion (forward bending), extension (backward bending), side bending, and rotation, but functionally, these movements often occur in combination. For example, in executing a tennis serve, the spine both extends and rotates. The spine is at risk for injury when movements are performed repetitively, performed beyond a joint's healthy range of motion, or performed under conditions of heavy or inefficient lifting.

The spinal column has an important role in bearing loads and protecting the back and neck from injury. The widest portion of each vertebra articulates with the intervertebral disc to form a strong pillar of support extending from the skull to the pelvis. The unique structure of the intervertebral discs is critical in distributing force and absorbing shock. The bony structure of the spine bears loads and provides protection to the spinal cord and spinal nerves. Poor posture and poor body mechanics can damage discs and vertebrae, resulting in pain and disability.

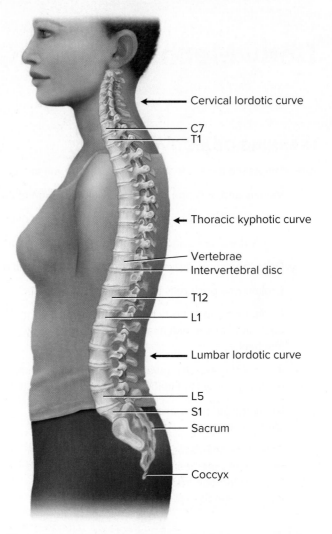

Cervical lordotic curve

C7
T1

Thoracic kyphotic curve

Vertebrae
Intervertebral disc

T12
L1

Lumbar lordotic curve

L5
S1
Sacrum

Coccyx

Figure 1 ▶ Curvatures of the spinal column.

Anatomy and Function of the Core Musculature

The core is composed of an integrated series of muscles. There is no definitive list of muscles belonging to the core. The core can be described as including as few as 6 or as many as 20 different muscle groups, depending on the source. Regardless, the muscles of the core all share common anatomical traits: their location and attachment to the spine, pelvis, or rib cage. Conceptually, the core can be described as a three-dimensional, cylindrical area of the body that encompasses the spine, abdominal cavity, and the body's center of gravity (see Figure 2). Its anatomical boundaries generally include the abdominal muscles (in front), the low back muscles (in back), the diaphragm (across the top), and the pelvic floor and hip muscles (across the bottom). However, it may also be described in broader terms and include other trunk muscles that have attachments to the shoulder or pelvic girdle.

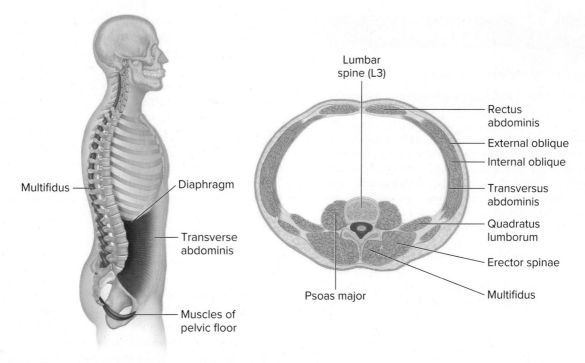

Figure 2 ▶ Cross section showing layers of core musculature.

The core muscles work together to provide the spine with optimal support and function. The core muscles play a key role in improving spinal stability, improving efficiency of movement, and aiding in force transmission. They help you walk, lift heavy objects, swing a bat, or kick a soccer ball. A strong core is believed to help protect the back from harm, improve daily function, and enhance athletic performance. Some describe core stability as the control of movement around a "neutral" postural zone, where the physiological stress and strain on the spine are minimized (e.g., squatting with good body mechanics). Others expand the definition of core stability to include the efficient and coordinated transfer of loads along the kinetic chain (e.g., the coordinated and fluid movement of legs, trunk, and arms during the act of swinging a golf club). The core muscles are essentially active during almost all functional movements.

The various core muscles can be categorized based on function. The core includes both superficial muscles that help move the trunk as well as deeply located muscles responsible for controlling intersegmental movements of the spine. They are often categorized 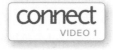 as core mobilizer muscles, core stabilizer muscles, or core transfer muscles, depending on their primary function. The distinctions are described in the following sections.

- **Core mobilizer muscles** typically produce concentric (shortening) contractions in order to generate movement of the trunk. Common examples of core mobilizers include the rectus abdominis (abdominal muscle) and erector spinae (back muscles). These muscles are capable of bending the trunk forward or backward when they contract. Examples of exercises that utilize the core mobilizers include the trunk curl-up and back extension exercises.

- **Core stabilizer muscles** use isometric (holding) and eccentric (braking) contractions to provide stiffness and stability to the spine. The stabilizers keep the individual spinal segments in "neutral" alignment and collectively provide a corset-like stiffness to the trunk. Core activation actually begins in anticipation and in preparation for movement, with muscles of the core contracting before those of the arms or legs. Examples of muscles that provide a role in core stabilization include the lumbar multifidus (the deepest back muscle) and the transverse abdominis (the deepest abdominal muscle). An example of an exercise that utilizes core stabilization is the plank exercise.

- **Core transfer muscles** transfer force from one region of the body to another. The premise is that power comes from a stable foundation. Thus, these muscles help stabilize the trunk in order to generate strong movements of the arms

Intervertebral Disc Spinal discs; cushions of cartilage between the bodies of the vertebrae. Each disc consists of a fibrous outer ring (annulus fibrosus) and a pulpy center (nucleus pulposus).

Core Mobilizer Muscles Superficial core muscles that produce trunk motion and also aid in stabilization.

Core Stabilizer Muscles Deep core muscles that provide stiffness and stability to the spine.

Core Transfer Muscles Superficial core muscles that help integrate trunk and limb function.

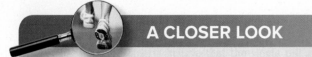

Functional Movement Tests

"Functional fitness" and "functional movements" are popular topics in the fitness world. The notion is that functional fitness training techniques better prepare the body to handle the forces, postures, and actions involved in real-life activities and sports and ultimately lead to reduced risk of injuries. A prominent assessment protocol called the Functional Movement Screen (FMS) has been widely marketed and used in fitness centers to try to predict potential risks for injury. Although identifying the potential for injuries before they occur is certainly appealing (and potentially important), the evidence in the literature has not supported the effectiveness of the FMS assessment. This does not mean that functional fitness isn't important, only that the FMS assessment doesn't presently work to screen for injury risk. (See link in Suggested Resources and Readings.)

Does it surprise you that assessments like this are promoted without sound evidence that they work?

connect
ACTIVITY

or legs. Examples of muscles involved in force transfer include trunk muscles with attachments to the shoulders or hips (e.g., latissimus dorsi, pectoral, and gluteus maximus muscles). An example of an exercise utilizing core force transfer would be the deadlift in weightlifting.

While this classification scheme is helpful to understanding the basic roles of the core muscles, core function is actually far more complex. For instance, muscles may serve multiple functions or work together in an integrated fashion rather than in an isolated role of "mover" or "stabilizer."

Causes and Consequences of Back and Neck Pain

Although back and neck pain are common, many cases stem from lifestyle choices or life experiences. Back and neck pain are common in today's society, with statistics suggesting that nearly 80 percent of Americans will experience an episode of low back pain sometime in life. Back pain is second only to headache as a common medical complaint, and an estimated 30–70 percent of the population experiences recurring back problems. The original cause (or causes) of back and neck pain is (are) often hard to identify since damage can build over time. Although back and neck problems can result from an acute injury (e.g., a diving accident or car accident), most are caused by accumulated stresses over a lifetime. These factors include the avoidable effects of poor posture and body mechanics as well as

questionable exercises that put the back at risk. (Exercises to avoid are discussed later in this Concept.)

To reduce risk for back pain, reduce the risk factors that you have control over. Modifiable risk factors (factors you can change) include regular heavy labor, use of vibrational tools, routines of prolonged sitting, smoking, a hypokinetic lifestyle, and obesity. A number of health conditions can also contribute to back problems, including depression, anxiety, cancer, infections, and some visceral diseases (kidney, pelvic organs). You may have some control over these health conditions that contribute to back pain. Nonmodifiable risk factors include a family history of joint disease, age, sex, genetics, congenital anomalies (including some forms of **scoliosis**), and direct trauma (e.g., a fall or rough athletic activity when young). Lab 23A provides a questionnaire for assessing your potential risk for back and neck pain.

The nervous system and various pain-sensitive structures contribute to back pain. Back pain can result from direct or indirect causes. Direct causes are typically the result of mechanical trauma to tissues in or around the spine. Damage to structures of the spinal column can occur slowly over time (degenerative changes) or from a single traumatic event (acute injury). Pain from back problems can arise from a variety of sources including the spine, discs, muscles, and nerves. Indirect causes of back pain can include local cellular changes in and around the injured tissues (e.g., presence of pain-sensitive chemicals) or changes in the type of messages being generated by the nervous system. With chronic pain, the nervous system may continuously resend pain signals in abnormal feedback loops that enhance or maintain the perception of pain, even when the original cause or problem is corrected.

The integrity of the back and neck are jeopardized by excessive stress and strain. Forces are constantly at work to bend, twist, shear, compress, or lengthen tissues of the body. Stress on these tissues may eventually create strain, a change in the tissue's size or dimension. Healthy tissues typically return to their normal state once the force is removed. Injury occurs when excessive stress and strain prevent the tissue from returning to its normal state. A number of specific contributors to stress and strain on the back are listed described in the following sections.

- *Poor posture can cause body segments to experience stress and strain.* When body segments are in poor alignment (e.g., slouching or forward head positions), the muscles in the back and neck must work hard to compensate. This creates excessive stress and strain in the affected area(s). Over time, tension in these muscles can lead to myofascial trigger points, which can cause headache or **referred pain** in the face, scalp, shoulder, arm, and chest. The chronic stress from poor alignment can also lead to other postural deviations and degenerative changes in the neck and back.

- *Bad body mechanics contribute to stress and strain on the spine.* Activities that involve heavy lifting, bending, or twisting present risks, as do repetitive motions and those that involve vibrations. The lumbar vertebrae and the sacrum are most vulnerable to this type of injury due to the significant weight they support and the thinner ligaments at this level.

- *Being overweight or obese increases the risk of back pain.* Obesity and overweight status are hard on the body because they overload the bones, discs, tendons, and ligaments. Added wear and tear on joint surfaces can lead to osteoarthritis. Postural changes accompany weight gain and create additional stress and strain on joints. For example, a large protruding abdomen often causes forward tipping of the pelvis and excessive arching of the low back that can lead to back pain. Studies confirm that the risk of back pain increases exponentially with higher levels of body mass, so keeping a healthy body weight is an important prevention strategy.

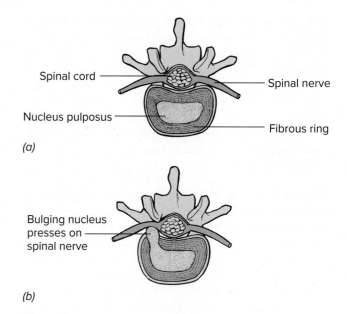

(a)

(b)

Figure 3 ▶ Normal disc (*a*) and herniated disc (*b*).

Some exercises and movements can produce microtrauma, which can lead to back and neck pain. Most people are familiar with acute injuries, such as ankle sprains. These injuries are associated with immediate onset of pain and swelling. **Microtrauma** is a "silent injury"—a subtle form of injury that results from accumulated damage over time. It can result from repetitive motion, repeated forceful exertion, long-term vibration, or working with awkward postures. When microtrauma occurs as the result of activities at work, it is often referred to by the medical terms *repetitive stress injury (RSI)* or *cumulative trauma disorder (CTD)*. One common example is carpal tunnel syndrome, a painful irritation of the median nerve at the wrist, often brought on by repetitive motion of the wrist during long and extended periods of typing, assembly line tasks, or construction work.

Microtrauma can also result from the repetitive performance of unsafe exercises or contraindicated movements. For example, regular performance of full deep knee squats or full neck circles may irritate the joint surfaces and eventually cause knee or neck pain. Repeated overhead lifting with excessive loads can irritate and damage the rotator cuff tendon of the shoulder. The initial wear and tear from microtrauma is not typically noticed but, over many years, microscopic changes occur in the joint. Examples include swelling, fibrosis of the synovial lining, abnormal thickening of the surrounding joint capsule, calcifications in the tendons, and thinning and roughening of the cartilage cushioning the joint surfaces. Because these changes are unseen and often unfelt, the offending exercise or activity is often viewed as harmless. However, later in life the effects from accumulated microtrauma become more apparent, manifesting in tendonitis, bursitis, arthritis, or nerve compression. Chances are when the injury reaches a painful stage, the cause is not identified and instead is attributed to aging.

The lumbar intervertebral discs are particularly susceptible to injury and herniation. The intervertebral discs located between the vertebrae of the spine are composed of a tire-like outer ring (annulus fibrosus) surrounding a gel-like center (nucleus pulposus). The greatest risk for injury to the discs occurs during excessive loading and twisting motions of the spine. Most people think that disc injuries occur from an acute injury, but herniation typically reflects a degenerative process that takes place over time. With repeated microtrauma, small tears begin to occur in the inner fibers of the annulus. The nucleus begins to move outward (**herniated disc**), much like toothpaste moving within a squeezed tube. Disc herniation is termed *incomplete* or *contained* as long as the migrating edge of the nucleus remains within the fibers of the annulus. As damage continues (often the result of years of cumulative microtrauma), the annular fibers may reach a point of rupture at their periphery (see Figure 3). At this point (termed *disc extrusion*), the nucleus pulposus moves into the space around the spinal cord or nerve root and herniation is termed *complete* or *noncontained*. A noncontained or complete disc herniation can irritate nerve tissue causing pain, numbness, or weakness in an arm or leg.

Scoliosis A curvature of the spine that produces a sideways curve with some rotation; while typically mild, this condition can sometimes be painful.

Referred Pain Pain that appears to be located in one area, though it originates in another area.

Microtrauma Injury so small it is not detected at the time it occurs.

Herniated Disc The soft center part of the spinal disc that squeezes out through a small tear in the outer boundary of the disc and leaks into the surrounding tissue; also called prolapse.

The risk of disc herniation is greater for younger adults. Disc herniation is frequently listed as a cause of back pain, but studies show that only 5–10 percent of persons with herniated discs experience pain. The reason is that pain is often not experienced until complete herniation occurs. Pain is felt as the nuclear material begins to press on pain-sensitive structures in its path. Interestingly, the risk for disc herniation is greatest for individuals in their 30s and 40s. Risk decreases with age as the disc degenerates and becomes less soft and less pliable.

Degenerative disc disease is a common part of aging and a source of back pain. Most adults tend to get shorter with age and this is attributable to degenerative changes within the vertebral bodies and discs. Specific changes include a loss of flexibility and a flattening of the discs as a result of lost water content. This reduces the space between vertebrae and increases the compressive forces on the small facet joints and the large vertebral bodies. The rubbing between the facets may cause an abnormal bony growth called a bone spur. Likewise, excess motion between spinal segments may cause thickening of ligaments lining the spinal canal. Bone spurs and thickened ligaments may lead to stenosis, or narrowing of the canal around the nerve roots or spinal cord, increasing the likelihood of nerve impingement, which then can contribute to back pain and disability (see Figure 4). In contrast to disc herniation, the risk of pain from degenerative disc disease increases with age due to accumulated wear and tear on our spines.

Injury to the spine negatively affects the function of the core musculature. One of the more important core muscles, the lumbar multifidus, is adversely affected by back pain. In the healthy individual, the multifidus is believed to be responsible for providing more than two-thirds of the dynamic rigidity to the lumbar spine and serves an important role in proprioception and kinesthetic awareness. Studies demonstrate that with low back pain, the muscle becomes more inhibited and

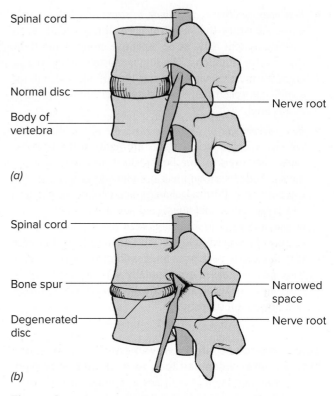

(a)

(b)

Figure 4 ▶ Normal disc (*a*) and degenerated disc with nerve impingement and arthritic changes (*b*).

exhibits decreased levels of activation and increased fatigability. It is also prone to atrophy and becomes infiltrated with fatty deposits with lack of use. Research studies have shown specific spinal stabilization exercises to be effective in reversing some of the adverse changes to the multifidus, including positive gains in cross-sectional area/muscle bulk and improved neural recruitment. Participation in a program of core training exercise has also been shown to improve pain tolerance and function. Rehabilitation of the lumbar multifidus appears critical in the recovery period following back pain.

Medical intervention is sometimes needed for neck or back pain. Most cases of back pain resolve spontaneously, with 70 percent having no symptoms at the end of 3 weeks and 90 percent recovered after 2 months. However, medical approaches have been shown to speed up recovery from acute back or neck pain and to improve pain tolerance and function in chronic cases. Conservative treatment typically involves the use of anti-inflammatory medications, muscle relaxants, traction, or electrical stimulation. It can involve application of heat or cold (e.g. cryotherapy) and may also include therapeutic exercise, massage, and joint mobilization. When this treatment is unsuccessful, referral to an alternative therapy, such as acupuncture, or to a pain clinic for steroidal anti-inflammatory injections may occur. As a last measure, surgery may be needed for removal of a herniated portion of a disc.

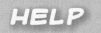

HELP **Health is available to Everyone for a Lifetime, and it's Personal**

Is Back Pain in Your Future?

According to the National Institutes of Health, the most common medical problem in the United States is back pain, which is very often caused by degeneration of the discs in the spine. Preventive measures include maintaining a healthy weight over the lifespan, using proper lifting techniques, and engaging in regular exercise, particularly strength training and flexibility exercises.

What steps are you taking today to help prevent back problems later in life?

connect ACTIVITY

Prevention and Rehabilitation of Back and Neck Problems

Exercise is a frequently prescribed treatment for back or neck pain. The integrity of individual vertebral segments of the spine is often compromised with injury to the back or neck. One or more components of the passive restraint system (ligaments, discs, vertebrae, or joints) may be damaged, creating a weak link in the stabilization system. In addition, optimal function of the dynamic and neural control systems is often adversely affected by injury. This may make a specific segment of the spine more vulnerable to delayed healing or further injury. Core training may enhance stability to the injured area by improving the function of the dynamic and neural control systems. Core training programs are also effective in treating low back pain. Studies have shown significant improvements in pain level and functional status following a program of spinal stabilization exercises, but positive results have also been obtained from more general exercise interventions. Future research may help identify subsets of people who may benefit from one type of exercise program over another.

Both resistance and aerobic exercises have been found to be helpful in treating many types of chronic pain. Exercises that are selected specifically to help correct pain-related problems are classified as therapeutic. These exercises are aimed at correcting the underlying cause of back or neck pain by strengthening weak muscles, stretching short ones, and improving circulation to and nourishment of tissues of the body. Both therapeutic and health-related fitness exercises may be considered preventive if done regularly, and with the appropriate FIT guidelines.

Core stabilization training refers to a variety of neuromuscular control exercises aimed at improving core muscle function. *Core stabilization training* is a popular buzz phrase found in both clinical and fitness-related settings. The phrase refers to a wide variety of interventions designed to improve the strength, endurance, and dynamic control of the core musculature. Core exercises can range from the static plank and dynamic curl-up exercise, to functional movements like performing medicine ball lifts in conjunction with active squatting. Beginner-level core stability exercises focus on promoting neuromuscular control and improving body awareness. For example, isometric contractions are first aimed at keeping the spine in "neutral" alignment since this typically requires active engagement of the core stabilizer muscles. As participants gain improved strength and control, exercises can be made more challenging by introducing graduated movements of the arms and legs while maintaining this "neutral" posture of the back. An example is tensing the abdominal muscles while raising one arm and the opposite leg from an all-fours position. This involves engagement of the overall core musculature since it combines mobilization and stabilization.

Use of specific core stabilization exercises can reduce low back pain and functional disability. In the clinical or rehabilitation setting, core training is used to help reduce pain, assist in recovery from injury, and improve function. In fitness and sports enhancement settings, it is used with the goal of improving core strength and athletic performance. The effectiveness of core stabilization exercises has been evaluated most frequently in terms of how well they reduce pain and disability. Core stabilization has been shown to reduce both pain and functional disability in those with low back pain, particularly those with pain lasting longer than 3 months. A recent systematic review demonstrated that stabilization-specific exercises are superior to a general exercise program in reducing pain and disability. However, other studies report no differences between the two forms of intervention. A challenge in this line of research is that there is little consensus regarding the most effective exercise approach.

While core training seems to provide benefits to some, many people continue to suffer from low back pain. Some experts suggest that not all subjects with back pain benefit from the same type of exercise. Future research may help identify subsets of people who may benefit from one type of exercise program over another. Other experts recommend a multimodal approach to treating back pain, one that trains the body to work as an integrated whole using functional movement patterns. Additional research is needed to identify

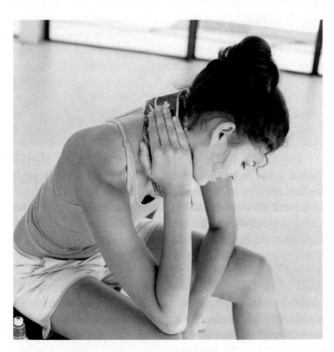

Following recommended preventive strategies can reduce the likelihood of back and neck pain.
George Doyle/Getty Images

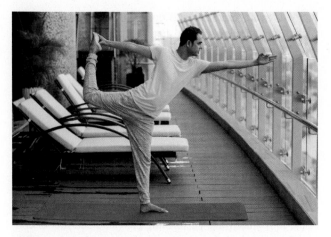

Movement disciplines like yoga can promote body awareness and contribute to back health; however some movements may be contraindicated and may not be appropriate for all.
Mangostar/Shutterstock

the most successful methods for preventing and treating chronic low back pain.

Use of mind–body exercise programs, such as yoga, tai chi, and Pilates, can reduce low back pain and functional disability. Muscular exercises can provide benefits for some individuals with low back pain, but the overall effectiveness is rather modest. A possible explanation for the small effect is that exercise-specific treatments do not address other psychosocial correlates of back pain. Exercise programs that incorporate education, breath control, and cognitive components (body awareness, relaxation) may actually be better suited at reducing pain and disability than exercise alone. Both the American College of Physicians and the American Pain Society have supported the use of mind–body exercises in treating chronic low back pain. Yoga and tai chi are theorized to affect back and neck pain by improving body awareness, proprioception, posture, and balance. Studies indicate that nearly 43 percent of those with low back pain who participated in yoga or tai chi found the exercises beneficial. Tai chi has also been shown to reduce depression, a common psychosocial outcome in those with chronic pain.

Correcting muscle imbalances can help address many postural and back problems. If the muscles on one side of a joint are stronger than the muscles on the opposite side, the body part is pulled in the direction of the stronger muscles. Corrective exercises are usually designed to strengthen the long, weak muscles and to stretch the short, strong ones in order to have equal pull in both directions. For example, people with lumbar lordosis may need to strengthen the abdominals and gluteal muscles and also stretch the lower back and hip flexor muscles.

Good Posture Is Important for Back and Neck Health

Posture is important for both health and wellness. Posture is critically important for back and neck health, but there is no universally accepted definition of optimal **posture**. Good posture is unique to each individual and dependent on variations in body structure. Most people know good posture when they see it but often have trouble perceiving their own posture. This has important implications because posture is an important part of nonverbal communication. The first impression a person makes is usually a visual one, and good posture can help convey an impression of alertness, confidence, and vitality. Thus, posture makes important contributions to both health and wellness.

Proper posture allows the body segments to be balanced. Ideal posture is one where forces acting across the body do no harm to the integrity of local body segments. The individual segments of the human body (i.e., the head, shoulder girdle, pelvic girdle, rib cage, and spine) are aligned in a vertical column and are supported by muscles and ligaments. Proper posture helps maintain an even distribution of force across the body, improve shock absorption, and minimize the degree of active muscle tension required to maintain upright posture. When viewed from the side, three normal curvatures of the spine are present, causing the vertebral column to appear S-shaped. These curvatures are created by the **lordotic (inward) curve** of the cervical and lumbar spines and the **kyphotic (outward) curve** of the thoracic spine (see Figure 1). The curves help balance forces on the body and minimize muscle tension. They are also responsible for humans' unique ability to walk upright on two legs while maintaining a forward gaze. The degree of curvature is influenced by the tilt of the pelvis. A forward pelvic tilt increases curvature in the neck and lower back, whereas a backward pelvic tilt flattens the lower back. The most desirable position is a **neutral spine** in which the spine has neither too much nor too little lordotic curvature. The forces across the spine are balanced, and muscular tension is at a minimum. Specific guidelines for standing and sitting posture are described in the following sections.

- When *standing*, the head should be centered over the trunk with forward gaze, the shoulders should be down and back but relaxed, with the chest high and the abdomen flat. The spine should have gentle curves when viewed from the side but should be straight when seen from the back. When the pelvis is tilted properly, the pubis falls directly underneath the lower tip of the sternum. The knees should be relaxed, with the kneecaps pointed straight ahead. The feet should point straight or slightly outward, and the weight should be borne over the heel, on the outside border of the sole, and across the ball of the foot and toes (see Figure 5).

- When *sitting*, the head should be centered over the trunk, the shoulders down and back. If one is using a computer, the screen should be positioned at arm's reach from your

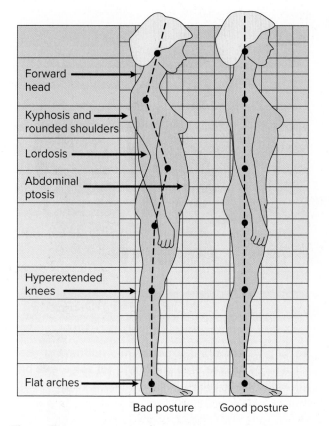

Figure 5 ▶ Comparison of bad and good posture.

Labels on figure (left to right): Forward head, Kyphosis and rounded shoulders, Lordosis, Abdominal ptosis, Hyperextended knees, Flat arches; Bad posture, Good posture

position of uneven loading, increasing pressure on the facet joints of the vertebrae. Over time, degenerative changes may occur, including a narrowing of the openings where spinal nerves exit, thus increasing risk for pain.

- *Flat back posture*, on the other hand, occurs when the pelvis is tipped backward from a position of neutral tilt. With this posture, the lumbar spine is flexed, the lower back muscles are in a lengthened (weak) position, and the hamstring muscles are shortened and tight. A reduced lumbar curvature increases pressure on the intervertebral bodies and decreases shock absorption capabilities. Relative differences in flexibility between tight hamstring and long trunk muscles may also increase risk for injury. Laws of physics demonstrate that the body takes the path of least resistance during a chain of movement (e.g., forward bending), with the most flexible segment (i.e., the back) providing a greater contribution to the total range of movement. It follows that regions of greater movement will experience greater tissue strain. In the case of flat back posture, tight hamstrings may limit the contribution of hip motion during forward bending tasks, thus predisposing the lower back to become the fulcrum for movement and the site of injury.

Poor posture can contribute to back and neck pain, but it also contributes to risks of injury. However, it is important to understand that static posture does not always predict dynamic posture. An example of this would be an older person who may be able to stand upright with good posture but, with walking, a forward stoop and lateral limp become apparent. Dynamic conditions typically place greater demands on the musculoskeletal system making it more difficult to control alignment, which increases the risk for injuries. Athletic trainers and coaches routinely evaluate dynamic posture in order to identify problems before injuries occur. For example, the risk of anterior cruciate ligament (ACL) injuries is more likely in individuals with poor dynamic posture of the lower leg. If a person's knee rolls inward excessively in the landing phase of a jump or drop test, it can indicate a greater risk for injury. Postural correction through improved dynamic control is warranted to then reduce the risk.

eyes or a little farther if using a large monitor. (The top of the screen should be 2 to 3 inches above the eyes.) The seat of the chair should be at an angle that allows the knees to be positioned slightly lower than the hips. The feet should be supported on the floor. Good seated posture decreases pressure within the discs of the lower back and reduces fatigue of lower back muscles. A large percentage of our day is spent sitting, so it is important to use good postural habits at work or when studying (see Figure 6).

Poor posture contributes to a variety of health problems. When posture deviates from neutral, weight distribution becomes uneven and tissues are at risk for injury. Examples of common postural deviations are described in Table 1 along with associated health problems. Two of those highlighted are lumbar lordosis (excessive curvature of the lower back) and flat back (reduced curvature of the lower back).

- *Lumbar lordosis posture* occurs when the pelvis is tipped forward from a position of neutral tilt. With this posture, the hip flexor muscles become shortened and tight while the abdominal muscles become weak and long (with a reduced ability to "hold" within inner range). This muscle imbalance shifts body segment alignment toward a

Posture The relationship among body parts, whether standing, lying, sitting, or moving. Good posture is the relationship among body parts that allows you to function most effectively, with the least expenditure of energy and with a minimal amount of stress and strain on the body.

Lordotic (Inward) Curve The normal inward curvature of the cervical and lumbar spine.

Kyphotic (Outward) Curve The normal outward curvature of the thoracic spine.

Neutral Spine Proper position of the spine to maintain a normal lordotic curve. The spine has neither too much nor too little lordotic curve.

Sitting

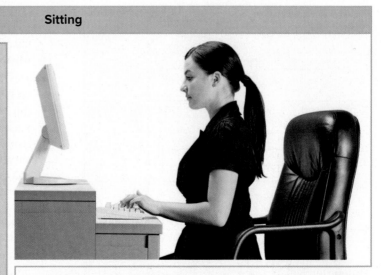

- Sit upright with eyes looking straight ahead, chest lifted, shoulders down and back, slight arch in lower back, knees slightly lower than hips, feet supported on a firm surface.
- If you cross your legs, alternate which leg is crossed on top.
- When sitting for longer periods of time, use chair with armrests, an adequate seat cushion, and lumbar support.
- When driving, adjust seat to allow easy reach of foot pedals with slight knee bend; recline seat to allow gentle arch in low back.
- Reading material should be elevated or supported at eye level.
- The office desk should be about 29 to 30 inches high for the average man and about 27 to 29 inches high for the average woman. The computer screen should be positioned at arm's reach from your eyes (or a little farther if using a large monitor) and slightly below eye level.

Elements of Good Posture

Standing

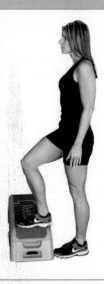

- Stand upright with forward gaze, shoulders down and back, chest raised, stomach pulled up and in, slight arch in the lower back, slight bend in the knees, feet shoulder width apart, and toes pointing straight ahead or slightly outward.
- If you stand with weight shifted to one side, alternate which leg you lean on.
- If you stand in one place for a prolonged time, prop one foot on small step stool.
- Height of work surface should be about 2 to 4 inches below the waist.

Lying

- Use a pillow between the knees when lying on your side and under the knees when lying on the back.
- Choose a pillow that supports the head and neck in neutral alignment.
- Avoid reading in bed.

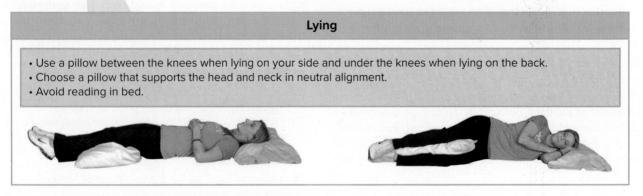

Figure 6 ▶ Characteristics of good posture for sitting, standing, and lying.

(Sitting): ©Jonathon Ross/Cutcaster; (Standing): ©Mark Ahn Creative Services; (Lying back) ©Mark Ahn Creative Services; (Lying side) ©Mark Ahn Creative Services

Table 1 ▶ Health Problems Associated with Poor Posture

Posture Problem	Definition	Health Problem
Forward head	The head aligned in front of the center of gravity	Headache, dizziness, and pain in the neck, shoulders, or arms
Kyphosis	Excessive curvature (flexion) in the upper back; also called humpback	Impaired respiration as a result of sunken chest and pain in the neck, shoulders, and arms
Lumbar lordosis	Excessive curvature (hyperextension) in the lower back (sway back), with a forward pelvic tilt	Back pain and/or injury, protruding abdomen, low back syndrome, and painful menstruation
Flat back	Reduced curvature in the lower back	Back pain, increased risk for injury due to reduced shock absorption
Abdominal ptosis	Excessive protrusion of abdomen	Back pain and/or injury, lordosis, low back syndrome, and painful menstruation
Hyperextended knees	The knees bent backward excessively	Greater risk for knee injury and excessive pelvic tilt (lordosis)
Pronated feet	The longitudinal arch of the foot flattened with increased pressure on inner aspect of foot	Decreased shock absorption, leading to foot, knee, and lower back pain

Correcting postural deviations begins with restoring adequate muscle fitness and muscle length. Lifestyle has a tremendous influence on posture, with most of us having a natural tendency to slouch when sitting and standing. We can correct 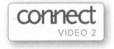 our posture with conscious effort; however, if poor posture is maintained for very long or very frequent periods of time, the body loses resiliency. Over time, muscles on one side of a joint or body segment can become shortened or tight while muscles on the opposite side can become lengthened and weak. Poor posture can also result following muscle injury. This may manifest itself in guarded postures or muscle dysfunction, which eventually leads to muscles on one side of the joint becoming inflexible due to facilitation and muscles on the opposite side becoming weak due to inhibition.

Improving posture can be challenging since it is determined by the body's structure and function, including passive elements (integrity of the joints), active elements (the muscles), and the neural system (signals from the nervous system). Postural correction can be achieved by improving body awareness, increasing flexibility of tight muscles, and improving strength of weak (inhibited) muscles. For example, a slouched posture with rounded and forward shoulders can be improved by elongating the pectoral (chest) and paraspinal (neck) muscles and strengthening muscles of the upper back. A lumbar lordosis posture can be improved by stretching the hip flexors and back extensors that keep the top of the pelvis tipped forward, followed by strengthening of the abdominal and gluteal muscles that help tip the pelvis backward (see Figure 7).

Awareness of posture is critical for prevention and treatment of back problems. Posture is largely maintained through the input of small sensors in our skin and joints that

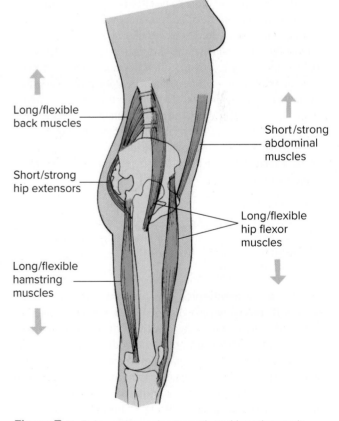

Long/flexible back muscles

Short/strong abdominal muscles

Short/strong hip extensors

Long/flexible hip flexor muscles

Long/flexible hamstring muscles

Figure 7 ▶ Balanced muscle strength and length permit good postural alignment.

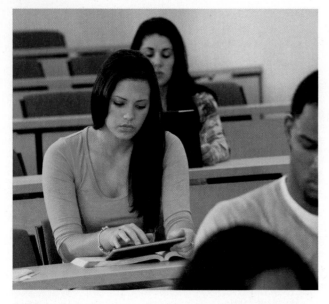

Taking a break when using a laptop or tablet helps reduce back and neck strain.

©Ariel Skelley/Blend Images LLC

reinforce our most frequent postures. Postural correction can be achieved by improving body awareness, increasing flexibility of tight muscles, and improving strength of weak (inhibited) muscles. However, in order to be effective, postural correction requires an ongoing use of body awareness and self-correction throughout the day. Studies have demonstrated that a focused stretching and strengthening program can improve posture only a little, at best. What is often missing in these interventions is the use of postural awareness. Poor posture must be corrected regularly in order to overcome the nervous system's memory of the faulty posture and to establish the improved postures as automatic. Both tai chi and yoga have been shown to be effective in improving dynamic postural control, perhaps in part related to the body awareness component of these mind–body disciplines.

Good Body Mechanics Are Important for Back and Neck Health

Proper body mechanics can prevent back and neck injury. Biomechanics is a discipline that applies mechanical laws and principles to study how the body performs more efficiently and with less energy. Good body mechanics, as applied to back care, implies maintaining a neutral spine during activities of daily living. A neutral spine maintains the normal curvature of the spine, thus allowing an optimal balance of forces across the spine, reducing compressive forces, and minimizing muscle tension. In the following sections, specific recommendations and examples of good body mechanics are provided for a variety of body positions.

Ergonomics is a discipline that uses biomechanical principles to develop tools and workplace settings that put the least amount of strain on the body. Many employers take an active interest in ergonomic principles, since repetitive motion injuries and other musculoskeletal conditions are the leading cause of work-related ill health. One application of ergonomics (also known as human factors engineering) is the design of effective workstations for computer users. Properly fitting desks and chairs and the effective positioning of computer screens and keyboards can minimize problems such as carpal tunnel syndrome.

Good lifting technique focuses on using the legs. The muscles of the legs are relatively large and strong compared with the back muscles. Likewise, the hip joint is well designed for motion. It is less likely to suffer the same amount of wear and tear as the smaller joints of the spine. 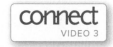 When lifting an object from the floor, straddle the object with a wide stance; squat down by hinging through the hips and bending the knees; maintain a slight arch to the lower back by sticking out the buttocks; test the load and get help if it is too heavy or awkward; rise by tightening the leg muscles, not the back; keep the load close to the waist; don't pivot or twist.

Poor body mechanics can increase risks for back pain. A common cause of backache is muscle strain, frequently precipitated by poor body mechanics in daily activities, such as lifting or exercising. If lifting is done improperly, great pressure is exerted on the lumbar discs, and excessive stress and strain are placed on the lumbar muscles and ligaments (see Figure 8). Many popular exercises involve poor body mechanics and should be viewed with caution.

Exercise Guidelines for Back and Neck Health

Some exercises and movements may put the back and neck at risk. The human body is designed for motion. Nevertheless, certain movements can put the joints and musculoskeletal system at risk and should therefore be avoided. 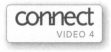 With respect to care of the spine, many **contraindicated** movements involve the extremes of hyperflexion and hyperextension. Hyperflexion, particularly in combination with rotation, causes increased pressure in the discs, potentially leading to disc herniation. Hyperextension causes compressive wear and tear on the facet joints

Contraindicated Not recommended because of the potential for harm.

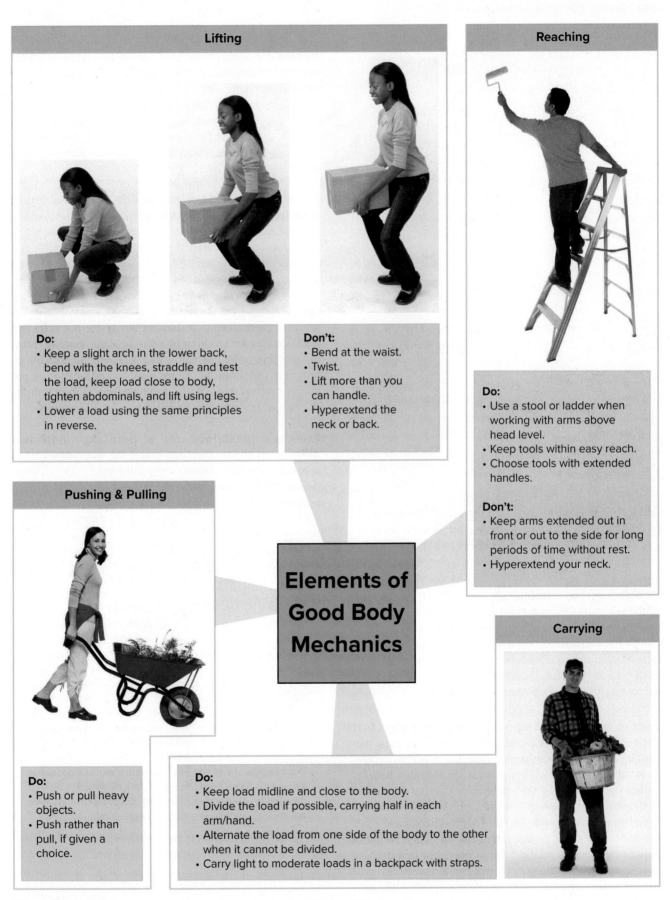

Lifting

Do:
- Keep a slight arch in the lower back, bend with the knees, straddle and test the load, keep load close to body, tighten abdominals, and lift using legs.
- Lower a load using the same principles in reverse.

Don't:
- Bend at the waist.
- Twist.
- Lift more than you can handle.
- Hyperextend the neck or back.

Reaching

Do:
- Use a stool or ladder when working with arms above head level.
- Keep tools within easy reach.
- Choose tools with extended handles.

Don't:
- Keep arms extended out in front or out to the side for long periods of time without rest.
- Hyperextend your neck.

Elements of Good Body Mechanics

Pushing & Pulling

Do:
- Push or pull heavy objects.
- Push rather than pull, if given a choice.

Carrying

Do:
- Keep load midline and close to the body.
- Divide the load if possible, carrying half in each arm/hand.
- Alternate the load from one side of the body to the other when it cannot be divided.
- Carry light to moderate loads in a backpack with straps.

Figure 8 ▶ Characteristics of good body mechanics for different lifestyle tasks.
(Lifting): Ken Karp/McGraw Hill; (Reaching): Ingram Publishing/SuperStock; (Pushing & Pulling): George Doyle/Stockbyte/Getty Images; (Carrying): Creatas/Getty Images

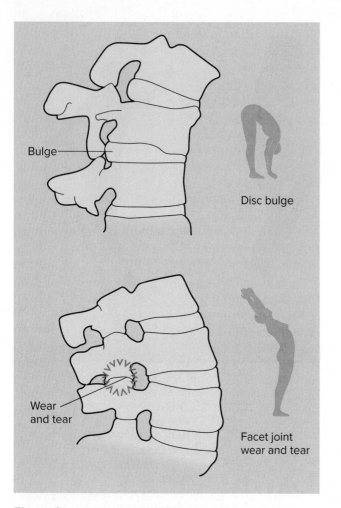

Bulge

Disc bulge

Wear
and tear

Facet joint
wear and tear

Figure 9 ▶ Risks of hyperflexion and hyperextension.

that join vertebral segments (see Figure 9). Hyperextension of the spine also causes narrowing of the intervertebral canal, potentially causing nerve impingement. Extremes of motion can be harmful to other joints as well. For example, knee hyperextension places excessive stress on structures at the back of the knee, whereas hyperflexion increases compressive forces under the kneecap (patello-femoral joint).

Following established exercise guidelines is important for safe exercise. "Safe" exercises are defined as those performed with normal body posture, mechanics, and movement in mind (see Table 2). They provide the intended benefits without compromising the integrity or stability of another body part. "Questionable" exercises, on the other hand, are exercises that may violate normal body mechanics and place the joints, ligaments, or muscles at risk for injury. No harm may occur from doing the exercise once, but repeated use over time can lead to injury. A number of commonly used exercises are regarded as poor choices (contraindicated) for nearly everyone in the general population due to the reasonable risk for injury over time. A separate category of

questionable exercises are poor choices for certain segments of the population because of a specific health issue or known physical problem.

Differentiating exercises as "safe" or "questionable" can be difficult—even experts in the field have different opinions on the subject. These views change over time as new knowledge and research findings reshape our understanding of the effect of exercise on the human body.

When considering the merits and risks of different exercises, it may be necessary to consult an expert. Professionals such as athletic trainers, biomechanists, physical educators, physical therapists, and certified strength and conditioning specialists typically have college degrees and 4–8 years of study in such courses as anatomy, physiology, kinesiology, preventive and therapeutic exercise, and physiology of exercise. On-the-job training, a good physique or figure, and good athletic or dancing ability are not sufficient qualifications for teaching or advising about exercise. Most fitness centers hire instructors and personal trainers with appropriate certifications. Unfortunately, certification is not always a requirement. When searching for advice on training or exercise, inquire about an individual's qualifications.

Exercises prescribed for a particular individual differ from those that are good for everyone (mass prescription). In a clinical setting, a therapist works with one patient. A case history is taken and tests are conducted to determine which muscles are weak or strong, long or short. Exercises

Technology Update

Breaking Bad Posture Habits

Back pain is a common and debilitating condition that afflicts most adults at some point in their lives. While the underlying causes of back pain are often not apparent, improving your posture and body mechanics remains one of the most proactive strategies for preventing back pain. Our posture is determined in part by factors such as flexibility and muscle imbalances, but it is also influenced by choices we make and by our habits. One device designed to break bad posture habits is Upright GO, which attaches to your back (and one version can be attached like a necklace) and vibrates to remind the user if posture is worsening. Since products like this are designed to be sold directly to consumers, carefully consider the relative advantages and disadvantages before purchasing.

Do you see merit in these types of technological approaches to posture? Would you benefit from efforts to improve your posture?

connect
ACTIVITY

are then prescribed for that person. For example, a wrestler with a recent history of shoulder dislocation would probably be prescribed specific shoulder-strengthening exercises to regain stability in the joint. Common shoulder-stretching exercises would likely be contraindicated. In this case, the muscles and joint capsule on the front of the shoulder are already quite lax to have allowed dislocation to occur in the first place.

Exercises prescribed or performed as a group cannot typically take individual needs into account. For example, when a physical educator, an aerobics instructor, or a coach leads a group of people in exercise, there may be little consideration for individual differences. Some of the exercises performed in this type of group setting may not be appropriate for all individuals. Similarly, an exercise that is appropriate for a certain individual may not be appropriate for all members of a group. Since it is not always practical to prescribe individual exercise routines for everyone, it is often necessary to provide general recommendations that are appropriate for most individuals. The classification of exercises in this Concept should be viewed in this context.

The risks associated with physical activity can be reduced by modifying the variables or conditions under which the activity is performed. Although some exercises are clearly contraindicated, risks are often associated with the frequency, intensity, and duration of the movement. *Frequency* may contribute to microtrauma of the back in a gymnast who repeatedly hyperextends the spine. *Intensity* may jeopardize the lower back of the power lifter who pushes too quickly. *Duration* may be a factor in the knee strain of a baseball catcher who spends sustained time in a deep squat. The speed of a movement and the movement quality may also influence the risk. In some cases, changing a single variable (*frequency, duration, intensity, speed,* or *movement quality*) may significantly reduce risk; but in other cases, multiple factors may need to be changed. In some cases, the best strategy

may be to look for a safer exercise or to modify the offending activity. (A variety of contraindicated exercises and safer alternatives are presented in Table 2 later in this Concept.)

Risks from exercise can't be avoided completely. Variables that are not always under the direct control of the participant include environmental conditions, such as temperature, humidity, or exercise surface. Likewise, the demands of sports and certain occupations may require individuals to train or work to the maximal limit of these variables (up to or just short of injury). Circumstances may not always permit every variable to be modified to suit an individual. However, making an active effort to adjust variables that are modifiable will make a difference in reducing injury risk.

Some additional general guidelines will help prevent postural, back, and neck problems. In addition to the suggestions for improving body mechanics noted in the previous sections, the following guidelines should be helpful:

- Establish a habit of aerobic activity for overall conditioning of the entire body.
- Maintain a healthy weight to reduce strain on the lower back.
- Do exercises to strengthen abdominal and hip extensors and to improve flexibility of the hip flexor and lumbar muscles if they are tight.
- Avoid hazardous exercises and sudden jerky movements of the trunk, especially twisting.
- Sleep on a moderately firm mattress and use chairs that promote good posture.
- Maintain good posture when carrying heavy loads; do not lean forward, sideways, or backward.
- Adjust sports equipment (e.g., bikes) to permit good posture and body alignment.
- Avoid long periods of sitting at a desk or driving.

In the News

Digital Eye Strain and Zoom Fatigue

Excessive sitting and staring at computer screens may not only lead to back problems and other metabolic risks. Digital eye strain is a condition characterized by physical eye discomfort felt after 2 or more hours in front of a digital screen. The majority of adults have likely experienced symptoms of digital eye strain due to prolonged use of electronic devices like laptops, tablets, and smartphones. If unresolved, symptoms can transition to blurred vision, burning eyes, headaches, and disrupted sleep. And as millions moved to virtual rather than in-person meetings, a new problem called "Zoom fatigue" has emerged. According to

scientists, the brain has to work harder to decipher information that normally can be inferred through nonverbal communication. To break up extended sitting and computer time, ophthalmologists recommend the "20/20/20" rule: for every 20 minutes spent using a screen, look away at something that is 20 feet away from you for a total of 20 seconds. This would also be a good time to stand up and move around.

Have you experienced digital eye strain or Zoom fatigue? What strategies can you use to manage these challenges?

connect
ACTIVITY

Using Self-Management Skills

Gaining performance skills related to posture and body mechanics is important for reducing risks of back and neck pain. Awareness of body posture is an important self-management skill that takes time to develop. Knowledge about posture and body mechanics is important, but the bigger challenge is to develop the discipline and body awareness needed to make corrections in posture during your daily life. Similarly, it is important to develop good habits and discipline to use good body mechanics when working, lifting, and carrying objects. These types of skills are called "performance skills" since it is important to apply them in practice. Like with other skills, you can improve your awareness and establish better postural habits to decrease your risks for future back and neck problems.

Building knowledge and changing your beliefs can help you avoid harmful exercises. As discussed, back and neck pain can result from accumulated damage (microtrauma) caused by performing unsafe exercises. There are clear risks associated with performing exercises that involve excess hyperflexion and hyperextension movements. Other exercises may put excess load on the spine. Thus, a key self-management skill for back health is to build sufficient knowledge so that you can identify harmful exercises and select safer alternatives. A variety of examples are provided in Table 2 for leg, arm, and trunk exercises. Changing your belief system regarding these exercises is also important. You may have learned these exercises from coaches or teachers, but that doesn't mean they are safe.

Applying self-assessment and self-planning skills can help prevent problems and enhance recovery. The exercises included in this Concept are aimed at building flexibility or promoting strength/muscle endurance; however, each is selected specifically to help correct a postural problem or to remove the cause of back and neck pain. Therefore, these exercises may be classified as therapeutic. The same exercises may be called preventive because they can be used to prevent postural or spine problems. Results from the Healthy Back assessment (See Lab 23A) can help inform needs, and it is important to use the information to identify exercises that can address those needs. The exercises in Tables 3, 4, 5, and 6 depict variations of exercises used to strengthen and stabilize the neck and back. Tables 4 and 5 illustrate core trunk variations that become progressively more difficult throughout the sequence. The beginning pose is appropriate for most people, whereas the last pose is more advanced. You can determine which level of difficulty is appropriate for you and begin there, progressing to the more advanced exercises as

you gain better strength and control. Individuals with back and neck pain are encouraged to seek the advice of a physician or physical therapist to guide these decisions.

Strategies for Action: Lab Information

An important step in taking action is assessing your current status. The Healthy Back Tests consist of eight pass or fail items that will give you an idea of the areas in which you might need improvement. The Healthy Back Tests are described in the Lab Resource Materials. You will take these tests in Lab 23A. Experts have identified behaviors associated with potential future back and neck problems. A questionnaire is also provided for assessing these risk factors.

Adopting and maintaining good posture promotes good back health. Lab 23B includes a posture test to help you evaluate your posture. Identify possible postural problems and take appropriate corrective action to reduce stress and strain on your back and neck.

Keep records of progress to maintain a back care program. Lab 23C provides an activity logging sheet for keeping records of your progress as you regularly perform exercises to build and maintain good back and neck fitness.

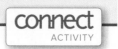

connect ACTIVITY

Suggested Resources and Readings

The websites for the following sources can be accessed by searching online for the organization, program, or title listed. Specific scientific references are available at the end of this edition of *Concepts of Fitness and Wellness*.

- Ingraham, P. (2021). "The Functional Movement Screen (FMS): The Benefits of the Popular Screening System for Athletes Might Be Over-Sold by Some Professionals." *PainScience.com*. Online commentary.
- Medline Plus. Back Pain.
- National Institute of Neurological Disorders and Stroke. *Low Back Pain Fact Sheet.*
- Richey, B. (2021). *Back Exercise: Stabilize, Mobilize, and Reduce Pain*. Champaign, IL: Human Kinetics.
- Spine-health. Specific Low Back Pain Exercises.
- WebMD. Understanding Back Pain—Symptoms.

Design Element: (*magnifying glass*): Siede Preis/Getty Images; (*runners shoes*): Maridav/Getty Images; (*tablet*): McGraw Hill; (*woman*): GlobalStock/Getty Images; (*blue sports shoes*): chictype/Getty Images; (*smartphone*): Alexey Boldin/Shutterstock; (*Why It Matters*): MHHE

Table 2

1. Questionable Exercise: The Swan

This exercise hyperextends the lower back and stretches the abdominals. The abdominals are too long and weak in most people and should not be lengthened further. Extension can be harmful to the back, potentially causing nerve impingement and facet joint compression. Other exercises in which this occurs include cobras, backbends, straight-leg lifts, straight-leg sit-ups, prone-back lifts, donkey kicks, fire hydrants, backward trunk circling, weight lifting with the back arched, and landing from a jump with the back arched.

Safer Alternative Exercise: Back Extension

Lie prone over a roll of blankets or pillows and extend the back to a neutral or horizontal position.

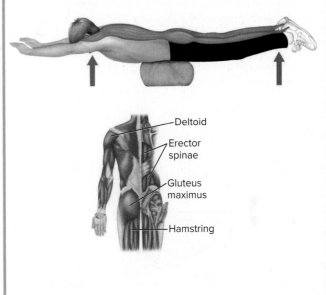

- Deltoid
- Erector spinae
- Gluteus maximus
- Hamstring

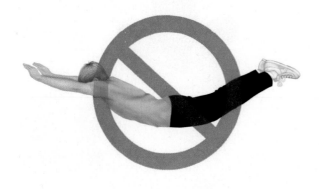

2. Questionable Exercise: Back-Arching Abdominal Stretch

This exercise can stretch the hip flexors, quadriceps, and shoulder flexors (such as the pectorals), but it also stretches the abdominals, which is not desired. Because of the armpull, it can potentially hyperflex the knee joint and strain neck musculature.

Safer Alternative Exercise: Wand Exercise

This exercise stretches the front of the shoulders and chest. Sit with wand grasped at ends. Raise wand overhead. Be certain that the head does not slide forward. Keep the chin tucked, neck straight, and spine erect. Bring wand down behind shoulder blades. Hold. Press forward on the wand simultaneously by pushing with the hands. Relax; then try to move the hands lower, sliding the wand down the back. Hold again.
Hands may be moved closer together to increase stretch on chest muscles.

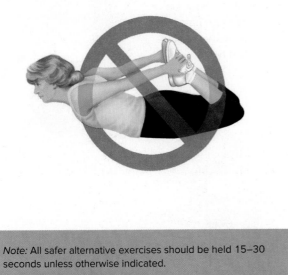

- Pectoralis minor
- Pectoralis major

Note: All safer alternative exercises should be held 15–30 seconds unless otherwise indicated.

Table 2

Table 2 Questionable Exercises and Safer Alternatives

3. Questionable Exercise: Seated Forward Arm Circles with Palms Down

This exercise (arms straight out to the sides) may cause pinching of the rotator cuff and biceps tendons between the bony structures of the shoulder joint and/or irritate the bursa in the shoulder. The tendency is to emphasize the use of the stronger chest muscles (pectorals) to perform the motion rather than emphasizing the weaker upper back muscles.

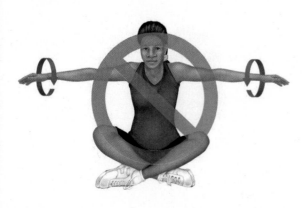

Safer Alternative Exercise: Seated Backward Arm Circles with Palms Up

Sit, turn palms up, pull in chin, and contract abdominals. Circle arms backward.

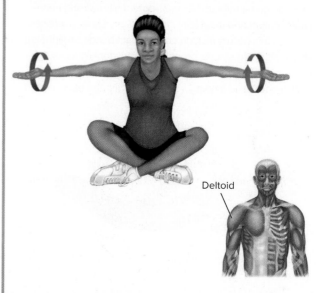

Deltoid

4. Questionable Exercise: Double-Leg Lift

This exercise is usually used with the intent of strengthening the abdominals, when in fact it is primarily a hip flexor (iliopsoas) strengthening exercise. Most people have overdeveloped the hip flexors and do not need to further strengthen those muscles because this may cause forward pelvic tilt. Even if the abdominals are strong enough to contract isometrically to prevent hyperextension of the lower back, the exercise produces excess stress on the discs.

Safer Alternative Exercise: Reverse Curl

This exercise strengthens the lower abdominals. Lie on your back on the floor and bring your knees in toward the chest. Place the arms at the sides for support. For movement, pull the knees toward the head, raising the hips off the floor. Do not let knees go past the shoulders. Return to starting position and repeat.

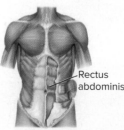

Rectus abdominis

5. Questionable Exercise: The Windmill

This exercise involves simultaneous rotation and flexion (or extension) of the lower back, which is contraindicated. Because of the orientation of the facet joints in the lumbar spine, these movements violate normal joint mechanics, placing tremendous torsional stress on the joint capsule and discs.

Safer Alternative Exercise: Back-Saver Toe Touch

Sit on the floor. Extend leg and bend the other knee, placing the foot flat on the floor. Bend at the hips and reach forward with both hands. Grasp one foot, ankle, or calf depending upon the distance you can reach. Pull forward with your arms and bend forward. Slight bend in the knee is acceptable. Hold. Repeat with the opposite leg.

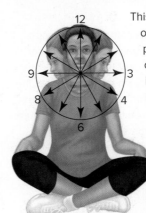

Erector spinae

Gluteals

Adductors

6. Questionable Exercise: Neck Circling

This exercise and other exercises that require neck hyperextension (e.g., neck bridging) can pinch arteries and nerves in the neck and at the base of the skull, cause wear and tear to small joints of the spine, and produce dizziness or myofascial trigger points. In people with degenerated discs, it can cause dizziness, numbness, or even precipitate strokes. It also aggravates arthritis and degenerated discs.

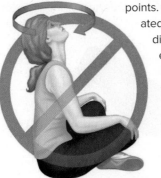

Safer Alternative Exercise: Head Clock

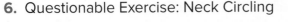

This exercise relaxes the muscle of the neck. Assume a good posture (seated with legs crossed or in a chair), and imagine that your neck is a clock face with the chin at the center. Flex the neck and point the chin at 6:00, hold, lift the chin; repeat pointing chin to 4:00, to 8:00, to 3:00 and finally to 9:00. Return to center position with chin up after each movement.

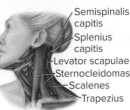

Semispinalis capitis
Splenius capitis
Levator scapulae
Sternocleidomastoid
Scalenes
Trapezius

Table 2 Questionable Exercises and Safer Alternatives

Table 2

7. Questionable Exercise: Shoulder Stand Bicycle

This exercise and the yoga positions called the plough and the plough shear (not shown) force the neck and upper back to hyperflex. It has been estimated that 80 percent of the population has forward head and kyphosis (humpback) with accompanying weak muscles. This exercise is especially dangerous for these people. Neck hyperflexion results in excessive stretch on the ligaments and nerves. It can also aggravate preexisting arthritic conditions. If the purpose for these exercises is to reduce gravitational effects on the circulatory system or internal organs, lie on a tilt board with the feet elevated. If the purpose is to warm up the muscles in the legs, slow jog in place. If the purpose is to stretch the lower back, try the leg hug exercise.

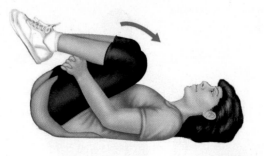

Safer Alternative Exercise: Leg Hug

Lie on your back with the knees bent at about 90 degrees. Bring your knees to the chest and wrap the arms around the back of the thighs. Pull knees to chest and hold.

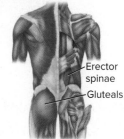

Erector spinae

Gluteals

8. Questionable Exercise: Straight-Leg and Bent-Knee Sit-Ups

There are several valid criticisms of the sit-up exercise. Straight-leg sit-ups can place extra stress on the lower lumbar vertebrae, causing back problems. A bent-knee sit-up creates less shearing force on the spine, but some recent studies have shown it produces greater compression on the lumbar discs than the straight-leg sit-up. Placing the hands behind the neck or head during the sit-up or during a crunch results in hyperflexion of the neck.

Safer Alternative Exercise: Crunch

Lie on your back with the knees bent more than 90 degrees. Curl up until the shoulder blades lift off the floor, then roll down to starting position and repeat. There are several safe arm positions. The easiest is with the arms extended straight in front of the body. Alternatives are with the arms crossed over the chest or the palms or fist held beside the ears.

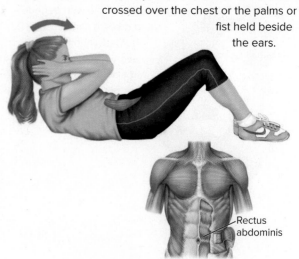

Rectus abdominis

9. Questionable Exercise: Standing Toe Touches or Double-Leg Toe Touches

These exercises—especially when done ballistically—can produce degenerative changes at the vertebrae of the lower back. They also stretch the ligaments and joint capsule of the knee. Bending the back while the legs are straight may cause back strain, particularly if the movement is done ballistically. If performed only on rare occasions as a test, the chance of injury is less than if incorporated into a regular exercise program. Safer stretches of the lower back include the leg hug, the single knee-to-chest, the back-saver hamstring stretch, and the back-saver toe touch.

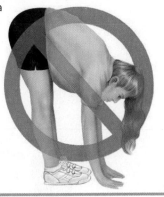

Safer Alternative Exercise: Back-Saver Hamstring Stretch

This exercise stretches the hamstring and lower back muscles. Sit with one leg extended and one knee bent, foot turned outward and close to the buttocks. Clasp hands behind back. Bend forward from the hips, keeping the low back as straight as possible. Allow bent knee to move laterally so trunk can move forward. Stretch and hold. Repeat with the other leg.

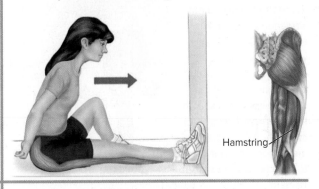

Hamstring

10. Questionable Exercise: Bar Stretch

This type of stretch may be harmful. Some experts have found that when the extended leg is raised 90 degrees or more and the trunk is bent over the leg, it may lead to **sciatica** and **piriformis syndrome**, especially in the person who has limited flexibility.

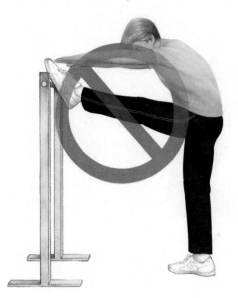

Safer Alternative Exercise: One-Leg Stretch

This exercise stretches the hamstring muscles. Stand with one foot on a bench, keeping both legs straight. Hinge forward from the hips keeping shoulders back and chest up. Bend forward until a pull is felt on the back side of the thigh. Hold. Repeat.

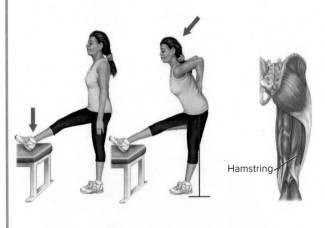

Hamstring

Sciatica Pain along the sciatic nerve in the buttock and leg.

Piriformis Syndrome Muscle spasm and nerve entrapment in the piriformis muscle of the buttocks region, causing pain in the buttock and referred pain down the leg (sciatica).

Table 2 Questionable Exercises and Safer Alternatives

11. Questionable Exercise: Shin and Quadriceps Stretch

This exercise causes hyperflexion of the knee. When the knee is hyperflexed more than 120 degrees and/or rotated outward by an external **torque**, the ligaments and joint capsule are stretched, and damage to the cartilage may occur. *Note:* One of the quadriceps, the rectus femoris, is not stretched if the trunk is allowed to bend forward because it crosses the hip as well as the knee joint. If the exercise is used to stretch the quadriceps, substitute the hip and thigh stretch. For most people it is not necessary to stretch the shin muscles, since they are often elongated and weak; however, if you need to stretch the shin muscles to relieve muscle soreness, try the shin stretch.

Safer Alternative Exercise: Hip and Thigh Stretch

Kneel so that the front leg is bent at 90 degrees (front knee directly above the front ankle). The knee of the back leg should touch the floor well behind the front foot. Press the pelvis forward and downward. Hold. Repeat with the opposite leg forward. Do not bend the front knee more than 90 degrees.

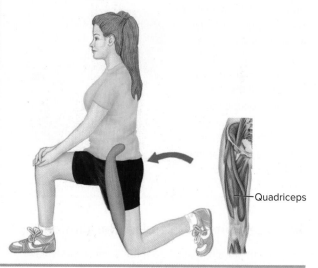

Quadriceps

12. Questionable Exercise: The Hero

Like the shin and quadriceps stretch, this exercise causes hyperflexion of the knee. It also causes torque on the hyperflexed knee. For these reasons the ligaments and joint capsule are stretched and the cartilage may be damaged. For most people it is not necessary to stretch the shin muscles since they are often elongated and weak; however, if you need to stretch the shin muscles, use the shin stretch. If this exercise is used to stretch the quadriceps, substitute the hip and thigh stretch.

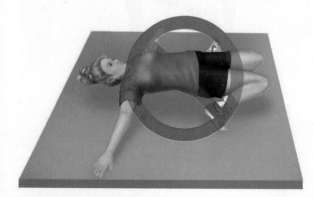

Safer Alternative Exercise: Shin Stretch

Kneel on your knees, turn to right and press down on right ankle with right hand. Hold. Keep hips thrust forward to avoid hyperflexing the knees. Do not sit on the heels. Repeat on the left side.

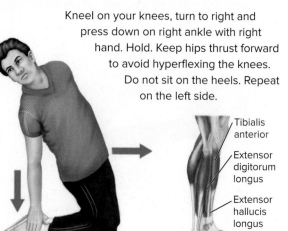

Tibialis anterior

Extensor digitorum longus

Extensor hallucis longus

Torque A twisting or rotating force.

13. Questionable Exercise: Deep Squatting Exercises

This exercise, with or without weights, places the knee joint in hyperflexion, compressing the joint surfaces, stretching certain ligaments, irritating the synovial membrane, and possibly damaging the cartilage. The joint has even greater stress when the lower leg and foot are not in straight alignment with the knee. If you are performing squats to strengthen the knee and hip extensors, try substituting the alternate leg kneel or half squat with free weight or leg presses on a resistance machine.

Safer Alternative Exercise: Half Squat

This exercise develops the muscles of the thighs and buttocks. Stand upright with feet shoulder width apart. Squat slowly by moving hips backward, then bending knees. Keep shins vertical. Bend knees 45–90 degrees. Repeat.

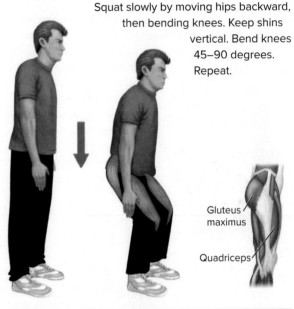

Gluteus maximus

Quadriceps

14. Questionable Exercise: Knee Pull-Down

This exercise can result in hyperflexion of the knee. The arms or hands placed on top of the shin places undue stress on the knee joint.

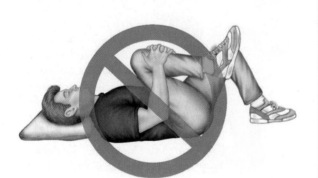

Safer Alternative Exercise: Single Knee-to-Chest

Lie down with both knees bent, draw one knee to the chest by pulling on the thigh with the hands, then extend the knee and point the foot toward the ceiling. Hold. Pull to chest again and return to starting position. Repeat with other leg.

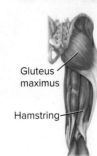

Gluteus maximus

Hamstring

Table 3

Table 3 Stretching and Strengthening Exercises for the Muscles of the Neck

These exercises are designed to increase strength in the neck muscles and to improve neck range of motion. They are helpful in preventing and resolving symptoms of neck pain and for relieving trigger points. Hold stretches for 15–30 seconds.

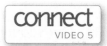

1. Upper Trapezius Stretch

This exercise stretches the upper trapezius muscle and relieves neck pain and headache. To stretch the right upper trapezius, place left hand on top of head, right hand behind back. Gently turn head toward left underarm and tilt chin toward chest. Increase stretch by gently drawing head forward with left hand. Hold. Repeat to opposite side.

— Trapezius

2. Chin Tuck

This exercise stretches the muscles at the base of the skull and reduces headache symptoms. Place hands together at the base of the head. Tuck in the chin and gently press head backward into your hands, while looking straight ahead. Hold.

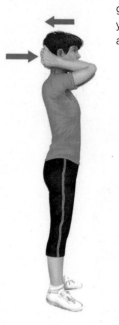

Deep extensors

3. Head Nod

Lie flat on the back without a pillow. Gently nod the head in a "yes" motion. Motion should result in the tightening of muscles deep in the front of the neck. Place two fingers over the sides of the neck to monitor for the undesirable substitution of stronger muscles in this region. Hold 10–30 seconds (or as long as can be maintained without substitution). Repeat 10 times. Progress this exercise by first nodding "yes" and then lifting the head ¼ inch to ½ inch off the surface.

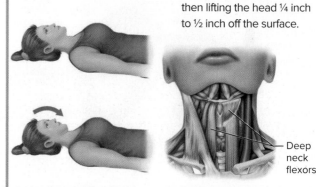

— Deep neck flexors

4. Isometric Neck Exercises

This exercise strengthens the neck muscles. Sit and place one or both hands on the head as shown. Assume good head and neck posture by tucking the chin, flattening the neck, and pushing the crown of the head up (axial extension). Apply resistance *(a)* sideward, *(b)* forward, and *(c)* backward. Contract the neck muscles to prevent the head and neck from moving. Hold contraction for 6 seconds. Repeat each exercise up to six times. *Note:* For neck muscles, it is probably best to use a less than maximal contraction, especially in the presence of arthritis, degenerated discs, or injury.

(a)

(b)

(c)

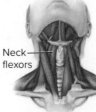

Neck flexors

Neck rotator and extensors

Table 4

Core Stabilization Exercise Variations   Table 4

These exercises are designed to help improve the ability of the core muscles to stabilize the trunk during dynamic movements of the arms and legs. The variations depict exercises of progressive difficulty. Many other variations exist along these same themes. Advance to the next exercise in each set only when the preceding level is mastered. Exercises can be performed in 2–3 sets of 10–20 repetitions.

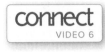

1. Front Plank Variations

(a) Begin by holding a plank position with support through the forearms and toes, keeping back straight and stomach pulled in. Hold for 20–30 seconds. *Variations:* Progress by performing plank with elbows extended and support through palms and feet *(b)*, by adding a single-arm raise with support through opposite forearm and feet *(c)*, or by adding a single-leg raise with support on both forearms *(d)*.

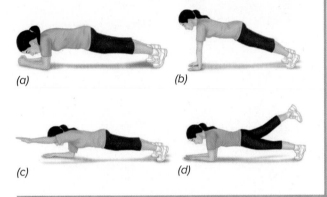

(a)

(b)

(c)

(d)

2. Side Plank Variations

(a) Begin by holding a side plank position with support through one forearm and lower legs, with knees bent. Lift hips off ground and keep back straight and stomach pulled in. Hold for 20–30 seconds. *Variations:* Progress by performing plank with elbow straight and support through palm *(b)*, by raising one arm straight over head with support through opposite forearm *(c)*, or by raising one leg upward with support through forearm *(d)*.

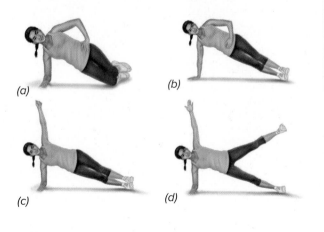

(a)

(b)

(c)

(d)

3. Superman Variations

(a) Begin on hands and knees. Tighten stomach and extend one leg behind you until it is parallel with the floor. Don't arch the back. Hold for 5 seconds. Relax and repeat. *Variations:* Progress by raising one arm and opposite leg parallel with the floor. Perform exercise while lying over a medicine ball *(b)*, while positioned on an unstable dome surface *(c)*, or while supported on an extended arm and leg *(d)*.

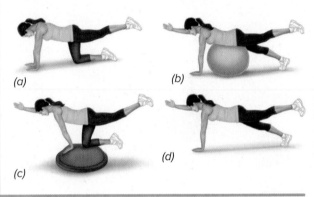

(a)

(b)

(c)

(d)

4. Abdominal Bracing Variations

(a) Begin by lying on back with stomach tightened. Raise one foot off the floor until hip and knee are bent 90 degrees and then slowly lower the foot back to the floor without letting back arch. *Variations:* Progress by raising/lowering arms and legs from the floor in alternate fashion, keeping back flat *(b)*; by raising/lowering arms and legs while lying on an unstable surface such as a foam roller *(c)*; or by adding resistance using a medicine ball, lowering ball overhead while extending one leg and then touching ball and knee together over midline *(d)*.

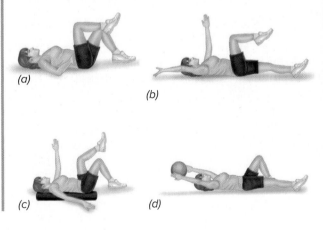

(a)

(b)

(c)

(d)

Table 4   Core Stabilization Exercise Variations

Table 4

5. Bridge Variations

(a) Begin by lying on back and lifting hips from the floor. Hold 5 seconds. Lower hips slowly and repeat. *Variations:* Progress by performing exercise with only one foot on the floor and opposite leg held in the air, knee bent *(b)*, or by performing exercise with only one foot on the floor and opposite leg extended straight *(c)*. Add complexity by holding a bridge while lying over an unstable medicine ball and moving a weighted ball in an arc overhead *(d)*.

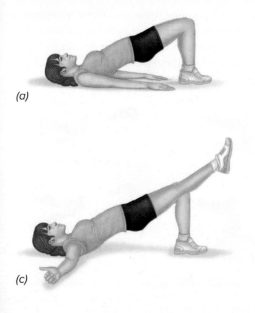

(a)

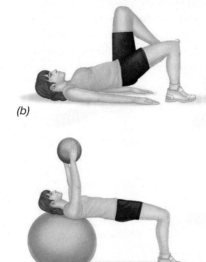

(b)

(c)

(d)

Table 5

Exercises for Muscle Fitness of Abdominals **Table 5** and Back Extensors

These exercises will increase the strength of the abdominal and back muscles. Strong trunk muscles are important for maintaining a neutral pelvis, maintaining good posture, and preventing backache.

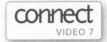

1. Abdominal Crunch Variations

(a) Curl-Up (develops the upper abdominal muscles): Begin by lying on the floor with knees bent. Hands can be progressed from arms extended to cross over chest to palms on ears. Curl up until shoulder blades leave the floor; then roll down. *Variations: (b) Crunch with Twist* (strengthens the oblique abdominal): Curl up while bringing one elbow toward opposite knee. Place feet on a bench to increase difficulty. *(c) Reverse Curl* (develops the lower abdominal muscles): Lie on back with arms at sides. Left knees to the chest, raising hips from floor. Do not let knees pass the shoulders. *(d) Sitting Tucks* (develops the lower abdominal muscles): Sit on the floor with feet raised, arms extended for balance. Alternately bend and extend legs without touching feet or back to the floor.

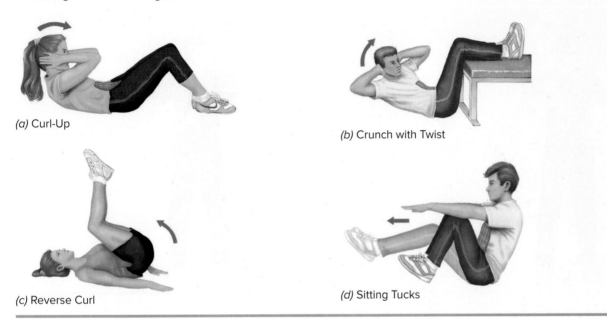

(a) Curl-Up

(b) Crunch with Twist

(c) Reverse Curl

(d) Sitting Tucks

2. Back Extension Variations

(a) Arm Lift (strengthens the scapular adductors): Lie on stomach with arms extended overhead. Raise arms 2–3 inches off the floor. Hold 5 seconds. Relax and repeat. *(b) Trunk Lift* (develops the muscles of the upper back and corrects rounded shoulders): Lie face down with hands behind neck. Raise head and chest from the floor. Relax and repeat. *(c) Upper Trunk Lift* (strengthens the muscles of the back): Lie over bench with upper half of body over the edge and partner stabilizing legs. Slowly raise trunk parallel to floor. Lower and repeat.

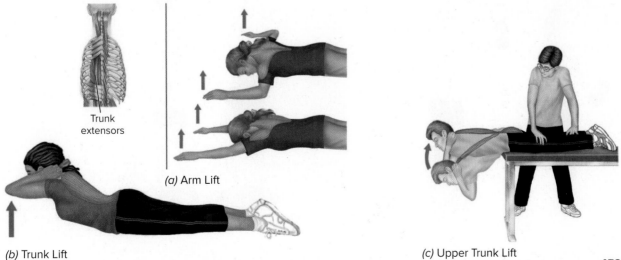

Trunk extensors

(a) Arm Lift

(b) Trunk Lift

(c) Upper Trunk Lift

Table 6

Table 6 Core Functional Movement Exercises

These exercises are designed to train the muscles of the core, arms, and legs by using functional movement patterns of the trunk and limbs.

1. Pulls and Lifts with Stabilization

(a) Pulls: Begin with elastic cord secured above shoulder height. Grasp free end and pull down across body, ending with hand at waist level on opposite side of body. Keep back and neck in a "neutral" posture and stomach tightened throughout. *(b) Lifts:* Begin with elastic cord secured below waist height. Cross arms toward opposite side of body and grasp free end. Pull upward, uncrossing arm as it is lifted overhead. Keep back and neck in a "neutral" posture and stomach tightened throughout.

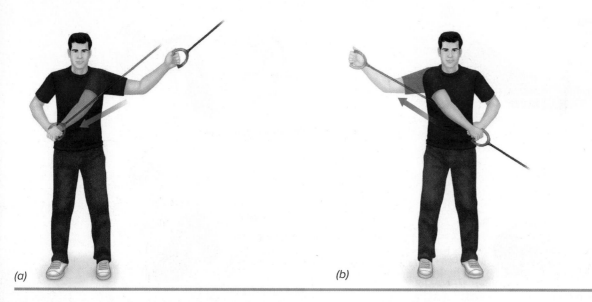

(a)   *(b)*

2. Weighted Lifts and Squats with Stabilization

(a) Forward Press: Begin by holding a weight plate at waist level, elbows bent. Tighten stomach and press plate out in front of you by straightening elbows. Return weight to starting position. Maintain low back in a "neutral" posture throughout. *(b) Overhead Lift:* Begin by holding weighted ball at chest level while squatting on an unstable surface such as a BOSU. Tighten stomach and lift ball overhead, straightening arms and legs. Return to starting position. Maintain balance and gentle arch in low back throughout.

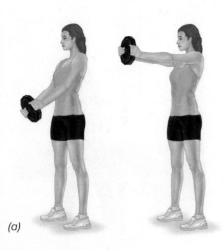

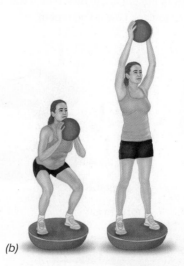

(a)   *(b)*

Lab Resource Materials: Healthy Back Tests

Chart 1 Healthy Back Tests

Physicians and therapists use these tests, among others, to make differential diagnoses of back problems. You and your partner can use them to determine if you have muscle tightness that may put you at risk for back problems. Discontinue any of these tests if they produce pain, numbness, or tingling sensations in the back, hips, or legs. Experiencing any of these sensations may be an indication that you have a low back problem that requires diagnosis by your physician. Partners should use *great caution* in applying force. Be gentle and listen to your partner's feedback.

FLEXIBILITY

Test 1—Straight-Leg Lift. Lie on your back with hands behind your neck. The partner on your left should stabilize your right leg by placing his or her right hand on your knee. With the left hand, your partner should grasp your left ankle and raise your left leg as near to a right angle as possible. In this position (as shown in the diagram), your lower back should be in contact with the floor. Your right leg should remain straight and on the floor throughout the test.

If your left leg bends at the knee, this indicates short hamstring muscles. If your back arches and/or your right leg does not remain flat on the floor, this indicates short lumbar muscles or hip flexor muscles. For you to pass the test, each leg should be able to reach approximately 90 degrees without the knee or back bending. (Both sides must pass in order to pass the test.)

Test 2—Thomas Test. Lie on your back on a table or bench with your right leg extended beyond the edge of the table (approximately one-third of your thigh off the table). Bring your left knee to your chest and pull your thigh down tightly with your hands. Lower your right leg. Your lower back should remain flat against the table, as shown in the diagram. For you to pass the test, your right thigh should be at table level or lower.

Test 3—Ober Test. Lie on your left side with your left leg flexed 90 degrees at the hip and 90 degrees at the knee. A partner should place your right hip in slight extension and right knee with just a slight bend (~20 degrees flexion). Your partner stabilizes your pelvis with the left hand to prevent movement. Your partner then allows the weight of the top leg to lower the leg to the floor. For you to pass the test, your knee or upper leg should be able to touch the table.

CORE TRUNK ENDURANCE TESTS

Test 4—Leg Drop Test.* Lie on your back on a table or on the floor with both legs extended overhead. Flatten your low back against the table or floor by tightening your abdominals. Slowly lower your legs while keeping your back flat.

If your back arches before you reach a 45-degree angle, your abdominal muscles are too weak and you fail the test. A partner should be ready to support your legs if needed to prevent your lower back from arching or strain to the back muscles.

*The Leg Drop Test is suitable as a diagnostic test when performed one time. It is not a good exercise to be performed regularly by most people. If it causes pain, stop the test.

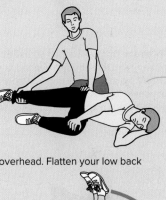

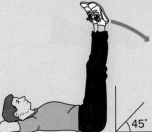

Chart 1 Healthy Back Tests (*Continued*)

Test 5—Isometric Abdominal Test. Lie supine with hips bent 45 degrees, feet flat on the floor, and arms by the side. Draw a line 4 1/2 inches beyond fingertips. Tuck chin and curl trunk forward, touching line with fingers. To pass, hold for 30 seconds.

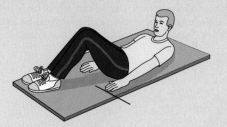

Test 6—Isometric Extensor Test. Lie on a table with upper half of the body hanging over the edge and arms crossed in front of chest. Have a partner stabilize your feet and legs. Raise your trunk smoothly until your back is in a horizontal position parallel to the floor. Do not arch the back. To pass the test, hold this position for 30 seconds.

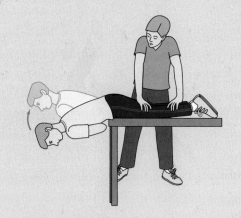

Test 7—Prone Bridge. Support yourself on the floor by resting on forearms and toes, body extended and back straight. Elbows are placed directly underneath shoulders. Look straight down toward hands. Do not arch the back. To pass the test, hold this position for 30 seconds.

Test 8—Quadruped Stabilization. Begin on hands and knees. Place hands directly below shoulders and knees directly below hips. Draw abdominals in. Extend one arm and opposite leg to a horizontal position. Do not allow back to arch or body to sway. To pass, hold position for 30 seconds.

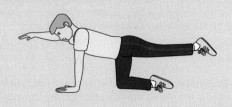

Test 9—Right Lateral Bridge. Lie on your right side with legs extended. Raise pelvis off the floor until trunk is straight and body weight is supported on arm and feet. Do not roll forward or backward. Do not arch back. To pass the test, hold this position for 30 seconds.

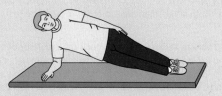

Test 10—Left Lateral Bridge. Lie on your left side with legs extended. Raise pelvis off the floor until trunk is straight and body weight is supported on arm and feet. Do not roll forward or backward or arch back. To pass the test, hold this position for 30 seconds.

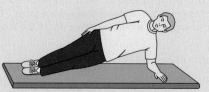

Chart 2 Healthy Back Test Ratings

Classification	Number of Tests Passed
Excellent	8–10
Very good	7
Good	6
Fair	5
Poor	1–4

Lab 23A The Back/Neck Questionnaire and Healthy Back Tests

Name	**Section**	**Date**

Purpose: To self-assess your potential for back problems using the Healthy Back Tests and the back/neck questionnaire.

Procedures

1. Answer the questions in the following Risk-Factor Questionnaire for Back and Neck Problems. Count your points for nonmodifiable factors, modifiable factors, and total score, and record these scores in the Results section. Use Chart 1 to determine your rating for all three scores and record them in the Results section.
2. With a partner, administer the Healthy Back Tests to each other (see Lab Resource Materials). Determine your rating using Chart 2. Record your score and rating in the Results section. If you did not pass a test, list the muscles you should develop to improve on that test.
3. Complete the Conclusions and Implications section.

Risk-Factor Questionnaire for Back and Neck Problems

Directions: Place an X in the appropriate circle after each question. Add the scores for each of the circles you checked to determine your nonmodifiable risk, modifiable risk, and total risk scores.

Nonmodifiable

1. Do you have a family history of osteoporosis, arthritis, rheumatism, or other joint disease?   (0) No   (1) Yes

2. What is your age?   (0) <40   (1) 40–50   (2) 51–60   (3) 61+

3. Did you participate regularly in these sports when you were young: gymnastics, football, weight lifting, skiing, ballet, javelin, or shot put?   (0) No   (1) Some   (3) Regularly

4. How many previous back or neck problems have you had?   (0) None   (1) 1   (2) 2   (5) 3+

Total Nonmodifiable Score = _____

Modifiable

5. Does your daily routine involve heavy lifting?   (0) No   (1) Some   (3) A lot

6. Does your daily routine require you to stand for long periods?   (0) No   (1) Some   (3) A lot

7. Do you have a high level of job-related stress?   (0) No   (1) Some   (3) A lot

8. Do you sit for long periods of time (computer operator, typist, or similar job)?   (0) No   (1) Some   (3) A lot

9. Does your daily routine require doing repetitive movements or holding something (e.g., baby, briefcase, suitcase) for long periods of time?   (0) No   (1) Some   (3) A lot

10. Does your daily routine require you to stand or sit with poor posture (e.g., sitting in a low car seat, reaching overhead with head tilted back)?   (0) No   (1) Some   (3) A lot

11. What is your score on the Healthy Back Tests?   (0) 9–10   (1) 7–8   (3) 5–6   (5) 0–4

12. What is your score on the posture test in Lab 23B?   (0) 0–2   (1) 3–4   (3) 5–7   (5) 8+

Total Modifiable Score = _____

Summary of Healthy Back Tests

	Pass	Fail	If you failed, what exercise should you do?
1. Straight-leg lift	○	○	
2. Thomas test	○	○	
3. Ober test	○	○	
4. Leg drop test	○	○	
5. Isometric abdominal test	○	○	
6. Isometric extensor test	○	○	
7. Prone bridge	○	○	
8. Quadruped stabilization	○	○	
9. Right lateral bridge	○	○	
10. Left lateral bridge	○	○	

Total ▢

Chart 1 Back/Neck Questionnaire Ratings

Rating	Nonmodifiable Score	Modifiable Score	Total Score
Very high risk	12+	7+	19+
High risk	8–11	5–6	13–17
Average risk	4–7	3–4	7–11
Low risk	0–3	0–2	0–5

Chart 2 Healthy Back Tests Ratings

Classification	Number of Tests Passed
Excellent	8–10
Very good	7
Good	6
Fair	5
Poor	1–4

Results

Back/Neck Questionnaire

Nonmodifiable Score ▢ + Modifiable Score ▢ = Total Score ▢ Rating ▢

Healthy Back Tests

Total Number of Tests Passed ▢ Classification ▢

Conclusions and Implications: In several sentences, discuss your need to do exercises for care of the back and neck. Include steps you might take to prevent future problems. Use your test results to answer.

Lab 23B Evaluating Posture

Name		**Section**	**Date**

Purpose: To learn to recognize postural deviations and thus become more posture conscious and to determine your postural limitations in order to institute a preventive or corrective program.

Procedures

1. Wear as little clothing as possible (bathing suits are recommended) and remove shoes and socks.
2. Work in groups of two or three, with one person acting as the subject while partners serve as examiners; then alternate roles.
   a. Stand by a vertical plumb line.
   b. Using Chart 1 and the figure, check any deviations and indicate their severity using the following point scale (0 = none, 1 = slight, 2 = moderate, and 3 = severe).
   c. Total the score and determine your posture rating from the Posture Rating Scale (Chart 2).
3. If time permits, perform back and posture exercises (see Lab 23C).
4. Complete the Conclusions and Implications section.

Results

Record your posture score (0–18):

Record your posture rating from the Posture Rating Scale in Chart 2:

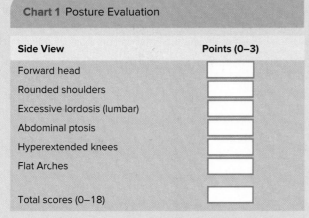

Chart 1 Posture Evaluation

Side View	Points (0–3)
Forward head	
Rounded shoulders	
Excessive lordosis (lumbar)	
Abdominal ptosis	
Hyperextended knees	
Flat Arches	
Total scores (0–18)	

Chart 2 Posture Rating Scale

Classification	Total Score (0–18)
Excellent	0–4
Very good	5–7
Good	8–10
Fair	11–13
Poor	14 or more

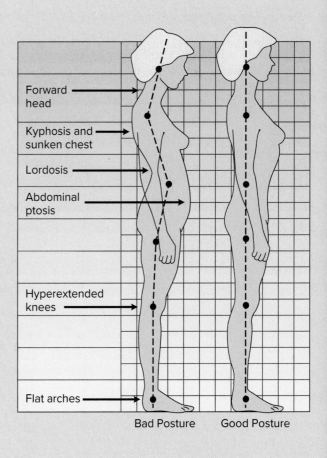

Forward head

Kyphosis and sunken chest

Lordosis

Abdominal ptosis

Hyperextended knees

Flat arches

Bad Posture   Good Posture

Conclusions and Implications

Were you aware of the deviations that were found?   Yes 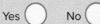   No

1. List the deviations that were moderate or severe (use several complete sentences).

2. In several sentences, describe your current posture status. Include in this discussion your overall assessment of your current posture, whether you think you will need special exercises in the future, and the reasons your posture rating is good or not so good.

Lab 23C Planning and Logging Core and Back Exercises

Name	Section	Date

Purpose: To select exercises for the back and neck that meet your personal needs and monitor progress.

Procedures

1. Using Chart 1, provide some background information about your experience with core and back exercise, your goals, and your plans for incorporating these exercises into your normal exercise routine.
2. Using Chart 2, choose one variation for each of the nine possible exercises listed. Refer to the core stabilization exercises on Table 4 (page 451), abdominal and back strengthening exercises on Table 5 (page 453), and functional core movements on Table 6 (page 454). Perform the exercises for at least 3 days over a weeklong period. If you are just starting out, it is best to start with the easier variations. If you are more experienced, try the more advanced variations.
3. Answer the questions in the Results and Conclusions and Implications sections.

Chart 1 Core and Back Exercise Survey

1. Determine your current stage for core and back exercise. Check only the stage that represents your current activity level.

◯ Precontemplation. I do not do core or back exercises and have not been thinking about starting.

◯ Contemplation. I do not do core or back exercises but have been thinking about starting.

◯ Preparation. I am planning to start doing core and back exercises.

◯ Action. I do core and back exercises but not that regularly.

◯ Maintenance. I regularly do core and back exercises.

2. What are your primary goals for core and back exercise?

◯ Prevention of back pain.

◯ Sports improvement (specify sport:_____).

◯ Better functional fitness.

3. Are you currently involved in a regular exercise program that includes resistance exercises?

◯ Yes

◯ No

Results

Did you do at least nine exercises at least 3 days in the week?   Yes ◯   No ◯

Conclusions and Implications: Were you able to find variations that provided an appropriate challenge? Do you feel that you will use core and back exercises as part of your regular exercise routine? Use several sentences to answer.

Chart 2 Core and Back Exercise Log

Check (√) at least one exercise variation from each of the nine categories and record the number of sets performed on at least 3 days over a 1-week period. Write the date (month/day) in the day column for the date you performed the exercise.

Table 4 Core Stabilization Exercise Variations

Front Plank Variations	Day 1	Day 2	Day 3	Day 4	Day 5	Day 6	Day 7
☐ A.							
☐ B.							
☐ C.							
☐ D.							
Side Plank Variations							
☐ A.							
☐ B.							
☐ C.							
☐ D.							
Superman Variations							
☐ A.							
☐ B.							
☐ C.							
☐ D.							
Abdominal Bracing Variations							
☐ A.							
☐ B.							
☐ C.							
☐ D.							
Bridge Variations							
☐ A.							
☐ B.							
☐ C.							
☐ D.							

Table 5 Abdominals and Back Extensors Exercise Variations

Abdominal Crunch Variations							
☐ A.							
☐ B.							
☐ C.							
☐ D.							
Back Extension Variations							
☐ A.							
☐ B.							
☐ C.							

Table 6 Core Functional Movement Exercise Variations

Pulls and Lifts with Stabilization							
☐ A.							
☐ B.							
Weighted Lifts and Squats with Stabilization							
☐ A.							
☐ B.							

Making Informed Consumer Choices

LEARNING OBJECTIVES

After completing the study of this Concept, you will be able to:

► Define quackery and fraud and outline steps that can be taken to avoid being susceptible to them.

► Evaluate the effectiveness of different physical activity programs and products.

► Select exercise equipment based on effectiveness, safety, and utility.

► Assess health clubs and exercise leaders (and their qualifications).

► Evaluate body composition and weight loss products for effectiveness and safety.

► Evaluate nutrition products for effectiveness and safety.

► Detect potentially fraudulent consumer products based on credibility, marketing/advertising strategies, and the nature of the claims.

"Let the buyer beware" is a good motto for the consumer seeking advice or planning a program for developing or maintaining health, wellness, and fitness.

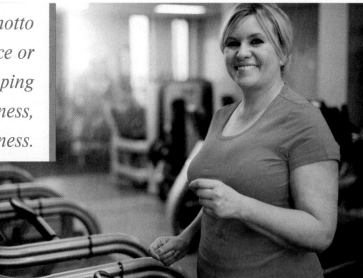

gpointstudio/Shutterstock

People have always searched for the fountain of youth and an easy, quick, and miraculous route to happiness and health. In current society, this search is often driven by goals related to fitness, nutrition, weight loss, or improved appearance. Products often promise easy weight loss, better health, or increased fitness—typically with little or no effort. The sale of many, if not most, products can be classified as either quackery or fraud since they simply do not work. The content throughout this edition is designed to help clarify facts and dispute myths. This Concept integrates information to help you build and reinforce your consumer skills so that you can avoid being a victim of quackery and make informed decisions about health, wellness, and fitness products.

Quacks and Quackery

Quacks can be identified by exaggerated claims, frequent use of testimonials, and gimmicks to support their products. The definition of *quack* is "a pretender of medical skill" or "one who talks pretentiously without sound knowledge of the subject discussed." This implies that the promotion of quackery involves

deliberate deception, but quacks often believe in what they promote. The consumer watchdog group Quackwatch defines quackery more broadly as "anything involving overpromotion in the field of health." This definition encompasses questionable ideas as well as questionable products and services. The word *fraud* is reserved for situations in which deliberate deception is involved. Look for these clues to identify quacks, frauds, and rip-off artists:

- Quacks rely on testimonials from paid athletes and celebrities to endorse their products.

- Quacks rely on anecdotal evidence and prey on consumer gullibility.

- Quacks sell products primarily through the mail or the Internet, which does not allow you to examine the products personally.

- Quacks promise quick, miraculous results and money-back guarantees.

- Quacks claim everyone can benefit from the product or service they are selling.

Quacks ignore scientific practice but often pretend to be scientists. Scientific research is a systematic search for truth, and specific procedures are used to control error and minimize bias. The peer-review process used to publish and share findings helps ensure that the design and methods were sound and that the conclusions are appropriate. The

standardized process helps ensure that the information in published research studies is scientifically sound and defensible.

Quack products are typically released without any scientific evidence of safety or efficacy. However, quacks know that people value the research process and they often mislead consumers by pretending to follow scientific methods. Occasionally, companies will mention that their product or program has been scientifically tested, but this does not necessarily mean that the results were positive. They may also cite irrelevant findings in obscure journals because they assume (correctly) that most consumers would not check the sources or the nature of the study. Even if a study did show positive results, the study may have been flawed. An article in a prominent scientific journal documented that results of studies, especially small studies that are not well controlled, are often found to be wrong or the effects are not as large as originally thought. The list below summarizes additional unscientific practices used by quacks:

- Quacks mix a little bit of truth with a lot of fiction to try to impress consumers with the use of scientific terms and mechanisms (even if they are not correct in their interpretation).

- Quacks misquote scientific research (or quote out of context) to mislead consumers.

- Quacks quote from individuals, journals, or institutions with questionable reputations.

- Quacks may claim to have the support of "experts," but the experts are not identified.

- Quacks often claim their products are based on "new" experimental discoveries, and they frequently discredit legitimate organizations such as the Food and Drug Administration (FDA) and the American Medical Association (AMA).

Experts have an educated, scientific base and meet other professional criteria. Unlike quacks, experts base their work on the scientific method. Some characteristics of professional experts are an extended education, an established code of ethics, membership in well-known associations, involvement in the profession as an intern before obtaining credentials, and a commitment to perform an important social service. Some experts require a license. Examples of experts in the health, wellness, and fitness area are medical doctors, nurses, certified fitness leaders, physical educators, registered dietitians, physical therapists, and clinical psychologists. In most cases, you can check if a person has the credentials to be considered an expert before obtaining services. The following list includes some things that can be done to determine a person's expertise:

- Determine the source of the person's education and the nature of the degree and/or certification.

- Check with the person's professional association, a government board, licensing agency, or certifying agency to

In the News

Operation Quack Hack: Targeting False COVID-19 Information

Operation Quack Hack is a joint venture of the Food and Drug Administration (FDA) and the Federal Trade Commission (FTC). The goal of this initiative is to target fake treatments and to protect the public from quacks and cons who sell products that can be harmful. The current law prohibits the use of words such as *diagnose, prevent, treat,* and *cure* in advertisements, yet many quacks use the terms anyway. The COVID-19 pandemic provided new opportunities for scammers, and in 2021 the FTC warned the public about intentional efforts to "cash in on COVID-19 confusion." According to the FDA, consumers were being targeted with unproven cures, illegitimate test kits, and substandard or counterfeit respirators. And thousands of newly registered Internet domain names in 2020 are considered as "high-risk" for potential fraud. The scams identified by Quack Hack illustrate how quacks and cons are quick to take advantage of health emergencies to bilk consumers.

Does the information about false COVID-19 information surprise you or anger you? Do you support broader efforts by the FTC and FDA to address quackery?

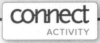

see if there are any complaints against the person; for example, you can contact your state's medical board to check complaints against physicians.

- Check if the person has credentials to provide the service you are seeking (e.g., a registered dietitian is qualified to give nutrition advice but not medical advice).

Physical Activity Quackery

There is no "effortless" way to get the benefits from physical activity. Advertisements for exercise that claim to "get you totally fit in 10 minutes" or "get you fit with little effort" are false. The only way to get fit is to follow the FIT formula for the type of exercise that you choose for meeting specific fitness goals. Claims for exercise that will effortlessly reduce weight or produce significant health benefits are equally false. One example is the false claims made by shoe manufacturers. Reebok International agreed to pay $25 million and Skechers paid $40 million to settle charges related to false claims that their shoes aid weight loss and strengthen and tone buttocks, leg, and abdominal muscles. As noted in previous Concepts, there are specific guidelines for physical activity designed for weight loss or maintenance and for achieving health benefits. Beware of those who claim otherwise.

Claims for many forms of exercise are overstated or unsubstantiated. New exercise programs or routines are often promoted as the complete answer for total fitness or a **panacea** for health. This is very similar to how new fad diets are promoted. With both diet and exercise, it is very unlikely that some new regimen will be discovered to have unique fitness or health benefits. The claims just spin the benefits of exercise in a new way to attract interest.

Similar hype may be used for promoting new pieces of exercise equipment. Each piece of equipment claims to be fun, easy to use, and more effective than other forms of exercise. The benefits from exercise depend on the relative intensity and duration of the activity—and whether it is done regularly over time. The best form of exercise is clearly the one that you are willing and able to do!

Contrary to claims, passive exercises do not provide any benefits for fitness or weight loss. For exercise to be beneficial, the work must be done by contracting skeletal muscles. A variety of **passive exercise** forms have been promoted to try to reduce the effort required to perform regular exercise. Some passive devices have value for people with special needs when administered by a qualified person, such as a physical therapist. However, passive devices sold for use by the general public are ineffective. The goal of sellers is to convince people that there is an effortless way to exercise—there is not. The fallacies associated with many past forms of passive exercise, such as fat rolling machines (purported to break up and redistribute fat), seem obvious today, but new approaches come out all the time with different marketing and promotions. The following list highlights some examples of passive exercise gimmicks and false claims:

- *Vibrating belts.* These wide canvas or leather belts are driven by an electric motor, causing loose tissue of the body part to shake. They have no beneficial effect on fitness, fat, or figure.

- *Toning tables.* Contrary to advertisements, these vibrating tables will not improve posture, trim the body, reduce weight, or develop muscle **tonus**.

Panacea A cure-all; a remedy for all ills.

Passive Exercise Exercise in which no voluntary muscle contraction occurs; an outside force moves the body part with no effort by the person.

Tonus The most frequently misused and abused term in fitness vocabularies. Tonus is the tension developed in a muscle as a result of passive muscle stretch. Tonus cannot be determined by feeling or inspecting a muscle. It has little or nothing to do with the strength of a muscle.

- *Continuous passive motion (CPM) tables.* These machines passively move body parts repeatedly through a range of motion. Because the muscles are not doing any work, these tables provide no real benefits. Hospitals and rehabilitation centers may use similar machines to maintain range of motion in patients, but a healthy person has nothing to gain from these devices.

- *Magnets.* A variety of magnets and ion balance bracelets have been marketed with many claims, but there is no evidence to support any benefits. To date, the FDA has not approved the marketing of any magnets for medical use, and sellers making medical claims for magnets are in violation of the law.

- *Electrical muscle stimulators.* Neuromuscular electrical stimulators cause the muscle to contract involuntarily. In the hands of qualified medical personnel, muscle stimulators are valuable therapeutic devices, but in a healthy person they do not have the same value. Spas and clinics often promote various muscle stimulators for fitness enhancement, but they have no value for healthy people.

- *Weighted belts.* Claims have been made that these belts reduce waists, thighs, and hips when worn under the clothing. In reality, they do none of these things and have been reported to cause physical harm.

- *Sauna belts and rubberized suits.* Various garments are marketed to promote weight loss, but they really just promote sweating. If exercise is performed while wearing such garments, the exercise, not the garment, may be beneficial. You cannot squeeze fat out of the pores, nor can you melt it.

- *Body wrapping.* Some reducing salons, gyms, and clubs advertise that wrapping the body in bandages soaked in a magic solution will reduce body girth. Tight, constricting bands can temporarily compress the skin and squeeze body fluids into other parts of the body, but the skin or body will regain its original size within minutes or hours. Users may temporarily deplete water, but the water is regained quickly. Body fat is not lost.

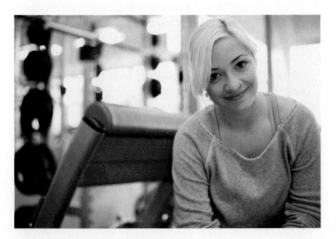

It is important to be an informed consumer when selecting a fitness center or joining a program.

Hero/Corbis/Glow Images

Considerations with Exercise Equipment and Fitness Programs

Home exercise machines can be convenient, but research options before making a purchase. When using a piece of equipment at a health club, you can change machines if you don't like the one you are using. However, if you buy the equipment, you are stuck with it even if you don't like it. Before purchasing, consider the following:

- *Is this the best piece of equipment for you?* Should you buy a resistance machine, a treadmill, an exercise bicycle, or some other equipment? Consider your goals and fitness needs to help you decide what equipment to buy.

- *Do you have space for it?* If you do not have a space where you can put the equipment and leave it, you will probably not use it regularly. Some equipment is "portable" so that it can be stored when not in use, but it is less likely to be used regularly than equipment that is readily available. Be sure all members of the family approve of the location of the equipment before purchasing it.

- *Will you use it?* Carefully consider how the equipment might help address barriers to your exercise program. Try out the equipment before you buy, especially when considering expensive machines.

- *Is the price appropriate?* In some cases, a simpler and less expensive device may be a good choice. However, with some equipment, it may be worth saving up for a higher-quality machine that is more durable or quieter to use. The quality of the experience can make you more likely to want to use it.

- *Is the equipment reliable?* Many organizations review fitness products and equipment, so look for a quality review to compare companies and products. Pay attention to various features as well as quality and reliability of various machines.

- *Is the equipment safe to use?* Check for standard safety features. For example, free weights should have quality safety collars and treadmills should have locks to prevent use by children and "kill switches" for stopping safely.

- *Is the dealer reputable?* Select a company or store that has been in business for a while and that has a good reputation. Compare prices for similar equipment. Beware of dealers who try to sell you extra attachments or accessories you won't use. Also consider the product warranty and the cost of repairs if you do not get a warranty.

Think carefully about your needs before enrolling in fitness programs. Fitness centers provide a range of fitness courses, but there are now many online options for group exercise programming. Regardless of the setting, it is

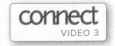

important to carefully consider whether it will be a good fit for you. Consider these questions:

- *What is your current state of fitness and your current level of physical activity?* It is important to find programming that caters to your level of fitness as well as to the type of activity that you enjoy.

- *What are your goals?* There are numerous options for programming, so search out options that address your personal fitness goals (e.g., muscle fitness vs. cardiorespiratory endurance).

- *Will you enjoy it?* A potential limitation of structured programs is that they may not be as fun as doing sports or other recreational activities. Consider your own preferences before committing to a program or service.

- *Will you stick with it?* Choose program options that enhance your personal motivation. Personal trainers and online exercise classes may provide short-term accountability; however, it is important to learn how to establish your own habits and motivation over time.

- *Is it safe?* Programs such as CrossFit and extreme forms of yoga may work well for some individuals but may be unsafe for others. Choose programming that you feel comfortable with and that considers your unique physical needs.

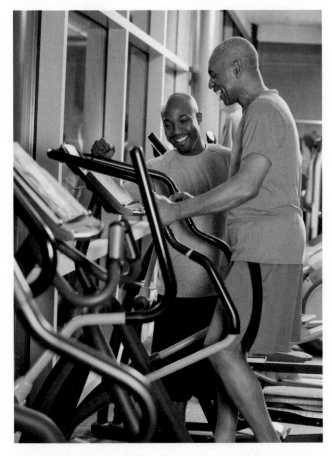

Take time to learn the features of exercise equipment.
Ariel Skelley/Getty Images

Consider the hype and exaggerated claims on devices, apps, and websites. Although exercise machines and apps can be useful in carrying out your personal exercise plan, they are not without limitations. It is important to develop good consumer skills and consider the facts instead of falling victim to the hype. The list below provides some considerations when interpreting fitness information:

- *No single device can provide a comprehensive fitness solution.* Fitness is multidimensional, so machines designed to enhance cardiorespiratory endurance may do little for muscle fitness or flexibility. Thus, be wary of overstated claims of simple solutions for fitness.

- *Estimates of caloric expenditure are often not very accurate.* Many devices and apps include built-in estimates to help track calories burned; however, these are rough estimates and may not reflect actual energy expenditure.

- *Notions of a "fat burning zone" are oversimplifications of weight control principles.* All forms of physical activity can contribute to weight control. Lower-intensity activity offers advantages since you can last longer and burn more calories.

- *Programs that promise more efficient paths to fitness or weight loss are exaggerations.* Regimens such as high-intensity interval training (HIIT) may hype the higher intensity as an advantage, but safety and long-term adherence are important considerations as well. Focus on ways to sustain lifestyles over time.

- *Avoid contraindicated exercises and approaches.* It is best to be skeptical of ideas and routines you may read about on fitness websites. A simple example is the common "recommendation" to carry hand weights while walking to burn more calories. While it may seem like a logical suggestion, experts have concluded that the benefit of added energy expenditure is not worth the added risk for injury. Ankle weights are also not recommended because they may alter your gait and stress the knees.

Considerations with Health Clubs and Spas

Consider the credentials of a fitness leader or personal trainer before making a selection. Individuals with a college degree in physical education, physical therapy, exercise science, or kinesiology are recommended, as well as certifications from reputable organizations, such as the American College of Sports Medicine (ACSM). The ACSM offers several certifications with differing levels of expertise and education ranging from certified personal trainer to registered clinical exercise physiologist. Not all certifications are equal. Some unreputable and unethical organizations require little more than an application and a fee payment.

Using the sauna, steam room, whirlpool, or hot tub at your local fitness center provides no significant health benefits. Baths do not melt off fat; fat must be metabolized. The heat and humidity from baths may make you perspire, but it is water, not fat, oozing from your pores. Any positive effect is largely psychological, although some temporary relief from aches and pains may result from the heat. Use of these facilities is not advised for people with health problems, such as high or low blood pressure, and should be limited for children, pregnant females, older adults, those who have consumed alcohol, and those who have recently finished a vigorous exercise bout. Skin infections can be spread in a bath; make certain it is cleaned regularly and that the hot tub or whirlpool has proper pH and chlorination. Additional guidelines include:

- Cool down after exercise before using a sauna or tub.
- Take a soap shower before and after use.
- Do not wear makeup, lotion, oil, or jewelry.
- Adhere to the posted temperature guidelines.
- Drink plenty of water before or during use.
- Do not sit on a metal stool; sit on a towel.
- Get out immediately if you become dizzy; feel hot, chilled, or nauseous; or develop a headache.

Sunlamp products, such as tanning beds and various suntanning products, can increase the risk of sun damage and skin cancer. Tanning salons often promise "safe tanning" because they tend to elicit UVA radiation instead of the more intense UVB. It was previously thought that UVA radiation was not as harmful as UVB since it is less intense and penetrates to deeper layers of the skin. However, new evidence suggests that it can significantly damage skin cells called keratinocytes in the basal layer of the epidermis, where most skin cancers occur. The dosage of UVA radiation from salons is also 12 times as strong as that of the sun. Not surprisingly, people who use tanning salons are 2.5 times more likely to develop squamous cell carcinoma than people who don't. As noted previously, the World Health Organization has classified all UV radiation as carcinogenic (cancer causing). The FDA also requires warnings to be placed on a variety of products classified as "suntanning preparations." This includes a variety of gels, creams, liquids, and other topical products marketed to provide cosmetic benefits or the appearance of a tan. The required warning statement conveys the important message for consumers: *"Warning—This product does not contain a sunscreen and does not protect against sunburn. Repeated exposure of unprotected skin while tanning may increase the risk of skin aging, skin cancer, and other harmful effects to the skin even if you do not burn."* It is wise to avoid tanning salons, pills, and other products designed to accelerate tanning.

Consider a number of factors before making decisions about a health or fitness club. In addition to having well-trained experts, there are other guidelines to consider when selecting a health and fitness club. Some of these guidelines are illustrated in Figure 1. You will have the opportunity to rate a health and fitness club using a comprehensive list of factors in Lab 24B.

Body Composition Quackery

Cellulite is not a special form of fat. Cellulite is ordinary fat with a fancy name. You do not need a special treatment or device to get rid of it. In fact, it has no special remedy. To decrease fat, reduce calories and do more physical activity.

Spot-reducing, or losing fat from a specific location on the body, is not possible. When you do physical activity, calories are burned and fat is recruited from all over the body in a genetically determined pattern. You cannot selectively exercise, bump, vibrate, squeeze, or freeze the fat from a particular spot. If you are flabby to begin with, localized exercise can strengthen the local muscles, causing a change in the contour and the girth of that body part, but exercise affects the muscles, not the fat on that body part. General aerobic exercises are the most effective for burning fat, but you cannot control where the fat comes off.

Surgically sculpting the body with implants and liposuction to acquire physical beauty will not give you physical fitness and may be harmful. Rather than doing it the hard way, an increasing number of people are resorting to surgery and muscle implants to improve their physique. Liposuction is not a weight loss technique but, rather, a contouring procedure. Like any surgery, it has risks, including risks for infection, hematoma, skin slough, other conditions, and death. Muscle implants give a muscular appearance, but they do not make you stronger or more fit. The implants are not really muscle tissue but, rather, silicon gel or saline, such as that used in breast implants or a hard substitute. Some complications can occur, such as infection and bleeding, and some physicians believe that calf implants may put pressure on the calf muscles and cause them to atrophy. A better way to improve physique and fitness is to engage in proper exercise. In recent years, buttocks augmentation has become a trendy cosmetic surgery procedure. Fat from the abdomen, hips, or thighs is relocated to "round out" the buttocks. Early procedures led to multiple deaths and many complications. While surgical rules and procedures have made it safer, surgical sculpting is not without risk, especially if performed by those lacking adequate credentials.

Weight loss quackery is the most common form of consumer fraud. The FTC indicates that nearly one-quarter of reported fraud cases involve weight loss products or

Questions to Ask

- Is the staff well qualified and available when you need help?
- Is the club well run (efficient in day-to-day operations)?

Facilities and Equipment

- Does the club meet your personal needs (e.g., offering equipment, classes, and services you want)?
- Is the facility convenient (near home or work)?
- Is the equipment up-to-date and well maintained?
- Is the facility clean?
- Are towels provided to wipe off machines?
- Are weights replaced after use?
- Are rules posted?
- Is there a time limit for using machines?
- Is there a dress code?

Quackery

- Are quack products sold and pushed?
- Do members speak well of the club and recommend it?
- Are you given promises of quick results?

Memberships

- Can your membership be sold, transferred, or canceled if you move?
- Is there a no-contract or monthly payment option available in case you change your mind?
- Are there hidden costs associated with membership (e.g., costs for testing, use of personal training)?

Other Important Questions

- Is the club well established (so it won't disappear overnight)?
- Can you make a trial visit during the hours when you would expect to use the facility to determine if it is overcrowded and if you would enjoy the atmosphere?
- Is the club well rated or have there been complaints? (Check the Better Business Bureau.)
- Is this club your best option? Have you investigated programs offered by the YMCA/YWCA, local colleges and universities, and municipal park and recreation departments?

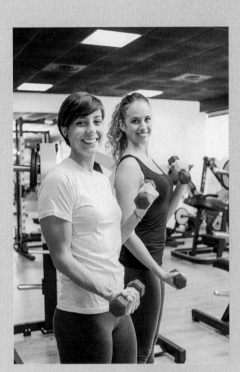

Figure 1 ▶ Questions to answer when choosing a health and fitness club.
Simone Becchetti/Getty Images

resources. Space does not allow a listing of all the common weight loss scams; however, following are two current scams that companies use to deceptively market products to gullible consumers:

- *Use of prescription drugs not approved for weight loss.* One example is hCG (human chorionic gonadotropin), a drug for the treatment of fertility. There is no scientific evidence of benefits for weight loss and the FTC and FDA have taken steps against those promoting its use for weight loss.

- *Acai berry scam.* Quacks have set up websites from fake news organizations (with graphics from a real news organization) to promote acai berry supplements for weight loss.

It is difficult for the FDA to keep up with the continual release of new health and weight loss supplements on the market; thus, consumers have to take responsibility for making sound decisions.

Nutrition Quackery

Diets are a major source of quackery. Recommendations for nutrition and healthy eating practices are summarized in established federally approved nutrition guidelines. Beware of diets that do not follow these guidelines. Avoid diets that emphasize one nutrient at the expense of others (unbalanced diets), require the purchase of special products, and are proposed by people lacking sound credentials.

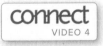

It is not true that if a little of something is "good," more is "better." The marketing of nutrition products often relies on convincing people that additional vitamins, minerals, or enzymes are beneficial. It is true that deficiencies of certain compounds may be harmful, but extra amounts don't always provide added protection or improved health. The

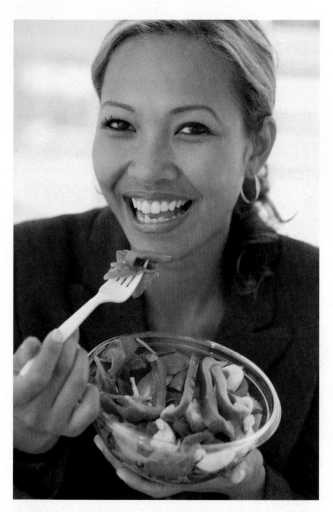

Vegetables provide many vitamins, minerals, and other essential nutrients.

©Stephen Welstead/Blend Images LLC

healthy. There are literally thousands of herbal products, and most medicines are derived from plants. However, the fact that herbs are natural does not mean they are safe. An herbal product known as kratom has been marketed with an array of claims (e.g., energy booster, mood enhancer, pain reliever, and an antidote for opioid withdrawal); however, it has many documented side effects and risks including seizures, coma, and death. The evidence has resulted in warnings from the FDA not to use the supplement; but consumers need to be aware since products may still contain this compound.

Many other supplements are marketed for losing weight. The herbal stimulant ephedra, which was used in many weight loss supplements, is one example. Over 150 deaths and thousands of adverse reactions were attributed to ephedra use before it could be officially banned. Several other prominent herbal products include saw palmetto, an herbal supplement touted as a preventive for prostate cancer, and echinacea, an herb widely used to reduce symptoms of the common cold. While early studies showed some promise for these products, subsequent studies have not supported claims for these supplements.

Some popular supplements from animal sources are also highly touted as having unique benefits. Glucosamine, for example, is made from shellfish, and chondroitin is made from the cartilage of sharks and/or cattle. Glucosamine and chondroitin are two of the most widely used supplements other than vitamins and minerals. They are often used to relieve symptoms and pain from osteoarthritis. Results of one large clinical trial suggested that the two supplements, taken together or separately, were no more effective than a placebo; however, a small group of people who had moderate to severe pain did experience some relief after using the supplements. These products probably do no harm, but they may also do little for clinical relief of joint problems.

Consumer Protections Against Fraud and Quackery

Current legislation makes it difficult to protect consumers against fraudulent dietary supplements. According to the FDA, a dietary supplement is a product taken by mouth that contains a "dietary ingredient" intended to supplement the diet. These ingredients include vitamins, minerals, herbs and other botanicals, amino acids, and other substances, such as enzymes, organ tissues, glandulars, and metabolites. Supplements come in many forms, including powders, tablets, softgels, capsules, gelcaps, and liquids. Consumers assume that supplements that are sold in stores (or online) are both safe and effective, but neither may be true. There are certainly many products sold in stores and online that are safe and effective, but careful research is necessary to be sure. The passage of the Dietary Supplements Health and Education Act (DSHEA) in the 1990s created loopholes that made it easy for companies to promote and sell untested products. Food supplements are typically not considered to

myth that vitamin C can cure the common cold is based on the fact that deficiencies of vitamin C can lead to scurvy. The same hype is used to sell consumers many other unnecessary supplements. For example, protein supplements are marketed with convincing (and honest) claims that the body needs amino acids to form muscle. The hidden truth is that the body cannot store or use more than it needs.

Beware of energy drinks with "boosts" sold at smoothie shops and fitness clubs. Many restaurants and shops now promote drinks containing "boosts" (a tablespoon or two of a food supplement). Health clubs that sell drinks with supplements are susceptible to the claim that they are selling products for financial gain rather than the best interests of clients. Even if some supplements are effective, which most are not, taking one dose in a drink would be ineffective and a waste of money.

The designations of "herbal" or "natural" on supplements do not ensure safety or efficacy. Many health and nutrition supplements emphasize the word *herbal* because it relates to plants, and people assume plants are natural and therefore

be drugs, so they are also not regulated. Unlike drugs and medicines, food supplements need not be proven effective or even safe to be sold in stores. To be removed from stores, they must be proven ineffective or unsafe. Unfortunately, it takes time and often extended court battles for the FDA and other agencies to get some products off the market.

When the DSHEA was passed in 1994, no provisions were included to ensure that dietary supplements contained the ingredients they claimed to contain. However, the FDA has since instituted a rule requiring supplement manufacturers to provide labels to ensure "a consistent product free of contamination, with accurate labeling." This is important because more than a few cases of product contamination have been reported. Under the new regulations, the manufacturer, not the FDA, has to test products to be sure that they are pure and accurately labeled. However, supplement companies are not required to document that their products are effective or even safe. It is not possible for the FDA to test all possible products so they monitor the safety of supplements through "adverse events monitoring." Thus, the only way that dangerous products and unscrupulous manufacturers can be identified is if consumers report problems to the FDA. The FDA has established a robust MedWatch alert system that allows consumers to report problems, symptoms, or spurious claims (see HELP feature for details). The "FDA 101" web page also provides information and tips to help avoid being a victim of fraud. (See Suggested Resources and Readings.)

Because supplements do not need approval of the FDA before they are marketed, consumers should be very cautious about any products they use. The following list represents a short summary of concerns and issues associated with unregulated supplements:

- Supplements can have unknown risks that are detected later. For example, hundreds of people died from consuming products containing ephedra before it could be banned.

- Supplements may include illegal or banned components. For example, an evaluation of more than 240 supplements detected that over 18 percent contained steroids.

- Supplements often contain drugs with chemical structures similar to banned drugs. For example, many weight loss/muscle supplements contain AMP citrate, a stimulant drug similar in chemical structure to an already banned stimulant known as DMAA.

- Supplements can have negative interactions with medicines or other treatments. For example, St. John's wort (a common herbal supplement used to treat depression) is thought to affect fertility and may lead to birth defects when used during pregnancy.

- Supplements can present unexpected risks due to contamination effects during production. For example, the FDA recently warned consumers about liver injuries and failure following use of the weight loss supplement Lipokinetix.

Consult labels for independently conducted quality checks to help you identify supplements that are what they say they are. The FDA's tainted supplement database lists over 100 companies that have been caught selling supplements spiked with drugs and chemicals that are banned or not listed as ingredients (search "FDA and Tainted Supplements"). However, as noted on its web page, *"the FDA is unable to test and identify all products marketed as dietary supplements that have potentially harmful hidden ingredients."* Several independent companies now assist by checking supplements for quality, safety, and compliance with FDA labeling and marketing requirements. The U.S. Pharmacopeial Convention (USP) and NSP International (NSP) are private nonprofit organizations that test supplements, while

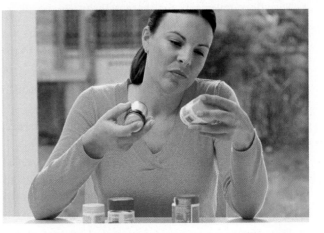

Good consumer skills are important for evaluating health products and for interpreting health claims.
Isadora Getty Buyou/Image Source

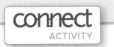

ConsumerLab (CL) is a for-profit group that also tests supplements. Products containing the USP, NSP, or CL labels provide some additional documentation that the products are what they say they are and contain no unspecified ingredients. However, these labels *do not* suggest that the products are recommended nor do they provide information about appropriate or inappropriate use of the products.

Most Americans favor increased regulation of the supplement industry. When informed that the FDA does not regulate supplements, more than 80 percent of adults indicate that the FDA should review supplements before they are offered for sale. More than half of adults want more regulation on advertising of supplements and better rules to ensure purity and accurate dosage. Despite the lack of regulation of supplements, nearly half of Americans routinely take supplements and slightly more than half believe in the value of supplements. Interestingly, 44 percent believe that physicians know little or nothing about supplements. More than a few critics point out that self-regulation within the industry has not worked well. To try to improve efforts to protect the public, the FDA has announced several initiatives to increase oversight of supplements, including modernization of DSHEA, enhanced enforcement actions against unlawful claims and ingredients, updated ingredient notifications, and development of a rapid notification system to alert the public about dangerous supplements. (See the Suggested Resources and Readings section in this Concept.)

Consumers should consult physicians about using vitamin supplements. A panel of experts with the National Institutes of Health (NIH) recently prepared a report noting the value of some vitamin and mineral supplements while not recommending others. Examples of vitamins and minerals that were endorsed include:

- Folic acid supplements for females of childbearing age.

- Calcium and vitamin D to protect against osteoporosis for postmenopausal females.

- Specific supplements for those with an eye condition called macular degeneration.

Examples of those that were *not* endorsed for health significant health benefits include:

- Beta-carotene (a form of vitamin A), as it was not found to be effective.

- Daily multivitamins. They were not found to be effective, although no evidence was found that they are harmful.

- Megadoses of vitamins and minerals. The board warned against taking very high levels of vitamins and minerals (megadoses), noting that they are not beneficial and can be dangerous.

These summaries are provided for general information. It is best to check with your physician about your personal needs.

Be wary of claims made for supplements, particularly in free pamphlets and handouts provided in stores. The DSHEA included regulations that prevent companies from making unsubstantiated claims on product labels. Unfortunately, the act failed to limit false claims that are not on the product label. Supplement makers circumvented the spirit of the rule by hinting at effects with clever names, through promotional ads, and most directly through a variety of quack pamphlets and publications. The literature is distributed separately from the product, thus allowing sellers to make unsubstantiated claims for products. (This is protected by free speech laws.) Also, the law does not prohibit unproven verbal claims by salespeople. Many medical experts feel that "alternative treatments" should be subjected to the same type of rigorous scientific testing used to evaluate other medicines. A prominent editorial suggested that "putting customers' health at risk is a high price to pay for a free market in diet supplements." In spite of difficulties in holding supplement companies accountable, the FTC has had some success in litigating against abusers. It won a judgment against the makers of the supplement ReJuvenation, which had been touted as an "antiaging wonder pill." It promised to reverse aging, repair the body, and treat disease. A multimillion-dollar settlement was reached and money from the settlement will be returned to customers.

Health Literacy and the Internet

Not all books provide information that is sound, reliable, and scientifically accurate. Some material is published on the basis of how popular, famous, or attractive the author is or how sensational or unusual his or her ideas are.
Very few movie stars, models, TV personalities, and Olympic athletes are experts in biomechanics, anatomy and physiology, exercise, and other foundations of physical fitness. Having a good figure or physique, being fit, or having gone through a training program does not, in itself, qualify a person to advise others.

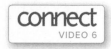

After reading the facts presented in this edition, you should be able to evaluate whether or not a book, a magazine, or an article on exercise and fitness is valid, reliable, and scientifically sound. To assist you further, Lab 24A lists 10 guidelines.

Not all websites provide information that is sound, reliable, and scientifically accurate. Currently, approximately three-fourths of all teen and young adult computer users seek health information on the Web. But many health websites contain misinformation. Studies show that Wikipedia is the most common source of health information for the general public. One report showed that as many as one-half of doctors surveyed used Wikipedia for health information. Many consumers, and some physicians, do not realize that Wikipedia can be edited by anyone and for this reason can contain erroneous information.

A research study directly compared information provided about prescription drugs on Wikipedia with similar content from a more credible site (Medscape Drug Reference). Not surprisingly, the Wikipedia site had incomplete answers, incorrect information about dosage, and errors of omission about side effects. The authors of the study concluded that Wikipedia should be used only as a supplemental source for drug information.

Improving health literacy is a public health goal. The Internet has made an almost unlimited amount of health information accessible, but it has proven difficult to ensure that the information is used wisely. The U.S. Public Health Service has established goals to improve public health literacy and the quality of health information on the Internet. The two goals are designed to work together: consumers need access to accurate information, but they also need to know how to interpret and use the information (health literacy). The content presented in this Concept provides a foundation for interpreting health information, but some additional guidelines are provided for effectively using the Internet.

One general rule is to consult at least two or more sources to confirm information. Getting confirmation of information from non-Web sources is also a good idea. Perhaps the most important recommendation is to consider the source of information. In general, government sites are valid sources that contain sound information prepared by experts and based on scientific research. Government sites typically include *.gov* as part of the address. Professional organizations and universities can also be good sources of information. Organizations typically have *.org* and universities typically have *.edu* as part of the address. However, caution should still be used with organizations because starting an organization and obtaining an *.org* address is easy. Your greatest trust can be placed in the sites of stable, credible organizations (see Suggested Resources and Readings). The great majority of websites promoting health products have *.com* in the address because these are commercial sites, which are in business to make a profit. Thus, although some contain good information, they may focus on selling products or services. Therefore, it is important to view content from these sites more critically.

Using Self-Management Skills

Reduce your susceptibility to quackery by being an informed consumer. Three characteristics that predispose people to health-related quackery are (1) a concern about appearance, health, or performance; (2) a lack of adequate knowledge; and (3) a desire for immediate results. Understanding the principles of exercise and nutrition will help you know when something sounds "too good to be true."

When evaluating health-related products or information, carefully consider the quality of your source. Common sources of misinformation are magazines, health food stores, and TV infomercials. These entities all have an economic incentive in promoting the purchase and use of exercise, diet, and weight loss products. Because of freedom of speech laws, it is legal to state opinion through these media. Note, however, that few companies make claims on product labels, since this is false advertising. Follow these additional guidelines to avoid being a victim of quackery:

- Read the ad carefully, especially the small print.
- Do not send cash; use a check, money order, or credit card so you will have a receipt.
- Do not order from a company with only a post office box, unless you know the company.
- When making decisions about products or services, begin your investigation well in advance of the day when a decision is to be made.
- Do not let high-pressure sales tactics make you rush into a decision.
- When in doubt, check out the company through the Better Business Bureau.

Understanding principles of persuasion can help you make more informed decisions. Making good consumer decisions requires critical thinking skills and discipline. Advertising and marketing campaigns can be highly persuasive; thus, it is important to learn to identify the strategies that companies

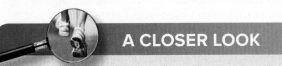

A CLOSER LOOK

College Students: Victims of Misinformation

Research indicates that teens and young adults rely heavily on the Internet when looking for health, wellness, and fitness information. This occurs in spite of evidence that much of the information that they view may be inaccurate or misleading. A recent study conducted at Stanford University found that college students have difficulty identifying if information on the Internet is accurate. Undergraduate college students were asked to assess the credibility of information in a news article and at a website. The news story was satire rather than factual information. Two-thirds of the students failed to realize that the story did not contain accurate news. Nine of ten students failed to recognize that the Internet article was created by a public relations firm and was not unbiased information. Many of the students failed to look at other websites or seek information to substantiate the contents on the website. The researcher recommends that people learn skills in fact-checking to avoid being deceived.

Do you have more confidence in your ability to know if news or Internet content is reliable and accurate? Do you agree that college students need to learn skills for assessing Internet content as it relates to health, wellness, and fitness?

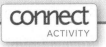
ACTIVITY

Technology Update

DNA Testing Services

Genetics have a major influence on health, and advances in genetic technology may make it possible for individuals to better understand inherited health risks as well as potential risks to offspring. A company called 23andMe provides a "DNA analysis service" that allows individuals to learn about and explore their DNA. Until recently, the company was able to provide only general information about genetic variants, but the FDA recently approved of "direct-to-consumer" genetic testing. The current approval is for "carrier testing," which determines whether a healthy person has a genetic variation that could lead to an offspring inheriting a potentially serious disorder. With this step, the FDA acknowledged that, in some cases, consumers should not have to go through a licensed medical provider to obtain information about their personal genetic information. The change will likely spur additional innovation and may open the door to broader access to genetic testing. However, reports from established public health agencies, such as the CDC, warn consumers about the limitations of these tests (see the article "Direct to Consumer Genetic Testing: Think Before You Spit, 2017 Edition!" in the Suggested Resources and Readings).

Do you support the use of this type of testing, or could it just lead to potential quackery? Would you value learning about your genetic predisposition if the information were available? Why or why not?

connect ACTIVITY

Suggested Resources and Readings

The websites for the following sources can be accessed by searching online for the organization, program, or title listed. Specific scientific references are available at the end of this edition of *Concepts of Fitness and Wellness.*

- American Council on Science and Health.
- Berezow, A. (2017). *Little Black Book of Junk Science.* New York: American Council on Science and Health.
- Bomey, N. (2020, October 19). "College Students Struggle to Spot Misinformation Online as 2020 Election Approaches." *USA Today.*
- Center for Science in the Public Interest.
- Centers for Disease Control and Prevention. "Direct to Consumer Genetic Testing: Think Before You Spit, 2017 Edition!"
- Cohut, M. (2019, December 3). "Study Outlines Concerns Around Natural Psychoactive Substances." *Medical News Today.*
- Federal Trade Commission:
  - Avoiding and Reporting Scams.
  - Bureau of Consumer Protection.
  - Consumer Information.

(and quacks) use to manipulate your beliefs and impulses. Robert Cialdini, a leading expert in consumerism, emphasizes that "persuasion is no longer just an art, it's an out-and-out science." For example, evidence clearly documents that individuals are more likely to follow through on a decision after they develop a personal commitment or internalized belief. Companies know this and frequently lure consumers with low-ball prices or promises that then are later retracted or softened. Once a person makes a preliminary decision to take an action, they tend to follow through, even after the costs (or value) of performing that action have been changed. Fortunately, evidence also suggests that awareness of these influences can help individuals detect when they are being influenced or manipulated into a decision or a purchase.

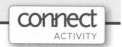

Strategies for Action: Lab Information

Being a good consumer requires time, information, and effort. Taking the time to investigate a product will help you save money and avoid making poor decisions that affect your health, wellness, and fitness. In Lab 24A you will evaluate an exercise device, a food supplement, a book, a magazine article, or a website. In Lab 24B you will evaluate a health, wellness, or fitness club to gain experience in what to look for.

connect ACTIVITY

- Dietary Supplements.
- "FTC Takes Action to Stop Anti-Aging 'Cure-All' Marketers from Making Baseless Health Claims." (2020, February 5).
- Indoor Tanning.
- McGrew, S., et al. (2019). "Improving University Students' Web Savvy: An Intervention Study." *British Journal of Educational Psychology, 89,* 485–500.
- MedlinePlus.
- Myer, Z. (2019, February 11). "Your Dietary Supplements Are about to Get Safer, as FDA Does First Overhaul in 25+ Years." *USA Today.*
- Quackwatch. Your Guide to Quackery, Health Fraud, and Intelligent Decisions.
- U.S. Department of Health and Human Services. MyHealthfinder.
- U.S. Food and Drug Administration:
  - FDA 101: Overview of FDA's Regulatory Review and Research Activities.
  - FDA Adverse Event Reporting System (FAERS) Public Dashboard.
  - MedWatch: The FDA Safety Information and Adverse Event Reporting Program.
  - Statement from FDA Commissioner Scott Gottlieb, M.D., on the Agency's New Efforts to Strengthen Regulation of Dietary Supplements by Modernizing and Reforming FDA's Oversight (2019, February 11).

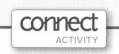

Lab 24A Practicing Consumer Skills: Evaluating Products

Name	**Section**	**Date**

Purpose: To evaluate an exercise device; a food supplement; a book, article, or advertisement; or a website.

Procedures

1. Select an appropriate product or promotional item to review from one of the following four categories: 1. Exercise Device, 2. Food Supplement, 3. Book, Article, or Advertisement, or 4. Website.
2. Complete Chart 1 to provide details of the product/item you reviewed. You should provide the specific name and manufacturer (if you selected an exercise device or food supplement) or a title/source/reference (if you reviewed a book, article, advertisement, or website), then the specific citation or source for a book, article, advertisement, or website. Finally, provide a description of the product in your own words.
3. Complete Chart 2 to evaluate the specific characteristics or qualities of the product or tool that you reviewed. Fill in circles for items that are "True" for the product or promotion you are evaluating.
4. Total the number of true statements out of 10 and report the total to compute an overall score for the item being evaluated. The higher the score, the more likely it is to be safe and/or effective.
5. Answer the questions in the Conclusions and Implications section.

Chart 1 Product Category _____ (I, 2, 3, or 4)

Name, Manufacturer, Source, or Reference	Brief Description of Product, Item, Book/Article/Advertisement, or Website

Conclusions and Implications: In several sentences, give your assessment of the product (be sure to refer to specific questions in Chart 2 that influenced your conclusion). Did it score well? Would you use/buy the product? Explain.

Results: Place an X over the circle by each true statement and summarize your score at the bottom by tallying the number of true statements.

Chart 2

Exercise Device

◯ 1. The exercise device requires effort consistent with the FIT fomula.

◯ 2. The exercise device is safe and the exercise done using the device is safe.

◯ 3. There are no claims that the device uses exercise that is effortless.

◯ 4. Exercise using the device is fun or is a type that you might do regularly.

◯ 5. There are no claims using gimmick words, such as *tone, cellulite, quick,* or *spot fat reduction*.

◯ 6. The seller's credentials are sound.

◯ 7. The product does something for you that cannot be done without it.

◯ 8. You can return the device if you do not like it (the seller has been in business for a long time).

◯ 9. The cost of the product is justified by the potential benefits.

◯ 10. The device is easy to store or you have a place to permanently use the equipment without storing it.

Food Supplement

◯ 1. The seller is not the prime source of product information.

◯ 2. The seller has been in business for a long time and has a good reputation.

◯ 3. There is scientific evidence of product effectiveness.

◯ 4. There is clear evidence about the side effects of the active ingredients.

◯ 5. The long-term effectiveness and safety of the product are cited.

◯ 6. You are sure of the content of the product.

◯ 7. You have information that the manufacturer is reputable.

◯ 8. The known benefits are worth the cost.

◯ 9. There is evidence that you can get benefits from this product that cannot be obtained from good food.

◯ 10. There are no claims that use quack words or claims about conspiracies against the product by reputable organizations.

Book/Article/Advertisement

◯ 1. The credentials of the author are sound. He or she has a degree in an area related to the content of the book or magazine.

◯ 2. The facts in the article are consistent with the facts described in *Concepts of Fitness and Wellness*.

◯ 3. The author does not claim "quick" or "miraculous" results.

◯ 4. There are no claims about the spot reduction of fat or other unfounded claims.

◯ 5. The author/advertisement is not selling a product.

◯ 6. Reputable experts are cited.

◯ 7. The article does not promote unsafe exercises or products.

◯ 8. New discoveries from exotic places are not cited.

◯ 9. The article/advertisement does not rely on testimonials by nonexpert, famous people.

◯ 10. The author/advertisement does not make claims that the AMA, the FDA, or another legitimate organization is trying to suppress information.

Website

◯ 1. The site does not sell products associated with information provided.

◯ 2. The provider is a person, an organization (.org), or a governmental agency (.gov) with a sound reputation.

◯ 3. The site does not use quack words.

◯ 4. The site does not try to discredit well-established organizations or governmental agencies.

◯ 5. The site does not rely on testimonials, celebrities, or people with unknown credentials.

◯ 6. The site is endorsed by, or linked to, credible agencies, associations, or experts.

◯ 7. The site has a history of providing good information.

◯ 8. The site provides complete information that is documented by research.

◯ 9. No claims of quick cures or miracle results are made.

◯ 10. The site provides information consistent with content provided in this Concept.

Summary Score: Total the number of Xs for the device, book/article/advertisement, food supplement, or website:

Lab 24B Evaluating a Health, Wellness, or Fitness Club

Name	**Section**	**Date**

Purpose: To practice evaluating a health club (various combinations of the words *health, wellness,* and *fitness* are often used for these clubs).

Procedures

1. Choose a club and make a visit.
2. Listen carefully to all that is said and ask many questions.
3. Look carefully all around as you are given the tour of the facilities. Ask what the exercises or the equipment will do for you, or ask leading questions such as, "Will this take inches off my hips?"
4. As soon as you leave the club, rate it using Chart 1.

Chart 1 Health Club Evaluation Questionnaire

Place an X over a "yes" or "no" answer.	Yes	No	Notes
1. Were claims for improvement in weight, figure/physique, or fitness realistic?	○	○	
2. Was a long-term contract (1–3 years) encouraged?	○	○	
3. Was the sales pitch high-pressure to make an immediate decision?	○	○	
4. Were you given a copy of the contract to read at home?	○	○	
5. Did the fine print include objectionable clauses?	○	○	
6. Did the club representative ask you about medical readiness?	○	○	
7. Did the club sell diet supplements as a sideline?	○	○	
8. Did the club have passive equipment?	○	○	
9. Did the club have cardiovascular training equipment or facilities (cycles, track, pool, aerobic dance)?	○	○	
10. Did the club make unscientific claims for the equipment, exercise, baths, or diet supplements?	○	○	
11. Were the facilities clean?	○	○	
12. Were the facilities crowded?	○	○	
13. Were there days and hours when the facilities were open but would not be available to you?	○	○	
14. Were there limits on the number of minutes you could use a piece of equipment?	○	○	
15. Did the floor personnel closely supervise and assist clients?	○	○	
16. Were the floor personnel qualified experts?	○	○	
17. Were the managers/owners qualified experts?	○	○	
18. Has the club been in business at this location for a year or more?	○	○	

Results

1. Score the chart as follows:

   A. Give 1 point for each "no" answer for items 2, 3, 5, 7, 8, 10, 12, 13, and 14 and place the score in the box.

   Total A ⬚

   B. Give 1 point for each "yes" answer for items 1, 4, 6, 9, 11, and 18 and place the score in the box.

   Total B ⬚

   Total A and B above and place the score in the box.

   Total A and B ⬚

   C. Give 1 point for each "yes" answer for items 15, 16, and 17 and place the score in the box.

   Total C ⬚

2. A total score of 12–15 points on items A and B suggests the club rates at least fair, compared with other clubs.

3. A score of 3 on item C indicates that the personnel are qualified and suggests that you could expect to get accurate technical advice from the staff.

4. Regardless of the total scores, you would have to decide the importance of each item to you personally, as well as evaluate other considerations, such as cost, location, and personalities of the clients and the personnel, to decide if this would be a good place for you or your friends to join.

Conclusions and Implications: In several sentences, discuss your conclusion about the quality of this club and whether you think it would fit your needs if you wanted to belong.

Toward Optimal Health and Wellness: Planning for Healthy Lifestyle Change

LEARNING OBJECTIVES

After completing the study of this Concept, you will be able to:

▶ Assess inherited health risks.

▶ Describe how to access and use the health-care system effectively.

▶ Explain the importance of environmental influences on lifestyle (as well as the impact of our lifestyles on our environment).

▶ List the key healthy lifestyles that influence health and wellness.

▶ Explain how personal actions and interactions influence the adoption of healthy lifestyles.

▶ Apply behavioral skills to plan and follow personal health and fitness programs.

In addition to healthy lifestyles, other factors such as heredity, health care, the environment, cognitions and emotions, and personal actions and interactions contribute to good health, wellness, and fitness.

©Andersen Ross/Media Bakery

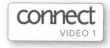

Why It Matters!

The broad vision of the national health goals is to create "a society in which all people live long, healthy lives." The focus is on *healthspan* (having many years of good health, wellness, and fitness), as well as *lifespan* (living a long life). Earlier, you were introduced to a comprehensive model that explained the many determinants of health, wellness, and fitness. You learned that you have the most control over the lifestyle you lead, reasonable control over your cognitions and emotions, some control over your environment and use of health care, but relatively little control over heredity factors. Lifestyle behaviors are emphasized because they are under your control. Self-management skills are also emphasized because they help you learn how to adopt and sustain healthy behaviors over time. This final Concept revisits the determinants model to enable you to address the many factors that influence your health, wellness, and fitness.

Understand Inherited Risks and Strengths

Learn about your family health history and take stock of inherited risk. As illustrated in Figure 1, biological determinants (such as heredity) influence health, wellness, and fitness status. If members of your immediate or extended family have had specific diseases or health problems, you may have a greater risk or likelihood of the same condition. Your DNA contains the instructions for building the proteins that control the structure and function of all the cells in your body. Abnormalities in DNA can provide the wrong set of instructions and lead to faulty cell growth or function. There are clear genetic influences on risks for obesity, cardiovascular disease risk factors, diabetes, and many forms of cancer. At present it is not possible for people to truly know their genetic risk profile, but it may be possible in the future with more comprehensive genetic testing.

Take action to diminish risk factors for which you have a predisposition. As mentioned, research shows strong familial aggregation of certain chronic disease risk factors (e.g., obesity, diabetes, cholesterol, blood pressure) as well as some cancers. While you cannot change your heredity risks, you can take steps to reduce your risks for certain inherited conditions (see lifestyle determinants in Figure 1). Specifically, adopting healthy lifestyles may significantly reduce inherited risks for certain diseases. Researchers have computed obesity risk scores based on the presence or absence of 32 genes known to increase weight status. The genetic risk score was associated with an individual's inherited risk for being overweight, but risk was influenced by lifestyle behaviors. An active lifestyle (marked by the presence of a brisk daily walk) reduced the genetic influence by

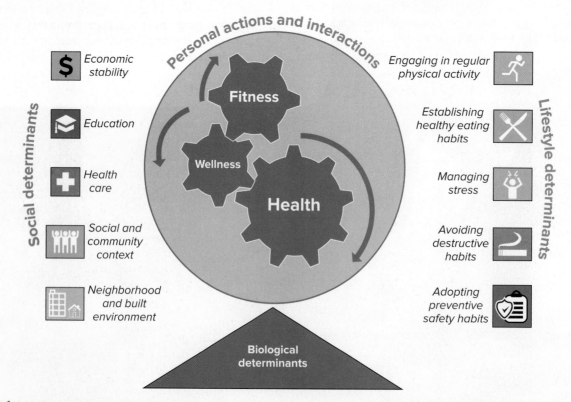

Figure 1 ▶ Influence of personal actions and interactions on health, wellness, and fitness.

50 percent, while a sedentary lifestyle (marked by watching television 4 hours a day) increased the genetic influence by 50 percent. Eating a healthy diet, managing stress, and not smoking are other important lifestyles that would likely contribute to lowering inherited risks for disease.

Make Effective Use of Health Care

Follow sound medical advice and recommendations. The medical system can provide individuals with supportive, personalized health care, but people have to seek consultation and follow advice for it to be effective (see Table 1). Some basic strategies for accessing the medical system effectively are summarized here:

- *Get medical insurance.* The rising costs of health care make health insurance more important than ever. However, recent CDC statistics indicate that young adults are most likely to be uninsured. Uninsured rates are highest for those aged 25–34 and second highest among those 18–24. Those who are poor and nearly poor are more than three times more likely to be uninsured than those who are not poor. A 2030 national health goal is to increase the number of people with health insurance. People who think they save money by avoiding the payment of insurance premiums place themselves (and their families) at risk and may not really save money.

- *Consider a health savings account (HSA).* An HSA, typically employee funded, allows you to set aside a portion of your earnings to pay future medical expenses. You do not pay tax on the money you set aside as long as you follow the rules. An HSA can save you money and encourages prevention and medical treatment.

- *Investigate and then identify a hospital and regular doctor.* Check with other physicians you know and trust for referrals. Check with your state medical board and national directories (e.g., Directory of Board Certified Medical Specialists, www.abms.org) for specialist certifications or fellowships. Choose an accredited emergency center near your home and a hospital that is accredited and grants privileges to your personal doctors.

- *Get periodic medical exams.* Do not wait until something is wrong before you seek medical advice. A yearly preventive physical exam is recommended for adults over the age of 40. Younger people should have an exam at least every 2 years.

- *Follow appropriate screening recommendations.* Many illnesses and chronic conditions can be treated effectively if they are identified early in the disease process. Following cancer screening guidelines is particularly important (e.g., mammograms for females and prostate tests for males). Breast and testicular self-exams are also important for detection.

- *Ask questions.* Do not be afraid to speak up. Prepare questions for doctors and other medical personnel. The American College of Surgeons suggests several questions before surgeries: What are the reasons for the surgery? Are there alternatives? What will happen if I don't have the procedure? What are the risks? What are the long-term effects and problems? How will the procedure impact my quality of life and future health?

- *Understand effects of medications.* Seek out information about medicines and supplements so you understand their intended effect. Read the inserts that come with the medicine and ask your doctor and pharmacist about correct dosage and information concerning when to take the medication. The FDA recently simplified drug inserts to help you understand the information that comes with medicine. Track your medicine and supplement use and share it with your physician.

- *Consider potential side effects of medicines you take.* Most medications are tested for use with certain populations, and they may not be safe or effective for all people. Consider the safety and potential risks. Side effects from preventable adverse reactions to medicines account for more than 1.5 million deaths each year. When medicine is prescribed, ask for details. Ask why the medicine was prescribed and the nature of side effects. Ask if the medicine interacts with other medicines or supplements.

- *If you have doubts about medical advice, get a second opinion.* Some estimates indicate that as many as 30 percent of original diagnoses are incorrect or differ from second opinions. Don't worry about offending your doctor by getting another opinion. Good doctors encourage this.

- *Make your wishes for health care known.* Have a medical power of attorney. This document spells out the treatments you desire in the case of severe illness. Without such a document, your loved ones may not be able to make decisions consistent with your wishes. Be sure your loved ones have a similar document so that you can also help them carry out their wishes.

Table 1 ▶ Facts about Health-Care Use

- More females than males have a regular physician.

- More than half of young males have no personal doctor.

- Three times more females than males have visited a doctor in the past year.

- Females are more aware of health issues than males.

- Nearly half of males wait a week or more to see a doctor when ill.

- Many males see sickness as "unmanly."

- Married males see doctors more frequently than single males because their spouses or partners prompt them.

- Lack of health insurance results in fewer doctor's visits, less frequent health screening, and less access to prescribed medicine.

Become a wise health- and medical-care consumer.
Medical illiteracy and lack of health-care information are
linked to higher than normal death rates. This is why improving medical literacy is such a high priority for public health
officials. Some strategies for becoming a better health- and
medical-care consumer are listed here.

- *Become familiar with the symptoms of common medical
  problems.* If symptoms persist, seek medical help. Many
  deaths can be prevented if early warning signs of medical
  problems are heeded.

- *Practice good hygiene.* The consensus among health experts is that hand washing is effective in flu prevention
  and is among the best defenses against the common cold
  and other respiratory illnesses (as reinforced during the
  COVID-19 pandemic). Always wash hands before preparing food or eating and after using the toilet, touching animals, handling garbage, coughing, or blowing your nose.
  Avoid sharing cups and utensils, and use hand sanitizers
  when you don't have access to water.

- *Stay home when you are sick.* Most companies urge sick
  employees to stay home to prevent spreading illness to
  others. Sickness (especially the flu) can spread rapidly in
  worksites or group settings, which is why quarantining
  during the pandemic was critical. Use your "sick days"
  or avoid interactions with others if possible. Sick workers
  are less productive, and working when sick lengthens recovery time.

Technology Update

Is the *Star Trek* Tricorder a Reality?

The science fiction television series *Star Trek* featured
many futuristic technologies. The physician in the 1960s
series used a fictional device called a "Tricorder" for medical testing and to diagnose health conditions. Interestingly,
several multiple-function health devices have recently
been developed—and they actually resemble the original
Tricorder. The MedWand, for example, can be used by physicians as a stethoscope, a thermometer, and an EKG/heart
rate/oxygen monitor, to name a few of its multiple functions. Another multiple-function health device is the DxtER,
which uses sensors and an iPad app to collect health data
from patients. The innovative aspect of these technologies
is that data can be transmitted electronically to clinicians
for virtual monitoring or evaluation.

*What are your reactions to devices that enable virtual
health monitoring? Would you feel comfortable using
such a device or having a physician use one?*

connect
ACTIVITY

- *Carefully review the credibility and accuracy of new health
  information.* There are many examples of misleading
  claims and fraud in the health and fitness industry. Even
  news reports from credible scientific studies can exert too
  much influence on consumer decisions. It takes years for
  scientific consensus to emerge, so carefully review new
  health claims.

Consider Environmental Influences on Your Health

**Understand how environmental factors shape your
behaviors.** As described throughout this edition, environmental factors influence your health and well-being (see
Figure 2). The term *obesogenic environments* has been used
to describe specifically how aspects of our environment
contribute to overeating and lack of physical activity. To
live healthy, it is important to understand how environmental settings and factors influence our lifestyles. Figure 2
summarizes the broad impact of physical, social, emo-
tional/mental, spiritual, and intellectual environments on
personal health and wellness. Specific environmental strategies that you can use for each dimension of wellness are
listed here:

- *Strategies for the physical environment.* Living healthy in
  our modern society can be challenging, but this can be
  overcome with good planning.
  Think ahead about ways to be sitting less during the day and how to
  add daily physical activity (e.g.,
  commuting and walk breaks). Plan your meals and dining
  choices to ensure you can make healthier food choices.
  Avoid smoke-filled establishments, highly polluted environments, and use of toxic products.

  connect
  VIDEO 2

- *Strategies for the social and emotional environments.* Find a
  social community that accommodates your personal and
  family needs; get involved in community affairs, including
  those that affect the environment; build relationships with
  family and friends; provide support for others so that their
  support will be there for you when you need it; and use
  time-management strategies to help you allocate time for
  social interactions.

- *Strategies for the spiritual environment.* Pray, meditate, read
  spiritual materials, participate in spiritual discussions,
  find a place to worship, provide spiritual support for others, seek spiritual guidance from those with experience
  and expertise, keep a journal, experience nature, honor
  relationships, and help others.

- *Strategies for the intellectual environment.* Make decisions
  based on sound information, question simple solutions to
  complex problems, and seek environments that stimulate
  critical thinking.

A positive *physical* environment helps make the healthy choice the easy choice.

- **Access to physical activity and healthy foods:** A healthy environment supports efforts to adopt healthy lifestyles by making it easier to be active and to eat healthy. Parks, trails, and green spaces provide opportunities to be active. Farmers' markets, health sections of grocery stores, and food co-ops make it easier to select healthy food.

- **Safe and clean communities:** A pleasant, clean, and safe environment encourages healthy living and the adoption of healthy lifestyles. Clean water and clean air are critical for good health.

A positive *spiritual* environment helps to support spiritual fulfillment.

- **Opportunities for spiritual development:** Reading spiritual materials, prayer, meditation, and discussions with others provide opportunities to clarify and solidify spiritual beliefs.

- **Access to spiritual community and leadership:** Finding a community for worship provides comfort and a path to fulfillment for many. Consider consultation with those with experience and expertise.

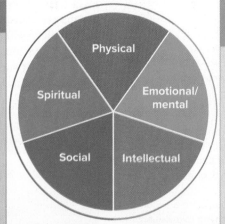

A positive *emotional* environment can help with adopting healthy lifestyles and managing stress.

- **Supportive personal relationships:** Support by others, especially family members, can help in managing stress and in adopting healthy lifestyles. Unhealthy relationships have the opposite effect.

- **Stress-management skills:** Friends, families, and coworkers can provide emotional support to assist in coping and stress management.

A healthy *social* environment enhances quality of life and supports wellness.

- **A sense of community:** Being a part of the greater community is important to social and mental health. Community-based groups are also important for planning and promoting healthy lifestyles for residents.

- **Social support:** A strong support network can help in times of need and provide advice, assistance, or support when needed.

A stimulating *intellectual* environment fosters learning and critical thinking.

- **Access to accurate information:** Whether the source is formal education or self-learning, access to accurate information is essential. Of course, good information is beneficial only if used.

- **Build and maintain cognitions:** A stimulating intellectual environment can promote self-discovery, build cognitive skills, and promote critical thinking.

Figure 2 ▶ The influence of environmental factors on dimensions of wellness.

Choose to live and work in places that support healthy living. Environmental factors are often out of a person's control. However, you do have some autonomy regarding where you choose to live and work. If physical activity is important to you, find a community with parks and playgrounds and accessible sidewalks, bike paths, jogging trails, swimming facilities, a gym, or health club. Avoid environments that have only fast food restaurants. Find a social environment that reinforces healthy lifestyles. If possible, work in businesses or settings that support healthy lifestyles. Ideally, the work environment should have adequate space, lighting, and freedom from pollution (tobacco smoke), as well as a healthy physical, social, spiritual, and intellectual environment. Considerable attention has been given recently to characteristics that define healthy work sites, communities, cities, and states. This is encouraging because the increased demand for healthy resources could lead to increased supply.

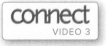

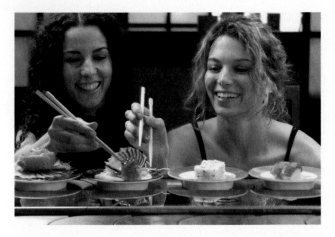

Being open to new experiences is important for optimal wellness.
Vision SRL/Getty Images

   Health is available to Everyone for a Lifetime, and it's Personal

A Planetary Health Pledge

The Hippocratic Oath taken by physicians is an ancient pledge that focuses on putting patients first: "do no harm." In 1948, the World Medical Association updated the oath with the Declaration of Geneva. Other health professionals have similar oaths that are periodically updated. Recently a group of health professionals proposed a "planetary pledge" that focuses on "committing to a vision of personal, community, and planetary health that will enable the diversity of life on our planet to thrive now and in the future." They advocate for "equity and justice by actively addressing environmental, social, and structural determinants of health" (as described in this edition). We are increasingly connected as a global society, thus, coordinated action is needed to support health and healthy environments for all.

Do you endorse the interconnectedness reflected by a planetary pledge? Would a personal pledge help you similarly achieve your personal wellness goals?

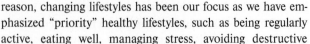
ACTIVITY

Adopt and Maintain Healthy Lifestyles

Consider strategies for adopting healthy lifestyles. Statistics show that more than half of early deaths are caused by unhealthy lifestyles. For this

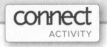
VIDEO 4

reason, changing lifestyles has been our focus as we have emphasized "priority" healthy lifestyles, such as being regularly active, eating well, managing stress, avoiding destructive

behaviors, and practicing safe sex, because they are factors over which we have some control, and if adopted, they have considerable impact on health, wellness, and fitness (see the right side of Figure 1). Being an informed consumer is another healthy lifestyle we have emphasized since it enables you to understand health information and take appropriate action. Other healthy lifestyles include adopting good health (e.g., getting adequate sleep), adopting safety habits (e.g., wearing seat belts and using bike helmets), and learning first aid. Examples of healthy lifestyles in these domains are highlighted in Table 2.

Consider the impact of your lifestyle on the health of the environment. The environment clearly influences your lifestyle, but your lifestyle can also have a damaging effect on the environment. Consider our use of fossil fuels. Burning fossil fuels has contributed to depletion of the ozone layer and the associated patterns of climate change. The changes in weather along with the pollution of our air and water compromise our agricultural systems, which in turn threatens our food and water supply. These are just a few examples of the complex ecological systems going on in the world. A number

Table 2 ▶ Other Healthy Lifestyles

Lifestyle	Examples
Adopting good personal health habits. Many of these habits, important to optimal health, are considered to be elementary because they are often taught in school or in the home at an early age. In spite of their importance, many adults regularly fail to adopt these behaviors.	• Brush and floss teeth. • Bathe and wash hands regularly. • Get adequate sleep. • Take care of ears, eyes, and skin. • Limit exposure to loud sounds, including live and recorded music. • Limit sun exposure (e.g., wear protective clothing, hats, and sunglasses) and use sunscreen with high SPF to reduce exposure to ultraviolet rays from the sun.
Adopting good safety habits. Thousands of people die each year and thousands more suffer disabilities or problems that detract from good health and wellness. Not all accidents can be prevented, but we can adopt habits to reduce risk.	• *Automobile accidents.* Wear seat belts, avoid using the phone while driving, do not drink and drive, and do not drive aggressively. • *Water accidents.* Learn to swim, learn cardiopulmonary resuscitation (CPR), wear life jackets while boating, and do not drink while boating. • *Others.* Store guns safely, use smoke alarms, use ladders and electrical equipment safely, and maintain cars, bikes, and motorcycles properly.
Learning first aid. Many deaths could be prevented and the severity of injury could be reduced if those at the sites of emergencies were able to administer first aid.	• Learn CPR. New research shows that chest compression alone saves lives even without mouth-to-mouth breathing. • Learn the Heimlich maneuver to assist people who are choking. • Learn basic first aid.

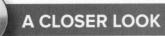

A CLOSER LOOK

Getting Enough Sleep? Turn Off Your Phone

According to the CDC, one in three adults fails to get the recommended 7 hours of sleep each night. Adults between the ages of 25 and 54 are least likely to get adequate sleep, followed by those 18–24. The CDC also indicates that "short sleepers" are more likely to be obese and to have hypokinetic conditions (e.g., heart disease, stroke, diabetes) than people who get adequate rest. A recent study of teens and their parents suggests that use of smartphones is one factor associated with inadequate sleep. Approximately 60–70 percent of adults report keeping their phone nearby when sleeping; about 25 percent wake up at least once in the night to check their phone. Of teens who have their phone with them at bedtime, 45 percent say they are using it only for personal use. Many (32 percent of teens and 23 percent of adults) check their phones within 5 minutes of waking up.

Do you get sufficient sleep for your health? Do you think smartphone use contributes to poor sleep habits?

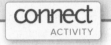

of promising strategies are being implemented to address these problems, including the use of alternative energy sources to reduce our consumption of fossil fuels. While technology can solve some of the problems, we cannot completely heal the environment without major efforts from large segments of the population. Individually we can't change the world, but if each person makes small changes, we can together have a big impact. For example, individual efforts to use your car less, recycle, and use less paper can add up to larger changes in society.

Importance of Personal Actions and Interactions

Consider strategies for taking action and benefiting from personal interactions. The diagram in Figure 1 includes the label "Personal actions and interactions" at the very top of the image. It is at the top for a reason—ultimately, it is what you do that counts. You can learn everything there is to know about health, wellness, and fitness, but if you do not take action and take advantage of your interactions with people and your environments, you will not benefit. As described in this Concept (and throughout this edition), your actions and interactions have a major influence on all aspects of wellness.

Commit to using this information to help plan your approaches for healthy living (see Table 3). People who plan are not only more likely to act, they are also more likely to act effectively and more proactively. Many people put off personal efforts to adopt healthier lifestyles, believing that they will eventually get around to making changes. Delaying action will only make it harder to change in the future. It is much easier to maintain a healthy weight than it is to lose weight after it is gained. This applies to all aspects of healthy living. "Do not put off until tomorrow what you can do today." We've discussed information to help you create plans for healthy living, but the decision to follow them is up to you.

Consider your cognitions and emotions when planning strategies for action. Much of the information in this edition is designed to help you make good decisions about health, wellness, and fitness. Using the guidelines and your

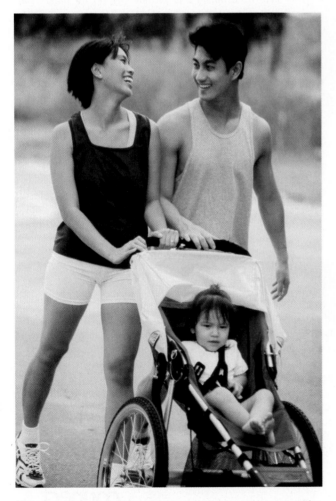

Make it a priority to find ways to remain active throughout your life.
Purestock/SuperStock

Table 3 ▶ Actions and Interactions That Influence Wellness

Dimension of Wellness	Influential Factors
Physical wellness	Pursuing behaviors that are conducive to good physical health (being physically active and maintaining a healthy diet)
Social wellness	Being supportive of family, friends, and coworkers and practicing good communication skills
Emotional wellness	Balancing work and leisure and responding proactively to challenging or stressful situations
Intellectual wellness	Challenging yourself to continually learn and improve in your work and personal life
Spiritual wellness	Praying, meditating, or reflecting on life
Total wellness	Taking responsibility for your own health

self-management skills can help you make good decisions. It is also important to consider your emotions when making decisions. Consider these guidelines:

- *Collect and evaluate information before you act.* Become informed before you make important decisions. Get information from reliable sources and consult with others you trust.

- *Emotions will influence certain decisions, but do not let them detract from sound decision-making processes.* Fear and anger are two emotions that can affect your judgment and influence your ability to make decisions. Even love for another person can influence your actions. Get control of your emotions, or seek guidance from others you trust, before making important decisions in emotionally charged situations.

- *Resist pressure to make quick decisions when there is no need to decide quickly.* Salespeople often press for a quick decision to get a sale. Take some time to think before making a quick decision that may be based on emotion rather than critical thinking. Of course, some decisions must be made when emotions are charged (e.g., medical care in an emergency), but, when possible, delaying a decision can be to your advantage.

- *Use stress-management techniques to help you gain control when you must make decisions in emotionally charged situations.* Practice stress-management techniques so that you can use them effectively when needed.

- *Honor your beliefs and relationships.* Actions and interactions that are inconsistent with basic beliefs and that fail to honor important relationships can result in reduced quality of life.

- *Seek help from others and provide support for others who need your help.* As already noted, support from friends, family, and significant others can be critical in helping you achieve health, wellness, and fitness. Get help. Do what you can to be there for others who need your help.

- *Consider using professional help.* Most colleges have health center programs that provide free, confidential assistance or referral. Many businesses have employee assistance programs (EAPs), providing counselors who will help you or your family members find ways to solve a particular problem. Other programs and support groups help with lifestyle changes. For example, most hospitals and many health organizations have hotlines that provide referral services for establishing healthy lifestyles.

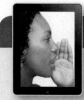

In the News

Healthy Lifestyles During the Pandemic

Numerous stories have commented on lifestyle changes caused by COVID-19. A survey conducted by the Cleveland Clinic (in cooperation with *Parade* magazine) evaluated whether people plan to sustain these lifestyle changes over time. Results showed that 87 percent have made a dietary change they plan to stick with, 76 percent have tried new coping techniques, and 65 percent say they have gained a new perspective on what really matters. These positive changes are important since 55 percent report an increase in mental stress during this period. People also identified changes in health care.

On the positive side, 41 percent reported that they are now more likely to comply with recommended health treatments and 25 percent said they were more likely to get a flu shot. Unfortunately, 38 percent skipped or delayed routine doctor's visits because of the pandemic. Some (27 percent) took advantage of telemedicine as an alternative to a face-to-face medical appointment.

What personal lifestyle changes have you made? Have you sustained them over time?

connect
ACTIVITY

Consider your personal beliefs and philosophy when making decisions. Though science can help you make good decisions and solve problems, most experts tell you that there is more to it than that. Your personal philosophy and beliefs play a role. The following are factors to consider:

- *Clarify your personal philosophy and consider a new way of thinking.* Health, wellness, and fitness are often subjective. Making comparisons to other people can result in setting personal standards impossible to achieve. For example, achieving the body fat level of a model seen on TV or performing like a professional athlete is not realistic for most of us. For this reason, the standards for health, wellness, and fitness in this edition are based on health criteria rather than comparative criteria. Adhering to the HELP philosophy can help you adopt a new way of thinking. This philosophy suggests that each person should use health (*H*) as the basis for making decisions rather than comparisons with others. This is something that everyone (*E*) can do for a lifetime (*L*). It allows each of us to set personal (*P*) goals that are realistic and possible to attain.

- *Allow for spontaneity.* The reliance on science we have emphasized can help you make good choices. But if you are to live life fully, you sometimes must allow yourself to be spontaneous. In doing so, the key is to be consistent with your personal philosophy so that your spontaneous actions will be enriching rather than a source of future regret.

- *Believe that you can make a difference.* As noted previously, you make your own choices. Though heredity and several other factors are out of your control, the choices that you make are yours. Believing that your actions make a difference is critical to taking action and making changes when necessary, allowing you to be healthy, well, and fit for a lifetime.

- *Be an optimist.* Optimism is a positive predictor of good physical health. This is the conclusion of a statistical review of 83 different studies. The analysis included studies of people with a variety of health conditions. In all cases, optimism was a predictor of positive health outcomes. Being optimistic, by itself, is not a treatment or a cure for physical health symptoms. However, maintaining an optimistic outlook and applying the HELP philosophy can go a long way toward maintaining health, wellness, and fitness throughout life.

Accepting personal responsibility is important for long-term health and well-being. Throughout this edition, we have placed emphasis on the fact that a healthy lifestyle is the most important determinant of good health. One of the five facets of a healthy lifestyle is adopting preventive safety habits. This includes complying with health screening guidelines and following medical advice. The Cooper Clinic in Dallas, Texas, specializes in preventive medical care and encourages personal responsibility in its patients. A staff physician (Dr. Tedd Mitchell) has categorized the types of

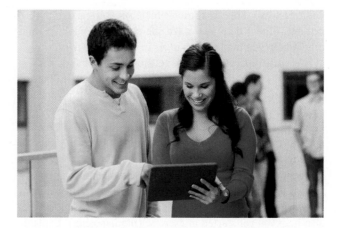

Support from friends can help you take action to achieve health, wellness, and fitness goals.
Syda Productions/Shutterstock

Table 4 ▶ Types of People Who Avoid Medical Checkups

- *Gamblers.* These people do not think about their health until a serious problem occurs.

- *Martyrs.* These people are so busy taking care of others that they fail to take care of themselves.

- *Economists.* These people think the cost of preventive exams is too high for the benefits received.

- *Shamans.* These people buy in to the latest health fad and self-diagnose, while avoiding regular medical care.

- *Informers.* These people have an ax to grind with health-care professionals and avoid health care for this reason.

- *Queens of denial (Cleopatra syndrome).* These people do not believe something could be wrong with them or do not want to know if there is.

- *Busy bees.* These people feel they are too busy to take the time to get regular medical care.

Source: Adapted from T. Mitchell, What's Your Excuse? 2002.

people by the reasons they give for not seeing a doctor or getting a regular medical checkup (see Table 4). According to Dr. Mitchell, there is no good reason to avoid your annual visit to the doctor. While it may be more difficult to do this during college years, make a commitment to establish plans for regular medical care and checkups in the future.

Using Self-Management Skills

Learning and adopting self-management skills can predispose and enable you to adhere to lifelong healthy behaviors and reinforce the behaviors once they are acquired. You have learned about the different self-management skills that help you adopt healthy lifestyles. For your review, these self-management skills are listed in

Table 5. Some skills are most useful to get you started (predisposing), others help you make the changes (enabling), and others help you maintain changes in behaviors (reinforcing). While each type of skill may be most influential at certain stages, *all* can be beneficial at any stage of change. For example, self-assessment is considered to be a predisposing factor because it provides you with the information about your personal needs. However, self-assessment can also be valuable in reinforcing behavior by providing a positive indicator of progress. Another example is using social support, which is considered to be reinforcing because having the support of friends and family can help you stick with a health behavior (e.g., regular exercise, healthy eating). But social support can also help you get started in exercise (predisposing). Explanations of how to apply various self-management skills have been included throughout the "Using Self-Management Skills" sections, but the summary in Table 5 will help remind you of the relevance of each one for lifestyle change.

Self-management skills, like all skills, must be practiced to be used effectively. All skills are best acquired through good practice. Good information, including good instruction with quality feedback, helps practice be effective. Many of the

lab activities in this edition are aimed at helping you practice self-management skills so that you can improve and perfect them. However, if you don't practice them regularly, your skills will eventually deteriorate. For this reason, regular use and practice of the self-management skills are encouraged.

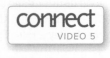

Formal steps for self-planning can become less formal with experience. Throughout this edition, we have presented a structured approach to self-planning that is designed to help you practice the various self-management skills required for effective planning (e.g., self-assessment, goal setting, self-monitoring). It is important to learn this process, but it is likely that you will eventually adopt less formalized procedures on your own. Few of us will go through life doing formal fitness assessments every month, writing down goals weekly, or self-monitoring activity daily. However, the more a person does self-assessments, the more he or she is aware of personal health, wellness, and fitness status. This awareness reduces the need for frequent testing. For example, a person

Table 5 ▶ Self-Management Skills and Relevance to Lifestyle Change	
Self-Management Skill	**Relevance to Lifestyle Change**
Predisposing Factors	
Overcoming Barriers	Adopting healthy lifestyles requires discipline, but you can learn to overcome barriers that make it difficult.
Building Confidence and Motivation	Focusing your efforts and progress can increase your confidence and motivation to change.
Balancing Attitudes	Adopting positive attitudes (and fighting negative ones) can increase the likelihood of making healthy changes.
Building Knowledge and Changing Beliefs	Distinguishing myths from facts can help with planning and behavior change.
Enabling Factors	
Goal-Setting Skills	Learning to set and follow reasonable goals can enable behavior change.
Self-Assessment Skills	Assessing your health, wellness, and fitness can help in determining needs and evaluating progress.
Self-Monitoring Skills	Learning to monitor your lifestyle behaviors can help you make healthier choices over time.
Self-Planning Skills	Following effective planning guidelines can increase your chances of being successful at behavior change.
Performance Skills	Applying and practicing various performance skills can increase your chances of success.
Coping Skills	Developing new ways of thinking can help you adapt to changing life circumstances.
Consumer Skills	Thinking critically about health, wellness, and fitness information can help you make better decisions.
Time-Managing Skills	Using time effectively can reduce stress and provide more time for physical activity and other healthy lifestyles.
Reinforcing Factors	
Using Social Support	Building strong support networks with friends and family members can help you adhere to and reinforce healthy habits.
Preventing Relapse	Preparing for challenges can increase your chance of overcoming them.

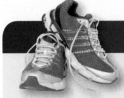

Strategies for Action: Lab Information

Doing a self-assessment of the factors that influence health, wellness, and fitness can identify needs for lifestyle change. The questionnaire in Lab 25A includes perceptions of your needs related to each of the five determinants described in Figure 1. An honest assessment of these items will help you determine factors that might be most important to change.

Following sound program planning skills can help you prepare a plan. In Lab 25B, you will have the opportunity to use the information gained from the self-assessment in Lab 25A to create a personal plan for appropriate changes aimed at improving health, wellness, and fitness. The lab guides you through appropriate steps to increase your chance of success.

Using the six steps in program planning can help you to prepare a comprehensive personal physical activity plan. In previous Concepts, you have had the opportunity to prepare plans for each of the different types of physical activity in the activity pyramid. Lab 25C provides you with the opportunity to use the self-management skills used in preparing these plans to provide a comprehensive plan for all types of physical activity.

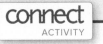

who does regular heart-rate monitoring knows when he or she is in the target zone without counting heart rate every minute. The same is true of other self-management skills. With experience, you can use the techniques less formally to manage your lifestyle in the future.

Building knowledge (a self-management skill) does not guarantee adherence to healthy behaviors, but it does provide the basis for making good decisions about future health behaviors. Throughout this edition, we have provided you with information that can be beneficial in making sound decisions about health, wellness, and fitness. But having the facts does not always lead to healthy decisions. For example, surveys consistently show that virtually all smokers know that tobacco use is unhealthy and leads to premature death. Yet people continue to start using tobacco, often at an early age and continue using throughout life. This example illustrates several important points. First, we sometimes make decisions at young ages, before we have all of the facts and when social and environmental factors have a larger impact on our decisions. We may know the facts, yet still not believe they will really impact us. Second, when unhealthy behaviors are adopted, they are often very difficult to change. Finally, we know that behaviors can change. With the use of self-management skills, even addictive behaviors can be changed. For example, social support from friends, loved ones, and professionals can help people, even smokers, change their behavior.

It is our hope that you will use the information (and self-management skills) learned from *Concepts of Fitness and Wellness* to help you adopt and sustain healthy behaviors throughout your life. Adopting a healthy lifestyle can be challenging, but you can hopefully rely on the strategies presented here to gradually shift your lifestyle toward behaviors more conducive to good health. We also hope that you will use your self-management skills to become a diligent and literate health consumer, seeking out the best and most current information about health, wellness, and fitness. New information becomes available daily, and being aware is critical to continuing to make sound decisions in the future.

Suggested Resources and Readings

The websites for the following sources can be accessed by searching online for the organization, program, or title listed. Specific scientific references are available at the end of this edition of *Concepts of Fitness and Wellness*.

- American College Health Association. Mental Health.
- American College of Sports Medicine. American Fitness Index.
- Centers for Disease Control and Prevention. Sleep and Sleep Disorders.
- Cleveland Clinic Newsroom. (2020, September 25). "Parade/Cleveland Clinic Survey Shows Americans Embracing Healthy Lifestyle Changes amid COVID-19 Pandemic."
- IQVIA Institute. (2017, November 7). *The Growing Value of Digital Health.* (pdf)
- Moschu, D. (2017). "How Close Are We to a Real *Star Trek*–Style Medical Tricorder?" *Scientific American*.
- Mullen, C. (2020, May 21). "Telemedicine Likely Here to Stay Post-Pandemic." *Bizwomen*.
- Robb, M. B. (2019). *The New Normal: Parents, Teens, Screens, and Sleep in the United States.* San Francisco, CA: Common Sense Media. (pdf)
- Sharecare. Well-Being Index.
- Trust for America's Health. Blueprint for a Healthier America.
- University of Wisconsin Population Health Institute. County Health Rankings & Roadmaps.
- Wabnitz, K., et al. (2020). "A Pledge for Planetary Health to Unify the Health Professions in the Anthropocene." *Lancet*, *396*, 1471–1473.

Design Element: (*magnifying glass*): Siede Preis/Getty Images; (*runners shoes*): Maridav/Getty Images; (*tablet*): McGraw Hill; (*woman*): GlobalStock/Getty Images; (*blue sports shoes*): chictype/Getty Images; (*smartphone*): Alexey Boldin/ Shutterstock; (*Why It Matters*): MHHE

Lab 25A Assessing Factors That Influence Health, Wellness, and Fitness

Name	Section	Date

Purpose: To assess the factors that relate to health, wellness, and fitness.

Chart 1 Assessment Questionnaire: Factors That Influence Health, Wellness, and Fitness

Factor	Very True	Somewhat True	Not True At All	Score
Heredity				
1. I have checked my family history for medical problems.	3	2	1	
2. I have taken steps to overcome hereditary predispositions.	3	2	1	
			Heredity Score =	
Health Care				
3. I have health insurance.	3	2	1	
4. I get regular medical exams and have my own doctor.	3	2	1	
5. I get treatment early, rather than waiting until problems get serious	3	2	1	
6. I carefully investigate my health problems before making decisions.	3	2	1	
			Health-Care Score =	
Environment				
7. My physical environment is healthy.	3	2	1	
8. My social environment is healthy.	3	2	1	
9. My spiritual environment is healthy.	3	2	1	
10. My intellectual environment is healthy.	3	2	1	
11. My work environment is healthy.	3	2	1	
12. My environment fosters healthy lifestyles.	3	2	1	
			Environment Score =	
Lifestyles				
13. I am physically active on a regular basis.	3	2	1	
14. I eat well.	3	2	1	
15. I use effective techniques for managing stress.	3	2	1	
16. I avoid destructive behaviors.	3	2	1	
17. I practice safe sex.	3	2	1	
18. I manage my time effectively.	3	2	1	
19. I evaluate information carefully and am an informed consumer.	3	2	1	
20. My personal health habits are good.	3	2	1	
21. My safety habits are good.	3	2	1	
22. I know first aid and can use it if needed.	3	2	1	
			Lifestyles Score =	
Personal Actions and Interactions				
23. I collect and evaluate information before I act.	3	2	1	
24. I plan before I take action.	3	2	1	
25. I am good about taking action when I know it is good for me.	3	2	1	
26. I honor my beliefs and relationships.	3	2	1	
27. I seek help when I need it.	3	2	1	
			Personal Actions/Interactions Score =	

Procedures

1. Answer each of the questions in Chart 1. Consider the information in this Concept as you answer each question. The five factors assessed in the questionnaire are from Figure 1.
2. Calculate the scores for heredity (sum items 1 and 2), health care (sum items 3–6), environment (sum items 7–12), lifestyles (sum items 13–22), and personal actions/interactions (sum items 23–27).
3. Determine ratings for each of the scores using the Rating Chart.
4. Record your scores and ratings in the Results chart. Record your comments in the Conclusions and Implications section.

Results

Factor	Score	Rating
Heredity		
Health Care		
Environment		
Lifestyles		
Personal Actions/Interactions		

Rating Chart

Factor	Healthy	Marginal	Needs Attention
Heredity	6	4–5	Below 4
Health Care	11–12	9–10	Below 9
Environment	16–18	13–15	Below 13
Lifestyles	26–30	20–25	Below 20
Personal Actions/ Interactions	13–15	10–12	Below 10

Conclusions and Implications

1. In the space provided, discuss your scores for the five factors (sums of several questions) identified in Chart 1. Use several sentences to identify specific areas that need attention and changes that you could make to improve.

2. For any individual item on Chart 1, a score of 1 is considered low. You might have a high score on a set of questions and still have a low score in one area that indicates a need for attention. In several sentences, discuss actions you could take to make changes related to individual questions.

connect
ACTIVITY

Lab 25B Planning for Improved Health, Wellness, and Fitness

Name	Section	Date

Purpose: To plan to make changes in areas that can most contribute to improved health, wellness, and fitness.

Procedures

1. Experts agree that it is best not to make too many changes all at once. Focusing attention on one or two things at a time will produce better results. Based on your assessments made in Lab 25A, select two areas in which you would like to make changes. Choose one from the list related to health care and environment and one related to lifestyle change. Place a check by those areas in Chart 1 in the Results section. Because Lab 25C is devoted to physical activity, it is not included in the list. You may want to make additional copies of this lab for use in making other changes in the future.

2. Use Chart 2 to determine your stage of change for the changes you have identified. Since you have identified these as an area of need, it is unlikely that you would identify the stage of maintenance. If you are at maintenance, you can select a different area of change that would be more useful.

3. In the appropriate locations, record the change you want to make related to your environment or health care. State your reasons, your specific goal(s), your written statement of the plan for change, and a statement about how you will self-monitor and evaluate the effectiveness of the changes made. In Chart 3, record similar information for the lifestyle change you identified.

Results

Chart 1

Check one in each column.

Area of Change	✓	Area of Change	✓
Health insurance		Eating well	
Medical checkups		Managing stress	
Doctor selection		Avoiding destructive habits	
Physical environment		Practicing safe sex	
Social environment		Managing time	
Spiritual environment		Becoming a better consumer	
Intellectual environment		Improving health habits	
Work environment		Improving safety habits	
Environment for lifestyles		Learning first aid	

Chart 2

List the two areas of change identified in Chart 1. Make a rating using the following diagram.

Identified Area of Change	Stage of Change Rating
1.	
2.	

Maintenance — "Regular participation for at least 6 months"

Action — "Regular participation but less than 6 months"

Preparation — "Some participation but not on a regular basis"

Contemplation — "Thinking about doing this but have not done it yet"

Precontemplation — "Don't want to change"

Note: Some of the areas identified in this lab relate to personal information. It is appropriate not to divulge personal information to others (including your instructor) if you choose not to. For this reason, you may choose not to address certain problems in this lab. You are encouraged to take steps to make changes independent of this assignment and to consult privately with your instructor to get assistance.

Chart 3 Making Changes for Improved Health, Wellness, and Fitness

Describe First Area of Change (from Chart 1)	**Describe Second Area of Change (from Chart 1)**
Step 1: State Reasons for Making Change	**Step 1: State Reasons for Making Change**
Step 2: Do Self-Assessment of Need for Change List your stage from Chart 2.	**Step 2: Do Self-Assessment of Need for Change** List your stage from Chart 2.
Step 3: State Your Specific Goals for Change State several specific and realistic goals.	**Step 3: State Your Specific Goals for Change** State several specific and realistic goals.
Step 4: Identify Activities or Actions for Change List specific activities you will do or actions you will take to meet your goals.	**Step 4: Identify Activities or Actions for Change** List specific activities you will do or actions you will take to meet your goals.

Step 5: Write a Plan; Include a Timetable
Expected start date:

Expected finish date:

Mon.	Tue.	Wed.	Th.	Fri.	Sat.	Sun.

Location: Where will you do the plan?

Step 5: Write a Plan; Include a Timetable
Expected start date:

Expected finish date:

Mon.	Tue.	Wed.	Th.	Fri.	Sat.	Sun.

Location: Where will you do the plan?

Step 6: Evaluate Your Plan
How will you self-monitor and evaluate to determine if the plan is working?

Step 6: Evaluate Your Plan
How will you self-monitor and evaluate to determine if the plan is working?

connect
ACTIVITY

Lab 25C Planning Your Personal Physical Activity Program

Name	Section	Date

Purpose: To establish a comprehensive plan of lifestyle physical activity and to self-monitor progress in your plan. (*Note:* You may want to reread the Concept on planning for physical activity before completing this lab.)

Procedures

Step 1. Establish Your Reasons

In the spaces provided, list several of your principal reasons for doing a comprehensive activity plan.

1.
2.
3.

4.
5.
6.

Step 2. Identify Your Needs Using Fitness Self-Assessments and Ratings of Stage of Change for Various Activities

In Chart 1, rate your fitness by placing an X over the circle by the appropriate rating for each part of fitness. Use your results obtained from previous labs or perform the self-assessments again to determine your ratings. If you took more than one self-assessment for one component of physical fitness, select the rating that you think best describes your true fitness for that fitness component. If you were unable to do a self-assessment for some reason, check the "No Results" circle.

Chart 1 Rating for Self-Assessments

	Rating			
Health-Related Fitness Tests	Good Fitness Zone	Marginal Fitness Zone	Low Fitness Zone	No Results
1. Cardiorespiratory: walking test (Chart 1, page 129)	◯	◯	◯	◯
2. Cardiorespiratory: step test (Chart 2, page 129)	◯	◯	◯	◯
3. Cardiorespiratory: bicycle test (Chart 5, page 131)	◯	◯	◯	◯
4. Cardiorespiratory: twelve-minute run (Chart 6, page 131)	◯	◯	◯	◯
5. Cardiorespiratory: swim test (Chart 7, page 132)	◯	◯	◯	◯
6. Strength: isometric grip (Chart 3, page 178)	◯	◯	◯	◯
7. Strength: 1RM upper body (Chart 2, page 176)	◯	◯	◯	◯
8. Strength: 1RM lower body (Chart 2, page 176)	◯	◯	◯	◯
9. Muscular endurance: curl-up (Chart 4, page 178)	◯	◯	◯	◯
10. Muscular endurance: 90-degree push-up (Chart 4, page 178)	◯	◯	◯	◯
11. Muscular endurance: flexed-arm support (Chart 5, page 178)	◯	◯	◯	◯

Chart 1 Rating for Self-Assessments, *continued* 495

Health-Related Fitness Tests	Rating			
	Good Fitness Zone	Marginal Fitness Zone	Low Fitness Zone	No Results
12. Power: vertical jump (Chart 6, page 178)	○	○	○	○
13. Power: medicine ball throw (Chart 6, page 178)	○	○	○	○
14. Flexibility: sit-and-reach test (Chart 1, page 216)	○	○	○	○
15. Flexibility: shoulder flexibility (Chart 1, page 216)	○	○	○	○
16. Flexibility: hamstring/hip flexibility (Chart 1, page 216)	○	○	○	○
17. Flexibility: trunk rotation (Chart 1, page 216)	○	○	○	○
18. Body Fat: Skinfolds (Chart 2, page 259)	○	○	○	○
19. Body Mass Index (Chart 8, page 265)				

Skill-Related Fitness and Other Self-Assessments	Excellent	Very Good or Good	Fair	Poor	No Results
1. Fitness of the back (Chart 2, page 456)	○	○	○	○	○
2. Posture (Chart 2, page 459)	○	○	○	○	○
3. Agility (Chart 1, page 235)	○	○	○	○	○
4. Balance (Chart 2, page 236)	○	○	○	○	○
5. Coordination (Chart 3, page 236)	○	○	○	○	○
6. Reaction time (Chart 4, page 237)	○	○	○	○	○
7. Speed (Chart 5, page 238)	○	○	○	○	○

Summarize Your Fitness Ratings Using the Previous Results	High-Performance Zone	Good Fitness Zone	Marginal Fitness Zone	Low Fitness Zone	No Results
Cardiorespiratory	○	○	○	○	○
Flexibility	○	○	○	○	○
Strength	○	○	○	○	○
Muscular endurance	○	○	○	○	○
Body fatness	○	○	○	○	○
Power	○	○	○	○	○

	Excellent	Very Good or Good	Fair	Poor	No Results
Skill-related fitness	○	○	○	○	○
Posture and fitness of the back	○	○	○	○	○

Rate your stage of change for each of the different types of activities from the physical activity pyramid. Place an X over the circle beside the stage that best represents your behavior for each of the five types of activity in the lower three levels of the pyramid. A description of the various stages is provided below to help you make your ratings.

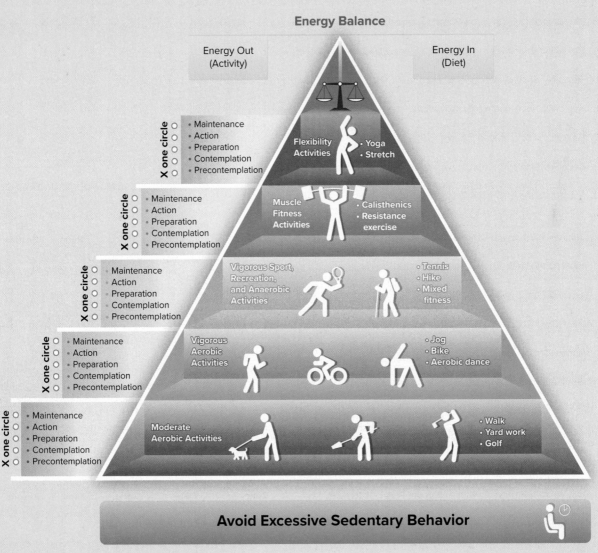

Energy Balance

Energy Out (Activity)

Energy In (Diet)

X one circle
- Maintenance
- Action
- Preparation
- Contemplation
- Precontemplation

Flexibility Activities
- Yoga
- Stretch

X one circle
- Maintenance
- Action
- Preparation
- Contemplation
- Precontemplation

Muscle Fitness Activities
- Calisthenics
- Resistance exercise

X one circle
- Maintenance
- Action
- Preparation
- Contemplation
- Precontemplation

Vigorous Sport, Recreation, and Anaerobic Activities
- Tennis
- Hike
- Mixed fitness

X one circle
- Maintenance
- Action
- Preparation
- Contemplation
- Precontemplation

Vigorous Aerobic Activities
- Jog
- Bike
- Aerobic dance

X one circle
- Maintenance
- Action
- Preparation
- Contemplation
- Precontemplation

Moderate Aerobic Activities
- Walk
- Yard work
- Golf

Avoid Excessive Sedentary Behavior

Source: Charles B. Corbin.

In step 1, you wrote down some general reasons for developing your physical activity plan. Setting goals requires more specific statements of goals that are realistic and achievable. For people who are at the contemplation or preparation stage for a specific type of activity, it is recommended that you write only short-term physical activity goals (no more than 4 weeks). Those at the action or maintenance level may choose short-term goals to start with, or if you have a good history of adherence, choose long-term goals (longer than 4 weeks). Precontemplators are not considered because they would not be doing this activity.

Step 3. Set Specific Goals

Chart 2 Setting Goals

Physical Activity Goals. Place an X over the appropriate circle for the number of days and weeks for each type of activity. Write the number of exercises or minutes of activities you plan in each of the five areas.

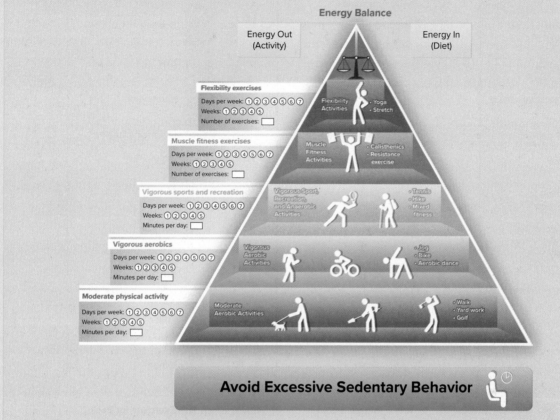

Flexibility exercises
Days per week: ① ② ③ ④ ⑤ ⑥ ⑦
Weeks: ① ② ③ ④ ⑤
Number of exercises: ☐

Muscle fitness exercises
Days per week: ① ② ③ ④ ⑤ ⑥ ⑦
Weeks: ① ② ③ ④ ⑤
Number of exercises: ☐

Vigorous sports and recreation
Days per week: ① ② ③ ④ ⑤ ⑥ ⑦
Weeks: ① ② ③ ④ ⑤
Minutes per day: ☐

Vigorous aerobics
Days per week: ① ② ③ ④ ⑤ ⑥ ⑦
Weeks: ① ② ③ ④ ⑤
Minutes per day: ☐

Moderate physical activity
Days per week: ① ② ③ ④ ⑤ ⑥ ⑦
Weeks: ① ② ③ ④ ⑤
Minutes per day: ☐

Energy Balance
Energy Out (Activity) — Energy In (Diet)

Flexibility Activities • Yoga • Stretch
Muscle Fitness Activities • Calisthenics • Resistance exercise
Vigorous Sport, Recreation, and Anaerobic Activities • Tennis • Hike • Mixed fitness
Vigorous Aerobic Activities • Jog • Bike • Aerobic dance
Moderate Aerobic Activities • Walk • Yard work • Golf

Avoid Excessive Sedentary Behavior

Source: Charles B. Corbin.

Physical Fitness Goals (for People at Action or Maintenance Only). Write specific physical fitness goals in the spaces provided. Indicate when you expect to accomplish the goal (in weeks). Examples include improving the 12-minute run to a specific score, being able to perform a specific number of push-ups, attaining a specific BMI, and being able to achieve a specific score on a flexibility test.

Part of Fitness	Description of Specific Performance	Weeks to Goal

Step 4. Select Activities

In Chart 3, indicate the specific activities you plan to perform from each area of the physical activity pyramid. If the activity you expect to perform is listed, note the number of minutes or reps/sets you plan to perform. If the activity you want to perform is not listed, write the name of the activity or exercise in the space designated as "Other." For moderate activities, active aerobics, and active sports and recreation, indicate the length of time the activity will be performed each day. For flexibility, muscle fitness exercises, and exercises for back and neck, indicate the number of repetitions for each exercise.

Chart 3 Lifetime Physical Activity Selections

✓	Moderate Activities	Min/Day	✓	Active Aerobics	Min/Day	✓	Active Sports and Recreation	Min/Day
	Active housework			Aerobic exercise machines			Basketball	
	Bicycling to work or store			Bicycling			Bowling	
	Gardening			Circuit training or calisthenics			Golf	
	Occupational activity			Dance or step aerobics			Karate/judo	
	Social dancing			Hiking or backpacking			Mountain climbing	
	Walking			Jogging or running (or walking)			Racquetball	
	Wheeling in wheelchair			Skating/cross-country skiing			Skating	
	Yard work			Swimming			Softball	
	Other:			Water activity			Skiing	
	Other:			Other:			Soccer	
	Other:			Other:			Volleyball	
	Other:			Other:			Other:	
	Other:			Other:			Other:	
	Other:			Other:			Other:	
	Other:			Other:			Other:	

✓	Flexibility Exercises	Reps/ Sets	✓	Muscle Fitness Exercises	Reps/ Sets	✓	Exercises for Back and Neck	Reps/ Sets
	Calf stretch			Bench or seated press			Back saver stretch	
	Hip and thigh stretch			Biceps curl			Single knee to chest	
	Groin stretch			Triceps curl			Spine twist	
	Hamstring stretch			Lat pull-down			Hip/thigh stretch	
	Back stretch (leg hug)			Seated rowing			Cobra/child's pose	
	Trunk twist			Wrist curl			Bridge variation	
	Pectoral stretch			Knee extension			Superman variation	
	Arm hug stretch			Side leg raise			Abdominal brace	
	Overhead arm stretch			Half squat			Neck rotation	
	Other:			Lunge			Isometric neck exercise	
	Other:			Push-up			Chin tuck	
	Other:			Crunch or reverse curl			Trapezius stretch	
	Other:			Plyometrics			Other:	
	Other:			Other:			Other:	
	Other:			Other:			Other:	

Step 5. Prepare a Written Plan

In Chart 4, place a check in the shaded boxes for each activity you will perform for each day you will do it. Indicate the time of day you expect to perform the activity or exercise (Example: 7:30 to 8 a.m. or 6 to 6:30 p.m.). In the spaces labeled "Warm-Up Exercises" and "Cool-Down Exercises," check the warm-up and cool-down exercises you expect to perform. Indicate the number of reps you will use for each exercise.

Chart 4 My Physical Activity Plan

✓	Monday	Time	✓	Tuesday	Time	✓	Wednesday	Time
	Moderate activity			Moderate activity			Moderate activity	
	Vigorous activity			Vigorous activity			Vigorous activity	
	Sports/Rec/Anaerobics			Sports/Rec/Anaerobics			Sports/Rec/Anaerobics	
	Flexibility exercises*			Flexibility exercises*			Flexibility exercises*	
	Muscle fitness exercises*			Muscle fitness exercises*			Muscle fitness exercises*	
	Back/neck exercises*			Back/neck exercises*			Back/neck exercises*	
	Warm-up exercises			Warm-up exercises			Warm-up exercises	
	Other:			Other:			Other:	

✓	Thursday	Time	✓	Friday	Time	✓	Saturday	Time
	Moderate activity			Moderate activity			Moderate activity	
	Vigorous activity			Vigorous activity			Vigorous activity	
	Sports/Rec/Anaerobics			Sports/Rec/Anaerobics			Sports/Rec/Anaerobics	
	Flexibility exercises*			Flexibility exercises*			Flexibility exercises*	
	Muscle fitness exercises*			Muscle fitness exercises*			Muscle fitness exercises*	
	Back/neck exercises*			Back/neck exercises*			Back/neck exercises*	
	Warm-up exercises			Warm-up exercises			Warm-up exercises	
	Other:			Other:			Other:	

✓	Sunday	Time	✓	Warm-Up Exercises	Reps	✓	Cool-Down Exercises	Reps
	Moderate activity			Walk or jog			Walk or jog	
	Vigorous activity			Grapevine			Calf stretch	
	Sports/Rec/Anaerobics			Knee stride and reach			Hamstring stretch	
	Flexibility exercises*			High skip and reach			Leg hug	
	Muscle fitness exercises*			Inchworm			Sitting side stretch	
	Back/neck exercises*			Calf stretch or hamstring stretch			Zipper	
	Warm-up exercises			Leg hug or seated side stretch			Other:	
	Other:			Other:			Other:	

*Perform the specific exercises you checked in Chart 3.

Step 6. Keep Records of Progress and Evaluate Your Plan

Make copies of Chart 4 (one for each week that you plan to keep records). Each day, make a check by the activities you actually performed. Include the times when you did the activities in your plan. Periodically check your goals to see if they have been accomplished. At some point, it will be necessary to reestablish your goals and create a revised activity plan.

Results

After performing your plan for a specific period of time, answer the question in the space provided.

How long have you been performing the plan? Please provide a short statement about your previous experience.

Conclusions and Implications

1. In several sentences, discuss your adherence to the plan. Have you been able to stick with the plan? If so, do you think it is a plan you can do for a lifetime? If not, why do you think you are unable to do your plan?

2. In several sentences, discuss how you might modify your plan in the future.

3. In several sentences, discuss your goals for your program. Do you think you will meet your goals? Why or why not?

Appendix A
Metric Conversion Charts

Chart 1 Traditional/Metric Measurement Conversions

	Metric to Traditional	Traditional to Metric
Length	centimeters to inches: cm × 0.39 = in	inches to centimeters: in × 2.54 = cm
	meters to feet: m × 3.3 = ft	feet to meters: ft × 0.3048 = m
	meters to yards: m × 1.09 = yd	yards to meters: yd × 0.92 = m
	kilometers to miles: km × 0.6 = mi	miles to kilometers: mi × 1.6 = km
Weight (Mass)	grams to ounces: g × 0.0352 = oz	ounces to grams: oz × 28.41 = g
	kilograms to pounds: kg × 2.2 = lb	pounds to kilograms: lb × 0.45 = kg
Volume	milliliters to fluid ounces: ml × 0.03 = fl oz	fluid ounces to milliliters: fl oz × 29.573 = ml
	liters to quarts: l × 1.06 = qt	quarts to liters: qt × 0.95 = l
	liters to gallons: l × 0.264 = gal	gallons to liters: gal × 3.8 = l

Chart 2 Isometric Strength Rating Scale (kg)—page 174

	Males			Females		
Classification	Left Grip	Right Grip	Total Score	Left Grip	Right Grip	Total Score
High-performance zone	57+	61+	118+	34+	39+	73+
Good fitness zone	45–56	50–60	95–117	27–33	32–38	59–72
Marginal fitness zone	41–44	43–49	84–94	20–26	23–31	43–58
Low fitness zone	<41	<43	<84	<20	<23	<43

Suitable for use by young adults between 18 and 30 years of age. After 30, an adjustment of 0.5 to 1 percent per year is appropriate because some loss of muscle tissue typically occurs as you grow older.

Chart 3 Rating Scale for Power—page 190

	Vertical Jump (centimeters)		Medicine Ball Throw (centimeters)	
Classification	Males	Females	Males	Females
High-performance zone	55+	39+	472+	307+
Good fitness zone	45–54	32–38	434–471	281–306
Marginal fitness zone	40–44	27–31	391–433	256–280
Low fitness zone	<40	<27	390 or less	255 or less

Chart 4 Reaction Time Rating Scale—page 237

Classification	Score in Inches	Score in Centimeters
Excellent	>21	>52
Very good	19–21	48–52
Good	16–18 ¾	41–47
Fair	13–15 ¾	33–40
Poor	<13	<33

Chart 5 Speed Rating Scale—page 238

	Males		Females	
Classification	Yards	Meters	Yards	Meters
Excellent	24+	22+	22+	20+
Very good	22–23	20–21.9	20–21	18–19.9
Good	18–21	16.5–19.9	16–19	14.5–17.9
Fair	16–17	14.5–16.4	14–15	13–14.4
Poor	<16	<14.5	<14	<13

Appendix B
Calories of Protein, Carbohydrates, and Fats in Foods

Food Choice	Total Calories	Protein Calories	Carbohydrate Calories	Fat Calories
Breakfast				
Scrambled egg (1 lg.)	111	29	7	75
Fried egg (1 lg.)	99	26	1	72
Pancake (6 inch)	146	19	67	58
Syrup (1 T)	60	0	60	0
French toast (1 slice)	180	23	49	108
Waffle (7-inch)	245	28	100	117
Biscuit (medium)	104	8	52	44
Bran muffin (medium)	104	11	63	31
White toast (1 slice)	68	9	52	7
Wheat toast (1 slice)	67	14	52	6
Peanut butter (1 T)	94	15	11	68
Yogurt (8 oz plain)	227	39	161	27
Orange juice (8 oz)	114	8	100	6
Apple juice (8 oz)	117	1	116	0
Soft drink (12 oz)	144	0	144	0
Bacon (2 slices)	86	15	2	70
Sausage (1 link)	141	11	0	130
Sausage (1 patty)	284	23	0	261
Grits (8 oz)	125	11	110	4
Hash browns (8 oz)	355	18	178	159
French fries (reg.)	239	12	115	112
Donut, cake	125	4	61	60
Donut, glazed	164	8	87	69
Sweet roll	317	22	136	159
Cake (medium slice)	274	14	175	85
Ice cream (8 oz)	257	15	108	134
Cream cheese (T)	52	4	1	47
Jelly (T)	49	0	49	0
Jam (T)	54	0	54	0
Coffee (cup)	0	0	0	0
Tea (cup)	0	0	0	0
Cream (T)	32	2	2	28
Sugar (t)	15	0	15	0
Corn flakes (8 oz)	97	8	87	2
Wheat flakes (8 oz)	106	12	90	4
Oatmeal (8 oz)	132	19	92	21
Strawberries (8 oz)	55	4	46	5
Orange (medium)	64	6	57	1
Apple (medium)	96	1	86	9
Banana (medium)	101	4	95	2
Cantaloupe (half)	82	7	73	2

Food Choice	Total Calories	Protein Calories	Carbohydrate Calories	Fat Calories
Grapefruit (half)	40	2	37	1
Custard pie (slice)	285	20	188	77
Fruit pie (slice)	350	14	259	77
Fritter (medium)	132	11	54	67
Skim milk (8 oz)	88	36	52	0
Whole milk (8 oz)	159	33	48	78
Butter (pat)	36	0	0	36
Margarine (pat)	36	0	0	36
Lunch				
Hamburger (reg. FF)	255	48	120	89
Cheeseburger (reg. FF)	307	61	120	126
Doubleburger (FF)	563	101	163	299
¼ lb burger (FF)	427	73	137	217
Doublecheese burger (FF)	670	174	134	362
Doublecheese baconburger (FF)	724	138	174	340
Hot dog (FF)	214	36	54	124
Chili dog (FF)	320	51	90	179
Pizza, cheese (slice FF)	290	116	116	58
Pizza, meat (slice FF)	360	126	126	108
Pizza, everything (slice FF)	510	179	173	158
Sandwich, roast beef (FF)	350	88	126	137
Sandwich, bologna	313	44	106	163
Sandwich, bologna-cheese	428	69	158	201
Sandwich, ham-cheese (FF)	380	91	133	156
Sandwich, peanut butter	281	39	118	124
Sandwich, PB and jelly	330	40	168	122
Sandwich, egg salad	330	40	109	181
Sandwich, tuna salad	390	101	109	180
Sandwich, fish (FF)	432	56	147	229
French fries (reg. FF)	239	12	115	112
French fries (lg. FF)	406	20	195	191
Onion rings (reg. FF)	274	14	112	148
Chili (8 oz)	260	49	62	148
Bean soup (8 oz)	355	67	181	107
Beef noodle soup (8 oz)	140	32	59	49
Tomato soup (8 oz)	180	14	121	45
Vegetable soup (8 oz)	160	21	107	32
Small salad, plain	37	6	27	4
Small salad, French dressing	152	8	50	94
Small salad, Italian dressing	162	8	28	126
Small salad, bleu cheese	184	13	28	143
Potato salad (8 oz)	248	27	159	62

The principal reference for the calculation of values used in this appendix was the *Nutritive Value of Foods*, published by the United States Department of Agriculture, Washington, DC, Home and Gardens Bulletin, No. 72, although other published sources were consulted, including Jacobson, M., & Fritschner, S. (1986). *The Fast-Food Guide.* New York: Workman.

Notes:
1. FF by a food indicates that it is typical of a food served in a fast food restaurant.
2. Your portions of foods may be larger or smaller than those listed here. For this reason, you may wish to select a food more than once (e.g., two hamburgers) or select only a portion of a serving (i.e., divide the calories in half for a half portion).
3. An ounce equals 28.35 grams.
4. T = tablespoon and t = teaspoon.

Food Choice	Total Calories	Protein Calories	Carbohydrate Calories	Fat Calories
Cole slaw (8 oz)	180	0	25	155
Macaroni and cheese (8 oz)	230	37	103	90
Beef taco (FF)	186	59	56	71
Bean burrito (FF)	343	45	192	106
Meat burrito (FF)	466	158	196	112
Mexican rice (FF)	213	17	160	36
Mexican beans (FF)	168	42	82	44
Fried chicken breast (FF)	436	262	13	161
Broiled chicken breast	284	224	0	60
Broiled fish	228	82	32	114
Fish stick (1 stick FF)	50	18	8	24
Fried egg	99	26	1	72
Donut	125	4	61	60
Potato chips (small bag)	115	3	39	73
Soft drink (12 oz)	144	0	144	0
Apple juice (8 oz)	117	1	116	0
Skim milk (8 oz)	88	36	52	0
Whole milk (8 oz)	159	33	48	78
Diet drink (12 oz)	0	0	0	0
Mustard (t)	4	0	4	0
Catsup (t)	6	0	6	0
Mayonnaise (T)	100	0	0	100
Fruit pie	350	14	259	77
Cheesecake (slice)	400	56	132	212
Ice cream (8 oz)	257	15	108	134
Coffee (8 oz)	0	0	0	0
Tea (8 oz)	0	0	0	0

Dinner

Food Choice	Total Calories	Protein Calories	Carbohydrate Calories	Fat Calories
Hamburger (reg. FF)	255	48	120	89
Cheeseburger (reg. FF)	307	61	120	126
Doubleburger (FF)	563	101	163	299
¼ lb burger (FF)	427	73	137	217
Doublecheese burger (FF)	670	174	134	362
Doublecheese baconburger (FF)	724	138	174	412
Hot dog (FF)	214	36	54	124
Chili dog (FF)	320	51	90	179
Pizza, cheese (slice FF)	290	116	116	58
Pizza, meat (slice FF)	360	126	126	108
Pizza, everything (slice FF)	510	179	173	158
Steak (8 oz)	880	290	0	590
Fried shrimp (6 oz)	360	133	68	158
Roast beef (8 oz)	440	268	0	172
Liver (8 oz)	520	250	52	218
Corned beef (8 oz)	493	242	0	251
Meat loaf (8 oz)	711	228	35	448
Ham (8 oz)	540	178	0	362
Spaghetti, no meat (13 oz)	400	56	220	124
Spaghetti, meat (13 oz)	500	115	230	155
Baked potato (medium)	90	12	78	0
Cooked carrots (8 oz)	71	12	59	0
Cooked spinach (8 oz)	50	18	18	14
Corn (1 ear)	70	10	52	8
Cooked green beans (8 oz)	54	11	43	0
Cooked broccoli (8 oz)	60	19	26	15
Cooked cabbage	47	12	35	0
French fries (reg. FF)	239	12	115	112
French fries (lg. FF)	406	20	195	191
Onion rings (reg. FF)	274	14	112	148
Chili (8 oz)	260	49	62	148
Small salad, plain	37	6	27	4
Small salad, French dressing	152	8	50	94
Small salad, Italian dressing	162	8	28	126
Small salad, bleu cheese	184	13	28	143
Potato salad (8 oz)	248	27	159	62
Cole slaw (8 oz)	180	0	25	155

Food Choice	Total Calories	Protein Calories	Carbohydrate Calories	Fat Calories
Macaroni and cheese (8 oz)	230	37	103	90
Beef Taco (FF)	186	59	56	71
Bean burrito (FF)	343	45	192	106
Meat burrito (FF)	466	158	196	112
Mexican rice (FF)	213	17	160	36
Mexican beans (FF)	168	42	82	44
Fried chicken breast (FF)	436	262	13	161
Broiled chicken breast	284	224	0	60
Broiled fish	228	82	32	114
Fish stick (1 stick FF)	50	18	8	24
Soft drink (12 oz)	144	0	144	0
Apple juice (8 oz)	117	1	116	0
Skim milk (8 oz)	88	36	52	0
Whole milk (8 oz)	159	33	48	78
Diet drink (12 oz)	0	0	0	0
Mustard (t)	4	0	4	0
Catsup (t)	6	0	6	0
Mayonnaise (T)	100	0	0	100
Fruit pie (slice)	350	14	259	77
Cheesecake (slice)	400	56	132	212
Ice cream (8 oz)	257	15	108	134
Custard pie (slice)	285	20	188	77
Cake (slice)	274	14	175	85

Snacks

Food Choice	Total Calories	Protein Calories	Carbohydrate Calories	Fat Calories
Peanut butter (1 T)	94	15	11	68
Yogurt (8 oz plain)	227	39	161	27
Orange juice (8 oz)	114	8	100	6
Apple juice (8 oz)	117	1	116	0
Soft drink (12 oz)	144	0	144	0
Donut, cake	125	4	61	60
Donut, glazed	164	8	87	69
Sweet roll	317	22	136	159
Cake (medium slice)	274	14	175	85
Ice cream (8 oz)	257	15	108	134
Softserve cone (reg.)	240	10	89	134
Ice cream sandwich bar	210	40	82	88
Strawberries (8 oz)	55	4	46	5
Orange (medium)	64	6	57	1
Apple (medium)	96	1	86	9
Banana (medium)	101	4	95	2
Cantaloupe (half)	82	7	73	2
Grapefruit (half)	40	2	37	1
Celery stick	5	2	3	0
Carrot (medium)	20	3	17	0
Raisins (4 oz)	210	6	204	0
Watermelon (4×6-in slice)	115	8	99	8
Chocolate chip cookie	60	3	9	48
Brownie	145	6	26	113
Oatmeal cookie	65	3	13	49
Sandwich cookie	200	8	112	80
Custard pie (slice)	285	20	188	77
Fruit pie (slice)	350	14	259	77
Gelatin (4 oz)	70	4	32	34
Fritter (medium)	132	11	54	67
Skim milk (8 oz)	88	36	52	0
Diet drink	0	0	0	0
Potato chips (small bag)	115	3	39	73
Roasted peanuts (1.3 oz)	210	34	25	151
Chocolate candy bar (1 oz)	145	7	61	77
Chocolate almond candy bar (1 oz)	265	38	74	164
Saltine cracker	18	1	1	16
Popped corn	40	7	33	0
Cheese nachos	471	63	194	214

References

This edition of *Corbin's Concepts of Fitness and Wellness* incorporates the latest updates in research as well as new developments in public health, medicine, and technology related to health, wellness, and fitness. Resources new to this edition include the following.

Concept 1

Arunachalam, P. S., Wimmers, F., Mok, C. K. P., Perera, R. A., Scott, M., Hagan, T., . . . & Pulendran, B. (2020). Systems biological assessment of immunity to mild versus severe COVID-19 infection in humans. *Science, 369*(6508), 1210-1220.

Aubertin-Leheudre, M., & Rolland, Y. (2020). The importance of physical activity to care for frail older adults during the COVID-19 pandemic. *Journal of the American Medical Directors Association, 21*(7), 973.

Chirikov, I., Soria, K. M, Horgos, B., & Jones-White, D. (2020). Undergraduate and graduate students' mental health during the COVID-19 pandemic. UC Berkeley: Center for Studies in Higher Education. Retrieved from https://escholarship.org/uc/item/80k5d5hw

Nieman, D. C. (2020). Coronavirus disease–2019: A tocsin to our aging, unfit, corpulent, and immunodeficient society. *Journal of Sport and Health Science, 9*(4), 293-301.

Piercy, K. L., Troiano, R. P., Ballard, R. M., et al. (2018). Physical Activity Guidelines for Americans. *JAMA, 320*(19), 2020-2028.

Sallis, J. F., Adlakha, D., Oyeyemi, A., & Salvo, D. (2020). An international physical activity and public health research agenda to inform coronavirus disease-19 policies and practices. *Journal of Sport and Health Science, 9*(4), S2095-S2546.

U.S. Department of Health and Human Services, Office of Disease Prevention and Health Promotion. (2021). *Healthy People 2030.* Retrieved [July, 15, 2021] from https://health.gov/healthypeople/objectives-and-data/social-determinants-health

Concept 2

Andrade, G. (2020, April 16). Medical conspiracy theories: Cognitive science and implications for ethics. *Medicine, Health Care and Philosophy,* 1-14.

Chen, X., Zhang, S. X., Jahanshahi, A. A., Alvarez-Risco, A., Dai, H., Li, J., & Ibarra, V. G. (2020). Belief in a COVID-19 conspiracy theory as a predictor of mental health and well-being of health care workers: Cross-sectional survey study. *JMIR Public Health and Surveillance, 6*(3), e20737.

Keralis, J. M., Javanmardi, M., Khanna, S., et al. (2020). Health and the built environment in United States cities: Measuring associations using Google Street View–derived indicators of the built environment. *BMC Public Health, 20*(1), 215.

Li, Y. (2020). Healthy lifestyle and life expectancy free of cancer, cardiovascular disease, and type 2 diabetes: Prospective cohort study. *BMJ, 368,* l6669.

Phan, L., Yu, W., Keralis, J. M., et al. (2020). Google Street View–derived built environment indicators and associations with state-level obesity, physical activity, and chronic disease mortality in the United States. *International Journal of Environmental Research and Public Health, 17*(10), 3659.

Concept 3

Aldenaini, N., Alqahtani, F., Orji, R., & Sampalli, S. (2020). Trends in persuasive technologies for physical activity and sedentary behavior: A systematic review. *Frontiers in Artificial Intelligence, 3,* 7.

Dunton, G. F., Wang, S. D., Do, B., & Courtney, J. (2020). Early effects of the COVID-19 pandemic on physical activity locations and behaviors in adults living in the United States. *Preventive Medicine Reports, 20,* 101241.

Lesser, I. A., & Nienhuis, C. P. (2020). The impact of COVID-19 on physical activity behavior and well-being of Canadians. *International Journal of Environmental Research and Public Health, 17*(11), 3899.

Concept 4

Tainio, M., Andersen, Z. J., Nieuwenhuijsen, M. J., Hu, L., de Nazelle, A., An, R., . . . & de Sá, T. H. (2021). Air pollution, physical activity and health: A mapping review of the evidence. *Environment International, 147,* 105954.

Zègre-Hemsey, J. K., Bogle, B., Cunningham, C. J., Snyder, K., & Rosamond, W. (2018). Delivery of automated external defibrillators (AED) by drones: Implications for emergency cardiac care. *Current Cardiovascular Risk Reports, 12*(11), 25.

Concept 5

Gronek, P., Balko, S., Gronek, J., Zajac, A., Maszczyk, A., Celka, R., . . . & Yu, F. (2019). Physical activity and Alzheimer's disease: A narrative review. *Aging and Disease, 10*(6), 1282.

Gronek, P., Wielinski, D., Cyganski, P., Rynkiewicz, A., Zając, A., Maszczyk, A., . . . & Celka, R. (2020). A review of exercise as medicine in cardiovascular disease: Pathology and mechanism. *Aging and Disease, 11*(2), 327.

Henriksson, H., Henriksson, P., Tynelius, P., Ekstedt, M., Berglind, D., Labayen, I., . . . & Ortega, F. B. (2020). Cardiorespiratory fitness, muscular strength, and obesity in adolescence and later chronic disability due to cardiovascular disease:

A cohort study of 1 million men. *European Heart Journal, 41*(15), 1503-1510.

Jiménez-Pavón, D., Carbonell-Baeza, A., & Lavie, C. J. (2020). Physical exercise as therapy to fight against the mental and physical consequences of COVID-19 quarantine: Special focus in older people. *Progress in Cardiovascular Diseases, 63*(3), 386.

Li, Y., Schoufour, J., Wang, D. D., et al. (2020). Healthy lifestyle and life expectancy free of cancer, cardiovascular disease, and type 2 diabetes: Prospective cohort study. *BMJ, 368,* l6669.

Wendt, A., da Silva, I. C. M., Gonçalves, H., Menezes, A., Barros, F., & Wehrmeister, F. C. (2020). Short-term effect of physical activity on sleep health: A population-based study using accelerometry. *Journal of Sport and Health Science.*

Zhao, M., Veeranki, S. P., Magnussen, C. G., & Xi, B. (2020). Recommended physical activity and all cause and cause specific mortality in US adults: Prospective cohort study. *BMJ, 370,* m2031.

Concept 6

Ding, E. Y., Marcus, G. M., & McManus, D. D. (2020). Emerging technologies for identifying atrial fibrillation. *Circulation Research, 127*(1), 128-142.

Dupont, F., Léger, P. M., Begon, M., Lecot, F., Sénécal, S., Labonté-Lemoyne, E., & Mathieu, M. E. (2019). Health and productivity at work: Which active workstation for which benefits: A systematic review. *Occupational and Environmental Medicine, 76*(5), 281-294.

Herold, F., Müller, P., Gronwald, T., & Müller, N. G. (2019). Dose-response matters!–A perspective on the exercise prescription in exercise-cognition research. *Frontiers in Psychology, 10.*

O'Donovan, G., et al. (2017). Association of "Weekend Warrior" and other leisure time physical activity patterns with risks for all-cause, cardiovascular disease, and cancer mortality. *JAMA Internal Medicine, 177*(3), 335-342.

Teo, J. (2020). Early detection of silent hypoxia in COVID-19 pneumonia using smartphone pulse oximetry. *Journal of Medical Systems, 44*(8), 1-2.

Tison, G. H., Avram, R., Kuhar, P., Abreau, S., Marcus, G. M., Pletcher, M. J., & Olgin, J. E. (2020). Worldwide effect of COVID-19 on physical activity: A descriptive study. *Annals of Internal Medicine, 173*(9), 767-770.

Varma, V. R., et al. (2017). Re-evaluating the effect of age on physical activity over the lifespan. *Preventive Medicine, 101,* 102-108.

Wasserlauf, J., You, C., Patel, R., Valys, A., Albert, D., & Passman, R. (2019). Smartwatch performance for the detection and quantification of atrial fibrillation. *Circulation: Arrhythmia and Electrophysiology, 12*(6), e006834.

Concept 7

Dempsey, P. C., Hadgraft, N. T., Winkler, E. A., Clark, B. K., Buman, M. P., Gardiner, P. A., . . . & Dunstan, D. W. (2018). Associations of context-specific sitting time with markers of cardiometabolic risk in Australian adults. *International Journal of Behavioral Nutrition and Physical Activity, 15*(1), 114.

Diamond, R., & Byrd, E. (2020). Standing up for health–improving mental wellbeing during COVID-19 isolation by reducing sedentary behaviour. *Journal of Affective Disorders, 277*, 232-234.

Hallgren, M., Owen, N., Stubbs, B., Vancampfort, D., Lundin, A., Dunstan, D., . . . & Lagerros, Y. T. (2020). Cross-sectional and prospective relationships of passive and mentally active sedentary behaviours and physical activity with depression. *The British Journal of Psychiatry, 217*(2), 413-419.

Loh, R., Stamatakis, E., Folkerts, D., Allgrove, J. E., & Moir, H. J. (2020). Effects of interrupting prolonged sitting with physical activity breaks on blood glucose, insulin and triacylglycerol measures: A systematic review and meta-analysis. *Sports Medicine, 50*(2): 295-330.

Meyer, J. D., Ellingson, L. D., Buman, M. P., Shook, R. P., Hand, G. A., & Blair, S. N. (2020). Current and 1-year psychological and physical effects of replacing sedentary time with time in other behaviors. *American Journal of Preventive Medicine, 59*(1), 12-20.

Pereira, M. A., Mullane, S. L., Toledo, M. J. L., Larouche, M. L., Rydell, S. A., Vuong, B., . . . & Carlson, N. G. (2020). Efficacy of the "stand and move at work" multicomponent workplace intervention to reduce sedentary time and improve cardiometabolic risk: A group randomized clinical trial. *International Journal of Behavioral Nutrition and Physical Activity, 17*(1), 1-11.

Concept 8

American College of Sports Medicine. (2022). *ACSM's Guidelines for Exercise Testing and Prescription* (11th ed.). Philadelphia: Wolters Kluwer.

Franklin, B. A. (2021). Evolution of the ACSM guidelines: Historical perspectives, new insights, and practical implications. *ACSM's Health & Fitness Journal, 25*(2), 26-32.

Gripp, F., Nava, R. C., Cassilhas, R. C., Esteves, E. A., Magalhães, C. O. D., Dias-Peixoto, M. F., . . . & Amorim, F. T. (2021). HIIT is superior than MICT on cardiometabolic health during training and detraining. *European Journal of Applied Physiology, 121*(1), 159-172.

Vellers, H. L., Verhein, K. C., Burkholder, A. B., Lee, J., Kim, Y., Lightfoot, J. T., . . . & Kleeberger, S. R. (2020). Association between mitochondrial DNA sequence variants and V̇O$_2$ max trainability. *Medicine and Science in Sports and Exercise, 52*(11), 2303-2309.

Concept 9

Bélanger, M., Gallant, F., Doré, I., O'Loughlin, J. L., Sylvestre, M. P., Abi Nader, P., . . . & Sabiston, C. M. (2019). Physical activity mediates the relationship between outdoor time and mental health. *Preventive Medicine Reports, 16*, 101006.

Hall, G., Laddu, D. R., Phillips, S. A., Lavie, C. J., & Arena, R. (2021). A tale of two pandemics: How will COVID-19 and global trends in physical inactivity and sedentary behavior affect one another? *Progress in Cardiovascular Diseases, 64*, 108.

Iannetta, D., Keir, D. A., Fontana, F. Y., Inglis, E. C., Mattu, A. T., Paterson, D. H., . . . & Murias, J. M. (2021, April 26). Evaluating the accuracy of using fixed ranges of METs to categorize exertional intensity in a heterogeneous group of healthy individuals: Implications for cardiorespiratory fitness and health outcomes. *Sports Medicine*, 1-11.

Thompson, W. R. (2021). Worldwide Survey of Fitness Trends for 2021. *ACSM's Health & Fitness Journal, 25*(1), 10-19.

Winter, P. L., Crano, W. D., Basáñez, T., & Lamb, C. S. (2020). Equity in access to outdoor recreation–informing a sustainable future. *Sustainability, 12*(1), 124.

Concept 10

Bohannon, R. W. (2019). Grip strength: An indispensable biomarker for older adults. *Clinical Interventions in Aging, 14*, 1681.

Gentil, P., Ramirez-Campillo, R., & Souza, D. (2020). Resistance training in face of the coronavirus outbreak: Time to think outside the box. *Frontiers in Physiology, 11*.

Kravitz, L. R. (2019). Developing a lifelong resistance training program. *ACSM's Health & Fitness Journal, 23*(1), 9-15.

Rowlands, A. V., Edwardson, C. L., Dawkins, N. P., Maylor, B. D., Metcalf, K. M., & Janz, K. F. (2020). Physical activity for bone health: How much and/or how hard? *Medicine & Science in Sports & Exercise, 52*(11), 2331-2341.

Ward, R. C., Janz, K. F., Letuchy, E. M., Peterson, C., & Levy, S. M. (2019). Contribution of high school sport participation to young adult bone strength. *Medicine & Science in Sports and Exercise, 51*(5), 1064.

World Health Organization. (2020). Global guidelines on physical activity and health. Retrieved from www.who.int/publications/i/item/9789241599979

Yang, J., Christophi, C. A., Farioli, A., Baur, D. M., Moffatt, S., Zollinger, T. W., & Kales, S. N. (2019). Association between push-up exercise capacity and future cardiovascular events among active adult men. *JAMA Network Open, 2*(2), e188341-e188341.

Concept 11

Nagarathna, R., Nagendra, H. R., & Majumdar, V. (2020). A perspective on yoga as a preventive strategy for coronavirus disease 2019. *International Journal of Yoga, 13*(2), 89.

Thomas, E., Bianco, A., Paoli, A., & Palma, A. (2018). The relation between stretching typology and stretching duration: The effects on range of motion. *International Journal of Sports Medicine, 39*(04), 243-254.

Zhu, F., Zhang, M., Wang, D., Hong, Q., Zeng, C., & Chen, W. (2020). Yoga compared to non-exercise or physical therapy exercise on pain, disability, and quality of life for patients with chronic low back pain: A systematic review and meta-analysis of randomized controlled trials. *PLOS One, 15*(9), e0238544.

Concept 12

Feiss, R., Lutz, M., Reiche, E., Moody, J., & Pangelinan, M. (2020). A systematic review of the effectiveness of concussion education programs for coaches and parents of youth athletes. *International Journal of Environmental Research and Public Health, 17*(8), 2665.

Wackerhage, H., & Schoenfeld, B. J. (2021, June 18). Personalized, evidence-informed training plans and exercise prescriptions for performance, fitness and health. *Sports Medicine*, 1-9.

Concept 13

Albano, D., Messina, C., Vitale, J., & Sconfienza, L. M. (2020). Imaging of sarcopenia: Old evidence and new insights. *European Radiology, 30*(4), 2199-2208.

Hales, C. M., Carroll, M. D., Fryar, C. F., and Ogden, C. L. (February 2020). Prevalence of obesity and severe obesity among adults: United States, 2017-2018. NCHS Data Brief, No. 360.

Hendren, N. S., de Lemos, J. A., Ayers, C., Das, S. R., Rao, A., Carter, S., . . . & Grodin, J. L. (2021). Association of body mass index and age with morbidity and mortality in patients hospitalized with COVID-19: Results from the American Heart Association COVID-19 Cardiovascular Disease Registry. *Circulation, 143*(2), 135-144.

Liu, B., Du, Y., Wu, Y., Snetselaar, L. G., Wallace, R. B., & Bao, W. (2021). Trends in obesity and adiposity measures by race or ethnicity among adults in the United States 2011-18: Population based study. *BMJ, 372*.

McLester, C. N., Nickerson, B. S., Kliszczewicz, B. M., & McLester, J. R. (2020). Reliability and agreement of various InBody body composition analyzers as compared to dual-energy X-ray absorptiometry in healthy men and women. *Journal of Clinical Densitometry, 23*(3), 443-450.

Popkin, B. M., Du, S., Green, W. D., Beck, M. A., Algaith, T., Herbst, C. H., . . . & Shekar, M. (2020). Individuals with obesity and COVID-19: A global perspective on the epidemiology and biological relationships. *Obesity Reviews, 21*(11), e13128.

Sung, H., Siegel, R. L., Rosenberg, P. S., & Jemal, A. (2019). Emerging cancer trends among young adults in the USA: Analysis of a population-based cancer registry. *The Lancet Public Health, 4*(3), e137-e147.

Ward, Z. J., Bleich, S. N., Cradock, A. L., Barrett, J. L., Giles, C. M., Flax, C., . . . & Gortmaker, S. L. (2019). Projected US state-level prevalence of adult obesity and severe obesity. *New England Journal of Medicine, 381*(25), 2440-2450.

Concept 14

Aridi, Y. S., Walker, J. L., Roura, E., & Wright, O. R. L. (2020). Adherence to the mediterranean diet and chronic disease in Australia: National Nutrition and Physical Activity Survey analysis. *Nutrients, 12*(5), 1251.

Butler, M. J., & Barrientos, R. M. (2020). The impact of nutrition on COVID-19 susceptibility and long-term consequences. *Brain, Behavior, and Immunity, 87*, 53–54.

Chlebowski, R. T., Aragaki, A. K., Anderson, G. L., et al. (2017). Low-fat dietary pattern and breast cancer mortality in the Women's Health Initiative Randomized Controlled Trial. *Journal of Clinical Oncology, 35*(25), 2919–2926.

Chlebowski, R. T., Aragaki, A. K., Anderson, G. L., et al. (2020). Dietary modification and breast cancer mortality: Long-term follow-up of the Women's Health Initiative Randomized Trial. *Journal of Clinical Oncology, 38*(13), 1419–1428.

Dietary Guidelines Advisory Committee. (2020). *Scientific Report of the 2020 Dietary Guidelines Advisory Committee: Advisory Report to the Secretary of Agriculture and the Secretary of Health and Human Services.* U.S. Department of Agriculture, Agricultural Research Service, Washington, DC.

Dumoitier, A., Abbo, V., Neuhofer, Z. T., & McFadden, B. R. (2019). A review of nutrition labeling and food choice in the United States. *Obesity Science & Practice, 5*(6), 581–591.

Grant, W. B., Lahore, H., McDonnell, S. L., Baggerly, C. A., French, C. B., Aliano, J. L., & Bhattoa, H. P. (2020). Evidence that vitamin D supplementation could reduce risk of influenza and COVID-19 infections and deaths. *Nutrients, 12*(4), 988.

Mariotti, F., Havard, S., Morise, A., Nadaud, P., Sirot, V., Wetzler, S., & Margaritis, I. (2021). Perspective: Modeling healthy eating patterns for food-based dietary guidelines–scientific concepts, methodological processes, limitations, and lessons. *Advances in Nutrition, 12*(3), 590–599.

Meier, B. P., Dillard, A. J., & Lappas, C. M. (2019). Naturally better? A review of the natural-is-better bias. *Social and Personality Psychology Compass, 13*(8), e12494.

Reedy, J., Pannucci, T., Herrick, K., Lerman, J., Shams-White, M., & Zimmer, M. (2021). Healthy Eating Index protocol: Review, update, and development process to reflect dietary guidance across the lifespan. *Current Developments in Nutrition, 5*(Suppl. 2), 447–447.

Shan, Z., Rehm, C. D., Rogers, G., Ruan, M., Wang, D. D., Hu, F. B., . . . & Bhupathiraju, S. N. (2019). Trends in dietary carbohydrate, protein, and fat intake and diet quality among US adults, 1999–2016. *JAMA, 322*(12), 1178–1187.

Stookey, J., et al., (2020). Underhydration is associated with obesity, chronic diseases, and death within 3 to 6 years in the U.S. population aged 51–70 years. *Nutrients, 12,* 905.

Vigar, V., Myers, S., Oliver, C., Arellano, J., Robinson, S., & Leifert, C. (2020). A systematic review of organic versus conventional food consumption: Is there a measurable benefit on human health? *Nutrients, 12*(1), 7.

Zabetakis, I., Lordan, R., Norton, C., & Tsoupras, A. (2020). COVID-19: The inflammation link and the role of nutrition in potential mitigation. *Nutrients, 12*(5), 1466.

Concept 15

Christensen, P., Meinert Larsen, T., Westerterp-Plantenga, M., Macdonald, I., Martinez, J. A., Handjiev, S., . . . & Pastor-Sanz, L. (2018). Men and women respond differently to rapid weight loss: Metabolic outcomes of a multi-centre intervention study after a low-energy diet in 2500 overweight, individuals with pre-diabetes (PREVIEW). *Diabetes, Obesity and Metabolism, 20*(12), 2840–2851.

Kalamov, Z. (2020). A sales tax is better at promoting healthy diets than the fat tax and the thin subsidy. *Health Economics, 29*(3), 353–366.

Masler, I. V., Palakshappa, D., Skinner, A. C., Skelton, J. A., & Brown, C. L. (2021). Food insecurity is associated with increased weight loss attempts in children and adolescents. *Pediatric Obesity, 16*(1), e12691.

Turnwald, B. P., Handley-Miner, I. J., Samuels, N. A., Markus, H. R., & Crum, A. J. (2021). Nutritional analysis of foods and beverages depicted in top-grossing US movies, 1994–2018. *JAMA Internal Medicine, 181*(1), 61–70.

Zhang, Y., Yang, J., Hou, W., & Arcan, C. (2021). Obesity trends and associations with types of physical activity and sedentary behavior in US adults: National Health and Nutrition Examination Survey, 2007–2016. *Obesity, 29*(1), 240–250.

Concept 16

Hallgren, M., Owen, N., Stubbs, B., Vancampfort, D., Lundin, A., Dunstan, D., . . . & Lagerros, Y. T. (2019). Cross-sectional and prospective relationships of passive and mentally active sedentary behaviours and physical activity with depression. *The British Journal of Psychiatry, 217*(2)1–7.

Kroencke, L., Geukes, K., Utesch, T., Kuper, N., & Back, M. D. (2020). Neuroticism and emotional risk during the COVID-19 pandemic. *Journal of Research in Personality, 89,* 104038.

McGinigal, K. (2016). *The upside of stress: Why stress is good for you, and how to get good at it.* New York: Penguin Random House.

Son, C., Hegde, S., Smith, A., Wang, X., & Sasangohar, F. (2020). Effects of COVID-19 on college students' mental health in the United States: Interview survey study. *Journal of Medical Internet Research, 22*(9). e21279

Storoni, M. (2017). *Stress proof: The scientific solution to protect your brain and body.* New York: Penguin Random House.

Teychenne, M., Stephens, L. D., Costigan, S. A., Olstad, D. L., Stubbs, B., & Turner, A. I. (2019). The association between sedentary behaviour and indicators of stress: A systematic review. *BMC Public Health, 19*(1), 1357.

Wingo, M. (2016). *The impact of the human stress response.* Austin, TX: Roxwell Waterhouse.

Concept 17

Behan, C. (2020). The benefits of meditation and mindfulness practices during times of crisis such as COVID-19. *Irish Journal of Psychological Medicine, 37*(4), 256–258.

Blease, C. R. (2015). Too many "friends," too few "likes"? Evolutionary psychology and "Facebook depression." *Review of General Psychology, 19*(1), 1–13.

Dominski, F. H., & Brandt, R. (2020). Do the benefits of exercise in indoor and outdoor environments during the COVID-19 pandemic outweigh the risks of infection? *Sport Sciences for Health, 16*(3), 583–588.

Greenberg, J. (2021). *Comprehensive stress management* (15th ed.). St. Louis: McGraw-Hill Higher Education.

Liu, J. J., Ein, N., Gervasio, J., & Vickers, K. (2019). The efficacy of stress reappraisal interventions on stress responsivity: A meta-analysis and systematic review of existing evidence. *PLOS One, 14*(2), e0212854.

Procaccia, R., Segre, G., Tamanza, G., & Manzoni, G. M. (2021). Benefits of expressive writing on healthcare workers' psychological adjustment during the COVID-19 pandemic. *Frontiers in Psychology, 12,* 360.

Tison, G. H., Avram, R., Kuhar, P., Abreau, S., Marcus, G. M., Pletcher, M. J., & Olgin, J. E. (2020). Worldwide effect of COVID-19 on physical activity: A descriptive study. *Annals of Internal Medicine, 173*(9), 767–770.

Yusufov, M., Nicoloro-SantaBarbara, J., Grey, N. E., Moyer, A., & Lobel, M. (2019). Meta-analytic evaluation of stress reduction interventions for undergraduate and graduate students. *International Journal of Stress Management, 26,* 132–145.

Concept 18

Alla, F., Berlin, I., Nguyen-Thanh, V., Guignard, R., Pasquereau, A., Quelet, S., . . . & Arwidson, P. (2020). Tobacco and COVID-19: A crisis within a crisis? *Canadian Journal of Public Health, 111*(6), 995–999.

Odani, S., et al., (2019). Tobacco and marijuana use among US college and noncollege young adults. *Pediatrics. 144,* 1–10.

van Zyl-Smit, R. N., Richards, G., & Leone, F. T. (2020). Tobacco smoking and COVID-19 infection. *The Lancet Respiratory Medicine, 8*(7), 664–665.

Williams, R. S., Derrick, J., & Ribisl, K. M. (2015). Electronic cigarette sales to minors via the internet. *JAMA Pediatrics, 169*(3), e1563.

Yach, D. (2020). Tobacco use patterns in five countries during the COVID-19 lockdown. *Nicotine & Tobacco Research, 22*(9), 1671-1672.

Concept 19

Chaney, B. H., Martin, R. J., Barry, A. E., Lee, J. G. L., Cremeens-Matthews, J., & Stellefson, M. L. (2019). Pregaming: A field-based investigation of alcohol quantities consumed prior to visiting a bar and restaurant district. *Substance Use & Misuse, 54*(6), 1017-1023.

Grossman, E. R., Benjamin-Neelon, S. E., & Sonnenschein, S. (2020). Alcohol consumption during the COVID-19 pandemic: A cross-sectional survey of US adults. *International Journal of Environmental Research and Public Health, 17*(24), 9189.

Jackson, K. M., Merrill, J. E., Stevens, A. K., Hayes, K. L., & White, H. R. (2021). Changes in alcohol use and drinking context due to the COVID-19 pandemic: A multimethod study of college student drinkers. *Alcoholism: Clinical and Experimental Research, 45*(4), 752-764.

Jaffe, A. E., Kumar, S. A., Ramirez, J. J., & DiLillo, D. (2021). Is the COVID-19 pandemic a high-risk period for college student alcohol use? A comparison of three spring semesters. *Alcoholism: Clinical and Experimental Research, 45*(4), 854-863.

Lucas, P., Boyd, S., Milloy, M. J., & Walsh, Z. (2020). Reductions in alcohol use following medical cannabis initiation: Results from a large cross-sectional survey of medical cannabis patients in Canada. *International Journal of Drug Policy, 86*, 102963.

Pollard, M. S., Tucker, J. S., & Green H. D. (2020). Changes in adult alcohol use and consequences during the COVID-19 pandemic in the U.S. *JAMA Network Open, 3*, e2022942.

Sugarman, D. E., & Greenfield, S. F. (2021). Alcohol and COVID-19: How do we respond to this growing public health crisis? *Journal of General Internal Medicine, 36*(1), 214-215.

Wood, A. M., Kaptoge, S., Butterworth, A. S., Willeit, P., Warnakula, S., Bolton, T., . . . Thompson, S. (2018). Risk thresholds for alcohol consumption: Combined analysis of individual-participant data for 599,912 current drinkers in 83 prospective studies. *The Lancet, 391*(10129), 1513-1523.

Concept 20

Bachhuber, M. A., Saloner, B., Cunningham, C. O., & Barry, C. L. (2014). Medical cannabis laws and opioid analgesic overdose mortality in the United States, 1999-2010. *JAMA Internal Medicine, 174*(10), 1668-1673.

Birnbaum, H. G., et al. (2011). Societal costs of prescription opioid abuse, dependence, and misuse in the United States. *Pain Medicine, 12*, 657-667.

Boyd, C. J., McCabe, S. E., Evans-Polce, R. J., & Veliz, P. T. (2021). Cannabis, vaping, and respiratory symptoms in a probability sample of U.S. youth. *Journal of Adolescent Health, 69*(1), 149-152.

Chihuri, S., & Li, G. (2019). State marijuana laws and opioid overdose mortality. *Injury Epidemiology, 6*(1), 1-12.

Johnston, L. D., Miech, R. A., O'Malley, P. M., Bachman, J. G., Schulenberg, J. E., & Patrick, M. E. (2021). *Monitoring the Future national survey results on drug use 1975-2020: Overview, key findings on adolescent drug use.* Ann Arbor: Institute for Social Research, University of Michigan.

Schulenberg, J. E., Johnston, L. D., O'Malley, P. M., Bachman, J. G., Miech, R. A. & Patrick, M. E. (2020). *Monitoring the Future national survey results on drug use, 1975-2019: Vol. II, College students and adults ages 19-60.* Ann Arbor: Institute for Social Research, University of Michigan. Retrieved from http://monitoringthefuture.org /pubs.html#monographs

Substance Abuse and Mental Health Services Administration. (2020). *Key substance use and mental health indicators in the United States: Results from the 2019 National Survey on Drug Use and Health* (HHS Publication No. PEP20-07-01-001, NSDUH Series H-55). Rockville, MD: Center for Behavioral Health Statistics and Quality, Substance Abuse and Mental Health Services Administration. Retrieved from https://www.samhsa.gov/data/

Concept 21

Davis, K. C., Gulati, N. K., Neilson, E. C., & Stappenbeck, C. A. (2018). Men's coercive condom use resistance: The roles of sexual aggression history, alcohol intoxication, and partner condom negotiation. *Violence against Women, 24*(11), 1349-1368.

Havlir, D., Lockman, S., Ayles, H., Larmarange, J., Chamie, G., Gaolathe, T., . . . & Universal Test, Treat Trials (UT3) Consortium. (2020). What do the Universal Test and Treat Trials tell us about the path to HIV epidemic control? *Journal of the International AIDS Society, 23*(2), e25455.

Ingram, L. A., Macauda, M., Lauckner, C., & Robillard, A. (2019). Sexual behaviors, mobile technology use, and sexting among college students in the American south. *American Journal of Health Promotion, 33*(1), 87-96.

World Health Organization. (2016). *Consolidated guidelines on the use of antiretroviral drugs for treating and preventing HIV infection: Recommendations for a public health approach,* 2nd ed. Geneva, Switzerland: World Health Organization.

Concept 22

Abdel-Latif, M. M. M. (2020). The enigma of health literacy and COVID-19 pandemic. *Public Health, 185*, 95.

Gregory, J. M., Slaughter, J. C., Duffus, S. H., Smith, T. J., LeStourgeon, L. M., Jaser, S. S., . . .

& Moore, D. J. (2021). COVID-19 severity is tripled in the diabetes community: A prospective analysis of the pandemic's impact in type 1 and type 2 diabetes. *Diabetes Care, 44*(2), 526-532.

Hendren, N. S., de Lemos, J. A., Ayers, C., Das, S. R., Rao, A., Carter, S., . . . & Grodin, J. L. (2021). Association of body mass index and age with morbidity and mortality in patients hospitalized with COVID-19: Results from the American Heart Association COVID-19 Cardiovascular Disease Registry. *Circulation, 143*(2), 135-144.

Klein, S. L., Dhakal, S., Ursin, R. L., Deshpande, S., Sandberg, K., & Mauvais-Jarvis, F. (2020). Biological sex impacts COVID-19 outcomes. *PLOS Pathogens, 16*(6), e1008570.

Paakkari, L., & Okan, O. (2020). COVID-19: Health literacy is an underestimated problem. *The Lancet. Public Health, 5*(5), e249.

Zare, M., Norouzi Roshan, Z., Assadpour, E., & Jafari, S. M. (2021). Improving the cancer prevention/treatment role of carotenoids through various nano-delivery systems. *Critical Reviews in Food Science and Nutrition, 61*(3), 522-534.

Concept 23

Dorrel, B., Long, T., Shaffer, S., & Myer, G. D. (2018). The functional movement screen as a predictor of injury in national collegiate athletic association division II athletes. *Journal of Athletic Training, 53*(1), 29-34.

Zhu, F., Zhang, M., Wang, D., Hong, Q., Zeng, C., & Chen, W. (2020). Yoga compared to non-exercise or physical therapy exercise on pain, disability, and quality of life for patients with chronic low back pain: A systematic review and meta-analysis of randomized controlled trials. *PLOS One, 15*(9), e0238544.

Concept 24

Nsoesie, E. O., & Oladeji, O. (2020). Identifying patterns to prevent the spread of misinformation during epidemics. *The Harvard Kennedy School Misinformation Review.*

Paige, S. R., Black, D. R., Mattson, M., Coster, D. C., & Stellefson, M. (2019). Plain language to communicate physical activity information: A website content analysis. *Health Promotion Practice, 20*(3), 363-371.

Thomas, J. D., & Cardinal, B. J. (2020). Analyzing suitability: Are adult web resources on physical activity clear and useful? *Quest, 72*(3), 316-337.

Thomas, J. D., & Cardinal, B. J. (2020). How credible is online physical activity advice? The accuracy of free adult educational materials. *Translational Journal of the American College of Sports Medicine, 5*(9), 82-91.

Concept 25

Aminuddin, H. B., Jiao, N., Jiang, Y., Hong, J., & Wang, W. (2021). Effectiveness of smartphone-based self-management interventions on self-efficacy, self-care activities, health-related quality of life and clinical outcomes in patients with type 2 diabetes: A systematic review and meta-analysis. *International Journal of Nursing Studies, 116*, 103286.

Bentley, C. L., Powell, L., Potter, S., et al. (2020). The use of a smartphone app and an activity tracker to promote physical activity in the management of chronic obstructive pulmonary disease: Randomized controlled feasibility study. *JMIR mHealth uHealth, 8*(6), e16203.

Bryson, W. J. (2021). Long-term health-related quality of life concerns related to the COVID-19 pandemic: A call to action. *Quality of Life Research, 30*(3), 643-645.

Franssen, W. M. A., Franssen, G. H. L. M., Spaas, J., Solmi, F., Eijnde, B. O. (2020). Can consumer wearable activity tracker-based interventions improve physical activity and cardiometabolic health in patients with chronic diseases? A systematic review and meta-analysis of randomised controlled trials. *International Journal of Behavioral Nutrition and Physical Activity, 17*(1), 57.

Simpson, R. J., Campbell, J. P., Gleeson, M., Krüger, K., Nieman, D. C., Pyne, D. B., . . . & Walsh, N. P. (2020). Can exercise affect immune function to increase susceptibility to infection? *Exercise Immunology Review, 26*, 8-22.

Thompson, W. R., Sallis, R., Joy, E., Jaworski, C. A., Stuhr, R. M., & Trilk, J. L. (2020). Exercise is medicine. *American Journal of Lifestyle Medicine, 14*(5), 511-523.

Wabnitz, K., et al. (2020). A pledge for planetary health to unify the health professions in the Anthropocene. *The Lancet, 396,* 1471-1473.

Wendt, A., da Silva, I. C. M., Gonçalves, H., Menezes, A., Barros, F., & Wehrmeister, F. C. (2020, May 15). Short-term effect of physical activity on sleep health: A population-based study using accelerometry. *Journal of Sport and Health Science.*

Index

Note: Page numbers in **boldface** refer to glossary terms; those followed by "f" refer to figures; those followed by "t" refer to tables

A

ABCDE self-exam, 414, 414f
ABC system for time management, 340, 340t
abdominal exercises. *See* core training
abdominal muscles, 173f, 174f
abdominal ptosis, 435f, 437t
abduction, 196, 196f
absolute muscle fitness, **157**
ACA (Patient Protection and Affordable Care Act), 20
academic performance
    alcohol use and, 370, 370f
    physical activity, 78
acai berry scam, 469
A1C blood test, 417
accidental injuries, 419–420, 420t
acclimatization, 52–53
ACEs (adverse childhood experiences), 320
acetaminophen, 57
achilles tendon, 174f
acquired aging, 70
acquired immune deficiency syndrome (AIDS). *See* HIV/AIDS
ACSM. *See* American College of Sports Medicine
ACTH (adrenocorticotropic hormone), 320
active assistance, in stretching, 201, **201**
active living
    moderate physical activity, 100–101
    physical activity pyramid, 100f
active stretching, 203. *See also* stretching
activity. *See* physical activity
activity monitoring apps, 147–148
activity neurosis, 232
activity patterns
    by age group, 144, 145f
    for cardiovascular endurance, 127
    during college, 127
    vigorous physical activity, 146–147
adaptations
    defined, **321**
    stress and, 320
Adderall, 380
addiction. *See also* alcohol use and abuse; tobacco use
    biopsychosocial model, 388
    genetics and, 388
    nicotine, 358
    treatment apps, 372
adduction, 196, 196f
adductor brevis, 184
adductors
    adductor longus, 173f
    adductor magnus, 174f
    exercising, 184, 445
    stretching, 212
adenocarcinomas (malignant tumors), 408
Adequate Intake (AI), 279
adherence, 28, 29
adherence questionnaire, 149–150
adolescents
    alcohol use, 369
    drug use, 383, 383f
    secondhand smoke susceptibility, 354

smoking, 356–357
    stress, 318
adoption, healthy behavior, 28
adrenocorticotropic hormone (ACTH), 320
advanced fitness training
    aerobic and anaerobic capacity, 224
    cardiorespiratory endurance, training for, 224–227
    functional fitness and flexibility, training for, 229–230
    "Heads Up" concussion awareness, 223
    high-level performance and training characteristics, 222–224
    high-level performance training, 231–232
    muscular endurance training, 226–227
    performance trends and ergogenic aids, 232–233
    performers training, 227
    power training, 226–227
    self-management skills, 233–234
    skill-related fitness and skill, 230–231, 230t
    strength training, 226–227
    training for speed and power, 228
    training for strength, muscular endurance and power, 226–227
adverse childhood experiences (ACEs), 320
aerobic activities. *See also* moderate physical activity; vigorous physical activity
    using hand weights during, 467
aerobic capacity, 118, 142, 143, 222, **223**
    assessments, 118, 120
    defined, 118
aerobic exercise, 222, **223**
    adaptations to, 118
    defined, 118
aerobic fitness. *See* cardiorespiratory endurance
aerobic intervals, 225
aerobic metabolism, 118
aerosols (inhalants), 382t
age and aging
    acquired aging, 70
    calcium intake, 287
    creeping obesity, 251, 251f
    degenerative disc disease, 432
    flexibility, 198
    functional fitness, 161
    muscle fitness, 158
    physical activity effects on, 332–333
    physical activity patterns, 144
    stress effect on, 320
    target heart rate zone and, 125f
    time-dependent aging, 70
agility, 10f
Agility Rating Scale, 235
AI (Adequate Intake), 279
AIDS. *See* HIV/AIDS
air pollution, and physical activity, 55
alarm reaction phase, 319f
alcohol expectancies, 369
alcoholic cirrhosis, 366, **367**
alcohol tolerance, 365, **365**
alcohol use and abuse
    accidents and, 419
    beverage contents, 364, 364f
    blood alcohol concentration, 364, 368t, 375–376
    in college students, 370–373, 370f, 370t
    consumption guidelines, 288
    consumption patterns, 365–373, 365t
    drug classification, 364, 380
    effects on body, 364

excessive intake, 288
    as gateway drug, 388
    health risks and benefits, 366–367, 366f
    impaired driving and, 368–369, 368t, 369f
    in military personnel, 372
    people who should abstain, 367t
    perceptions about, 377–378
    prevention and treatment, 372
    problem drinking risk factors, 369
    self-monitoring, 373
    smoking and, 358
alcohol use disorders (AUD), 365, **365**, 365t
alcohol withdrawal, **365**, 365–366
all-or-none thinking, 336t
altitude, and physical activity, 55
Alzheimer disease, 77, 78, 418
amenorrhea, 246, **247**
American Cancer Society (ACS), 78
American College of Sports Medicine (ACSM), 88
American Fitness Index, 5
American Psychological Association (APA), 18–19
amino acids, 283, **283**
amphetamines, 380–381, 381t
anabolic steroids, 165, **165**
anaerobic capacity, 142, 143, 223, **223**
anaerobic exercise, 143, 222, **223**
anaerobic intervals, 225
anaerobic metabolism, 118
anaerobic threshold, 223, **223**
android (upper body) fat, 249
androstenedione (andro), 165
anemia, 116
ankle weights, 467
anorexia athletica, 255
anorexia nervosa, 81, 255
antagonist muscles, 157, **157**, 157f
anthocyanins, 289t
antibodies, 396, **397**
antioxidants, 285, **285**
antiretroviral (ART) drugs, 397–398
anxiety, 77
    in college students, 317
    muscle fitness and, 159
    physical activity and, 332
    as response to stress, 320
appetite, 303
appetite suppressants, 309
apple shape, 249
appraisal-focused coping, 334–335, **335**, 335t, 336
apps (applications)
    activity monitors, 147–148
    addiction treatment, 372
    environmental monitors, 55
    role in STIs, 402
    smoking cessation, 360
    stress management, 339
    stretching prompts, 198
    target heart rate calculators, 124t
arm circles, 444
arm lift (back exercise), 453
arm stretches, 213
ART (antiretroviral) drugs, 397–398
arteries, healthy, 116
arteriosclerosis, **73**, 116
arthritis, 79
artificial sweeteners, 308
assertiveness, 340–341
asthma, 79

Astrand-Ryhming Bicycle Test, 127, 129–130
atherosclerosis, **73**, 116
  blood coagulants, 73
  defined, 72
  HDL in blood, 73
  lowering blood lipid levels, 72–73
  monitoring lipid profiles, 72
athletic performance. *See* high-level performance
at-risk drinking, 365t
attitude balance
  lifestyle change and, 488t
  to moderate stress, 324
  physical activity and, 58–59, 59t
attitude questionnaire, 64–65
AUD (alcohol use disorders), 365, **365**, 365t
automated external defibrillators (AEDs), 56
automatic (distorted) thinking, 336t, 337, 337t
avoidant coping strategies, 334, **335**, 335t

B

BAC (blood alcohol concentration), 364, 368t, 375–376
back-arching abdominal stretch, 443
back extension exercises, 443, 453
back extensor muscles, exercising, 184
back pain or problems
  body mechanics and, 430–431, 438
  causes and consequences, 430–432
  exercise guidelines, 438–441
  exercise planning and logging, 461–462
  exercises for, 453
  healthy back test, 455–456
  muscle fitness and, 161
  posture and, 434–438, 437t
  prevention and treatment, 432, 433–434
  questionnaire, 457–458
  stretching for, 199
back problems, 77
back-saver hamstring stretch, 211, 447
back-saver toe touch, 445
back scratcher stretch, 213
backward jog, 64
balance (skill-related fitness)
  as dimension of fitness, 10f
  in muscle fitness, 158
balance of energy. *See* caloric (energy) balance
Balance Rating Scale, 236
ballistic stretching, 202f, 203
barbiturates, 380, 380t
barriers, overcoming, 24, 488t
bar stretch, 447
basal metabolic rate (BMR), 251, **251**, 302, **303**
Bass test, of dynamic balance, 235
bath salts (cathinones), 384
BED (binge eating disorder), 254–255
beer, 364f, 367
behavioral goals, 305, **305**
behavior change. *See* lifestyle changes
beliefs
  drug use and, 388
  health decisions and, 486, 487
  lifestyle change and, 488t
Belviq, 309
bench press, 179
benign tumors, 78, 408, **409**
bent-knee situps, 446
beta-carotene, 289t, 472
beverages, 288
BIA (bioelectric impedance analysis), 248
biceps brachii
  exercising, 179, 181
  location, 173f
biceps curl
  free-weight, 179
  machine, 181

biceps femoris, location, 174f
bicycle exercise, 446
bicycle test, 120, 127–128
Bicycle Test Rating Scale, 131
Bikram (hot) yoga, 205
binge drinking, 365, 370, 370t, 372
binge eating disorder (BED), 254–255
bioelectric impedance analysis (BIA), 248
biofeedback, 339
biological determinants
  at birth, 18–19
  disabilities types, 19
  effects on aging, 19
biopsy, 408, **409**
biopsychosocial model of addiction, 388
black beauties (amphetamines), 381t
blame, 336t
blood alcohol concentration (BAC), 364, 368t, 375–376
blood pressure. *See* high blood pressure (hypertension)
blood sugar levels, 417
blood vessels, 119f
Bloomberg Global Health Index, 21
blow (cocaine), 381t
blunt (marijuana), 382t
BMI. *See* Body Mass Index
BMR (basal metabolic rate), 251, **251**, 302, **303**
Bod Pod, 247
body awareness, for posture correction, 437–438, 442
bodybuilding, 159
body composition
  assessment methods, 246
  as dimension of fitness, 9f
  evaluating, 267–272
  indicators and standards, 245–246, 246f
  quackery in, 468–469
  self-assessment, 255
  in weight loss, 252
body fatness. *See also* weight control
  evaluating, 257–263
  fitness and, 120
  health risks of, 248
  muscle fitness and, 158
  reducing, 252, 468
  standards for, 245–246
Body Mass Index (BMI)
  calculating, 264, 271
  defined, 246
  disease risk and, 266
  standards for, 246, **247**
body mechanics. *See also* posture
  back or neck pain and, 430–431, 438
  core musculature and, 428–430, 429f
  proper techniques, 439f
  spinal anatomy and, 428, 428f
body neurosis, 81
body sculpting, surgical, 468
body types, 250
body weight exercises, 145t, 166, 440
body wrapping, 466
bone integrity, 12
brachialis, 173f, 174f
brachioradialis, 173f, 174f
brain, 78
breakfast, in sound nutrition, 291
breast cancer, 79t, 409–410, 411t
breast self-exam, 425–426
breathing exercises, for stress management, 338
bridge variations, 452
brown sugar (heroin), 381t
Buettner, Dan, 29
built environment, 19, 21
bulimia, 255
buttock stretch, 212

C

caffeic/ferulic acids, 289t
caffeine, 288
calcium, 284, 286t, 287, 472
calf stretch, 64, 211
calisthenics, 183–184, 193–194
calorie sparing, 308
caloric (energy) balance
  defined, **251**
  for fat and weight loss, 252
calories
  daily expenditure calculation, 273
  deficit for weight loss, 252
  defined, 251
  expenditures by activity, 109t, 253t
  for healthy weight, 279
Canadian 24-Hour Movement Guidelines, 103
cancer
  alcohol use and, 367
  Big 4, 408
  breast self-exam, 425–426
  described, 408
  HPV and, 398–399, 413
  incidence and death rates, 408–409, 409f
  major types, 409–415
  physical activity and, 79t
  prevention of, 415–416, 416t
  risk assessment, 423–424
  screening guidelines, 411t, 412
  spread of, 408, 408f
  testicular self-exam, 425–426
  tobacco use and, 353, 355t
candy (drugs), 380t
cannabis
  decriminalization, 385
  drug class, 382, 382t
  use prevalence and consequences, 383, 385–386
  vaping technology, 389
Cannon, Walter, 318
capillaries, healthy, 116
carbohydrates, 308
  dietary recommendations, 280–282, 286t
  DRI value, 280f
  physical performance and, 292
carbohydrate loading, 292, **293**
carbon monoxide, 55, 352
carcinogens
  cancer prevention and, 415
  defined, **353**
  in tobacco, 352
carcinomas (malignant tumors), 408
cardiac muscle, 156
cardiopulmonary resuscitation (CPR), 56
cardiorespiratory endurance, 119f, 222, **223**
  as dimension of fitness, 9f
  elements of, 116
  FIT formula for, 121–123
  moderate physical activity and, 102
  muscular endurance and, 158
  non-exercise estimate of, 132
  term, 116
  threshold, target zones for, 123–126, 124t, 125f
cardiorespiratory endurance, training for, 224–227
cardiovascular disease
  alcohol use and, 367
  casual participation, *versus* regular, 144
  dietary habits and, 283
  extreme exercise and, 50
  inactivity and, 120
  risk factor assessment, 83–84
carotenoids, 289t
carotid pulse, 126
carpal tunnel syndrome, 431
cathinones (bath salts), 384
CAUTION acronym, 416, 416f
CD4 helper cells (T helper cells), 395, **395**
cellulite, 468

Centers for Disease Control and Prevention (CDC), 18
cervical cancer, 399, 411t, 413
cervical spine, 428, 428f
chancre, 400, **401**
chancroid, 401, 401t
change. *See* lifestyle changes
chest press, 181
chewing tobacco, 355. *See also* tobacco use
children
    physical activity patterns, 89
    secondhand smoke susceptibility, 354
child's pose, 210
chin tuck, 209, 450
chlamydia, 398t, 399, 400, **401**
cholesterol, 73t, 282-283
chondroitin, 470
chronic diseases, 70
    muscle fitness and, 158
cigarette smokers. *See* tobacco use
cigar smokers, 353. *See also* tobacco use
circuit resistance training (CRT), 166
cirrhosis, alcoholic, 366, **367**
cities, healthiest, 5
CL (ConsumerLab), 470
clinical exercise tes, 48
clothing, athletic, 50, 50t
cobra pose, 210
cocaine, 380, 381t, 385, 386
coccyx, 428, 428f
codeine, 380, 381t
cognitions, 24, 485
    determinant interactions, 24
cognitive function
    cannabis use and, 385
    physical activity, 77
cognitive reappraisal, 336
coke (cocaine), 381t
cold, exercising in, 53-54
college students
    activity patterns, 127
    alcohol use, 370-372, 370f, 370t
    condom use, 401-402
    drug use, 383f, 384
    mental health problems, 317
    sleep habits, 333
    STI risk, 401-102
    stress, 316t, 317
    stress-management resources, 334
    time use, 340f
    weight gain, 244
colonoscopy, 410
colon-rectal cancer, 79t, 410-412, 411t
combo aerobic classes, 141
competitive events, 222
compression of illness, 70
concentric muscle contractions, 161, **161**
condom use, 401-402, 404
conduction, 52
conscientiousness, 324, **324**
ConsumerLab (CL), 470
consumer skills, 13, 234
    consumer protections and, 470-472
    diet and nutrition evaluation, 469-470
    as enabling factor, 30t
    exercise equipment evaluation, 466-467
    expert identification, 464-465
    fat and weight loss evaluation, 468
    in health and medical care, 482
    health club evaluation, 467-468, 469f, 477-478
    information source evaluation, 465
    knowledge building, 25
    lifestyle change and, 488t
    nutrition supplement evaluation, 470-472
    product evaluation form, 475-476
    quack identification, 464
continuous passive motion (CPM) tables, 466
contract-relax-antagonist-contract (CRAC), 203

contraindicated exercises, defined, **438**
convection, 52
cool-down, 52, **53**
coordination, 10f
    stick test of, 236
Coordination Rating Scale, 236
coping skills and strategies
    coping defined, 334
    as enabling factor, 30t
    lifestyle change and, 488t
    for quitting smoking, 359t, 360
    for stress management, 334-340, 335t
core musculature
    anatomy and function, 428-430, 429f
    muscle types, **429**, 429-430, 429f
    spinal injury and, 432
core training
    for back pain, 433, 453
    body-weight exercises, 440
    core stabilization, 433, 451-452
    functional movements, 454
    for muscle fitness, 185-186
    planning and logging, 193-194, 461-462
coronary collateral circulation, 74, **75**
corticotropin-releasing hormone (CRH), 319
cortisol, 320
cotton, for athletic wear, 50
COVID-19 pandemic, 3, 22, 68, 70, 71, 78
    complications, 420
    health status, 2
    healthy lifestyles, 486
    lifespan (life expectancy) of Americans, 5
    lifestyle determinants, 22
    long-term effects on health, 80
    mental health, 8
    personal actions and interactions, 24
    personal health *versus* public health, 420
    personal responsibility, 3
    Quack Hack, 485
    symptoms of, 420
    threat to public health, 421
    vaccines, 421
CPM (continuous passive motion) tables, 466
crab lice, 400, 401t
CRAC (contract-relax-antagonist- contract), 203
crack (cocaine), 381t
crank (methamphetamine), 381t
C-reactive protein (CRP), 73
creatine, 169-170, 233
CRH (corticotropin-releasing hormone), 319
critical thinking, 24
CrossFit, 166
CRT (circuit resistance training), 166
crunches, 183, 185, 446, 453
crystal methamphetamine, 381, 381t, 384
CTD (cumulative trauma disorder), 431
cumulative trauma disorder (CTD), 431
curl-ups, 183, 453
cystic fibrosis, 79

D

dance aerobics, 140
date-rape drugs, 383t, 386
death, actual causes, 21-22
decision-making, 94, 485
deep breathing, 338
deep neck flexors, stretching, 450
deep squats, 449
definition, in muscles, **157**
definition of muscle, 226, **227**
degenerative disc disease, 432, 432f
dehydration, 53, **53**
delayed-onset muscle soreness (DOMS), 57
deltoid
    exercising, 161f, 179, 181, 183, 443

location, 173f, 174f
    stretching, 213
dementia, 77
    physical activity, 77
    symptoms and treatment, 418
depressant drugs, 364, 380, 380t
depression, 77
    in college students, 317
    physical activity and, 332
    treatment of, 419
designer drugs, 382-383, 383t, 384, 386
determinant interactions
    cognitions and emotions, 24
    personal actions and, 24
determinants of health. *See also* specific determinants
    actions and interactions as, 485-487, 486t
    assessing, 490-491
    biological determinants, 18-19
    interactions, 24
    lifestyle determinants, 21-23
    social determinants, 19-20
diabetes, 76, 120
    associated health problems, 417
    prevention of, 417-418, 418t
    types of, 416-417
diaphragmatic breathing, 338
diastolic blood pressure, **73**
Dietary Guidelines for Americans, 278
dietary patterns, defined, 279
Dietary Reference Intake (DRI), 279, 280f, 286t
dietary supplements. *See* nutritional supplements
Dietary Supplements Health and Education Act
    (DSHEA), 470
diet, defined, 252
diet pills, 381t
digital eye strain, 441
dimagery, 147-148
dimensions of wellness, 483
diphtheria, 22
dips, 183
disabilities
    as health determinant, 19
    wellness and, 8
discounting the positives, 336t
discrimination, and stress, 318
disease limitations, 79
distorted thinking, 336t, 337, 337t
distress, 321, **321**
dithiolthiones, 289t
diverse mind-body movement, 205
diversity, equity, and inclusion (DEI) issues, 244
DMAA (dimethylamylamine), 169
DNA testing, 18
DNA testing services, 474
doctors, 481
DOMS (delayed-onset muscle soreness), 57
dorsiflexion, 196, 196f
dose-response relationship, 86
double-leg lift, 444
double progressive system, 168
downers (depressant drugs), 364, 380, 380t
DRI (Dietary Reference Intake), 279, **279**, 280f, 286t
drinking age, 371
drinking games, 371. *See also* alcohol use and abuse
driving while impaired, 368-369, 368t, 369f
drug-impaired driving, 388
drug use and abuse. *See also* alcohol use and abuse;
    prescription drugs; tobacco use
    avoiding drug problems, 389-390
    causes of, 388-389
    consequences and costs, 385-388, 385f
    drug classifications, 380-382, 380t, 381t, 382t,
        383t
    drug defined, **353**, 365
    evaluating, 391-392
    help resources, 390
    prevalence and trends, 383-388, 383f, 386f

drug use and abuse (*continued*)
    smoking and, 358
    for sports performance, 165
drunk driving, 368-369, 368t, 369f
DSHEA (Dietary Supplements Health and Education Act), 470
dual-energy absorptiometry (DXA), 247
dumbbell rowing, 180
duration of physical activity. *See* time (duration) of physical activity
DXA (dual-energy absorptiometry), 247
dynamic balance, Bass test of, 235
dynamic flexibility, 197
dynamic muscular endurance, 160, **161**
dynamic strength, 160, **161**
dynamic stretching, 203, 229, 230
dynamic warm-up, 51, 64

E

eating
    guidelines for, 307
    strategies for, 311-312
eating disorders, 245, 254-255
eating patterns, changes in, 307-308
eccentric muscle contractions, 160
echinacea, 470
e-cigarettes, 354, 357
economic costs
    health insurance, 481, 483
    illicit drug use, 384-385, 385f
    mental disorders, 419
    tobacco use, 354
ecstasy (designer drug), 384, 385, 386
ectomorph body type, 251
egg consumption, 282
EIM (Exercise Is Medicine), 145t
electrical muscle stimulators, 466
emotion(s), 24
    decision-making and, 85
    determinant interactions, 24
    as health determinant, 24, 483, 484f
    stress management and, 339
emotional eating, 303
emotional reasoning, 336t
emotional stressors, 316
emotion-focused coping, 334-335, **335**, 335t, 337
employees. *See* workplace issues
empty calories, 308, **309**
enabling factors, 30t, 488t
endometrial cancer, 413
endomorph body type, 251
endurance sports
    success in, 222
endurance training, 164
energy balance. *See* caloric (energy) balance
energy bars, 233
energy drinks
    with "boosts," 470
    mixing with alcohol, 371
energy expenditure, 107-108. *See also* calories
    calorie needs calculation, 273-276
    calories used by activity, 109t, 253t
energy intake, 302
environment
    in alcohol problems, 369
    as cancer risk, 416
    as health determinant, 21, 482-484, 484f
    lifestyle impacts on, 484-485
    obesogenic, 482
    physical activity and, 24, 52
    plant-based diets and, 291
    as stressor, 316
environmental conditions, 55
Environmental Protection Agency, 55
ephedra, 470

erector spinae
    exercising, 186, 443, 445, 446
    location, 429f
    stretching, 210
ergogenic aids, 232, **233**
    advanced fitness training, 232-233
ergonomics, 438
essential amino acids, 283, **283**
essential fat, 245, **245**
ethanol, in alcoholic beverages, 364
eustress, 321, **321**
evaporation of sweat, 52
eversion, 196, 196f
exceptional performance, 222
exercise. *See also* physical activity
    back and neck health guidelines, 438-441
    calisthenics, 183-184
    core training, 161, 185, 193-194, 440
    and extreme, 50
    free-weight resistance, 179-180, 191-192
    as health determinant, 23
    neck muscles, 450
    quackery in, 465-466
    questionable *versus* safe, 440, 442, 443-449
    resistance machines, 181-182, 191-192
    stretches, 209-213
    warm-up, 64
exercise equipment and fitness programs, 466-467
Exercise Is Medicine (EIM), 145t
exercise machines, 141
    advantages/disadvantages, 165t
    determining type to use, 466-467
    limitations of, 467-468
    purchasing, 466
    resistance, 165, 181-182, 191-192
exercise warm-up guidelines, 51t
exhaustion phase, 319f
experts, identifying, 464-465
extension, 196, 196f
extensor digitorum longus
    location, 173f
    stretching, 448
extensor hallucis longus, 448
external abdominal oblique
    exercising, 183
    location, 173f, 174f, 221f, 429f
external respiration, 116
external rotation, 192, 192f
extreme exercise, 224
eye strain, 441

F

fad diets, 308-309
FAS (fetal alcohol syndrome), 367
fast food, 291
fast food restaurants, evaluation, 313-314
fasting plasma glucose (FPG) test, 417
fast-twitch (Type II) muscle fibers, 156
fat control, factors influencing, 302-303
fat, dietary
    dietary recommendations, 282-283, 286t
    DRI value, 280f
    reducing intake, 279
fatigue, from stress, 320
fatness. *See* body fatness
fatty liver, 366, **367**
fecal immunochemical test (FIT), 10, 410
fecal occult blood test (FOBT), 410
female athlete triad, 255
fetal alcohol syndrome (FAS), 367
fiber, dietary, 281, **281**, 286t
fibrin, **73**
fight-or-flight response, 318
FIT (fecal immunochemical test), 104, 410
fitness. *See* physical fitness
FitnessGram (skinfold method), 257, 258, 260

fitness leaders, evaluating, 467
fitness ratings, 19
fitness tests
    cardiorespiratory endurance, 128-136
    flexibility, 215-218
    muscle fitness, 175-178, 187-190
fitness trends, 144, 145t
fitness zones, 94
FITT, FIT formula
    for cardiorespiratory endurance, 121-123
    components of, 88
    defined, 88
    for progressive resistance exercise, 162-165, 163t
flat back posture, 435
flavanones, 289t
flavonoids, 289t
flavonols, 289t
flexibility
    for advanced fitness training, 229-230
    as dimension of fitness, 9f
    exercise plan for, 208-209
    factors influencing, 196-198
    FIT formula for, 199t
    fitness tests, 215-218
    and flexibility activities, 205-206
    guidelines for, 206-207
    injury risk and, 198
    in physical activity pyramid, 200, 200f
    self-management skills, 207-208
    static *versus* dynamic, 197
    stretching methods, 201-204, 202f
flexibility activities, 91
    flexibility and, 205-206
flexion, 192, 192f
fluid replacement beverages, 50, 53, 233
foam rolling (FR), 207
FOBT (fecal occult blood test), 410
folic acid, 472
food
    fortified, 285, 287
    organic, 289-290
    quality comparison, 291t
food insecurity, and obesity, 305
food labels
    bolder statements and communication on, 305
    GMO debate, 290
    "healthy" and "natural," 290
    reading, 293
forearm stretch, 213
fortified foods, 285, 287
forward press, 454
FPG (fasting plasma glucose) test, 417
frame size, 263
fraud, defined, 464
free play, 334
free weights
    advantages/disadvantages, 165t
    controversial use of, 466
    described, 164
    exercises using, 179-180
    planning and logging exercise, 191-192
frequency of physical activity
    for cardiorespiratory endurance, 122
    in FITT formula, 87-88
    injury prevention and, 441
    for progressive resistance exercise, 162-165, 163t
    for stretching, 203, 204t
Fresh Food Farmacy, 281
freshman 15 (weight gain), 244, 245
fruit and vegetable consumption, 281
full flip, 236
functional balance training, 229
functional fitness, **12**
    for advanced fitness training, 229-230
    described, 12, 161
    for older adults, 164
    testing, 430

functional foods, 288–289, 289t
fusion inhibitors, 397

G

gastrocnemius
  exercising, 161f
  location, 173f, 174f
  stretching, 211
Gatorade, 50
gender, 19
gender differences
  alcohol effects, 364
  body fatness standards, 246f
  cancer incidence and deaths, 409f
  doctors, 481
  health care use, 481t
  injury rates, 419
  stress, 317
  suicide, 419
gender identity, 19
general adaptation syndrome, 319, 319f
generational forgetting, 384, **385**
genetically modified organism (GMO), 290
genetics
  advanced fitness training, 224
  alcohol problems and, 369
  cancer and, 415
  drug addiction and, 388
  flexibility and, 198
  as health determinant, 479–480
  muscle fitness and, 157
  obesity and, 250
genetic testing, 18, 480
genital herpes, 398t, 399, **400, 401**
genital warts, 400, 401t
Gen Xers, stress in, 317, 317f
Georgia homeboy (drug), 383t
gestational diabetes mellitus, 417
GHB (drug), 383t, 386–387
GI (glycemic index), 280
glucosamine, 470
gluteal muscles
  exercising, 161f, 180, 184, 186, 445, 446, 449
  gluteus maximus, 174f, 180, 184, 209, 210, 449
  gluteus medius, 174f, 184
  stretching, 210
gluten intolerance, 290
glycemic index (GI), 280
glycemic load, 280
glycogen, 292, **293**
GMO (genetically modified organism), 290
goal setting
  as enabling factor, 30t
  lifestyle change and, 488t
  for moderate physical activity, 110
  in time management, 341
gonorrhea, 398, 398t, 400, **401**
good skill-related fitness, 230
gracilis
  exercising, 184
  location, 173f, 174f
grapevine exercise, 64
grapevine movement, 229
grass (marijuana), 382t
grip strength, testing, 176, 187
groin stretch, 212
group exercise classes, 145t
gyms, evaluating, 467–468, 469f, 477–478
gynoid (lower body) fat, 250

H

habit
  formation, 23
  for optimal health, 23t
  for physical activity, 60

half flip (coordinated test), 236
half squat, 180, 449
hallucinations, 381, **381**
hallucinogens, 381–382, 382t
hamstrings
  exercising, 182, 443, 449
  stretching, 64, 211, 447
hand weight use, 467. *See also* free weights
hand position, 236
hardiness, 324, **324**, 329–330
hCG (human chorionic gonadotropin), 469
HDL (high-density lipoprotein), 73t
head clock exercise, 445
head nod, 450
"heads up" concussion awareness, 223
Health Apps, 34
health. *See also* determinants of health; healthy
    lifestyles; lifestyle changes; physical fitness
  dimensions of, 7, 7f
  national goals, 419, 473
  wellness integration, 8
health and medical care
  effective use of, 481–482
  emergency care, 419
  gender differences in, 481t
  as health determinant, 20–21
  regular checkups, 421–422, 481
  screening tests, 411t, 481
health-based criterion-referenced standards, 93–94
health benefits, 88
health-care costs. *See* economic costs; health
    insurance
health-care system. *See* health and medical care
health clubs, evaluating, 467–468, 469f, 477–478
health determinants. *See* determinants of health
health disparities, 5, 18, 19
healthiest places to live, 5
health information. *See* consumer skills;
    misinformation
health insurance
  Fresh Food Farmacy, 281
  as health determinant, 20–21
  saving money and, 481
health literacy, 472, 482
health-related fitness, 9f
health-related quality of life, 7, 22
health savings account (HSA), 481
healthspan
  muscle fitness and, 159
health standards
  blood pressure, 74t
  body composition, 245–246, 246f
  physical fitness, 94t
healthy food
  in schools, 305
"healthy" food labels, 291
healthy lifestyle questionnaire, 27–28
healthy lifestyles. *See also* lifestyle changes
  during COVID-19 pandemic, 486
  effects on aging, 19
  HELP philosophy, 2
  personal actions, interactions and, 485–487, 486t
  strategies for, 484–485, 484t
Healthy People 2030, 3–5
  health equity, 5
  health goals, 3t–4t
  health, wellness, and healthy behaviors, 6
  social, physical, and economic environments, 6
healthy shopping
  guidelines for, 307t
heart disease. *See* cardiovascular disease
heart health
  cardiorespiratory endurance and, 116
heart rate
  fitness improvement and, 126
  monitoring, 126
  target zone, 123–126, 124t, 125f

heart rate reserve (HRR), 122, 124t
heart rate variability, 231
heat, exercising in, 52–54
heat index, **53**, 54t
heat-related illnesses, 53, 53t
heavy-episodic drinking, 365t
height-weight measurements, 263–264, 271
HELP philosophy, 2
  adopt, 2
  healthy behaviors, 2
  healthy lifestyle, 2
  lack of equity, 2
  personal needs, 2
hemoglobin, **116**
hepatitis B (HPB), 398t, 400, **401**
herb (marijuana), 382t
herbal supplements, 470
heredity. *See* genetics
herniated disc, **431**, 431–432, 432f
hero exercise, 448
heroin, 380, 381t
herpes, genital, 398t, 399, **401**
HGH (human growth hormone), 169
high blood pressure (hypertension), 74t, 288
high-density lipoprotein (HDL), **73**, 73t
high-intensity interval training (HIIT), 123, 145t,
    226
high-level performance, 222–224
  advanced fitness training, 231–232
  nutrition for, 290
  skill-related fitness and skill for, 12
high skip and reach, 64
HIIT (high-intensity interval training), 123, 145t
hip and thigh stretches, 211, 212, 448
HIV/AIDS
  as cause of death, 23
  definitions, **395**
  prevalence, 394–395
  prevention and treatment, 396–397
  replication cycle, 397f
  testing for, 396
  transmission routes, 395, 395f
  types of, 396
holistic health, 9
hook-up apps, 402
hormone replacement therapy (HRT), 416
hospitals, 481
hot tubs, 468
hot (Bikram) yoga, 205
HPA (hypothalamic-pituitary-adrenal) axis, 319–320
HPV (hepatitis B), 400, **401**
HPV (human papillomavirus), 394, **395**, 398–399,
    398t, 413
HRR (heart rate reserve), 122, 124t
HRT (hormone replacement therapy), 416
HSA (health savings account), 481
huffing (inhalant abuse), 381–382, 382t, 386
human biology. *See* genetics
human chorionic gonadotropin (hCG), 469
human factors engineering (ergonomics), 438
human growth hormone (HGH), 169
human papillomavirus (HPV), 394, **395**, 398–399,
    398t, 413
humidity, and exercise, 53
hunger, 303, 309
hybrid exercise, 142
hybrid shoes, 49
hydration. *See* fluid replacement beverages; water
hygiene, for good health, 482
hyperextension, 438–440, 440f
hyperflexion, 438–440, 440f
hyperkinetic conditions, 81
hypermobility, 198, **199**
hypertension, 73, **73**, 74
hypertension (high blood pressure), 74t, 288
hyperthermia, 53, **53**
hypertrophy, **157**

hypokinetic diseases, **9**, 70
  cardiorespiratory endurance and, 116t, 120
  physical activity, 70–71
  physical activity and, 86
hypostress, 321, **321**
hypothalamic-pituitary-adrenal (HPA) axis, 319–320
hypothetical periodization cycle, 232
hypothermia, **53**

I

ibuprofen, 57
ice (methamphetamine), 381t
iliopsoas, stretching, 211
iliotibial tract
  location, 174f
  stretching, 211, 212
illinois agility run, 235
illness
  defined, 7
  wellness and, 8
  working during, 482
imagery, 338
immune system, 78
  alcohol use and, 366
  stress effects on, 320
impaired driving, 368–369, 368t, 369f
inactivity
  cardiovascular disease risk and, 120
  as cause of death, 23
  defined, 100
inchworm exercise, 64
individuality principle, 87
indoor tanning, 415, 468–469
infectious diseases, 25
inferior gemellus, stretching, 212
information sources. *See* consumer skills;
  misinformation
infraspinatus, 174f
inhalant abuse, 381–382, 382t, 386
injuries (accidents), 419–420, 420t
injuries (activity-related)
  flexibility and, 198–200
  most common, 56–57
  muscle fitness and, 158
  overuse injuries, 56–57
  resistance exercise and, 170, 170t
  treatment for, 57
injuries, in physical activity
  minor soft tissue injuries, 57
  muscle cramps, 58
  muscle soreness, 57–58
  types of, 56–57
injury prevention
  exercise variables in, 441
  safe exercises for, 440, 443–449
inner thigh stretch, 212
insomnia, 419
instructor evaluation, 208
insulin, **417,** 418
intellectual environment, 482, 484f
intellectual wellness, 69–70
international health rankings, 21
intensity of physical activity
  for cardiorespiratory endurance, 122
  classification of, 101t
  in FITT formula, 87–88
  injury prevention and, 441
  for progressive resistance exercise, 162–163, 163t
  for stretching, 204
  target heart rate zone, 125f
intermediate (Type IIa) muscle fibers, 156
intermittent activity, 105
internal abdominal oblique
  exercising, 183
  location, 429f

internal respiration, 117
internal rotation, 192, 192f
Internet resources
  credible websites, 13
  evaluating, 472
interpreting online information, challenges, 324
interval training, 224, **225**
interval-training workouts
  work and rest bouts for different types of, 225t
intervertebral discs, 428, 428f, **429,** 431
intoxication, **365**
intramural sports, 142
intrinsic motivation, 94
inversion, 192, 192f
IQOS cigarettes, 354
iron, dietary, 287
isokinetic exercises, 159t, 161
isometric exercises, 159t, 160
isometric neck exercises, 450
isothiocyanates, 289t
isotonic exercises, 159, **159**

J

jackets (high-tech fabric), 50
Jackson-Pollock method, 257, 260–262
Jacobson's progressive relaxation method, 338
Jenny Craig programs, 309
jog, backward, 64
joint laxity, 192, 192f
jumping to conclusions (distorted thinking), 336t
junk (heroin), 381t

K

K2 (drug), 382t
Kaposi's sarcoma, 396, **397**
Kennedy, John F., 68
ketamine, 383t
kettlebells, 166
knee extension, 182
knee hyperextension, 435f, 437t
knee pull-down, 449
knee stride and reach, 64
knee-to-chest, 449
knowledge building
  in decision-making, 77, 94, 489
  harmful exercises and, 442
  lifestyle change and, 488t
  physical activity adherence and, 128
kyphotic (outward) spinal curve, 434, **435,** 435f, 437t

L

labeling (distorted thinking), 336t
lactic acid, 57, 142, 143, 222, **223**
lacto-ovo vegetarians, 289, **289**
lateral trunk stretch, 209
latissimus dorsi
  exercising, 180
  stretching, 210, 213
lat pull-down, 182
lavator scapulae, stretching, 445
laxity of joints, 196, **197**
LDCT (low-dose computed tomography), 412
LDL (low-density lipoprotein), 73t
leg hug, 64, 210, 446
leg stretches, 211–212
leisure, 333, **333,** 334
leverage, in muscle movement, 156–157
lifelong habits, 2
lifespan (life expectancy)
  muscle fitness and, 159
  obesity and, 248

lifestyle behaviors, 22
lifestyle changes
  adoption and maintenance of, 30
  for cancer prevention, 415, 416t
  for diabetes prevention, 417–418, 418t
  enabling factors, 32, 33t
  as health determinant, 22, 484–485, 484t
  personal commitment, 34
  personal factors, 31
  personal responsibility, 29
  planning worksheet, 492–493
  predisposing factors, 32, 32t
  reinforcing factors, 32, 33
  self-management skills, 29–30, 30t
  self-management skills for, 487–489, 488t
  stages of change model, 28–29
  stages of change questionnaire, 39–42
lifestyle determinants, 18
  and COVID-19, 22
  disease and early death, impact for, 22–23
  health and well-being, impact on, 21–23
  healthy habits, 23, 23t
lifestyle physical activities, 109t
lifetime sports, 143
lifting technique, 438, 439f
lifts with stabilization exercises, 454
ligaments, 196, **197**
light activity, 102
  accumulation of, 303
  advantage of, 103
  classification by fitness level, 102t, 102t
  non-exercise activity thermogenesis (NEAT), 103
  replacing sedentary time, 104
  versus sedentary, 101t
light physical activity (LPA), 101
lipids, **73**
Lipokinetix, 471
lipoproteins, **73**
liposuction, 468
liquid ecstasy, 383t
liquor, 364f
liver disease, 366
location, and health, 5
locus of control, **323,** 323–324, 329–330
longissimus capitis, stretching, 209
long-slow distance (LSD) training, 224, **225**
long-term weight control, 302, 309
lorcaserin, 309
lordotic (inward) spinal curve, 434, **435,** 435f, 437t
losing body fat
  guidelines for, 305–308, 306t, 307t
low-calorie diet, 306
low-density lipoprotein (LDL), **73,** 73t
low-dose computed tomography (LDCT), 412
lower body (gynoid) fat, 250
LSD (drug), 381, 382t
lumbar lordosis posture, 435
lumbar spine, 428, 428f, 429f
lung cancer, 411t, 412
lunge, 180
lunge walks, 184
lutein, 289t
lycopene, 289t
lycra body suits, 232
lying posture, 436f

M

magnesium, 286t
magnets, medicinal, 466
magnification, 336t
mainstream smoke, 353, **353**
maintenance goals, 34
malignant tumors (carcinomas), 78, 408, **409**
mammograms (breast X-rays), 409, **409**
MapMyRun/Ride, 50

martial arts, 140
massage rollers, 207
maximal heart rate (maxHR), 122
maximum oxygen update (V̇O₂ max), 118, 120.
    See also aerobic capacity
MDMA (ecstasy), 383t
Mebaral, 380t
mechanical ergogenics, 232-233
media influence
    sexual behavior, 401
    tobacco use, 356, 356f
medical care. *See* health and medical care
medical illiteracy, 482
medical insurance. *See* health insurance
medical model, 21
medical power of attorney, 481
melanoma, 414, 414f, **415**
melt away fat, 308
memory, and physical activity, 332
memprobamate, 380t
men. *See* gender differences
mental filter, 336t
mental health. *See also* stress; stress management
    anxiety, 159, 317, 320, 332
    common disorders and costs, 419
    COVID-19, 8
    depression, 317, 332, 419
    muscle fitness and, 159
    physical activity and, 332
    problems in college students, 317
    public health goals, 419
    secondhand smoke and, 353
    sleep disorders, 419
    suicide prevention, 419
mental imagery, 338
mental wellness, 69
mesomorph body type, 251
metabolic fitness, 12, 76
metabolic fitness benefits, 104
metabolic health
    physical activity, 75-76
metabolic syndrome
    cardiorespiratory endurance and, 120
    diabetes, 76
    metabolic fitness, 76
    physical activity, 75-76
metastasis, 408, **409**
methadone, 380, 381t, 387
methamphetamines (meth), 380-381, 381t, 385, 386
methaqualone, 380t
microtrauma, 431, **431**
middle-distance events, 224
military personnel, 372
Millennials, stress in, 316, 317, 317f
mind-body awareness, 208
mind-body exercises, 434
mindfulness meditation, 339
minerals, 286t, 287-288
mineral supplements, 287, 472
minimization, 336t
minority populations
    cancer in, 409, 410, 413
    diabetes in, 417
    HIV/AIDS in, 395
    injury rates, 419
12-Minute Run Test, 128, 131
12-Minute Swim Test, 128, 132
misinformation. *See also* consumer skills
    avoiding, 13
    in online sources, 473
    superhighway, 342
mixed fitness activities, 142
mobilizer muscles, 429, **429,** 429f
moderate aerobic activity, 90-91. *See also* moderate
    physical activity
moderate drinking, 365t
moderate physical activity, 101, 105, 303

benefits, 104
classification by fitness level, 102t, 102t
combining with vigorous activity, 153-154
FIT formula, 104, 104t
goal setting, 110
guidelines, 105
vs. light or vigorous, 101t
metabolic fitness, 104
monitoring, 106f, 106f, 109t
physical activity guidelines, 105
physical activity pyramid, 100f
soreness and injuries from, 57
warm-up guidelines, 51t
wellness benefits, 104
moisture-wicking fabrics, 50
mole self-exam, 414, 414f
Molly (ecstasy), 386
mono-unsaturated fats, 282
morphine, 380, 381t
motivation
    effects on fitness tests, 128
    intrinsic, 94
    lifestyle change and, 488t
multiple-joint exercises, 226
motivational interviewing, 309
motor fitness, 12, 230, **231**
motor vehicles. *See* impaired driving
MTU (muscle-tendon unit), 196, **197**
multifidus, 429f
multivitamins, 472
muscle dysmorphia, 255
muscle fitness, 226, **227**
    cardiorespiratory endurance and, 117
    factors influencing, 156-158
    fitness tests, 175-178, 187-188
    loss of, 158
    self-assessments, 171
muscle fitness activities, 91
muscle fitness exercise, 303
muscle implants, 468
muscles
    balanced strength, 434
    core muscles, 429, **429,** 429f
    cramps in, 58, 199
    definition in, **157**, 226
    fiber types, 156
    full body diagram, 173-174
    hypertrophy, **157**
    movements of, 157
    soreness in, 57
    tissue types, 152
    tonic (postural), 197
    viscoelasticity, 197
muscle-tendon unit (MTU), 196, **197**
muscular endurance
    defined, 152
    as dimension of fitness, 9f
    dynamic, 160, **161**
    factors influencing, 156-158
    fitness tests for, 176-177, 178, 189-190
    static, 160, **161**
    training for, 162, 226-227
muscular power. *See* power
muscular strength. *See* strength
musculoskeletal health
    physical activity, 76-77
mushrooms (psychedelic), 381
myofascial trigger points, 199, **199**
MyPlate, 278, 292

N

narcotics, 380, 381t, 387
National Academy of Medicine (NAM), 222
national health goals, 3-5
National Weight Control Registry (NWCR), 306

"natural" food labels, 470
NEAT (non-exercise activity thermogenesis), 303,
    303
neck circling, 445
neck flexors, 450
neck pain
    body mechanics and, 438
    causes and consequences, 430-432
    exercise guidelines, 438-441
    exercises for, 450
    posture and, 434-438, 437t
    prevention and treatment, 432, 433-434
    questionnaire, 457-458
    stretching for, 199
neck rotator and extensors, 450
neck stretch exercise, 209, 450
negative attitudes, toward physical activity, 57
negative (distorted) thinking, 336t, 337, 337t
Nembutal, 380t
neuromuscular exercise. *See* functional fitness
neutral spine, 434, **435**
nicotine, 352, 358-359
Nike Alphafly model, 233
nitrites (inhalants), 382t
nonessential fat, 246, **247**
non-exercise activity thermogenesis (NEAT), 103,
    303, **303**
nonsteroidal anti-inflammatory drugs (NSAID), 57
NSP International (NSP), 471
nutrient-dense food, 279
nutrition. *See also* weight control
    analysis of, 295-299
    for cancer prevention, 415t
    carbohydrates, 280f, 281, 292
    as cause of death, 23
    fats, 279
    food quality comparisons, 291t
    food selection worksheet, 299-300
    as health determinant, 23
    healthy eating guidelines, 278-280, 278f, 280f, 286t
    minerals, 287-288
    physical performance and, 292-293
    proteins, 280f, 283-284, 292
    quackery in, 469-470
    self-management skills, 293-294
    sound eating practices, 291-292
    terms and trends, 288-290, 289t
    vitamins, 285, 287
    water and fluids, 288
nutritional content, 305
nutritional supplements
    fraud and quackery in, 470-472
    issues and concerns with, 471
    protein supplements, 284
    regulation of, 470-471
    vitamins and minerals, 287, 472
NWCR (National Weight Control Registry),
    306

O

obesity, 244-245
    food insecurity and, 305
    personal health and well-being, 244-245
    public health challenge, 244
obesity and overweight. *See also* weight control
    back pain and, 431
    causes of, 250-251
    defined, 246
    dietary habits and, 280, 283
    fear of, 254
    genetic risk scores, 480
    health risks of, 248-250
    physical activity and, 332
    prevention and treatment, 252
obesogenic, 482

obesogenic environment, 482
   confronting, 304–305, 304f
obturator internus, stretching, 212
occupational safety, 419
OGTT (oral glucose tolerance test), 417, **417**
older adults. *See* age and aging
omega-3 fats, 282, 283
omega-6 fats, 282, 283
one-leg stretch, 447
online dating apps, 402
online resources, evaluating, 472
opiate narcotics, 380, 381t, 387
opioid crisis, 387
opportunistic infections, 395, **395**
optimism, 323, **323,** 487
oral glucose tolerance test (OGTT), 417, **417**
organic foods, 289–290
Orlistat, 309
osteoporosis, 76–77, 76f
outcome goals, 36, 305, **305**
ovarian cancer, 413
overgeneralization, 336t
overhead arm stretch, 213
overhead lift, 454
overhead press
   free-weight, 179
   machine, 181
overload principle, **87,** 167
overload syndrome, 231
overtraining, 231
   identifying symptoms of, 241–242
overweight, 246, **246.** *See also* obesity and overweight
oxycontin, 381t, 387
oxygen debt, 142, 143, 223, **223**
ozone, 55

P
panacea, defined, 465, **465**
pap tests, 413, **413**
paralysis by analysis, **147**
parasympathetic nervous system (PNS), 319, **319**
PAR-Q+ (Physical Activity Readiness Questionnaire
   for Everyone), 62
participation, in physical activity. *See* activity patterns
party hosting, responsible, 373
passive assistance, in stretching, 202, 203
passive exercise, 465, **465**
Patient Protection and Affordable Care Act (ACA),
   21
patterns of activity. *See* activity patterns
PCP (drug), 381, 382t
pectineus, exercising, 184
pectoralis major
   exercising, 173f, 179, 181, 182, 183, 443
   location, 173f
   stretching, 209
pectoralis minor
   exercising, 183, 443
   stretching, 208, 209
pedometer step counts, 107t
Peleton, 50
pelvic floor muscles, 429f
pelvic inflammatory disease (PID), 400, **401**
pep pills (amphetamines), 381t
percent body fat, 245, **245**
performance, athletic. *See* high-level performance
performance skills (self-management)
   as enabling factor, 30t
   lifestyle change and, 488t
   posture-related, 442
performance trends
   advanced fitness training, 232–233
periodization, 169, 232, **233**
peroneus longus, 173f, 174f
personal actions, interactions, 24, 480, 485–486, 486t

personality types
   drug use and, 388
   stress and, 322–323
personalization (distorted thinking), 336t
personal philosophy, 2, 487
personal trainers, 145t, 467
persuasion, 473
peyote cactus buttons, 381
phenolic acids, 289t
phenterimine, 309
Phillip Morris International, 354
phosphorus, 286t, 287
physical activity. *See also* high-level performance;
      moderate physical activity; vigorous physical activity
   activity classification by, 102
   adherence questionnaire, 149–150
   air pollution and, 55
   attitudes toward, 58, 60, 64–65
   back problems, reduces risks of, 77
   benefits of, 69
   for cancer prevention, 415t
   cardiorespiratory system, 68
   cardiovascular adaptations, 117–120
   and cardiovascular health, 72–73
   casual *versus* regular, 144
   circulatory control and regulation, 75
   classification of, 101
   in cold or wet conditions, 50
   components of, 64
   consistent patterns of, 88
   delays aging, 70
   effects of inherited risk, 70
   emergencies and handling injuries, 56–58
   emotional/mental wellness, 69
   energy expenditure, 107–108
   FITT-VP, 88
   fluid-replacement beverages, 50
   functioning effectively, 68
   guidelines for, 105
   handling emergencies, 68
   harmful radiation, 55–56
   health and wellness, 80–81
   health benefits, 78–79
   as health determinant, 23
   heart attack, 74–75
   heart attack, reduce risks of, 74–75
   in heat and cold, 52–54
   at high altitude, 55
   hyperkinetic conditions, 81
   hypertension, 73–74
   immune system, 68
   informed decisions, 58
   intellectual wellness, 69–70
   intensity classifications, 101t
   lifespan and health span, increase, 70–71
   lifestyle medicine, 79–81
   light physical activity (LPA), 101
   mental health, 77–78
   metabolic health, 75–76
   metabolic syndrome, 75–76
   metabolic system, 68
   moderate physical activity (MPA), 101
   monitoring, 106f, 106f, 109t
   musculoskeletal health, 76–77
   musculoskeletal system, 68
   nervous system, 68
   physical wellness, 69
   planning for, 50
   prevention of chronic disease, 79–80
   prevention strategies, 50
   principles of, 86–87
   program planning, 494–501
   quackery in, 465–466
   quality of leisure time, 68
   recommendations for, 50–54
   reduce fibrin levels, in blood, 73
   reduce risks for hypokinetic diseases, 70–71

   shoes and clothing for, 50, 50t
   shoes, role of, 49
   sleep and, 333
   social wellness, 70
   soreness, 57–58
   spiritual wellness, 70
   stress and, 332–333
   technology for monitoring, 50
   trends in, 144, 145t, 146
   vigorous physical activity (VPA), 101
   warm-up guidelines, 51t
   "weekend warrior" approach, 93
   weight control, 302–303
   working efficiently, 68
   worksite and school health promotion programs, 80
Physical Activity Attitude Questionnaire, 64–65
Physical Activity Guidelines for American, 87, 93
physical activity level (PAL), 302
physical activity plan, 110
physical activity pyramid
   classification, 85
   described, 89–92, 90f
   energy balance, 91
   factors, 91–92
   flexibility activities, 91
   moderate aerobic activities, 90–91
   muscle fitness activities, 91
   vigorous aerobic activities, 91
   vigorous sports, recreation, and anaerobic activities,
      91
Physical Activity Readiness Questionnaire for
      Everyone (PAR-Q+), 62
physical dependence
   defined, **353**
   in tobacco use, 352
physical environment
   as health determinant, 483, 484f
   in public health goals, 6
physical fitness
   activity classification by, 102t, 102t
   bone integrity, 12
   components of, 12
   defined, **9**
   determinants of, 18f
   dimensions of, 9f, 10f
   functional fitness, 12
   good fitness, 12
   health-related dimensions of, 9, 9f
   heart rate and, 126–127
   metabolic fitness, 12
   obesity and, 248–249
   skill-related dimensions of, 9, 10f
   standards of, 93–94, 94t
physical wellness , 69
physiological fatigue, 320, **321**
physiological stressors, 316
PID (pelvic inflammatory disease), 400, **401**
Pilates, 205
pill, exercise in, 89
pipe smokers, 353. *See also* tobacco use
piriformis, stretching, 212
piriformis syndrome, 447
plank exercises, 451
planning, in time management, 341
plantar flexion, 196
plant-based diets, 289t, 291
plant-based foods, 284
plant-based protein, 284
play, 334, **335**
plough position, 446
plough shear position, 446
plyometric exercises, 160, **161**
   advantages/disadvantages, 159t
   described, 158
   equipment for, 166
   example of, 164, 165f
   planning and logging, 193–194

plyometrics, 228, 228t, **229**
    safety guidelines for, 228
PNF (proprioceptive neuromuscular facilitation), 203, **203**
PNS (parasympathetic nervous system), 319, **319**
polyunsaturated fats, 282, 283
poppers (inhalants), 382t
positive attitudes, toward physical activity, 58
positive thinking, 9
posterior cuff, stretching, 213
postmenopause, and calcium intake, 287, 288
post-traumatic stress disorder (PTSD), 320
postural (tonic) muscles, 197
posture
    back or neck pain and, 430
    correcting, 437-438, 437f
    defined, 434, **435**
    evaluating, 459-460
    guidelines for, 434-435, 435f, 436f
    health problems and, 435, 437t
    muscle fitness and, 158
pot (cannabis), 382t
potassium, 287
power
    advanced fitness training, 226-228
    defined, 158
    as dimension of fitness, 9f
    factors influencing, 156-158
    FIT formula for, 163
    fitness tests for, 189-190
    stretching and, 201
Powerade, 50
powerlifting, 159
power of attorney, medical, 481
PRE. *See* progressive resistance exercise
pre-contraction stretch, 202f, 203
pre-diabetes, **417,** 417-418
predisposing factors, 488t
pregnancy, 78-79
    alcohol use and, 288, 366
    calcium intake and, 288
    diabetes in, 417
    drug use during, 388
    physical activity, 78-79
    smoking during, 354
    St. John's wort and, 471
premenstrual syndrome (PMS), 79
pre-participation screening, 59
prescription drugs, 308. *See also* drug use and abuse
    effects and side effects, 481
    misuse prevalence, 383-384, 387-388
    overdose deaths, 387
    for smoking cessation, 360
    stimulants, 380-381
    use during pregnancy, 388
principle of diminished returns, 87
principle of rest and recovery, 87
priorities, in time management, 340t, 341
proanthocyanidins, 289t
problem-focused coping, 334-335, **335,** 335t, 339
process (behavioral) goals, 305
processed food, 291, 294
procrastination, 341, 341f
product (outcome) goals, 305
professional help, 343, 486
progression principle, 87, **87,** 167-168
progressive relaxation method, 338
progressive resistance exercise (PRE)
    defined, **157,** 159
    FIT formula for, 162-165, 163t
    guidelines for, 170-170
    sets and repetitions in, 164
    types of, 159
progressive resistance training programs, 226
proprioception, 229, **229**
proprioceptive neuromuscular facilitation (PNF), 203, **203**

prostate cancer, 79t, 411t, 412
prostate-specific antigen (PSA) blood test, 412
protease inhibitors, 397
protective gear, 50
proteins, 183-185, 280f, 286t, 292
protein supplements, 284
PRT (progressive resistance training), 159-162
PSA (prostate-specific antigen) blood test, 412
psoas major, 429f
psychedelics, 381-382, 382t
psychoactive drug, **381**
psychological ergogenics, 233
psychological fatigue, 320, **321**
psychosocial stressors, 316, 320
PTSD (post-traumatic stress disorder), 320
pubic crab lice, 400, 401t
public health
    anti-tobacco efforts, 357
    goals of, 3-5, 419, 473
pulls with stabilization exercise, 454
pull-ups, modified, 183
pulse rate, counting, 126
purging disorder, 255
push-ups, 183
pyramid models
    physical activity pyramid, 100f

quacks and quackery. *See also* consumer skills
    defined, 464
    fat and weight loss, 468
    identifying, 464
    nutritional supplements, 470-472
    physical activity, 473-474
    susceptibility to, 473-474
quadratus lumborum, 429f
quadriceps
    exercising, 158, 182, 182t, 184, 449
    stretching, 210, 211, 448
quality of life
    defined, 7
    muscle fitness and, 159
Qsymia, 309

radial pulse, 126
range of motion (ROM), 196, **197,** 206
ratings of perceived exertion (RPE), 123, 133
RDA (Recommended Dietary Allowance), 279, 286t
reaching technique, 439f
reaction time, 10f
reaction time rating scale, 237
reciprocal inhibition, 201, 201f
Recommended Dietary Allowance (RDA), 279, 286t
recreation activities
    stress management and, 333, **335,** 341
    vigorous, 144
rectal cancer, 79t
rectus abdominis
    exercising, 173f, 183, 185, 186, 444, 446
    location, 173f, 221f, 429f
rectus femoris
    exercising, 180, 184
    location, 173f
reduced-calorie diets, 306
Reebok International, 465
referred pain, 430, **431**
reinforcing factors, 30t, 488t
relapse prevention, 30t, 33, 488t
relationships, and health decisions, 486
relative muscle fitness, 157, **157**
relaxation techniques, 337-339, 347-348
1 repetition maximum (1 RM), 163, **163,** 187-188, 226

repetitions, in progressive resistance exercise, 164, 164f
repetitive stress injury (RSI), 431
resilience, 323, **323**
resistance exercise
    benefits of, 158-159
    circuit training, 166
    endurance training and, 166
    equipment for, 166
    fallacies and facts, 163t
    free-weight exercises, 179-180
    guidelines for, 170-171
    plan for, 171
    planning and logging, 191-194
    principles of, 167-168
    progressive resistance, **157,** 159-162, 160f
    resistance machine exercises, 181-182
    as trend, 145t
    warm-up guidelines, 51t
resistance phase, 319f
respiratory system, 116
responsible party hosting, 373
rest and recovery
    defined, 87
    described, 87
    resistance exercise, 164-165, 169
restaurants
    fast food, 294
    posting nutritional content, menus in, 305
resting heart rate (RHR)
    normal, 116
    target heart rate zone and, 124, 125f
reverse curls, 185, 444, 453
reverse transcriptase inhibitors, 397
reversibility principle, **87**
rhomboideus
    exercising, 180, 182, 183
    location, 174f
    rhomboid minor, 182
RHR. *See* resting heart rate
Ritalin, 380, 381t, 387
rohypnol, 383t, 386
ROM (range of motion), 196, **197**
RPE (ratings of perceived exertion), 123
RSI (repetitive stress injury), 431
rubberized suits, 466
running test, 128
rush (inhalants), 382t

sacrum, 428, 428f
safe sex, 403-405
safety concerns
    activity environments, 24
    occupational safety, 419
    questionable exercises, 440, 442, 443-449
salt (sodium) intake, 279, 288
sarcomas (malignant tumors), 408
sarcopenia, 157, **157**
sartorius, 173f, 174f
saturated fats, 282, **283**
sauna belts, 466
saunas, 468
saw palmetto, 470
Saxenda, 309
scalenes, stretching, 445
schools, access to healthy food in, 305
sciatica, 447
scoliosis, 431
screening
    professional screening, 48-49
    self-screening, 48
screening tests
    cancer, 411t
    for optimal health, 481

seated rowing, 182
seated side stretch, 64
secondhand smoke, 352, **353**, 353–355
sedatives, 364, 380, 380t
sedentary behavior, 102
  defined, 100
  issues of isolation, 103
  versus light activity, 101t, 102
  and mental health, 101
  monitoring, 106f, 106f, 111–112
  standardization of research, 102
self-affirmations, 339
self-assessment
  back and neck health, 442
  body composition and weight, 255
  cardiovascular endurance, 127–128
  defined, 12
  as enabling factor, 30t
  lifestyle change and, 488t
  muscle fitness, 171
  of stress, 324
self-confidence, 32
  lifestyle change and, 488t
  physical activity and, 94
self-efficacy, 32, 324, **324**
self-management skills, 18. *See also* specific skills
  for adopting active lifestyle, 110
  for adopting healthy lifestyle, 25, 487–489, 488t
  advanced fitness training, 233–234
  characteristics, 29
  clarifying reasons, 35
  consumer skills, 13
  defined, 2
  as enabling factor, 30t
  evaluating progress, 38
  factors, 31f
  flexibility, 207–208
  identifying needs, 35
  personal commitment and, 34
  practice and implement, 29
  program components, 37
  reinforcing factors related to, 30t
  self-planning, 34
  setting personal goals, 35–37
  using effectively, 12
  written plan, 37–38
self-monitoring
  activity intensity, 123–126
  alcohol use, 373
  as enabling factor, 30t
  lifestyle change and, 488t
  sedentary behaviors, 110
  time usage, 341
self-planning skills
  for back and neck health, 442
  as enabling factor, 30t
  less formal use of, 488
  lifestyle change and, 488t
self-promoting activities, 147
self-screening, PAR-Q+, 48
Selye, Hans, 319
semimembranosus exercising, 180, 184
semitendinosus, 174f
sensation seeking, and drug use, 388
serial monogamy, 401–403
serostatus, 395, **395**
serratus anterior, 173f
serratus, exercising, 173f
set-point, 250, **250**
sets, in progressive resistance exercise, 164
sex, 19
sexting, 403
sexual behavior, 394, 401–402
sexually transmitted infections
  CDC campaigns, 396
  common, 398–401, 398t, 399f

defined, **395**
general facts, 394
HIV/AIDS, 394–398, 395f, 397f
lesser-known, 400, 401t
prevention and intervention, 396, 403–404
risk factors, 401–403
risk questionnaire, 405–406
STI hotline, 403
term, 394
testing for, 396
vaccines for, 398, 399, 400
sexual misconduct, 402
shin and quadriceps stretch, 448
shin stretch, 211, 448
shoes, features of
  cushioning, 49
  flexibility, 49
  hybrid shoes, 49
  support, 49
  traction, 49
shoe technology, 233
short-length intervals, 225
shoulder stand bicycle, 446
"should" statements (distorted thinking), 336t
shrooms (psychedelic mushrooms), 381
sick days, 482
side leg raises, 184
side plank, 451
sidestream smoke, 353, **353**
side stretch, seated, 64
SIDS (sudden infant death syndrome), 353
sigmoidoscopy, 410
single knee-to-chest, 449
sitting, excessive, 102
sitting posture, 434–435, 436f
sitting tucks, 185, 453
sit-ups, bent-knee, 446
skeletal muscle, 156
skill-related fitness, 222
  advanced fitness training, 230–231, 230t
  dimensions of, 10f
  evaluation, 239–240
  performance, 9
  physical fitness, 235–236
  in sport performance, 12
skin cancer, 411t, 414–415, 414f, 468
skinfold measurements, 247–248, 257, 267–269
sleep, 77
sleep disorders, 419
sleep habits
  guidelines for, 333t
  smartphones, 485
  stress effects on, 321
  for stress management, 333
sleeping pills, 380t
slow-twitch (Type I) muscle fibers, 156, 197
smack (heroin), 381t
SMART (Stress Management and Resiliency Training), 339
smartphone apps. *See* apps (applications)
  weight control, 310
smartphone use, 318
smallpox, 22
smokeless tobacco, 355, 355t. *See also* tobacco use
smoking and smoking cessation. *See* tobacco use
smooth muscle tissue, 156
snacks, health, 291
sniffing inhalants, 381–382, 382t, 386
snow (cocaine), 381t
SNS (sympathetic nervous system), 318, **319**
snuff, 355
social determinants
  environment, influence of, 21
  health-care system, 20–21
  health disparities, 19
  and social justice, 20

Social-Ecological Model, 304
social environment
  drug use and, 389
  as health determinant, 483, 484f
  in public health goals, 6
social media
  for social support, 342
  as stressor, 318
social smokers, 353
social support, 33
  for avoiding alcohol-related problems, 373
  COVID-19 pandemic, 343
  defined, **343**
  evaluating, 349–350
  finding ways, 339f
  health decisions and, 488
  for healthy lifestyle, 25
  lifestyle change and, 488t
  as reinforcing factor, 30t
  for stress management, 342–343
  types of, 342
social wellness, 70
sodium intake, 279, 288
soft drink consumption, 281
software applications. *See* apps (applications)
soleus, 173f, 174f
somatotype, 250, **250**
soy-based foods, 284
soybeans, 284
spas, evaluating, 467–468, 469f, 477–478
Special K (drug), 383t
specificity of exercise, 86, **87**, 164
speed advanced fitness training, 228
speed (amphetamines), 381t
speed (velocity), dimension of fitness, 10f
speed rating scale, 238
speed-related power, 228
spice (drug), 382t
spinal column. *See also* back pain or problems
  anatomy and function, 428, 428f
  normal curvatures, 434
spine twist, 210
spinning classes, 140
spirituality
  as health determinant, 483, 484f
  for stress management, 339
spiritual wellness, 70
splenius capitis, stretching, 209, 445
spontaneity, 487
sports, 222
  skill-related requirements of, 230
sports activities
  improving skills in, 147–148
  participation patterns, 144
  skill-related fitness and skills for, 12
  warm-up guidelines, 51t
sports drinks, *versus* water, 53
sports fitness, 9, 230, **231**
sport-specific warm-up, 51
spot-reducing, 468
squats, 449, 454
stabilizer muscles, 429, **429**, 429f
stages of change
  action, 29
  contemplation, 29
  defined, 28, 29
  maintenance, 29
  preparation, 29
standing posture, 434, 435f, 436f
Star Trek, 482
static flexibility, 197
static muscular endurance, 160, **161**, 178
static strength, 160, **161**
static stretching, 201–203
steam rooms, 468

step counts, 110
step test, 127
step-ups, 184
sternocleidomastoid
    location, 173f, 174f
    stretching, 445
stick drop test, 237
stick test of coordination, 236
stiffness, defined, 197
stimulant drugs, 380–381, 381t, 386
St. John's wort, 471
strains and sprains, 56–57
strength
    defined, 156
    as dimension of fitness, 9f
    dynamic, 161
    factors influencing, 156–158
    fitness tests for, 175–176, 178, 187–188
    static, 160, **161**
    stretching and, 201
    training for, 163
strength-related power, 228
stress
    appraisal of, 321, 322f, 324
    in college students, 316t, 317, 336
    defined, 316, **317**
    effects on health, 320–321
    eustress versus distress, 321, 321f
    evaluating, 324, 327–328
    gender differences in, 317
    individual differences in responses to, 321–324
    personal characteristics and, 322–324
    physical reactions to, 318–320, 319f, 322f
    reduces in exercise, 333
    sources and types, 316–318, 316t
stress management
    coping strategies for, 335t, 336–340
    decision-making and, 486
    as health determinant, 23
    online resources, 339
    physical activity and, 332–333
    principles of, 334–335
    professional help for, 343
    recreation and leisure for, 333–334
    sleep habits for, 333, 333t
    time management for, 340–341, 340t
Stress Management and Resiliency Training
    (SMART), 339
stressors, defined, 316, **317**
stretching
    apps for, 198
    arm exercises, 213
    do and don't list for, 206t
    exercise, 199, **199**
    for injury treatment, 199
    leg exercises, 211–212
    methods of, 201–204, 202f
    neck exercises, 450
    semispinalis capitus, 209, 445
    semispinalis cervicis, 209
    for stress management, 338
    trunk exercises, 209–210
stretch-shortening cycle, 160
stretch tolerance, 197
stretch warm-up, 51, 64
stroke (brain attack)
    alcohol use and, 367
    sodium intake and, 288
substance use disorders, 384, **385**
sudden infant death syndrome (SIDS), 353
sudden sniffing death, 386
sugar consumption, 279, 282
suicide, 321, 419
sulfides, 289t
sulforaphane, 289t
Sun Protection Factor (SPF), 56

sunscreen, 415
superior gemellus, stretching, 212
superman exercise variations, 451
surgical body sculpting, 468
swan exercise, 443
sweat rate, and dehydration, 53
swim test, 128
sympathetic nervous system (SNS), 318, **319**
synergistic effect, 380, **381**
synthetic cannabinoids, 382t
synthetic opiates, 381t
syphilis, 398t, 400, **401**
systematic problem solving, 339
systemic racism and stress, 319
systolic blood pressure, **73**

T
T helper cells (CD4 helper cells), 395, **395**
tai chi applications, 204
    back and neck pain, 434
    posture correction, 438
Tanaka formula, 124
tanning devices, 414, 415, 468
tapering, 232, **233**
target heart rate zone, 124, 124t, 125f
target zone
    for body fat reduction, 252t
    defined, **88**, 88f
    resistance training, 163t
team sport participation patterns, 144
technology. See also apps (applications)
    drug misuse solution, 387
    obesity and, 251
    online health information, 472
    as stressor, 318
teens. See adolescents
temperature, and flexibility, 193–194, 197–198
tender points, 200
tendons, 196, **197**
tend or befriend model, 342
tensor fasciae latae, exercising, 184
teres major
    exercising, 180, 182, 183
    location, 174f
testicular cancer, 411t, 415
testicular self-exam, 425–426
thermogenesis, 302
thigh and hip stretches, 211, 212, 448
thiols, 289t
thirdhand smoke, 354
thoracic spine, 428, 428f
threshold of training, 86, 88
    for body fat reduction, 252t
    for muscle fitness, 163t
3-second run, 238
tibialis anterior
    location, 173f
    stretching, 448
time-dependent aging, 70
time management
    ABC system, 340, 340t
    as enabling factor, 30t
    for healthy lifestyle, 25
    lifestyle change and, 488t
    procrastination and, 341, 341f
    for stress management, 340–341
    worksheet, 345–346
time (duration) of physical activity
    as activity monitor, 108
    for cardiorespiratory endurance, 123
    in FITT formula, 87
    injury prevention and, 441
    for stretching, 204
time use, by college students, 340f

tobacco taxes, 357
tobacco use, 23
    as cause of death, 23, 355
    e-cigarettes, 354, 357
    economic costs, 354
    as gateway drug, 358, 388
    health risks, 352–353, 353f, 355t, 361–362
    nicotine and, 352
    prevalence and trends, 356–357, 356f
    promotion and prevention, 356–357, 356f
    quitting, 352–353, 358–359, 359t
    reasons for starting, 358
    secondhand smoke, 352, 353–355
    smokeless tobacco, 355, 355t
    smoking bans, 357
toe touches, 447
Tolerable Upper Intake Level (UL), 286t
tone, 227
tonic (postural) muscles, 197
toning tables, 465
tonus, 465, **465**
traditional medicine, 20
traffic crashes, alcohol-related, 367–368, 368t, 369f
TrailLink, 50
training, 222, **223**
training stimulus, 232
    for different resistance training programs, 227
tranks (drugs), 380t
tranquilizers, 380, 380t
trans fats, 283
transfer muscles, **429,** 429–430, 429f
Transtheoretical Model, 28, 30
transversus abdominis
    exercising, 161f, 185
    location, 429f
trapezius
    exercising, 161f, 182
    location, 173f, 174f
    stretching, 209, 445, 450
treadmills, 141
triceps brachii
    exercising, 179, 181, 183
    stretching, 213
triceps curl (free-weight), 179
triceps dips, 183
triceps press (machine), 181
triglycerides, **73**
trunk exercises
    muscle fitness, 186
    stretching, 209
trunk lateral flexors, stretching, 209
trunk lift (back exercise), 184, 453
trunk twist, 210
TRX Suspension Trainer, 162
tumors
    benign, 408, **409**
    malignant, 408, **409**
Tylenol (acetaminophen), 57
Type A behavior pattern, **323,** 323–324
Type D behavior pattern, 323, **323**
Type 1 diabetes, 8, 417, **417**
Type 2 diabetes, 417, **417**
type of physical activity, in FITT formula, 87

U
UL (Tolerable Upper Intake Level), 286t
underfat, 246, **247**
underwater weighing, 247
unhealthy lifestyles, cumulative effects of, 2
uninsured individuals, 20
online health information, 472
unsaturated fats, 282, **283**
upper body (android) fat, 249
uppers (amphetamines), 381t
upper trapezius/neck stretch, 209, 450

upper trunk lift, 453
U.S. Pharmacopeial Convention (USP), 471
uterine cancer, 411t, 413

V

vaccines, for STIs, 398, 399, 400
Valium, 380t
vaping, 358, 389
vascular system, 116
vastus lateralis
  exercising, 180, 184
  location, 173f, 174f
vastus medialis, 173f
vegans, 289, **289**
vegetable consumption, 281
vegetarian diets, 289
veins, healthy, 116
vertebrae, 428, 428f
vibrating belts, 465
Vicodin, 381t
vigorous activity, 105
vigorous aerobic activities, 91, 142, 143. *See also*
    vigorous physical activity
  cardiorespiratory endurance, 139–140
  continuous aerobic activity, 140
  in group setting, 140–141
  intermittent aerobic activity, 140
vigorous anaerobic activities, 142, 143
vigorous physical activity (VPA), 101, 303
  benefits of, 139t
  boost metabolism, 139
  classification by fitness level, 102t, 102t
  combining with vigorous activity, 153–154
  guidelines for, 146–147
  versus moderate or light, 101t
  patterns of, 144, 145f
  in physical activity pyramid, 138f
  planning and logging, 151–152
  warm-up guidelines, 51t
vigorous recreational activities, 143–144
vigorous sport
  cardiorespiratory endurance, 142
  recreation, and anaerobic activities, 91
viral load, 396, **397**
virtual racing, 141
visceral (abdominal) fat, 250
visualization (mental imagery), 338
vitamins, 285, 286t, 287
vitamin supplements, 287, 472–473
volume of physical activity, 88
$\dot{V}O_2$ max. *See* aerobic capacity

W

waist circumference, 266, 272
waist-to-hip ratio, 265, 266, 272
walking, 105
  environments for, 24
  with hand weights, 467
  popularity of, 100–101

walking test, 127
wand exercise, 443
warm-up
  defined, 50
  described, 50–51
  exercises in, 63–64
  guidelines for, 51t
  stretch warm-up, 51
water
  dietary guidelines, 288
  versus sports drinks, 53
water-based classes, 140–141
water sports, 50
wearable technology, 92, 144, 145t, 146
Weathering, 334
websites, credible, 13
weed (cannabis), 382t
weekend warrior, 93–94
weight control
  calorie needs, 302
  energy (caloric) balance for, 252
  energy expenditure, 302
  exercise programming for, 145t
  exercise type for, 158
  factors influencing, 302–303
  fad diets and clinical approaches, 308–309
  fast food option, evaluating, 313–314
  food insecurity and obesity, 305
  lab information, 310
  light physical activity, accumulation of, 303
  losing body fat, guidelines for, 305–308,
    306t, 307t
  managing eating, selecting strategies for, 311–312
  muscle fitness and, 158
  obesogenic environment, confronting, 304–305,
    304f
  paying attention, 303
  physical activity, 302–303
  quackery and fraud in, 473–474
  regulatory processes in, 250–251
  self-management skills, 309–310
  smartphone apps, 310
  weighing and, 255
weight discrimination, 245
weighted belts, 466
weighted lifts, 454
weighted squats, 454
weight gain
  in college students, 244
  nutrition for, 292
weight lifting (sport), 156
weight loss, 302
  fad diets and clinical approaches to, 308–309
  guidelines for, 306
weight maintenance, 302
Weight Watchers (WW), 309
well-being index, 9
wellness, 9
  benefits, 104
  defined, 7
  characteristics, 6
  debilitating conditions, 8–9
  determinants of, 18f

  dimensions, 6, 7–8, 7f, 7t
  emotional/mental wellness, 69
  health integration, 8
  integration of, 8
  intellectual wellness, 69–70
  muscle fitness and, 159
  physical activity and, 69–70
  physical wellness, 69
  self-perceptions assessment, 15–16
  services and products, 9
  social, 70
  spiritual, 70
whirlpools, 468
windchill factor, 54f
windmill exercise, 445
wine, 364f
withdrawal
  alcohol, **365,** 365–366
  cannabis, 386
  defined, **353**
  nicotine, 352
women. *See also* gender differences
  alcohol effects in, 367, 371
  HIV/AIDS in, 395
  secondhand smoke susceptibility, 354
  social support importance, 342
workouts, 52, **53**
workplace issues
  hours worked, 333
  occupational safety, 419
  sick employees, 482
  smoking policies, 357–358
wrist curl, 180
wrist flexors, exercising, 180
writing, for stress management, 339
written plans, 37–38

X

X (ecstasy), 383t
Xanax, 380t

Y

yoga, 205
yoga applications
  back and neck pain, 434
  posture correction, 438
  stress management, 338
  as trend, 145t
youth sports, 231
yo-yo dieting, 308

Z

zeaxanthin, 289t
zinc, 287
Zumba, 140
Zwift, 50